Tutorial on Neural Systems Modeling

Tutorial on
Neural Systems Modeling

Thomas J. Anastasio

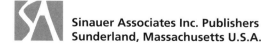
Sinauer Associates Inc. Publishers
Sunderland, Massachusetts U.S.A.

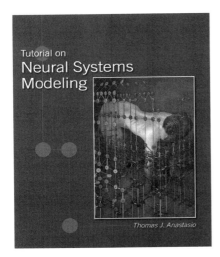

About the Cover

The picture on the cover, by artist Alan Larkin, is entitled *The Birth of Madness*. It depicts a structure that is simultaneously simple and complex, and a person who is simultaneously newborn and mature. The structure is self-revealing, and the inexperienced but perceptive person examines it intently. She has not seen it before, but she seems confident that she can understand the structure by exploring it. To the author, the structure represents neural systems modeling, and the person represents the intended readers of this book. Others will no doubt discover their own interpretations. For the author, the pursuit of neural systems modeling has been a kind of madness, but in the sense of a consuming excitement. His hope is to transfer some of that excitement to his readers. *The Birth of Madness* hangs at the Beckman Institute for Advanced Science and Technology, located on the campus of the University of Illinois at Urbana-Champaign. The Beckman Institute is where the author works and also where he wrote this book. He has long admired this picture.

Address inquiries and orders to
    Sinauer Associates, Inc.
    23 Plumtree Road
    Sunderland, MA 01375 USA
    www.sinauer.com
    FAX: 413-549-1118
    orders@sinauer.com
    publish@sinauer.com

MATLAB® is a trademark of The MathWorks, Inc. and is used with permission. The MathWorks does not warrant the accuracy of the text or exercises in this book. This book's use of MATLAB® software does not constitute endorsement or sponsorship by The MathWorks of a particular pedagogical approach or particular use of the MATLAB® software.

Library of Congress Cataloging-in-Publication Data

Anastasio, Thomas J.
Tutorial on neural systems modeling / Thomas J. Anastasio.
    p. cm.
Includes bibliographical references and index.
ISBN 978-0-87893-339-6 (hardcover : alk. paper)
1. Computational neuroscience. 2. Neural networks (Neurobiology) I. Title.
QP357.5.A53 2010
612.8'2--dc22
                                        2009008416

Printed in U.S.A.
5 4 3 2 1

This book is dedicated to my wife,
Anne Elizabeth McKusick

Brief Contents

Contents

Preface

Tutorial on Neural Systems Modeling is a textbook for students beginning their study of computational neuroscience. More generally, it is intended for readers who want to develop an understanding of neural systems modeling, but who lack specialized backgrounds in mathematics, computer programming, or neuroscience. The world of neural systems modeling is home to elegant and beautiful conceptual tools that provide real and satisfying insight into the workings of the brain. Although there are many excellent books on computational neuroscience and related areas, most of these are written at a mathematical level that is inaccessible to readers with predominantly biological backgrounds. Other excellent books assume prior knowledge of neuroscience, which makes them inaccessible to readers with predominantly computer science or engineering backgrounds. This book provides an entry point for nonspecialists into the world of neural systems modeling. Its goal is to make this wonderful world accessible to as many readers as possible.

Tutorial on Neural Systems Modeling is designed to give the reader a quick, basic, and usable understanding of the mathematical forms of various neural systems modeling paradigms, their implementations as computer programs, and their applications as models of real neural systems. All of the elements: actual listings of programs, figures showing real data or modeling results, and the relevant mathematics are interrelated by a narrative that carries the reader through the tutorial. The modeling paradigm covered in each chapter is broken down into a set of related computations. The objective is to show readers how a computer program that implements a computation can simulate aspects of the behavior of a real neural system. This leads to the hypothesis that the computer model and the neural system are implementing analogous computations. The narrative attempts to guide the reader to a deeper understanding of brain function by describing the mathematical and conceptual basis of each modeling paradigm, and by presenting the neurobiological evidence that the computations included under the paradigm actually occur in real neural systems.

The purpose is not to provide a survey of the field, but to select illustrative modeling examples and explore them in depth. The goal is to give readers full exposure to the mathematical, computational, and neurobiological aspects of each modeling paradigm. In all examples, the description begins from the most basic levels so as not to exclude readers who lack extensive background in any particular area. The expectation is that readers will run the computer code and develop their own "feel" for each modeling paradigm. This will provide readers with actual experience in neural systems modeling, which they can apply to other examples of their own specific interest.

The field of neural systems modeling has experienced vibrant growth over the past several decades. It is most readily applied in the area of systems neuroscience, which concerns the function of specific systems such as the visual system or the motor system. Neural systems modeling is now an integral part of systems neuroscience research, and many of the most recent models build on the classic paradigms. The modeling paradigms presented in this book span the range from the classic to the most recent. The book provides readers with experience using the main paradigms in neural systems modeling, and prepares them to engage with, and contribute to, ongoing modeling efforts across the spectrum of research in systems neuroscience.

Approach

Tutorial on Neural Systems Modeling is indeed a tutorial. It provides step-by-step instruction in the methods of neural systems modeling. It is structured around various modeling paradigms, and around examples in which they are used to simulate real neural systems. The approach taken is to provide readers with the background that is essential for understanding the mathematical basis, the computational implementation, and the application to real neural systems of each paradigm. The relevant neuroscience is briefly presented in the context of each modeling example, so prior knowledge of neuroscience is not required. The mathematics is kept to a minimum, with relevant but inessential math presented in Math Boxes.

The focal point for each modeling example is its computer program. The detailed instruction provided in the use of the programs ensures that all readers will be able to understand and run them. All computer programs are available for free download from the book Web site, www.sinauer.com/anastasio. Most of the programs are self-contained, making it easy for readers to see how the various parts fit together. The programs are all written in MATLAB® (which is a registered trademark of The MathWorks, Inc.), and the code is intended to be easy to follow and is abundantly commented. Programming code is listed in special MATLAB Boxes which appear in the context of the modeling example in which they are used. Prior experience with MATLAB programming is not a prerequisite for reading or using this book. The first chapter actually introduces readers to MATLAB using simple examples. The exercises at the end of each chapter are deliberately made easy, and are meant as invitations to explore the programs.

In this book a neural system is defined as a system composed of a number of interconnected neuron-like elements, which are referred to as units. The units can represent single neurons or small groups of similar neurons. For simplicity in this book, the units do not produce neural impulses (action potentials, or spikes). Instead, their activities are just numbers (binary or real) that represent the firing rates of actual neurons. The use of such simplified model neurons is consistent with the goal of bringing the main ideas to readers with the minimum of detail, and to prepare them for more advanced treatments, many of which do consider models composed of spiking neural elements.

All the models presented as examples in this book not only simulate the properties of a real neural system, but they also perform a useful computation. That computation may be as simple as prolonging an input signal in time, or as complicated as predicting the future value of a variable given current inputs. The theme that unifies all of the models is that the response properties of the units, which are compared with those of real neurons, emerge as a consequence of the computation being performed. The link between observable properties and useful computations provides insight into the ways in which real neural systems may actually work.

The book is designed for self-study, and it would be ideal for readers wishing to gain first-hand experience in neural systems modeling. Ample explanation for using each program is provided in the text. The correct parameter values for the current example are often repeated, even if they are the same values used in the previous example. In this way readers can freely change parameter values and explore model behavior on their own, but then easily regain the thread of the narrative. Frequent reference is made to earlier chapters that are relevant to material presented later in the book, so readers can dive in at any point and be guided back to more introductory material if necessary.

The book was written with instructors in mind. The MATLAB programs have been field tested in a computer lab setting, and the tutorial format of the book facilitates the setting of assignments. Instructors can use the examples and exercises as starting points for more in-depth treatment of specific topics. At fourteen chapters, the book is the ideal length for use as the textbook for a semester-long course in computational neuroscience. It could also be recommended by graduate advisors who would like their students to learn more about neural systems modeling.

Acknowledgments

I am grateful to the many individuals who, over the years, have encouraged and supported my development in the area of neural systems modeling. They include: Nanda Alapati, Michael Arbib, Andrew Barto, Jared Bronski, Manning Correia, Ehtibar Dzhafarov, Steven Grossberg, Simon Haykin, Robert Kearney, Stephen Levinson, William Lytton, Lee Moore, Pierre Moulin, Michael Paulin, Maxim Raginsky, Jesse Reichler, David Robinson, Sylvian Ray, Shihab Shamma, Terrence Sejnowski, Christoph von der Malsburg, and David Zipser. I would also like to thank the many individuals whose identities are unknown to me, but who have supported me with their constructive reviews, letters of support, and other good words.

This book is the outgrowth of a course in neural systems modeling that I taught for many years at the University of Illinois at Urbana-Champaign. I am grateful to the many students who took the course. They taught me a lot, including many slick programming tricks, and exposed many bugs in my computer programs.

I deeply appreciate the help of many colleagues who read and critically commented on parts of the book. They include: Andrew Barto, Jared Bronski, Jay McClelland, Sheryl Coombs, Lawrence Eshelman, Stephen Levinson, Paul Patton, Michael Paulin, Maxim Raginsky, Rajesh Rao, Fredrick Rothganger, Shihab Shamma, and David Zipser. I also appreciate the comments on earlier drafts of the book provided by reviewers whose identities are unknown to me.

I would like to thank the professionals at Sinauer Associates who helped put this textbook together: Graig Donini, the editor for the project; Chris Small, Janice Holabird, Joanne Delphia, and The Format Group for their superb design ideas, book layout, and artwork; and Sydney Carroll and Laura Green for their impressive editorial and organizational skills, and especially for their patience. Throughout the entire process, I felt that this group cared about the book as much as I did.

Vectors, Matrices, and Basic Neural Computations

The brain is the most complex organ known to exist, yet mathematical and computational methods can be used to simulate many aspects of neural systems function

Throughout this book we will use one computational device, the computer, to model another, the brain. As a machine constructed by humans, the computer is well understood. It is relatively easy for us to program computers for various computational purposes. But the brain, as an organ evolved over eons, is not well understood. Our goal is to write simple computer programs, with clear conceptual bases, which will simulate certain aspects of real brain function. These computer models will be abstract and relatively simple, but they will perform interesting, useful, and often sophisticated computations, and in so doing will reproduce the salient properties of the neural systems under study. The validity of the simulations will be evaluated through comparison with neurophysiological data. To the extent that the simulations are valid, the computations performed by our models will reflect those occurring in real neural systems, and the conceptual understanding we develop through modeling will translate into a deeper understanding of brain function.

Because models are really hypotheses that need to be tested experimentally, the understanding we develop will be provisional. Still, the insight we can attain through modeling will have a depth that could not be reached through experiment alone.

1.1   Neural Systems, Neural Networks, and Brain Function

The brain, as a whole, defies comprehension. It is likely to be capable of forms of processing that we, currently, cannot even imagine. Still, some of the functions of the brain are apparent and many, to a limited extent, are understood. Obviously, the brain must enhance the survivability of its organism, and to do that it must obtain information from the environment and use it to produce advantageous behaviors. Experiments in neuroscience, combined with computational modeling, have increased our knowledge about the brain. Many of its functions have been described and even simulated. Perhaps it is fair to say that a rough outline of brain function is emerging.

The brain uses its sensory systems to extract specific features from the environment, and it constructs internal representations of those features that contain much of the information available in the environment. These representations take the form of patterns of active neurons, and the brain can store some of those patterns for later retrieval. The brain uses the information it represents to make inferences about the configuration of the environment, and to make decisions based on those inferences. It also acts on the information it represents by producing behaviors that are ultimately driven by commands to the motor system. We will explore models of all these brain functions in this book. Our focus will be on the level of systems of neurons.

Brain function spans levels from molecules (such as neurotransmitters and ion channels) to membranes (via passive electrical properties) to synapses (transmitter release) to parts of neurons (dendritic processing) to whole neurons (generation of action potentials) to neural networks (systems of neurons in specific brain regions) to networks-of-networks (as between brain regions) and on to the behavior that results from these multilevel interactions (Churchland and Sejnowski 1992; Purves et al. 2008). A neural system is a set of neurons that interact together in a network. In this book we will focus on neural function occurring at the network level, because it is at this level that the relationship between computational function and the behavior of real neurons can be understood most clearly through modeling. The purpose of this book is to give the reader an understanding of this relationship for a wide range of different neural systems, with the goal of leaving the reader with deeper insight into brain function in general.

A case in point, and a unifying theme in the book, involves internal representations of the world by the brain. In order for it to process sensory inputs, recognize objects, evaluate situations, store and retrieve memories, control movements, and learn from experience, the brain must form internal representations of the world and use them to perform computations. Perhaps the greatest challenge faced by the brain in making useful computations is the uncertainty associated both with the world and with its own neural elements. One way in which the brain deals with this uncertainty is by accessing its representations. Recent evidence suggests that the brain perceives the world though a combination of its sensory input and its internal representations (Gilbert and Sigman 2007). A model we will explore later in this book will demonstrate how certain neurons could track moving, visible objects by combining sensory input with an internal representation of object motion. The model will offer an explanation for why these neurons continue to respond, but at a reduced level, even after the object is rendered invisible. By constructing and running this simulation, and by comparing the modeling results with real data, the reader will develop insight into how visual perception is a combination of what we actually see and what we expect to see.

Throughout this book we will model neural systems as neural networks. We will see how relatively small neural network models, composed of idealized neural units whose outputs are simple functions of their inputs, can nevertheless produce amazing behaviors. Through computer simulation, we will explore how neural systems in the spinal cord and brainstem could control movement by transforming sensory signals into motor commands. We will see how certain forms of sensation and perception, such as the detection of edges, the retrieval of signals from noise, or the prediction of future sensory inputs could occur in the retina or the tectum. We will show how the complex responses of neurons in the tectum to sensory inputs of two or more modalities could be understood as probability computations. We will also demonstrate how neural networks that dynamically settle down to two or more stable states could simulate memory storage and recall as it might occur in the hippocampus, or parts of cerebral cortex.

The functions of the networks arise from their structures and from the weights of the connections between their units. In some cases we will explicitly set these weights, but in most cases we will use adaptive algorithms to learn them. We will show how some forms of learning could produce the map-like representations of sensory input found in certain brain regions, and also increase the information that these brain regions contain about the sensory environment. Other forms of neural network adaptation reproduce the complex, diverse representation patterns found in many regions of the brain. We will consider neural network learning algorithms in light of the learning mechanisms that are thought to occur in the real brain, and will show how one form of learning through time could explain the responses of certain midbrain neurons that are involved in reward processing. We will also explore the role of evolution in shaping both the structures of neural networks and the mechanisms by which they learn to adjust their connection weights.

The purpose of this book is to give readers direct, hands-on experience with neural systems models, and through that experience to develop insight into how the computations performed by networks of neurons could underlie brain function. In all cases our network models will be of the same general type. The networks constructed in later chapters will build from those constructed in earlier chapters. Most of the examples presented in the book will be accompanied by computer code that you can use to run your own simulations. For convenience, the code is printed in the book and can also be downloaded from the book Web site (www.sinauer.com/anastasio).

1.2   Using MATLAB: The Matrix Laboratory Programming Environment

We will use the MATLAB® programming environment for our simulations. You should have access to a computer running MATLAB, and should familiarize yourself with the specifics of the MATLAB programming environment before you begin. The name MATLAB is short for "matrix laboratory," and the matrix is the basis for computation in MATLAB. Commands in MATLAB operate on matrices, and can include everything from simple arithmetic to complicated numerical computations. MATLAB offers an ideal programming environment for simulating neural systems, because most neural systems models are also based on matrices. The purpose of this chapter is to get you started with using MATLAB, and to present some very simple neural systems models.

MATLAB is an interpreted programming language, meaning that MATLAB commands will be interpreted and run as you enter them from the command line. In computing, code segments are variously described using terms such as statement, function, and command, but in this book we will generally use the term "command" to refer to any code segment that could be interpreted and run when entered at the MATLAB command line (or entered as part of an m-file, see Section 1.4). This chapter will introduce MATLAB commands for elementary arithmetic functions and special functions, vector and matrix operations, vector and matrix manipulations, graphics, and simple programming techniques such as for-loops. To distinguish them from the rest of the text, all MATLAB commands (and the variable names associated with those commands) will appear in `monotype` font. Only minimal explanation of MATLAB commands will be given in this book. Typing the command `help` followed by the name of another command in MATLAB (with a space in between) will display a more detailed description of that command.

Our first example does not involve a neural system model, but it nicely illustrates the style of computing with MATLAB. We will explore a simple calculation that, according to legend, was given as busywork by a stern schoolmaster to his pupils. The incident supposedly occurred around 1780 in provincial Germany. The busywork was to add up the integers from 1 to 100. The teacher figured that this problem would occupy his students for a good long while, but one of the youngsters surprised him. His name was Karl Friedrich Gauss (see Hayes 2006 for the sources of this famous tale).

1.3 Imitating the Solution by Gauss to the Busywork Problem

To begin our exploration of this calculation we will use vectors. A vector is a linear array of numbers. The easiest way to solve the busywork problem in MATLAB is simply to construct a vector of the series of integers from 1 to 100 and add up the elements in the vector. This can be done in one step in MATLAB. Of course, young Gauss did not have access to a computer, much less to MATLAB, but he solved the problem in under a minute by constructing the vector in his head, and by cleverly manipulating it so that the problem was greatly simplified. According to legend, the insightful method used by young Gauss was mentally to "fold" the series of numbers in the middle and add them in pairs: 1 + 100, 2 + 99, 3 + 98, …, 50 + 51. All the pairs sum to 101 and, because there are 50 pairs, the sum is equal to 50 times 101 or 5050. To introduce MATLAB, we will use it to imitate the mental manipulation that has been attributed to young Gauss.

To solve the busywork problem we can construct a vector whose elements are the series of integers from 1 to 100, and sum its elements. The most general way to construct a series of numbers in MATLAB is to use the `linspace` command. The command `x=linspace(1,100,1000);` will create a vector **x** containing an equally spaced series of 1000 elements from 1 to 100. In this case the numbers in **x** will have a spacing of less than 0.1. To solve the busywork problem we need a vector **x** of the integers from 1 to 100, so we want a spacing of 1. The MATLAB command `x=linspace(1,100,100);` will give us this vector. Notice that each command is followed by a semicolon. The semicolon is a signal to MATLAB that you do not want the results of the command to be displayed on the monitor. For clarity we will omit the semicolons henceforth, but you should use them in your own commands whenever you do not want the results to be displayed on the monitor.

A shorthand way in MATLAB to generate a series of integers from 1 to 100 is to use the colon command `x=1:100`. The command `sum` will compute the sum of the elements in a vector. To solve the busywork problem we can issue the command `sum(x)` or, without even constructing a vector **x**, we can solve it in one step with `sum(1:100)`. The result, as you will see if you run `sum(1:100)` (without a semicolon), is the number 5050. This solution is correct, but the method lacks the elegance of the solution by young Gauss. Properly imitating his solution will involve matrix construction and manipulation.

In MATLAB the basic element is the matrix. We generally think of a matrix as a rectangular (possibly square) array of numbers. The numbers of rows and columns of a rectangular matrix are its dimensions. We will use the rectangular matrix extensively in this book, and will also have occasion to use cuboidal matrices, which can be thought of as a "deck" of rectangular matrices (like a deck of cards). A linear array of numbers is called a vector. A single number is called a scalar. Vectors and scalars can be considered as special types of rectangular matrices where one (for a vector) or both (for a scalar) of the dimensions equal 1.

The `linspace` command, and the simpler colon command, both generate row vectors. If you neglected to follow your `linspace` or colon commands with semicolons, they would have displayed their results on the monitor. You would have seen the row vector as a series of horizontal arrays of numbers, listed out by column. (Of course, each column in a row vector has only one element.) By convention, most vectors are column vectors. In this book we will use either row or column vectors, depending on which format is the more convenient or natural under the circumstances.

We will use conventional mathematical notation throughout this book. Scalar variables (representing single numbers) will be denoted by lowercase or uppercase italic letters (e.g., x or X), vectors will be denoted by lowercase non-italic letters in bold (e.g., **x**), and matrices will be denoted by uppercase non-italic letters in bold (e.g., **X**). These conventions will be dropped whenever the variable names are expressed as parts of MATLAB commands, in which case they will appear in `monotype` font. Variable names are chosen to make it as easy as possible to remember the quantities they represent. Because many different quantities are represented in this book, the same variable name will sometimes be used to represent different quantities in different sections. The local usage of a variable name should always be clear from its context. So as not to confuse them with variable names, acronyms and abbreviations will be written in uppercase letters that are neither italic nor bold (e.g., MATLAB).

The transpose operator will convert the rows of a rectangular matrix to columns, or vice-versa. The transpose operator is denoted by an uppercase non-italic T in superscript (e.g., the transpose of matrix **X** is $\mathbf{X}^T$). The transpose symbol in MATLAB is an apostrophe. For example, `Y=X'` will make a matrix **Y** whose rows are the columns of a matrix **X**. The transpose command can also be used to convert a row vector into a column vector, or vice-versa. The command `y=x'` will produce a column vector **y** containing the series of integer elements from 1 to 100 from the row vector **x** constructed using `x=1:100`.

To imitate the solution by Gauss to the busywork problem we want to manipulate the vector **y** and represent it in a matrix. MATLAB provides many mechanisms for matrix manipulation. Some of these require that matrix elements be indexed individually or in matrix pieces (submatrices). The command `y(50)` will pluck the fiftieth element from **y** and show it on the monitor. The command `y(51:100)` will access the second half of column vector **y**. The

TABLE 1.1	Imitating the solution by young Gauss to the busywork problem	
1	100	101
2	99	101
3	98	101
4	97	101
5	96	101
6	95	101
7	94	101
8	93	101
9	92	101
10	91	101
11	90	101
12	89	101
13	88	101
14	87	101
15	86	101
16	85	101
17	84	101
18	83	101
19	82	101
20	81	101
21	80	101
22	79	101
23	78	101
24	77	101
25	76	101
26	75	101
27	74	101
28	73	101
29	72	101
30	71	101
31	70	101
32	69	101
33	68	101
34	67	101
35	66	101
36	65	101
37	64	101
38	63	101
39	62	101
40	61	101
41	60	101
42	59	101
43	58	101
44	57	101
45	56	101
46	55	101
47	54	101
48	53	101
49	52	101
50	51	101

command Z=reshape(y,50,2) will make a matrix **Z** having 50 rows and 2 columns, in which the first column contains the integers from 1 to 50, and in which the second column contains the integers from 51 to 100. The command Z(:,2)=flipud(Z(:,2)) will take the second column of **Z** and flip it from top to bottom. Note that the colon by itself in the previous command designates all of the row numbers (indices). (The first coordinate is the row's place, the second coordinate is the column's place.) In this case, the colon designates all the row elements in column 2 of **Z**. What we have with matrix **Z** is a column of integers from 1 to 100 that is "folded" onto itself, creating the column of pairs 1 and 100, 2 and 99, 3 and 98, …, 50 and 51. Now we need to sum the pairs.

When its argument is a matrix, sum will compute the sum over the columns of the matrix. We want to sum over the rows of **Z**, so we must first transpose matrix **Z** before we issue sum. For purposes of comparison with matrix **Z**, we want the resulting vector of sums to be a column vector, so we will have to transpose the result of the summing operation. The command s=sum(Z')' will do this, and store the result as column vector **s**. Because vector **s** holds the sums of the pairs, sum(s) will compute the total sum of the integers from 1 to 100. This also solves the busywork problem but, again, it is not the solution method we wish to imitate. Further matrix manipulation is needed.

Matrices can be composed in MATLAB by enclosing submatrices (such as single numbers, vectors, and other submatrices) within square brackets, provided that the dimensions of the submatrices are compatible. The command G=[Z s] will create a matrix **G** in which the first two columns are the columns of **Z** and the third column is the column vector **s**. We can compose matrix **G** of these submatrices in column-wise fashion because they all have the same number of rows. To find the dimensions of a matrix (or vector) use the size command. The command size(G) will display the dimensions of matrix **G** to be 50 rows and 3 columns.

To see how Gauss solved the busywork problem we can display **G** itself, simply by issuing the variable name G as a command (without a semicolon). This command will display a 50-by-3 rectangular array of numbers. The matrix **G** is reproduced in Table 1.1. Basically, Gauss visualized the vector of integers from 1 to 100 in his head, divided it in half lengthwise, flipped the

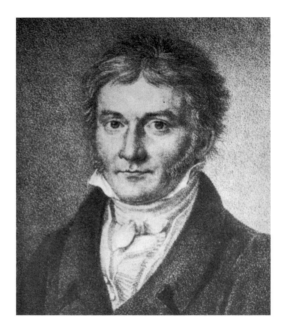

FIGURE 1.1   Karl Friedrich Gauss (after he grew up!) Portrait by S. Bendixen.

second half (from 100 to 51) and laid it next to the first half, thereby making 50 pairs of integers. He realized, as you can see from matrix **G**, that the sum of each pair of integers is 101. Since there are 50 pairs, the solution to the problem is 101 times 50, or 5050.

In doing this problem you should be able to see, literally, how Gauss completed this busywork, in his head, in under a minute. It is even more amazing to realize that Gauss not only solved the problem in under a minute, but that he also conceived the method in such a short period of time. This simple example illustrates how genius often involves the ability to see a problem from a different perspective. Gauss was probably younger than ten years old when this famous episode occurred. He went on to become one of the world's greatest mathematicians (Figure 1.1). In many places throughout this book we will use the Gaussian probability distribution, which was first defined by Gauss and named in his honor.

Despite the fact that Gauss did the problem in his head, the Gauss busywork problem is not an example of neural systems modeling. It simply illustrates the use of vectors (and matrices) in a fun and semi-biographical way. Vectors are used in many ways in neural systems modeling. Neural systems, or networks, are sets of interconnected neural elements, or units, which receive and process inputs to produce outputs. Vectors can be used to represent the activation states of the units, the weights of the connections to a unit, and the inputs and outputs of the network. The use of vectors to store inputs and outputs can be illustrated using the simplest neural system: a single unit that receives a weighted input and produces an output.

1.4 Operation and Habituation of the Gill-Withdrawal Reflex of *Aplysia*

A diagram of the simplest neural system is shown in Figure 1.2. In this diagram, x represents the input to the unit, y represents the state of the unit, and v represents the weight of the input connection to the unit. The input x could be sent from a separate input unit. In many models in this book we will represent input units explicitly, but in other models we will omit them for simplicity. We omit the input unit from the simplest neural model to emphasize its single-unit character. Obviously, this single-neuron model simplifies a lot of neurobiology (see Purves et al. 2008 for details).

Real neurons, or nerve cells, are like other cells in that they have a roundish cell body. What distinguishes neurons from other cells is that most of them send a long, thin process, known as an axon, to other neurons (and to other cell types as well, such as muscle cells). Neurons use their axons to transmit signals from one to another (and to other types of cells). Axons contact other cells at synapses. The pre-synaptic axon terminal releases chemical neurotransmitter in an amount proportional to the activity level of the pre-synaptic cell. Neurotransmitter flows across the synaptic space from the pre-synaptic cell to the post-synaptic cell. Binding of neurotransmitter to specialized receptors (the neurotransmitter-gated ion channels) on the post-synaptic cell can increase or decrease the activity level of the post-synaptic cell. The effect depends specifically on which one of the many different neurotransmitters is being secreted, and on the nature of the receptor. Thus, synapses can be excitatory (producing an increase in post-synaptic activity) or inhibitory

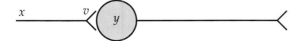

FIGURE 1.2   The simplest neural system
Input x contacts unit y with connection weight v.

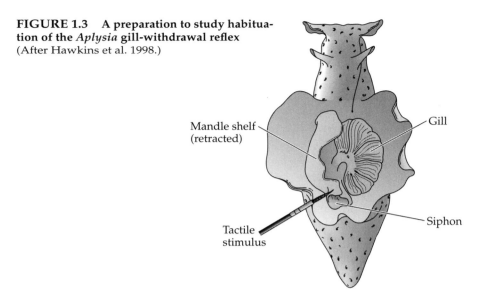

FIGURE 1.3   A preparation to study habituation of the *Aplysia* gill-withdrawal reflex (After Hawkins et al. 1998.)

Mandle shelf (retracted)

Gill

Tactile stimulus

Siphon

(producing a decrease in post-synaptic activity). In this book we will model synapses simply as the weights, either positive or negative, of the connections between neural units.

The simple neural model shown in Figure 1.2 could represent a monosynaptic reflex. The term "reflex" denotes a neural system that, relatively quickly and directly, transforms a sensory input into a motor output. Sensory afferents, which are neurons that transmit signals from sensory receptors into the nervous systems, form the input stage of a reflex pathway. Motoneurons, which are neurons that activate muscle cells, form the output stage of a reflex pathway. Interneurons are neurons that are situated between sensory afferent neurons and motoneurons on the reflex pathway. In a polysynaptic reflex, sensory afferents synapse on interneurons, and interneurons synapse on other interneurons or on motoneurons. More than simple relays, interneurons mediate interesting forms of signal processing, some of which we will study in later chapters. In a monosynaptic reflex, which is less common, sensory neurons synapse directly onto motoneurons. We will use the simple neural model shown in Figure 1.2 to simulate a monosynaptic reflex.

A well studied example of a monosynaptic reflex is the gill-withdrawal reflex of *Aplysia* (Kandel 1976). *Aplysia* is a sea slug, which is like a snail without a shell. A drawing of an *Aplysia* is shown in Figure 1.3. The body of *Aplysia* is rather tough, but its exposed gill is soft and is a favorite food for fish. To protect this sensitive structure, *Aplysia* has evolved a reflex to withdraw the gill in response to tactile stimulation. If we use the system of Figure 1.2 to model the *Aplysia* gill-withdrawal reflex, then input x would represent the axon and synaptic terminal of the gill sensory afferent neuron, and output unit y would represent the motoneuron of the muscle that retracts the gill. The weight of the sensory neuron to motoneuron synapse v would determine the sensitivity of the reflex, which is the ratio of the amount of gill withdrawal to the amount of sensory input. Input x and weight v determine the state of unit y. In this simple case the state of unit y will be the output of the neural model.

The activity level, or state, of most real neurons is expressed in terms of firing rate, which is the frequency at which a neuron produces action potential discharges. Neurons, like most other cells, have a membrane potential (voltage), which is a separation of ionic charge between the inside and the outside of the cell membrane (see Purves et al. 2008 for details). Unlike other cells, most neurons can produce action potentials when their membrane voltage exceeds a threshold. The membrane voltage of a post-synaptic neuron can be brought toward (or away from) threshold by the binding, to neurotransmitter-gated ion channels, of excitatory (or inhibitory) neurotransmitter released from pre-synaptic neurons. Such binding changes the membrane potential by allowing ions to flow across the membrane through the channels.

Ions can also flow through voltage-gated ion channels, which open or close according to the level of membrane potential. Action potentials, which are commonly called impulses or spikes, are temporally and spatially circumscribed reversals in the axonal membrane potential that are caused by flow of ions through voltage-gated ion channels. The frequency of spikes generated by a neuron is roughly proportional to the amount of supra-threshold input it receives from other neurons. The action potentials (spikes) generated by a neuron then propagate down its axon to its axon terminals, where the spikes cause neurotransmitter release in amounts proportional to their frequency. Sophisticated methods exist for simulating in detail the biophysical properties of real neurons (e.g., Koch and Segev 1989). Because a huge range of interesting and important neural systems phenomena can be simulated using simple neural elements having scalar state values, we will not model spiking neurons in this book, but will simply represent neural firing rate as the scalar value of the state of any neural unit.

We can use the neural system of Figure 1.2 to model the response of the *Aplysia* gill-withdrawal reflex to a series of stimuli that occur one after another in time, and we can use a vector to represent the input time series. First, make a pulse input using `pls=[0 0 1 0 0]`. Next, compose input **x** as a series of six pulses using `x=[pls pls pls pls pls pls]`. Constructed this way, vector **x**, which is our input time series, is a row vector. Since time series tend to be relatively long they are more naturally represented as rows than as columns, so we will usually represent time series as row vectors in this book.

The output of the single unit will also be a time series, and we will need to store the output in a (row) vector **y** that is as long as our input vector. Because we know the composition of our input we could easily compute this length, but in general it is easier to use the `size` command in MATLAB. The command `[nRows nCols]=size(x)` will give us the number of rows and columns of our input. Because time series **x** is a row vector, `nRows` will equal 1, but `nCols` will equal the number of time steps in our input. To help us remember that the number of time steps equals the number of columns, we can set a new variable `nTs=nCols`. Although it is not necessary to define, or pre-allocate, variables in MATLAB it is good practice to do so anyway, and we can define the output vector **y** using `y=zeros(1,nTs)`. This makes **y** a row vector of zeros having length `nTs`. Set the input weight value v to 4: `v=4`.

Now we need to compute the state of y for each state of x on each time step t. Note that time for this model is discrete (rather than continuous) in that it occurs in a series of individual steps. We will use the variable t to represent discrete time throughout this book. On each discrete time step, all that the simple reflex model does to form its output is to scale its input by the input weight. This can be expressed mathematically as in Equation 1.1:

$$y(t) = vx(t) \qquad\qquad \textbf{1.1}$$

Because vector **x** is arranged as a time series that is the same in length as the vector **y** that we wish to compute, we can express Equation 1.1 in vector notation as $\mathbf{y} = v\mathbf{x}$, which means that vector **y** is equal to vector **x** after it has been "scaled" by scalar v. In other words, $\mathbf{y} = v\mathbf{x}$ means that every element of **y** is equal to the corresponding element of **x** multiplied by v. In MATLAB this is done using `y=v*x` where the symbol * signifies multiplication, and the command multiplies every element in x by v. In general, neural models are more complicated than the simple reflex model and it is necessary to evaluate the output sequentially on each time step. One way to do that is to use a loop structure. The following commands use a for-loop to implement Equation 1.1 and find the output of the simple reflex model.

```
>> for t=1:nTs,
y(t)=v*x(t);
end
```

Note that `t=1:nTs` makes `t` the vector of time points, which is also the vector of indices of vectors x and y. Then `x(t)` and `y(t)` are the elements at time (or index) `t` of x and y, respectively. The loop command is carried out for each element of `t`. The loop takes each individual element $x(t)$ of **x**, for each time step t in the sequence, multiplies $x(t)$ by v, and stores the result as the corresponding element $y(t)$ of **y**. In entering these commands from the MATLAB command line you will have noticed that MATLAB waited for you to enter the statement internal to the loop, and executed the loop only after you entered `end`. We will use loops for more complicated processes later on, but this simple loop illustrates the principle.

For this simulation of the *Aplysia* gill-withdrawal reflex you now have both the input and output vectors, which can be plotted. The command `figure(1)` will open a plotting window. The command `clf` will clear an already open plotting window. The command `subplot(2,1,1)` will divide the plotting window into two subplots (one atop the other) and prepare to draw in the top subplot. The command `plot(x)` will plot the elements of vector **x** against their indices, which are the same as the time steps. The command `subplot(2,1,2)` followed by `plot(y)` will plot the vector **y** below the plot for vector **x**. The command `xlabel('time step')` will label the x axis of the currently open, second subplot. Similarly `ylabel('output')` will label the y axis. The command `text(1,3.5,'B')` will place the letter B in the upper-left corner of the second subplot. Issue `subplot(2,1,1)` again to reopen the first subplot and label its axes and assign its letter designation as you did for the second subplot. The resulting plots are shown in Figure 1.4.

The plots in the book are slightly stylized versions of the plots you will generate using MATLAB, so the pulse inputs and outputs you plotted will not look exactly like Figure 1.4. MATLAB gives the user a great deal of control over its graphic output (use `help plot` for a list of specifications), but issuing a simple plot command such as `plot(x)`, without specifying line or

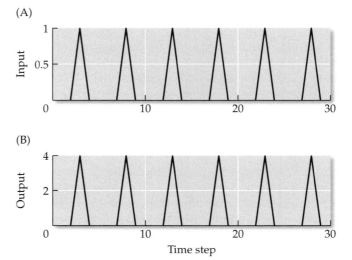

FIGURE 1.4   Behavior of the simple reflex model The output (B) is a scaled version of the input (A), which is a series of six pulses.

marker types, will simply plot the values of x without markers and connect them with a line. Each of our pulse inputs transitions from 0 to 1 and back to 0 over three time steps, so they appear as triangles when plotted with a line connecting them. The entire input to our simple reflex model is a series of six pulses of height 1 separated by 0s, as shown in Figure 1.4A. The output is also a series of six pulses, as shown in Figure 1.4B, but the pulses have been scaled by the weight of the sensory neuron to motoneuron synapse, which is 4 in this case. Thus, this simple reflex model has simply scaled the input to produce the output.

The *Aplysia* gill-withdrawal reflex is significant in neurobiology because it was used to demonstrate that learning involves changes in synaptic weights. The simplest form of learning is habituation, which is a decrease in the sensitivity of a reflex due to repeated stimulation. Habituation of the gill-withdrawal reflex would cause it to produce less gill withdrawal with repeated stimulation, such as buffeting in turbulent surf that does not pose a real threat to the slug or to its gill (but see Exercise 1.2). Eric Kandel and co-workers (Kandel 1976) demonstrated that habituation of the *Aplysia* gill-withdrawal reflex is mediated by a decrease in the weight of the sensory neuron to motoneuron synapse. We can use our simple reflex model to simulate habituation. Set a new variable for the unhabituated value of the sensory neuron to motoneuron synapse *v*, which can be thought of as the start value: `stv=4`. Also set a decrement by which the weight will be reduced on each stimulus presentation: `dec=0.7`. Now the for-loop can be modified to produce habituation by decrementing the weight on each input presentation. Note that this involves an if-then conditional structure, which checks to determine whether an input is present, and if it is, then it decrements the weight.

```
>> v=stv;
>> for t=1:nTs,
y(t)=v*x(t);
if x(t)>0, v=v*dec; end
end
```

The input to and output from the reflex model, with habituation, are plotted in Figure 1.5. As before, the input and output are series of six pulses. The output is scaled by the weight of the sensory neuron to motoneuron synapse,

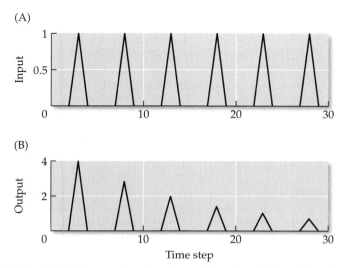

FIGURE 1.5 Simulating a simple reflex undergoing habituation The size of the output (B) decreases with each input (A).

MATLAB® BOX 1.1   **This script implements a simple simulation of habituation of the *Aplysia* gill-withdrawal reflex.**

```
% habituationGWR.m

stv=4; % set start weight value

dec=0.7; % set weight decrement

pls=[0 0 1 0 0]; % set up a pulse

x=[pls pls pls pls pls pls]; % set up a series of pulses as the input

[dum nTs]=size(x); % find the size of the input time series

y=zeros(1,nTs); % set up (define) a vector for the output time series

v=stv; % set weight to start weight value

for t=1:nTs, % for each time step do
    y(t)=v*x(t); % find the output
    if x(t)>0, % if the input is present
        v=v*dec; % then decrement the weight
    end % end the conditional
end % end the for-loop

clf % clear the plotting window
subplot(2,1,1) % set up the top subplot
plot(x) % plot out the input time series
axis([0 nTs 0 1.1]) % reset the axis limits
xlabel('time step') % label the x axis
ylabel('input') % label the y axis
text(1,1,'A') % place the letter A near the top-left
subplot(2,1,2) % set up the bottom subplot
plot(y) % plot out the output time series
axis([0 nTs 0 stv+0.5]) % reset the axis limits
xlabel('time step') % label the x axis
ylabel('output') % label the y axis
text(1,4,'B') % place the letter B near the top-left
```

but the weight decreases on each input presentation. The weight decrement is multiplicative in the example, resulting in a geometric decay of the output (see Section 1.5). The output response corresponds to the activation of the motoneuron in the reflex. Because the motorneuron controls the muscle that retracts the gill, the amount of gill withdrawl would be proportional to the activity level of the motorneuron. Actual habituation probably does not follow exactly the progression shown in Figure 1.5, but the model nicely captures its basic features (Pinsker et al. 1970; Kandel 1976). Data on habituation of the real *Aplysia* gill-withdrawal reflex is shown in Figure 1.6.

For the example without habituation (see Figure 1.4) we did not need a loop, but for the example with habituation (see Figure 1.5) we did, because we needed to include a conditional that checked for the presence of input on each iteration. Loops can be entered from the command line, but it is more convenient to place them in MATLAB programs called "scripts." For MATLAB, a script must be saved in a type of text file known as an m-file. All m-files must

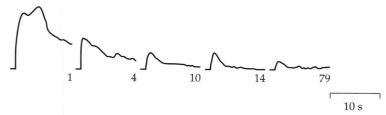

FIGURE 1.6   Habituation of the real *Aplysia* gill-withdrawal reflex The traces indicate the amount of gill withdrawal observed in a series of 80 sequential reflex activations. Selected activations are shown. (From Pinsker et al. 1970.)

have the suffix `.m`. A script file can be written using any editor, (provided it has the `.m` suffix) but it is convenient to use the editor that is supplied with MATLAB. You should store your scripts in a directory that is on the MATLAB path. The path can be set from the MATLAB command window. Any script stored in a directory that is on the MATLAB path can be run simply by typing the name of the script on the command line in the MATLAB command window. When using the name of a script as a command the `.m` suffix is omitted. A script that implements the simulation of habituation of the *Aplysia* gill-withdrawal reflex, called `habituationGWR.m`, is listed in MATLAB Box 1.1. We included the `.m` suffix here but will omit it henceforth for clarity.

1.5   The Dynamics of a Single Neural Unit with Positive Feedback

The function of a neural system, like that of many other kinds of systems, is to transform inputs into outputs. Input–output transformations can be static or dynamic. In a static transformation, the output at any time point depends only on the input at a corresponding time point. The simple reflex model we studied in the previous section, composed of a single unit receiving a weighted input, produces a static input–output transformation because the output $y(t)$ depends only on the input $x(t)$ at any time point t.

The simple reflex model is a neural system with two variables, input variable x and unit state variable y, and one parameter, input weight v. When we simulated habituation, we caused the value of the weight parameter v to decrease with each input pulse. Thus, the simple reflex model is a neural system with a time-varying parameter (Luenberger 1979), but we still consider its input–output transformation to be static because, for any specific value of v, its output at any time point depends only on the input at a corresponding time point. Habituation in the simple reflex model is considered adaptive because it simulates a decrease in a reflex response when such a response is not needed (but see Exercise 1.2). Thus, habituation is a simple form of adaptive weight change, or learning, in a neural system. We will study many neural systems in this book, both static and dynamic, whose connection weights can be changed through learning. What distinguishes a static from a dynamic neural system is not the modifiability of its connection weights but the nature of the temporal dependencies of its output.

In a dynamic neural system, the output depends both on the input and on the previous states of its constituent units. In principle, a single, real neuron is capable of dynamic processing. Because of the intrinsic electrical properties of its membrane, which are called passive properties because they do not involve voltage-gated ion channels, a real neuron would transform an impulse input into an exponentially decaying membrane voltage. The time constant of this

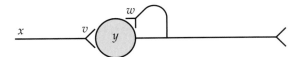

FIGURE 1.7   Simple neural system with feedback Input x, with feedforward connection weight v, contacts unit y, and unit y feeds back on itself with feedback weight w.

decay (i.e., the time it would take for the membrane voltage to decay to about 37% of its maximal value) is about 5 milliseconds in most neurons (Purves et al. 2008). This time is short enough that we can ignore it in this book.

Dynamic processing in systems of simple neural units requires interconnections between the units that form closed loops, or circuits. The simplest neural system capable of dynamic processing that we will study is composed of a single unit that receives an input and sends a positive feedback connection to itself. Most real neurons probably do not send excitatory connections directly to themselves, but many do so indirectly through interneurons. We will consider more complex forms of positive feedback in detail in Chapters 2 and 10, but we will often use positive self-connections for the purpose of dynamic processing in this book. A diagram of the single unit with positive feedback is shown in Figure 1.7. It is identical to the monosynaptic reflex model shown in Figure 1.2, with the addition of a feedback connection from the unit onto itself with weight w. Again, such a feedback connection probably would occur indirectly through interneurons in the real nervous system (see Chapter 2 for further discussion). We represent it as a direct connection because that simplification makes its functional role clearer.

We will use the simple system in Figure 1.7 to simulate the response to an input pulse of a neuron that receives an excitatory (positive) connection from an input neuron and sends a positive feedback connection to itself. The system (network) in Figure 1.7 has only two parameters. These are the connection weights v and w, where v is the weight of the input connection and w is the weight of the feedback connection. Equation 1.2 describes the responses of the simple network on each discrete time step:

$$y(t) = wy(t-1) + vx(t-1) \qquad \textbf{1.2}$$

Equation 1.2 specifies that the state of the unit on the current time step is the weighted sum of the input and the unit state on the previous time step. This dependence, not only on the input but also on the previous state of the unit, is what allows the single unit with positive feedback to produce dynamic input–output transformations. Equation 1.2 can be evaluated using a for-loop, in which the unit state on any time step is determined from the input and the unit state on the previous time step. The initial value of the unit state is 0. We can use this network to explore the effects of positive feedback weights of different strengths on the response properties of a neuron.

A script that implements this simulation, called `oneUnitWithPosFB`, is provided in MATLAB Box 1.2. As in the monosynaptic reflex model, the input to and output from the network will be sequences of values that vary in time (time series). Script `oneUnitWithPosFB` will generate either a pulse input, which takes value 1 on only one time step, or a step input, which takes value 1 and then maintains that value for the duration of the input time series. We will focus on pulse responses (but see Exercise 1.3). With `inFlag=1` the script sets up a pulse input as vector **x** with 101 elements, one element for each discrete time step from 0 to 100 in steps of 1. All elements of **x** are 0 except for one element, on time step 10, which is equal to 1. The script sets **x** up using `x=zeros(1,nTs)` and `x(start)=1`, where `nTs` is equal to 101 and `start=11`, which places the pulse on time step 10 (note that the time series starts on time step 0, so element 11 of the series corresponds to time step 10). The output of the network will be held in vector **y**, which will also have 101 elements, and is defined using `y=zeros(1,nTs)`. Thus, vectors **x** and **y** both have one element for each discrete time step t from 0 to 100 in steps of 1. Script `oneUnitWithPosFB` implements Equation 1.2 in a loop on each time step using `y(t)=w*y(t-1)+v*x(t-1)`.

MATLAB® BOX 1.2   **This script simulates the pulse or step response of a single neuron with positive feedback.**

```
% oneUnitWithPosFB.m

% set input flag (1 for pulse, 2 for step)
inFlag=1;

cut=-Inf; % set cut-off
sat=Inf; % set saturation

tEnd=100; % set last time step
nTs=tEnd+1; % find the number of time steps

v=1; % set the input weight
w=0.95; % set the feedback weight

x=zeros(1,nTs); % open (define) an input hold vector
start=11; % set a start time for the input
if inFlag==1, % if the input should be a pulse
    x(start)=1; % then set the input at only one time point
elseif inFlag==2, % if the input instead should be a step, then
    x(start:nTs)=ones(1,nTs-start+1); % keep it up until the end
end % end the conditional

y=zeros(1,nTs); % open (define) an output hold vector

for t=2:nTs, % on every time step (skipping the first)
    y(t)=w*y(t-1) + v*x(t-1); % compute the output
    if y(t)<cut, y(t)=cut; end % impose the cut-off constraint
    if y(t)>sat, y(t)=sat; end % impose the saturation constraint
end % end the for-loop
```

The script `oneUnitWithPosFB` allows you to set various parameters that are useful for exploring the single-unit with feedback model. We will first explore the effects on the pulse response of the unit due to positive feedback that is slightly less than 1. Set the feedback weight at $w = 0.95$ (w=0.95 in script `oneUnitWithPosFB`), and the input weight at $v = 1$ (v=1). The pulse response with $w = 0.95$ is shown in Figure 1.8. The output is clearly prolonged in time relative to the input. Technically, the output is a geometric decay, at a rate determined by the weight of the positive feedback connection (see Math Box 1.1). The main point of the simulation is to show that positive feedback can prolong the duration of the response of a neuron to a transient input.

Keeping all other parameters the same, change the feedback weight value to $w = 1$ (w=1) and recompute the output. The result is shown in Figure 1.9. The output is a step. Thus, with a feedback weight of 1, the simple network converts an input pulse into an output step. Technically, the single unit, with positive feedback weight $w = 1$, has temporally integrated the input, since the integral of a pulse is a step.

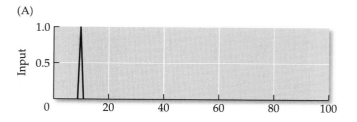

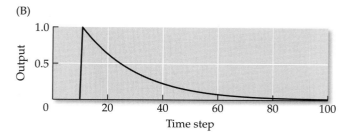

FIGURE 1.8   Behavior of the single-unit with positive-feedback model when the feedback weight is slightly less than 1 The input (A) is a pulse of 1 and the output (B) is a geometric decay from 1 to a 0 asymptote.

MATH BOX 1.1   GEOMETRIC DECAY OF THE DISCRETE PULSE RESPONSE

Consider the single unit with positive feedback in Figure 1.7 with response described by $y(t) = wy(t-1) + vx(t-1)$. If the unit receives a pulse of 1 on only one time step (after which the input goes back to 0) the unit will continue to activate itself through its own positive feedback. Thus, after the pulse, the state of the unit y on each time step t is the product of its previous state and its positive feedback weight: $y(t) = wy(t-1)$. To take some specific examples, assume that $y(0) = 0$, input weight $v = 1$, and the unit receives a pulse input of 1 on time step 0 ($x(0) = 1$) so that $y(1) = 1$. The input then goes back to 0, so the unit responses on time steps 2–4 are: $y(2) = wy(1)$, $y(3) = wy(2)$, and $y(4) = wy(3)$. By back substitution, we find that the response on time step 4 following a pulse response of 1 on time step 1 is $y(4) = wwwy(1) = w^3$ (since $y(1) = 1$). If its positive feedback connection has weight 0.95, then

$y(4) = 0.86$. In general, if the initial pulse response of 1 occurs on time step $t = 1$, then the response of the unit on any subsequent time step t will be w^{t-1}, where w is the positive feedback connection weight. The time axis can be shifted if the pulse occurs on some other time step. If the feedback weight w is a positive number between 0 and 1 ($0 < w < 1$), then the response will decrease with every subsequent time step and will approach 0. This geometric decay in discrete time is analogous to an exponential decay in continuous time (see Math Box 2.1). There are sophisticated mathematical techniques for analyzing both continuous and discrete-time systems (e.g., Luenberger 1979), but their usefulness is limited for complicated and nonlinear systems such as neural systems. Computer simulation is a viable technique for studying neural systems.

Neural systems, and models thereof, that have net positive feedback between 0 and 1 are often referred to as "leaky" (imperfect) integrators. The single unit with positive feedback of 0.95, whose pulse response is shown in Figure 1.8, is an example of a leaky integrator. Leaky integrators may be important components of neural systems in general, and may be of particular importance for motor control. We will explore the use of leaky integrators as components of models of motor control networks in the next chapter.

In the single-unit models we have studied so far, whether static or dynamic, the state is simply equal to the weighted sum of the inputs to the unit. As such, the output of the unit is linearly related to its weighted input sum over the entire range of the input. Because the connection weights can be positive or negative, the weighted input sum can take any value—positive, negative, or zero, and so the states of these linear units can similarly take any value. Linear units are often useful in modeling neural systems, but real neurons are not linear, since their action potential firing rates cannot take any value but are bounded between zero and some saturation level of firing rate. (Saturation is

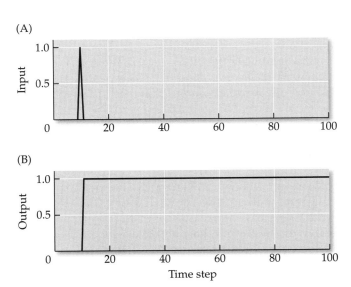

FIGURE 1.9   Behavior of the single-unit with positive-feedback model when the feedback weight equals 1 The input (A) is a pulse of 1 and the output (B) is a step of 1.

(A)

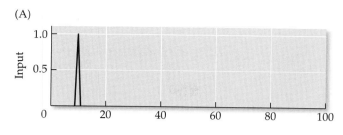

(B)

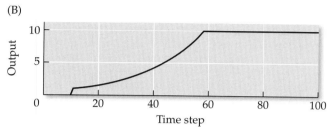

Time step

FIGURE 1.10   Behavior of the single-unit with positive-feedback model when the feedback weight is slightly greater than 1 Cut-off and saturation limits have been imposed. The input (A) is a pulse of 1 and the output (B) is a geometric rise from 1 to the saturation limit.

around 1000 spikes per second for the fastest-firing neurons; see Purves et al. 2008.) It is often necessary to model the neural nonlinearity.

One way to account for the neural nonlinearity is simply to bound the state of a unit between a cut-off level of 0 and some saturation level. This can be accomplished in MATLAB using the following conditionals: `if y(t)<cut, y(t)=cut; end` and `if y(t)>sat, y(t)=sat; end`, where `cut` is set to the cut-off level (generally 0) and `sat` is set to the saturation level. These commands are included in the for-loop in script `oneUnitWithPosFB` (see MATLAB Box 1.2). Note that these more expressive conditional commands can be replaced with more efficient commands using `max` and `min`: `y(t)=max(y(t),cut)` and `y(t)=min(y(t),sat)`. The more efficient versions are used in later MATLAB scripts.

Bound the state of unit y between a cut-off of 0 and a saturation level of 10. This can be done in `oneUnitWithPosFB` by setting `cut=0` and `sat=10`. Now change the feedback weight w from 1 to 1.05 (`w=1.05`) and find the pulse response to this new weight configuration. The results are shown in Figure 1.10. The output is a geometric rise (as opposed to a geometric decay as in Figure 1.8) from 1 up to the saturation level of 10.

These pulse-response results illustrate how the discrete-time dynamics of a simple neural system are governed by the strength of its positive feedback. For feedback connection weights between 0 and 1 the pulse response would decay, but the stronger the weight the more prolonged the response. When the feedback connection weight equals 1, the pulse response endures forever. For any feedback connection weight greater than 1 the pulse response would grow, and the rate of growth is proportional to the strength of the feedback weight.

Technically, a discrete-time system is unstable when the strength of its positive feedback is greater than 1. The state of an unstable system will grow to infinity, or to an upper bound such as a saturation limit. A system is stable if its positive feedback is less than 1 and greater than or equal to 0. A system is considered marginally stable if its positive feedback weight equals 1, because a small perturbation of the weight above 1 will cause the system to become unstable. While a marginally stable system can function as a perfect integrator, a leaky (imperfect) integrator may be preferred because of its comparative stability, provided the response prolongation it produces is sufficient. We will revisit these issues in the next chapter.

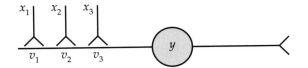

FIGURE 1.11   A model of a single neuron with three inputs The unit (model neuron) y has an "axon" (sending end) that is opposite its "dendrite" (receiving end). It receives three inputs, x_1, x_2, and x_3, which contact its dendrite with weights v_1, v_2, and v_3, respectively.

1.6   Neural Networks: Neural Systems with Multiple Interconnected Units

Of course, most real neural systems are composed of more than one neuron, and most real neurons receive more than one or two inputs. The human brain is estimated to contain on the order of 10^{11} neurons, and each neuron is estimated to receive about 10,000 inputs. To accommodate this huge number of synaptic inputs, most neurons have an extensive "tree" of dendrites, which are neural processes that extend from the cell body in a direction roughly opposite the axon (see Purves et al. 2008). The dendrites greatly expand the surface area of the neuron that is available for the synapses from other neurons to make contact. The dendrites do not merely collect the synaptic inputs to a neuron but are capable of complex forms of input processing known as synaptic integration. For simplicity in this book we will not attempt to simulate dendritic processing in detail. Instead, our neural units will approximate dendritic processing simply by computing the weighted sum of their inputs.

Compared with the actual brain, our neural network models will contain few neural units, and each unit will receive few inputs. Still, our models will have sufficiently many neural units and inputs that treating them individually would be impractical. We will use vectors and matrices to describe the inputs and outputs of a network, the states of the units in a neural network, and the weights of the connections from the external inputs to the units or between the units themselves. The computation by the units of the weighted sums of their inputs can be described using vector and matrix multiplication. This is demonstrated using the single unit with three inputs shown in Figure 1.11.

Unit y has a "dendrite" (its receiving end) that extends from it in the direction opposite its "axon" (its sending end). The three inputs, x_1, x_2, and x_3, make synaptic contact with the dendrite, and the corresponding synaptic weights are v_1, v_2, and v_3. Unit y computes the weighted sum of its inputs as $y = v_1 x_1 + v_2 x_2 + v_3 x_3$. If we express the weights and inputs as vectors, then the weighted input sum is the inner (dot) product between the weight vector and the input vector. By convention, vectors are arranged as columns, but on the page they are more naturally written as rows. The transpose operator T will change a row vector to a column vector. Thus, the weight and input vectors, as columns, can be written as $\mathbf{v} = [v_1\ v_2\ v_3]^{\mathrm{T}}$ and $\mathbf{x} = [x_1\ x_2\ x_3]^{\mathrm{T}}$.

In multiplying vectors (and matrices), their order and dimension are important (see Math Box 1.2). To compute the inner (or dot) product between two vectors, the first vector must be arranged as a row, and the second as a column. Thus, computation of the weighted input sum by unit y can be described as the inner product between its weight vector $\mathbf{v}$ and the input vector $\mathbf{x}$, as in Equation 1.3:

$$y = \mathbf{v}^{\mathrm{T}}\mathbf{x} = \begin{bmatrix} v_1 & v_2 & v_3 \end{bmatrix}\begin{bmatrix} x_1 \\ x_2 \\ x_3 \end{bmatrix} = v_1 x_1 + v_2 x_2 + v_3 x_3 \qquad \textbf{1.3}$$

MATH BOX 1.2   VECTOR AND MATRIX MULTIPLICATION: ACROSS THE ROW AND DOWN THE COLUMN

The rule for vector and matrix multiplication can be summarized by the phrase "across the row and down the column" (Noble and Daniel 1988). Two vectors can be multiplied if they have the same dimension (i.e., the same number of elements). Then the inner (or dot) product between the two vectors can be computed if the first vector is a row and the second a column (in which case they are conformable). Computation of the inner product is carried out by multiplying the corresponding pairs of elements in the vectors and summing the products. For example:

$$\begin{bmatrix} a & b & c \end{bmatrix} \begin{bmatrix} x \\ y \\ z \end{bmatrix} = ax + by + cz \qquad \text{B1.2.1}$$

Note that in finding the pairs of elements to be multiplied we moved across the row vector and down the column vector. The inner product between the vectors is a scalar (a single number) rather than another vector. The process can be extended to multiplication of a matrix and a column vector (in that order), provided that the matrix and the column vector are conformable (i.e., that the number of columns of the matrix equals the number of elements in the vector). For example:

$$\begin{bmatrix} a & b & c \\ d & e & f \\ g & h & i \end{bmatrix} \begin{bmatrix} x \\ y \\ z \end{bmatrix} = \begin{bmatrix} ax + by + cz \\ dx + ey + fz \\ gx + hy + iz \end{bmatrix} \qquad \text{B1.2.2}$$

Note that in finding the pairs of elements to be multiplied we moved across each row of the matrix and down the column vector. The result is a column vector that has as many elements as there are rows of the matrix. The same process can be extended to the multiplication of two conformable matrices (where the number of columns of the first equals the number of rows of the second), in which case the result is another matrix (see Math Box 4.3).

Computation of the inner product in MATLAB simply involves multiplication of two vectors, provided they are of the same dimension and the first vector is a row and the second a column. The commands v=[1 2 3]' and x=[3 2 1]' will make column vectors **v** and **x** with the elements as indicated. Recall that the apostrophe signifies the transpose in MATLAB. Then the inner product y can be computed as y=v'*x. The result of performing this operation in MATLAB is shown in Table 1.2. Note that the multiplication symbol * that we use here to multiply two vectors (and in this case to find their inner product) is the same as the one we used above to multiply two scalars, or a scalar and a vector. The multiplication symbol * in MATLAB is general and can be used to multiply scalars, vectors, and matrices in any pairwise combination, provided they are conformable (see Math Box 1.2).

Unit responses in neural systems having more than one unit can be computed by multiplication of a matrix and a vector, where the matrix holds the weight values and the vector holds the input values. This is demonstrated using the network shown in Figure 1.12. This network has three inputs, x_1, x_2, and x_3, but also has three output units, y_1, y_2, and y_3. Each unit has a long dendrite (as in Figure 1.11), and there is a synapse at the intersection of each input axon and unit dendrite. The individual weights are not labeled, for clarity. In the system

TABLE 1.2   Computing the inner (or dot) product between two vectors using MATLAB

```
>> v=[1 2 3]'    >> x=[3 2 1]'    >> y=v'*x

v =              x =              y =
    1                3                10
    2                2
    3                1
```

FIGURE 1.12   A model of three neurons, each receiving three inputs The inputs are x_1, x_2, and x_3 and the units are y_1, y_2, and y_3. Input x_j ($j = 1, 2, 3$) connects to unit y_i ($i = 1, 2, 3$) with weight v_{ij}. The v_{ij} are not shown for clarity.

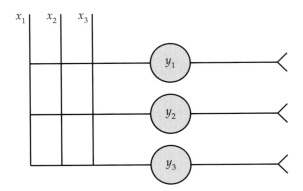

composed of only one unit (see Figure 1.11), it was obvious that the inputs had only one unit to project to. In the single-unit case the weight variable names had only one subscript, and that subscript designated the input number. In networks with more than one unit, both the input number and the receiving unit number must be designated.

By convention, the weight variables are subscripted with the receiving unit number first and the input number second. The order of the subscripts is like that of a letter, as in To John, From Mary. Thus, the input weight v_{12} denotes the weight to unit 1 from input 2. Also by convention, the first subscript corresponds to a row of the weight matrix, while the second subscript corresponds to a column of the weight matrix. Thus, each row of the input weight matrix holds the weights to a specific unit from all inputs, while each column holds the weights to all units from a specific input. The input weight matrix **V** for the network in Figure 1.12 is shown in Equation 1.4:

$$\mathbf{V} = \begin{bmatrix} v_{11} & v_{12} & v_{13} \\ v_{21} & v_{22} & v_{23} \\ v_{31} & v_{32} & v_{33} \end{bmatrix} \qquad \textbf{1.4}$$

Simply stated, each row of the input weight matrix **V** is the vector of weights to a specific unit. Thus, multiplication of the input vector by matrix **V** will yield a vector of inner products, which are the weighted input sums to each unit in the network. This is shown mathematically in Equation 1.5:

$$\mathbf{y} = \mathbf{V}\mathbf{x} = \begin{bmatrix} v_{11} & v_{12} & v_{13} \\ v_{21} & v_{22} & v_{23} \\ v_{31} & v_{32} & v_{33} \end{bmatrix} \begin{bmatrix} x_1 \\ x_2 \\ x_3 \end{bmatrix} = \begin{bmatrix} v_{11}x_1 + v_{12}x_2 + v_{13}x_3 \\ v_{21}x_1 + v_{22}x_2 + v_{23}x_3 \\ v_{31}x_1 + v_{32}x_2 + v_{33}x_3 \end{bmatrix} = \begin{bmatrix} y_1 \\ y_2 \\ y_3 \end{bmatrix} = \mathbf{y} \qquad \textbf{1.5}$$

TABLE 1.3   Computing the product of a matrix and a vector using MATLAB

`>> V=[1 2 3;4 5 6;7 8 9]`	`>> x=[3 2 1]'`	`>> y=V*x`
`V =`	`x =`	`y =`
`1  2  3`	`3`	`10`
`4  5  6`	`2`	`28`
`7  8  9`	`1`	`46`

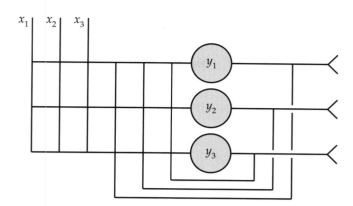

FIGURE 1.13 **A model of three neurons, each receiving three inputs, and each feeding back on themselves and on each other**
Input x_j ($j = 1, 2, 3$) connects to unit y_i ($i = 1, 2, 3$) with input weight v_{ij}, and unit y_l ($l = 1, 2, 3$) connects to unit y_k ($k = 1, 2, 3$) with feedback weight w_{kl}. The input (feedforward) and feedback weights are not shown for clarity.

The commands V=[1 2 3;4 5 6;7 8 9] and x=[3 2 1]' (with no semicolons following the commands) will make matrix **V** and vector **x** containing the elements as indicated. Note that the semicolons separating certain elements in V=[1 2 3;4 5 6;7 8 9] designate row breaks. Because no semicolons follow the commands, their results are displayed on the monitor. Now the product **y** can be computed as y=V*x and displayed on the monitor (again with no semicolon following the command). The results are shown in Table 1.3. Note that the first element of **y** is 10, which is the value of its response in the single-unit case as shown in Table 1.2.

The network in Figure 1.12 is capable only of static processing, in that the responses of the units at any point in time depend only on their inputs at a corresponding time point. The addition of feedback connections makes the network capable of dynamic input–output transformations. The modified network is shown in Figure 1.13. As before, we label input weights as v and feedback weights as w. Because the network has three inputs and three units, the input weight matrix **V** is the same as before (see Equation 1.4). The feedback weight matrix **W** will connect the three units to themselves. Subscripting the elements of **W** follows the same convention as described previously for the input weights. Thus, w_{12} denotes the weight to unit 1 from unit 2. The weight matrix **W** is shown in Equation 1.6:

$$\mathbf{W} = \begin{bmatrix} w_{11} & w_{12} & w_{13} \\ w_{21} & w_{22} & w_{23} \\ w_{31} & w_{32} & w_{33} \end{bmatrix} \qquad \textbf{1.6}$$

With feedback connections the network becomes dynamic, and the responses of the units are described using a matrix version of Equation 1.2, shown in Equation 1.7:

$$\mathbf{y}(t) = \mathbf{W}\mathbf{y}(t-1) + \mathbf{V}\mathbf{x}(t-1) = \begin{bmatrix} w_{11} & w_{12} & w_{13} \\ w_{21} & w_{22} & w_{23} \\ w_{31} & w_{32} & w_{33} \end{bmatrix} \begin{bmatrix} y_1(t-1) \\ y_2(t-1) \\ y_3(t-1) \end{bmatrix} + \begin{bmatrix} v_{11} & v_{12} & v_{13} \\ v_{21} & v_{22} & v_{23} \\ v_{31} & v_{32} & v_{33} \end{bmatrix} \begin{bmatrix} x_1(t-1) \\ x_2(t-1) \\ x_3(t-1) \end{bmatrix} \quad \textbf{1.7}$$

In modeling neural systems, it is sometimes convenient to concatenate the input and feedback matrices into a connectivity matrix **M**, and the input and unit vectors into a state vector **z**. This construction is shown in Equation 1.8:

$$\mathbf{y}(t) = \mathbf{M}\mathbf{z}(t-1) = \begin{bmatrix} v_{11} & v_{12} & v_{13} & w_{11} & w_{12} & w_{13} \\ v_{21} & v_{22} & v_{23} & w_{21} & w_{22} & w_{23} \\ v_{31} & v_{32} & v_{33} & w_{31} & w_{32} & w_{33} \end{bmatrix} \begin{vmatrix} x_1(t-1) \\ x_2(t-1) \\ x_3(t-1) \\ y_1(t-1) \\ y_2(t-1) \\ y_3(t-1) \end{vmatrix} \qquad \textbf{1.8}$$

We will use the construction of Equation 1.8 in later chapters, but for now we will stay with the separate construction of Equation 1.7. When using separate **V** and **W** weight matrices we can also refer to input weight matrix **V** as the feedforward weight matrix, to contrast it with the feedback weight matrix **W**. We will set up a network having ten inputs and ten units. Just for fun, we will randomize all of the feedforward and feedback weights. Since there are ten inputs and ten units, the feedforward and feedback matrices **V** and **W** both have dimensions of 10-by-10. A 10-by-10 matrix **V** having elements drawn from a mean 0, variance 1 Gaussian distribution can be constructed using `V=randn(10,10)`. Alternatively, random square matrices such as **V** and **W** can be constructed using the shorthand commands `V=randn(10)` and `W=randn(10)`.

Because the network has feedback connections and produces dynamic input–output transformations, its inputs and unit responses (outputs) will all be time series. We will set up the input as an array x having 10 rows and 101 columns, in which each column corresponds to a time point from 0 to 100 in steps of 1, and each row corresponds to 1 of the 10 inputs. To have all inputs deliver the same pulse, we set the values of all inputs at all time points to 0, except at time point 10, which we set to a pulse of 1 for all inputs. The command `x=zeros(10,101)` will set up the input array of all zeros, and `x(:,11)=ones(10,1)` will put a 1 at time point 10 in each input time series (note that time point 10 corresponds to column 11 of x). The 10 output responses are stored in an array y of the same dimensions as the input array. The command `y=zeros(10,101)` will define the output array. Input and output arrays of this form, and random feedforward and feedback matrices, are set up in script `BigMess`, which is listed in MATLAB Box 1.3.

The response of the units to this input can be found by evaluating Equation 1.7 at each time point. This can be done using a for-loop as in the case with only one unit feeding back onto itself (see the script `oneUnitWithPosFB` in MATLAB Box 1.2). To make the unit responses in the big network less unstable, and therefore more interesting, first scale the feedback weights by half. This is done in `BigMess` by setting the weight scale as `scw=0.5` and scaling matrix **W** with it after randomizing **W**. The script implements Equation 1.7 using `y(t)=W*y(t-1)+V*x(t-1)`. It also nonlinearly bounds the unit responses on each time step *t* between a cut-off of 0 and a saturation level of 1000 using `y(:,t)=max(y(:,t),cut)` and `y(:,t)=min(y(:,t),sat)`, with `cut=0` and `sat=1000`.

The script `BigMess` (see MATLAB Box 1.3) will compute the responses of the network and save them in array y. The weight matrices, the inputs, and the unit responses in this example can be plotted in three dimensions using the `mesh` command in MATLAB. Specifically, `mesh(V)`, `mesh(W)`, `mesh(x)`, and `mesh(y)` will provide 3D perspective plots of the feedforward weights, feedback weights, input states, and output states, respectively. They could all be placed in the same figure using the `subplot` command. For example, `subplot(2,2,1)` will divide the figure window into four quadrants and open the top-left quadrant for plotting.

MATLAB® BOX 1.3   **This script simulates the pulse or step response of a neural network with ten input and ten output units that are randomly connected.**

```
% BigMess.m

nIn=10; % set number of input units
nOut=10; % set number of output units

scw=0.5; % enter scale for feedback weights

inFlag=1; % set input flag (1 for pulse, 2 for step)

cut=0; % set cut-off
sat=1000; % set saturation

tEnd=100; % set the last time step value
nTs=tEnd+1; % find the number of time steps

x=zeros(nIn,nTs); % open (define) an input hold array
start=11; % set a start time for the input
if inFlag==1, % if the input should be a pulse
    x(:,start)=ones(nIn,1); % then set input at only one time point
elseif inFlag==2, % if the input instead should be a step, then
    x(:,start:nTs)=ones(nIn,nTs-start+1); % keep it up until the end
end % end the conditional

y=zeros(nOut,nTs); % open (define) an output hold array

V=randn(nOut,nIn); % construct random feedforward weight matrix
W=randn(nOut)*scw;% construct and scale random feedback weight matrix

for t=2:nTs, % on every time step (skipping the first)
    y(:,t)=W*y(:,t-1) + V*x(:,t-1); % compute the output
    y(:,t)=max(y(:,t),cut); % impose the cut-off constraint
    y(:,t)=min(y(:,t),sat); % impose the saturation constraint
end % end the for-loop
```

The connection weights, pulse inputs, and responses of the units in the 10-by-10 network with random input (feedforward) and feedback connections that are computed using script `BigMess` are shown in Figure 1.14. Figure 1.14A and B shows the feedforward and feedback matrices, respectively, which have all random elements. Figure 1.14C and D shows the pulse inputs and the unit responses, respectively. The responses are a mess! Some units saturate, some cut-off, and others assume intermediate values that may or may not remain constant over the time series. The actual form taken by the responses depends on the particular random elements in the connectivity matrices. In some cases all of the responses die down before the end of the time series, while different patterns of active and inactive units develop in other cases. You might want to run `BigMess` several times in order to observe the types of messes it is capable of producing.

The responses from a network with random connection weights, such as those illustrated in Figure 1.14, would not be very useful for computational purposes. Throughout the rest of this book we will develop networks with structures similar to the one studied in this example, but with non-random

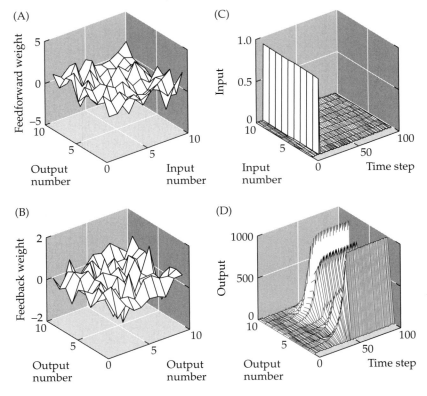

(A)

(B)

(C)

(D)

FIGURE 1.14   Behavior of a larger neural network model   Random feedforward weights (A), feedback weights (B), pulse input (C), and messy output (D) from a neural network as in Figure 1.13 but with ten inputs and ten units.

connection weights that make them much more useful computationally. We will explore networks that can shape signals in time and space, produce oscillations, exhibit multiple stable states, and predict the future values of inputs. We will also explore adaptive networks that can learn to memorize, categorize, classify, evaluate, and increase the amount of information they contain about their inputs. Most critically for our purposes in this book, all of these networks will resemble real neural systems in interesting and important ways.

Exercises

1.1   The Gauss busywork solution outlined at the beginning of the chapter works only for even integers, but would it work for any even integer? Try using the method to sum the integers from 1 to 2000. Does it work? Could you find a simple formula that would allow you to compute the sum of integers from 1 to any arbitrary integer?

1.2   Once habituated, the *Aplysia* gill-withdrawal reflex will dishabituate with time, but it also can be rapidly dishabituated through the process of sensitization (Kandel 1976). Sensitization occurs when an intense stimulus is applied to some body part of the *Aplysia* other than the gill or mantle, such as the tail. Model sensitization by modifying the script `habituationGWR` (see MATLAB Box 1.1) to include an input from the tail that, when activated, restores the sensory neuron to motoneuron synapse to its original value.

1.3 The script `oneUnitWithPosFB` (see MATLAB Box 1.2) allows the user to switch the input to the single unit with positive feedback from a pulse to a step. Set the feedback weight `w` to some positive value less than 1, and find the response to the step input. How would you describe the response? Both the pulse and the step responses move from 1 to some asymptotic level. Is the rate of movement toward their respective asymptotes the same for both the pulse and step responses?

1.4 The script `BigMess` (see MATLAB Box 1.3), which implements a one-layered neural network with positive feedback, will also allow the user to switch the input from a pulse to a step. How would you compare the step and pulse responses of this network?

References

Churchland PS, Sejnowski TJ (1992) *The Computational Brain.* MIT Press, Cambridge, MA.

Gilbert CD, Sigman M (2007) Brian states: Top down influences in sensory processing. *Neuron* 54: 677–696.

Hawkins RD, Cohen TE, Greene W, Kandel ER (1998) Relationships between dishabituation, sensitization, and inhibition of the gill- and siphon-withdrawal reflex in *Aplysia californica*: Effects of response measure, test time, and training stimulus. *Behavioral Neuroscience* 112: 24–38.

Hayes B (2006) Gauss's Day of Reckoning. *American Scientist* 94: 200–206.

Kandel ER (1976) *Cellular Basis of Behavior: An Introduction to Behavioral Neurobiology.* WH Freeman, San Francisco, CA.

Koch C, Segev I (eds) (1989) *Methods in Neuronal Modeling: From Synapses to Networks.* MIT Press, Cambridge, MA.

Luenberger DG (1979) *Introduction to Dynamic Systems: Theory, Models, and Applications.* John Wiley and Sons, New York.

Noble B, Daniel JW (1988) *Applied Linear Algebra: Third Edition.* Prentice Hall, Englewood Cliffs, NJ.

Pinsker H, Kupfermann I, Castellucci V, Kandel E (1970) Habituation and dishabituation of the gill-withdrawal reflex in *Aplysia. Science* 167: 1740–1742.

Purves D, Augustine GJ, Fitzpatrick D, Hall WC, LaMantia A-S, McNamara JO, White LE (eds) (2008) *Neuroscience: Fourth Edition.* Sinauer, Sunderland, MA.

Recurrent Connections and Simple Neural Circuits

Networks with recurrent connections, forming circuits, and containing only a few neural units can shape signals in time, produce oscillations, and simulate certain forms of low-level motor control

Brain function ranges from high-level cognition down to relatively simple forms of sensory processing and motor control. The processing associated with low-level motor control involves shaping the temporal characteristics of signals in various ways that include prolonging, foreshortening, and combining them. It can also involve the generation of oscillations that drive rhythmic movement patterns. A wide range of motor behaviors (including reflex responses and locomotion) can be explained in terms of such relatively simple forms of signal processing and temporal pattern generation (Gallistel 1980).

Many forms of motor control involve the transformation of a transient sensory input into a prolonged response. We observe this every time we try to swat a fly but fail. The fly transforms a brief visual input, from our rapidly moving hand or rolled-up newspaper, into an escape jump that is followed by rhythmic movements of its wings that continue long enough for it to fly away to safety (Holmqvist and Srinivasan 1991). Seminal

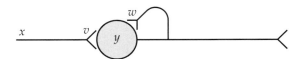

FIGURE 2.1   A single-unit leaky integrator A leaky integrator can be modeled as a single unit y that receives input x with weight v and sends an excitatory, recurrent (feedback) connection to itself with positive weight w.

studies of another insect, the locust, reveal that rhythmic wing movements are driven by neural systems that can generate sustained oscillations (Wilson 1961).

Prolonged responses are essential for the most basic types of motor control. The vestibular system maintains the stability both of the posture of an organism and of its retinal image by controlling movements of the body, limbs, head, and eyes (Wilson and Melvill Jones 1979). To do this, the system must transform often transient inputs from the vestibular receptors into motor commands that not only stretch out the response in time but also preserve the sharp onset of the sensory input. Surprisingly, prolonged responses in combination with other signals may actually foreshorten vestibular motor control commands in some cases.

In this chapter we will study neural systems models that can simulate these dynamic transformations. They will include, as a component, the single-unit leaky integrator that we studied in Chapter 1. This versatile neural subsystem can be used as a building block in dynamic signal processing neural networks. As you will recall from Chapter 1, the leaky integrator is composed of a single linear unit that receives an input connection and sends an excitatory, recurrent (positive feedback) connection to itself. As explained in Chapter 1, most real neurons probably do not send excitatory, recurrent connections directly to themselves (but see Section 2.5). In contrast, many real neurons probably do exert an excitatory influence on themselves indirectly through interneurons. These interneurons no doubt modulate the positive feedback in neural systems and therefore play important computational roles. In Chapter 10 we will explore an example in which positive feedback to some neural units is modulated by recurrent connections through other units. In this chapter (and in some later chapters) we will study networks containing units with positive self-connections because they are easy to construct and analyze. The single-unit with positive-feedback system is schematized in Figure 2.1.

As described in Chapter 1, the simple network in Figure 2.1 has only two parameters. These are the connection weights v and w, where v is the weight of the input (forward) connection and w is the weight of the recurrent connection. The input and output as functions of discrete time t can be designated as $x(t)$ and $y(t)$, respectively. The equation that describes the (discrete-time) responses of this simple network is shown in Equation 2.1:

$$y(t) = wy(t-1) + vx(t-1) \qquad \textbf{2.1}$$

Equation 2.1 specifies that the state of the unit on the current time step is the weighted sum of the input and unit state on the previous time step. This can be computed using a for-loop, in which the unit state on the previous time step is saved and used, along with the corresponding input value on the previous time step, to compute the unit state on the current time step. The single-unit leaky integrator model is implemented using the script `oneUnitWithPosFB`, which is listed in MATLAB® Box 1.2 (see Chapter 1).

Whereas the response to an input pulse of a perfect integrator would persist as a step (see Figure 1.9), the leaky response of a leaky integrator would decay (see Figure 1.8). As explained in Chapter 1, a single real neuron, even without positive feedback onto itself, could be considered a leaky integrator. Due to the passive electrical properties of its membrane, the membrane voltage increase due to a pulse of input current would not return immediately to baseline following the pulse but would decay exponentially. The time constant of this exponential decay, which is the time it takes for the membrane voltage to decay to about 37% of the maximal value of the pulse response, is called the membrane time constant. It is equal to the product of the resistance and the capacitance of the membrane, which is about 5 ms for most neurons (Purves et al. 2008). The exponential decay is a continuous-time phenomenon. For simplicity in this book, we will treat time in discrete time steps only. The geometric decay, which we encountered in Chapter 1, is the discrete-time analog of the continuous-time exponential decay, as explained in Math Box 2.1.

The dynamic effects of the membrane time constant could be simulated in discrete time using the single-unit with positive-feedback model (Math Box 2.2). However, the integrating properties of a real neuron with a membrane time constant of about 5 ms would be insignificant on the time scales of many seconds that will concern us here. Leaky integration on time scales of seconds probably requires some form of positive feedback in the real brain, and we will model it as such. For simplicity, we can assume that any effects due to membrane time constants, or to other dynamic properties of real neurons, are subsumed under the weight of the positive feedback connection.

Leaky integrators may be important components of neural systems in general, and may be of particular importance for motor control. In this chapter we will explore the use of leaky integrators as components of dynamic neural networks. While we will consider the benefits of nonlinearity in later chapters, we will use only linear units in this chapter (but see Exercise 2.4 for an example involving nonlinear units). For our first example, we will explore the behavior of a simple neural network model composed of two, linear, leaky integrators in series.

MATH BOX 2.1   THE GEOMETRIC DECAY IS THE DISCRETE-TIME ANALOG OF THE EXPONENTIAL DECAY

Continuous-time systems are evaluated at any time, where time is expressed as a real number, while discrete-time systems are evaluated only on integer-valued time steps. A simple comparison illustrates the difference between continuous- and discrete-time systems. Consider the following differential equation in continuous time $\hat{t}$

$$y'(\hat{t}) = -\frac{1}{\tau}y(\hat{t}) + x(\hat{t}) \qquad \text{B2.1.1}$$

where y' is the rate of change of y. Equation B2.1.1 says that y decreases at a rate proportional to its state and increases at a rate proportional to its input. If its input x is the unit impulse at time 0, which essentially imparts to y a state of 1 at time 0 ($y(0) = 1$), then the response of Equation B2.1.1 is the exponential decay

$$y(\hat{t}) = e^{-\hat{t}/\tau} \qquad \text{B2.1.2}$$

which decays with time constant τ that has dimensions of seconds. Now consider the following equation in discrete

time t. (We will use symbol t for discrete time throughout this book.)

$$y(t) = wy(t-1) + x(t-1) \qquad \text{B2.1.3}$$

Equation B2.1.3 says that the state of y at time t depends both on its own state and on the input on the previous time step. If $0 < w < 1$ and the input is a unit pulse delivered on time step –1 so that $y(0) = 1$, then the response of Equation B2.1.3 is the geometric decay

$$y(t) = w^t \qquad \text{B2.1.4}$$

If we disallow negative times, then an input pulse on time step 0 causes $y(1) = 1$ and the response is $y(t) = w^{t-1}$ (see Math Box 1.1). The exponential and geometric decays can be considered as the continuous-time and discrete-time analogs of one another.

MATH BOX 2.2   DISCRETE APPROXIMATION OF A CONTINUOUS DIFFERENTIAL EQUATION MODEL OF A SINGLE NEURON

The dynamic behavior of neurons is generally described using differential equations in continuous time (e.g., Dayan and Abbott 2001). Various numerical methods exist for accurately integrating differential equations (e.g., Hultquist 1988). We will not consider detailed simulation of single neuron dynamics in this book, but we can sketch out a rough correspondence between continuous-time models and our discrete-time approximations. The simplest continuous-time, differential equation model of a single neuron is:

$$\tau y'(\hat{t}) + y(\hat{t}) = \hat{v}x(\hat{t}) \qquad \text{B2.2.1}$$

where the caret denotes variables that are specific to the continuous-time case, such as weight $\hat{v}$ and continuous time $\hat{t}$. Variable y represents neural firing rate, which is proportional to membrane potential. In words, Equation B2.2.1 implies that both y and its rate of change (or first derivative) y' are proportional to input x weighted by $\hat{v}$, and the dynamics are governed by membrane time

constant τ. Equation B2.2.1 (a continuous-time differential equation) can be very roughly approximated using a difference equation:

$$\tau\left(\frac{y(t) - y(t-1)}{\Delta t}\right) + y(t-1) = \hat{v}x(t-1) \qquad \text{B2.2.2}$$

where t represents discrete time that occurs in steps of Δt, and Δt can take any real, positive value. (Since we use discrete time only in this book we will designate it using variable t.) Equation B2.2.2 can be written as

$$y(t) = wy(t-1) + vx(t-1) \qquad \text{B2.2.3}$$

where $w = (1 - \Delta t/\tau)$ and $v = (\Delta t/\tau)\hat{v}$. Thus, the self-weight w can represent the dynamic effects of the membrane time constant, as well as the weight of a connection from the unit onto itself. Equation B2.2.3 is the same as Equation 2.1 in the main text.

2.1   The Dynamics of Two Neural Units with Feedback in Series

We will begin by simulating the responses of two neurons connected in series, in which both neurons exert positive feedback on themselves. We will configure this neural network so that unit 2 (y_2) receives input from unit 1 (y_1), and unit 1 (y_1) receives an input connection from outside the network. This simple network is schematized in Figure 2.2.

The network composed of two leaky integrators in series (two-leak series) can be thought of as a member of the class of two-unit recurrent networks, in which each unit potentially can send a recurrent connection to itself or to the other unit, and can receive an input from outside the network. The general equation, in matrix format, that describes the discrete-time responses of the units in a recurrent, two-unit network that receives one input is shown in Equation 2.2:

$$\begin{bmatrix} y_1(t) \\ y_2(t) \end{bmatrix} = \begin{bmatrix} w_{11} & w_{12} \\ w_{21} & w_{22} \end{bmatrix}\begin{bmatrix} y_1(t-1) \\ y_2(t-1) \end{bmatrix} + \begin{bmatrix} v_1 \\ v_2 \end{bmatrix}x(t-1) \qquad \textbf{2.2}$$

where t denotes discrete time. We will use this equation to configure various two-unit recurrent networks, starting with the two-leak series, by setting the values of the individual v_i and w_{kl} weights (note that some weights can take value 0). We will generally use i ($i = 1, 2$) to index the units y_i, but we can also use k ($k = 1, 2$) and l ($l = 1, 2$) to index them. Then the input (forward or feedforward) weights v_i connect the single input x to the units y_i, and the recurrent weights w_{kl} connect units y_l to units y_k. Using such an abundance of indices will be especially useful later to avoid ambiguities when we describe larger networks.

In the small networks we consider in this chapter, a forward connection is directed from an external input to a unit, while a recurrent connection is directed from a unit to another unit within the network. Recurrent connections

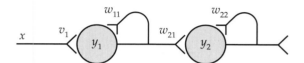

FIGURE 2.2   Two leaky integrators in series Both units y_1 and y_2 send excitatory, recurrent (positive feedback) connections to themselves with weights w_{11} and w_{22}, respectively. Unit y_1 receives input x from outside the network, with weight v_1, while unit y_2 receives input from unit y_1 with weight w_{21}. Note that unit y_2 does not also receive input x.

can form closed loops, or circuits. The simplest circuit is formed by a unit that sends a recurrent connection to itself, such as the single unit with positive feedback shown in Figure 2.1. Recurrent connections between units do not necessarily form circuits, because a unit can send connections to other units but not receive any connections in return. More generally, recurrent connections among the same set of units can form circuits of various sizes, the largest being the circuit that includes every unit in the network. We will consider some simple recurrent connectivity patterns in this chapter.

In Equation 2.2, the matrix of recurrent weights w_{kl} can be denoted by **W**, and the column vector of input weights v_i can be denoted by **V**, since a vector can be considered as a type of matrix (see Chapter 1). The column vector of unit states y_i can be denoted by **y**. Then the responses **y**(t) at any time t are described by $\mathbf{y}(t) = \mathbf{W}\mathbf{y}(t-1) + \mathbf{V}x(t-1)$, which is the sum of two column vectors. The product of matrix **W** and vector **y**$(t-1)$ produces one column vector (see Math Box 1.2), while the product of matrix (column vector) **V** and scalar $x(t-1)$ produces the other column vector. Note that multiplying a matrix (or vector) by a scalar is done simply by multiplying every individual element of the matrix (or vector) by the scalar. Summing two vectors (or matrices) is accomplished by summing corresponding elements. Summing is a valid operation only when the vectors (or matrices) to be summed are of the same size. These computations are illustrated with a numerical example.

To configure Equation 2.2 to represent the two units with positive feedback in series, some of the connection weight values will be 0. For our specific numerical example we will set the connection weights at $v_1 = 1$, $v_2 = 0$, $w_{11} = 0.95$, $w_{12} = 0$, $w_{21} = 0.5$, and $w_{22} = 0.6$. Note that the weights of disallowed connections, here v_2 and w_{12}, are simply set to 0. Thus, unit y_1 receives input x over weight $v_1 = 1$, but unit y_2 does not receive input x because $v_2 = 0$. Similarly, unit y_2 receives an input from y_1 over weight $w_{21} = 0.5$, but y_1 does not receive an input from y_2 because $w_{12} = 0$. Both units send an excitatory recurrent connection to themselves but y_1, with $w_{11} = 0.95$, exerts stronger positive feedback on itself than y_2, with $w_{22} = 0.6$. Thus, y_1 is a less leaky integrator than y_2 (see Chapter 1 for background on the leaky integrator, and for weight subscript conventions).

Given the weights as assigned, the response of y_1 is the weighted sum of the input and its own state on the previous time step, while the response of y_2 is the weighted sum of its own state and the state of y_1 on the previous time step. We can express **V** and **W** as $\mathbf{V} = [v_1 \, v_2]^T$ and $\mathbf{W} = [w_{11} \, w_{12}; w_{21} \, w_{22}]$, where the symbol ; in the expression for **W** signifies separate rows (semicolons are used to separate rows in MATLAB, as noted below in this section). Substituting the assigned weight values, $\mathbf{V} = [1 \, 0]^T$ and $\mathbf{W} = [0.95 \, 0; 0.5 \, 0.6]$. Now the responses of y_1 and y_2 can be computed using the matrix computations described above for Equation 2.2.

In this example we will study the leaking (or decaying) pulse responses of units y_1 and y_2. A discrete unit pulse is a signal that has value 1 on one time step, and has value 0 otherwise. To continue the numerical example, assume

MATLAB® BOX 2.1 **This script implements a model having two units in series, each with recurrent, excitatory self-connections allowing the units to exert positive feedback on themselves (the two units are leaky integrators).**

```
% twoLeakSeries.m

v1=1; v2=0; % set weights from the input
w11=0.95; w12=0; % set feedback weights to unit one
w21=0.5; w22=0.6; % set feedback weights to unit two

V=[v1;v2]; % compose input weight matrix (vector)
W=[w11 w12; w21 w22]; % compose feedback weight matrix

tEnd=100; % set end time
tVec=0:tEnd; % set time vector
nTs=tEnd+1; % find number of time steps
x=zeros(1,nTs); % zero (and define) the input vector
start=11; % set the input start time
x(start)=1; % set the input pulse at start time

y=zeros(2,nTs); % zero (and define) the output array
for t=2:nTs, % do for each time step
    y(:,t)=W*y(:,t-1) + V*x(t-1); % compute output
end   % end loop

[eVec,eVal]=eig(W); % find eigenvalues and eigenvectors
eVal=diag(eVal); % extract eigenvalues
magEVal=abs(eVal); % find magnitude of eigenvalues
[eVec eVal magEVal] % show eigenvectors, eigenvalues, stability
```

that the pulse input has already been applied, so that input $x(t-1)$ is now 0, and that the previous state values of the units, $y_1(t-1)$ and $y_2(t-1)$, are 0.63 and 0.89, respectively. Because the previous input is now 0, the product $Vx(t-1)$ is 0, so the current values of the units, $y_1(t)$ and $y_2(t)$, are found by multiplying weight matrix W and the vector $[0.63\ 0.89]^T$ (see Math Box 1.2 for multiplication of a matrix and a vector). The results for $y_1(t)$ and $y_2(t)$ are 0.60 and 0.85, respectively. Thus, the states of both y_1 and y_2 have decayed. This decay continues ad infinitum and approaches 0 asymptotically. While the pulse response of y_1 is a pure decay (as in Figure 1.8), the pulse response of y_2 is not a pure decay, as we will see.

The script twoLeakSeries, listed in MATLAB Box 2.1, implements the two leaky integrators in series network model. Set the weights as in the example above using the commands v1=1, v2=0, w11=0.95, w12=0, w21=0.5, and w22=0.6. The script makes matrices V and W using V=[v1;v2] and W=[w11 w12;w21 w22] (note that, in MATLAB, a comma or space separates elements while a semicolon separates rows). Because we are interested in studying the dynamic properties of this network, its input and output must be sequences of values that vary in time. We will set up an input that runs from 0 to 100 in steps of 1. The end time is set using tEnd=100. Since we include 0, the number of time steps is set as nTs=tEnd+1. The script will define and zero the input vector (array) using x=zeros(1,nTs). (To "zero" a vector means to set all of its elements to 0.) The script will set a start time of 10 using start=11 (since the time series starts at 0, element 11 corresponds to the time of 10), and will set the pulse ampli-

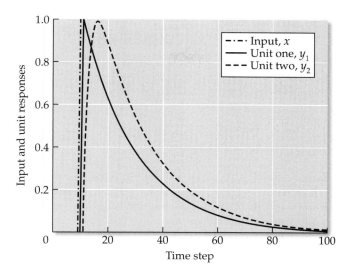

FIGURE 2.3   The pulse responses of two units, each with positive feedback, in series The excitatory, recurrent (positive feedback) weight value is less than 1 for both units, so they are each leaky integrators. The input (dot-dashed line, x) is a pulse with duration of one time step. The first unit (solid line, y_1) leaky integrates the input pulse, while the second unit (dashed line, y_2) leaky integrates the response of the first unit.

tude to 1 using $x(\text{start})=1$. The output of the network will be held in array y, which will have two rows (one for each unit), and nTs columns (one for each time step). Array y is defined (and zeroed) using $y=\text{zeros}(2,nTs)$. The response of the network is computed in a for-loop for each time step t, from 2 to nTs, using $y(:,t)=W*y(:,t-1)+V*x(t-1)$, which implements Equation 2.2. Since the loop starts on time step 2 (see script twoLeakSeries) the initial values of units y_1 and y_2 are 0.

The resulting pulse responses of the two units are shown in Figure 2.3. The responses can be plotted against the time vector $tVec$ using $\text{plot}(tVec,y)$. The response of unit y_1 is a geometric decay, as for the leaky integrator by itself that we studied in Chapter 1 (see Figure 1.8). The response of unit y_2 is prolonged in time relative to y_1, which provides the input to y_2. Also the response of y_2 does not rise instantaneously, but builds up over several time steps, so that the sharp, initial response of unit y_1 is rounded by y_2. The response of y_2 could be described as a sluggish (or rounded) version of its input from y_1. Basically, the response of y_1 is a pulse that has been leaky-integrated once, and the response of y_2 is a pulse that has been leaky-integrated twice. The twice leaky-integrated pulse response of y_2 appears as a lopsided bump, but this seemingly lowly response is actually quite useful for signal processing in neural systems, and we will make use of it throughout the rest of this chapter.

There are many ways in which two neurons in a network could be configured with regard to the input, and coupled, or connected, to each other. The two leaky-integrator units we just studied were connected in series because one unit received input from outside the network, and sent its output to the other unit, which did *not* receive input from outside the network (see Figure 2.2). The two units would be configured in parallel if they both received the same input from outside the network. In the two leaky-integrator example, both units exerted positive feedback on themselves directly. (A small part of this positive feedback could simulate the effects of the membrane time constants of real neurons; see Math Box 2.3 for a two-unit example.) But feedback needs not be limited to unit self-connections in a network. Each unit could also

MATH BOX 2.3   DISCRETE APPROXIMATION OF A SYSTEM OF TWO COUPLED, CONTINUOUS DIFFERENTIAL EQUATIONS THAT MODEL TWO INTERCONNECTED NEURONS

A simple, continuous-time differential equation model of two interconnected neurons is:

$$\tau y_1'(\hat{t}) + y_1(\hat{t}) = \hat{w}_{12} y_2(\hat{t}) + \hat{v}_{11} x_1(\hat{t}) + \hat{v}_{12} x_2(\hat{t})$$
$$\tau y_2'(\hat{t}) + y_2(\hat{t}) = \hat{w}_{21} y_1(\hat{t}) + \hat{v}_{21} x_1(\hat{t}) + \hat{v}_{22} x_2(\hat{t})$$

B2.3.1

where the caret denotes variables that are specific to the continuous-time case, such as weights $\hat{v}_{ij}$ and $\hat{w}_{kl}$ and continuous time $\hat{t}$. Inputs x_j (j = 1,2) connect to neurons y_i (i = 1,2) over weights $\hat{v}_{ij}$, and neurons y_l (l = 1,2) connect to neurons y_k (k = 1,2) over weights $\hat{w}_{kl}$. Specifically, neuron y_1 is coupled to neuron y_2 via connection weight $\hat{w}_{21}$ and y_2 is coupled to y_1 via connection weight $\hat{w}_{12}$. Equations B2.3.1 can be written in matrix form as:

$$\tau \begin{bmatrix} y_1'(\hat{t}) \\ y_2'(\hat{t}) \end{bmatrix} + \begin{bmatrix} y_1(\hat{t}) \\ y_2(\hat{t}) \end{bmatrix} = \begin{bmatrix} 0 & \hat{w}_{12} \\ \hat{w}_{21} & 0 \end{bmatrix} \begin{bmatrix} y_1(\hat{t}) \\ y_2(\hat{t}) \end{bmatrix} + \begin{bmatrix} \hat{v}_{11} & \hat{v}_{12} \\ \hat{v}_{21} & \hat{v}_{22} \end{bmatrix} \begin{bmatrix} x_1(\hat{t}) \\ x_2(\hat{t}) \end{bmatrix}$$

B2.3.2

Equation B2.3.2 can be approximated in discrete time t as a difference equation (see Math Box 2.2):

$$\tau \begin{bmatrix} \dfrac{y_1(t) - y_1(t-1)}{\Delta t} \\ \dfrac{y_2(t) - y_2(t-1)}{\Delta t} \end{bmatrix} + \begin{bmatrix} y_1(t-1) \\ y_2(t-1) \end{bmatrix} = \begin{bmatrix} 0 & \hat{w}_{12} \\ \hat{w}_{21} & 0 \end{bmatrix} \begin{bmatrix} y_1(t-1) \\ y_2(t-1) \end{bmatrix} + \begin{bmatrix} \hat{v}_{11} & \hat{v}_{12} \\ \hat{v}_{21} & \hat{v}_{22} \end{bmatrix} \begin{bmatrix} x_1(t-1) \\ x_2(t-1) \end{bmatrix}$$

B2.3.3

Equation B2.3.3 can be written (again in discrete time) as:

$$\begin{bmatrix} y_1(t) \\ y_2(t) \end{bmatrix} = \begin{bmatrix} w_{11} & w_{12} \\ w_{21} & w_{22} \end{bmatrix} \begin{bmatrix} y_1(t-1) \\ y_2(t-1) \end{bmatrix} + \begin{bmatrix} v_{11} & v_{12} \\ v_{21} & v_{22} \end{bmatrix} \begin{bmatrix} x_1(t-1) \\ x_2(t-1) \end{bmatrix}$$

B2.3.4

where $w_{11} = w_{22} = (1 - \Delta t / \tau)$, $w_{12} = (\Delta t / \tau)\hat{w}_{12}$, $w_{21} = (\Delta t / \tau)\hat{w}_{21}$, and $v_{ij} = (\Delta t / \tau)\hat{v}_{ij}$. Equation B2.3.4 is the same as Equation 2.4 in the main text. Equation B2.3.4 can be written succinctly as:

$$\mathbf{y}(t) = \mathbf{W}\mathbf{y}(t-1) + \mathbf{V}\mathbf{x}(t-1)$$

B2.3.5

in discrete time t where $\mathbf{y}$ is the vector of unit states, $\mathbf{x}$ is the vector of inputs, $\mathbf{W}$ is the matrix of the weights of the connections among the units in $\mathbf{y}$ (recurrent connection weights), and $\mathbf{V}$ is the matrix of the weights of the connections to units in $\mathbf{y}$ from the inputs in $\mathbf{x}$ (forward, or feedforward, connection weights). Equation B2.3.5 is the same as Equation 2.3 in the main text (see also Equation 1.7). All of the equations in the main text of this chapter are of the form of Equation B2.3.5 (and Equation 2.3), and can be analyzed using dynamic systems theory (see Math Box 2.4).

exert positive (or negative) feedback on itself through the other unit. Networks of more than two units offer many possible configurations. We will use several different network configurations to simulate neural systems in this chapter.

In general, the (discrete-time) response of a network of units with states in vector $\mathbf{y}$, which can each potentially connect to themselves and to each other (over recurrent connections) and receive inputs from vector $\mathbf{x}$ (over forward connections), can be described according to Equation 2.3:

$$\mathbf{y}(t) = \mathbf{W}\mathbf{y}(t-1) + \mathbf{V}\mathbf{x}(t-1)$$

2.3

where $\mathbf{W}$ is the matrix of interconnection weights between the units with states in $\mathbf{y}$, and $\mathbf{V}$ is the matrix of their connection weights from the inputs in

MATH BOX 2.4   EIGENMODE ANALYSIS OF DISCRETE, LINEAR DYNAMIC SYSTEMS

The theory of dynamic systems (e.g., Luenberger 1979) can be used to analyze networks of linear units. For linear networks evaluated in discrete time, the responses of the units on discrete time step t are computed from their inputs and their responses on time step $t - 1$ according to:

$$\mathbf{y}(t) = \mathbf{W}\mathbf{y}(t-1) + \mathbf{V}\mathbf{x}(t-1) \qquad \text{B2.4.1}$$

where $\mathbf{y}$ is the vector of unit states, $\mathbf{x}$ is the vector of inputs, $\mathbf{W}$ is the matrix of recurrent weights (weights of the connections among the units in $\mathbf{y}$), and $\mathbf{V}$ is the matrix of forward weights (weights of the connections to units in $\mathbf{y}$ from the inputs in $\mathbf{x}$). We find this response computationally at each time step but, since the system is linear, its response at any time t can be found analytically. Assuming the initial unit states $\mathbf{y}(0)$ are 0s, the response of the system to inputs $\mathbf{x}$ delivered over the series of discrete time steps from $\tilde{t} = 1$ to $\tilde{t} = t$ is:

$$\mathbf{y}(t) = \sum_i \sum_{\tilde{t}=1}^{t} \lambda_i^{t-\tilde{t}} \mathbf{e}_i \left[\mathbf{f}_i^{\mathrm{T}} \left(\mathbf{V}\mathbf{x}(\tilde{t}-1) \right) \right] \qquad \text{B2.4.2}$$

In Equation B2.4.2 the $\mathbf{e}_i$ are the system eigenvectors, the $\mathbf{f}_i$ are the adjoint eigenvectors, and the λ_i are the system eigenvalues, which satisfy the eigenvalue equations:

$$\mathbf{W}\mathbf{e}_i = \lambda_i \mathbf{e}_i \qquad \text{B2.4.3}$$

$$\mathbf{f}_i^{\mathrm{T}}\mathbf{W} = \lambda_i \mathbf{f}_i^{\mathrm{T}} \qquad \text{B2.4.4}$$

(The solution in Equation B2.4.2 is subject to the further condition that matrix $\mathbf{W}$ is diagonalizable which, among other important properties, means that the eigenvectors and adjoint eigenvectors satisfy the biorthogonality relation whereby $\mathbf{f}_k^{\mathrm{T}}\mathbf{e}_l = 0$ for all $k \neq l$.)

Each eigenvalue λ_i and its associated eigenvector $\mathbf{e}_i$ constitute a dynamic mode of the system, and each mode contributes a response component. Equation B2.4.2 shows how the modes together determine the response of the system. Each eigenvector $\mathbf{e}_i$ determines a response pattern among the system states in $\mathbf{y}$. Each adjoint eigenvector $\mathbf{f}_i$ determines the amount by which the input $\mathbf{V}\mathbf{x}$ will activate its associated eigenvector $\mathbf{e}_i$ (by the scaling term in square brackets in Equation B2.4.2). Each eigenvalue λ_i determines the temporal properties of the response pattern due to its eigenvector $\mathbf{e}_i$. In the linear networks we study, the eigenvectors determine the patterns of responses among the neural units in $\mathbf{y}$, while the eigenvalues determine their temporal properties.

Eigenvalues, and their associated eigenvectors, can be real or complex. Complex eigenvalues and eigenvectors occur in complex-conjugate pairs. Eigenvalue λ can be expressed as $\lambda = \mu + j\omega$, where μ and ω are the real and imaginary parts of λ and j is $\sqrt{-1}$. Alternatively, λ can be expressed as $\lambda = re^{j\theta}$ where e is the base of natural logarithms, and r is the length (magnitude, or absolute value) and θ the angle of the vector representing λ in the complex plane. The temporal sequence λ^t, in which λ is raised to powers of discrete time t, is

$$\lambda^t = r^t e^{jt\theta} = r^t \left(\cos t\theta + j \sin t\theta \right) \qquad \text{B2.4.5}$$

This eigenvalue term multiplies its associated, scaled eigenvector (see Equation B2.4.2) and determines the temporal properties of its response component. If λ is real and positive then $\theta = 0$, and its response component is the geometric sequence r^t that will grow, remain constant, or decay as $r > 1$, $r = 1$, or $r < 1$, respectively. If λ is real and negative the response is an alternating geometric sequence. If λ and its conjugate are complex then the response component due to both is an oscillation $r^t (A \sin t\theta + B \cos t\theta)$ at frequency θ radians per time step. Constants A and B depend on specific parameter values, but the oscillation amplitude will grow, remain constant, or decay as $r > 1$, $r = 1$, or $r < 1$, respectively. Modes with $r > 1$, $r = 1$, or $r < 1$, are considered unstable, marginally stable, or stable, respectively. It is critically important to point out that these stability criteria, along with the general solution described in this Math Box, apply only to *discrete-time* linear dynamic systems. The stability criteria and general solution for continuous-time linear dynamic systems are analogous but distinct (see Luenberger 1979 for further details on both kinds of systems).

$\mathbf{x}$. Equation 2.3 can be solved iteratively (in a loop) at each time step, as we did in the previous example using script `twoLeakSeries`. When the units (or system elements) are linear, it is also possible to solve Equation 2.3 analytically in terms of the network (or linear system) dynamic modes. A very brief description of linear systems analysis is provided in Math Box 2.4.

The dynamic modes of a linear system are properties of its system matrix. For the neural systems models we consider here, the system matrix is the matrix $\mathbf{W}$ of the weights of the recurrent connections that connect the units

TABLE 2.1   Eigenmode analysis for two leaky integrators in series

Eigenvector	0.5735	0.0000
	0.8192	1.0000
Eigenvalue	0.9500	0.6000
Magnitude	0.9500	0.6000

Eigenvectors, eigenvalues, and eigenvalue magnitude (stability) for each of the two dynamic modes are listed. The four-place precision is needed to properly represent the results of eigenmode analysis in this example and in the other examples in this chapter.

to themselves and to each other. Each dynamic mode of a linear system consists of an eigenvector and its associated eigenvalue. MATLAB has specialized commands for finding eigenvectors and eigenvalues. The command `[eVec,eVal]=eig(W)` will find the eigenvectors and store them as columns in matrix `eVec`, and will also find the associated eigenvalues and store them along the diagonal of matrix `eVal` (in which all off-diagonal elements are 0). The eigenvalues can be extracted from this diagonal matrix using `eVal=diag(eVal)`, which essentially replaces the diagonal matrix with a column vector of the same name (`eVal`) that holds only the eigenvalues. These commands are given in script `twoLeakSeries` (see MATLAB Box 2.1). The script also finds the magnitude of each eigenvalue using `magEVal=abs(eVal)`. (Note that the magnitude of an eigenvalue is the same as its absolute value.) The magnitude of an eigenvalue determines the stability of its associated dynamic mode (see Math Box 2.4).

In simplest terms, the dynamic modes are the components of the responses of the elements of a system, such as the units in a neural system model. The eigenvectors are the possible patterns that the unit responses can form, while the eigenvalues determine the temporal properties of the response component due to a dynamic mode. Eigenvalues (and eigenvector elements) can be real numbers or complex numbers. We will discuss complex modes in Section 2.7. Negative real eigenvalues, which occasionally arise, produce alternating sequences. Positive real eigenvalues produce the simplest responses, because they are just the geometric series (rising, constant, or decaying), that we have already studied using the single unit with positive feedback in Chapter 1. Eigenvalue magnitude determines the stability of a mode, but because the magnitude of an eigenvalue is its absolute value, the magnitudes of positive, real eigenvalues are just the eigenvalues themselves. The pattern of unit responses due to the eigenvector of such a dynamic mode will grow, stay constant, or decay accordingly as its real, positive eigenvalue is greater than, equal to, or less than 1. A linear system will have as many dynamic modes as it has elements, but it is essential to realize that modes and elements are different entities altogether. The dynamic modes are the ways in which the states of the elements can change. The same set of elements (or linear units in a network) can simultaneously express multiple dynamic modes (superimposed response components).

These ideas can be illustrated with the two leaky integrators in series example (see Figure 2.2). Because this linear network (system) has two elements (units y_1 and y_2), it also has two dynamic modes. The eigenvectors, eigenvalues, and eigenvalue magnitudes of the two modes, which are computed in script `twoLeakSeries`, are listed in Table 2.1. Note that both modes have positive, real eigenvalues less than 1, so they are both stable, decaying modes. They are responsible for the "leaks" we have been studying through simulation. The closer a real, positive eigenvalue is to 0 the faster its mode decays (or leaks). These eigenvalues determine the temporal properties of the response of each mode in the two-leak series network. The associated eigenvectors determine the patterns of response between the two units in the network.

The first mode has eigenvector $[0.5735\ 0.8192]^T$. This mode represents the pattern in which the responses of both units change together. Its associated eigenvalue is 0.9500, which corresponds to the slower leak. Thus, the first dynamic mode governs the relatively slow decays of the responses of both units in the network. The second mode has eigenvector $[0.0000\ 1.0000]^T$. This mode represents the pattern in which the response of y_2 changes while that of y_1 does not. Its associated eigenvalue is 0.6000, which corresponds to the faster leak. Thus, the second dynamic mode governs the rounded rise of the response of y_2, which y_1 does not share, and the slightly more prolonged decay of y_2 relative to y_1.

Note that each eigenvalue equals the weight of the single excitatory, recurrent connection to one of the two leaky-integrator units ($w_{11} = 0.95$ and $w_{22} = 0.60$). Indeed, the single eigenvalue of the single-unit leaky integrator we studied in Chapter 1 is equal to the value of its positive feedback weight (and its associated eigenvector is simply the number 1). This one-to-one correspondence between eigenvalue and feedback weight does not obtain in networks with more complicated recurrent structures, as we will see. Still, the magnitude of an eigenvalue and the positive feedback weight of the single-unit leaky integrator are analogous in the sense that they both determine stability. Whether for the positive feedback weight of a single-unit leaky integrator, or for the magnitude of a dynamic mode in a more complicated, discrete-time linear system, the associated response will grow, decay, or stay the same according to whether that weight or magnitude is greater than, less than, or equal to 1. (Note that these stability criteria apply specifically to discrete-time, as distinct from continuous-time, linear systems. See Math Box 2.4 for further details.)

Eigenmode analysis is an extremely powerful analytical tool, especially for linear systems (Luenberger 1979). We only touch on it in this book, but we also point out that in many neural systems, neurons operate approximately linearly in that their activity (firing rate) is linearly related to system variables over the operational range of the system. The vestibular and oculomotor systems, which we consider in detail in the next four sections of this chapter, are important examples of neural systems in which many neurons operate over an approximately linear range (Robinson 1981). Eigenmode analysis can be applied in cases where linear models provide valid approximations to real neural systems (e.g., Anastasio 1998; Barreiro et al. 2009).

As mentioned above, we restrict ourselves in this book to discrete-time, rather than continuous-time systems (see Luenberger 1979 for many examples of both types of systems). The unit pulse input, which we applied in the two leaky integrators in series example, is the simplest discrete input. While eigenmode analysis provides a quantitative description of the dynamics of a network of linear units, the pulse response provides a qualitative picture, and both are useful for studying neural systems models. We will use pulse responses to characterize the dynamics of networks of linear and of nonlinear units in this chapter and in Chapter 10, respectively.

The pulse input we have been using is, of course, an idealization. The elements of real physical systems, including input elements, generally do not come on and go off again instantaneously. More commonly, they might begin with an abrupt onset, but their return to baseline will be prolonged in time. In other words, the responses of many real systems, and system components, can be described roughly as leaky integrations.

A good example of this is the relatively simple neural system known as the vestibulo-ocular reflex (VOR). The VOR is a classic polysynaptic reflex pathway (see Chapter 1) composed of sensory neurons, interneurons, and motoneurons. The responses of the sensory neurons could be described as those of a leaky integrator. Rather than simply pass this signal on to the motoneurons, the interneurons process this signal and shape it into a motor command that better suits the behavioral needs of the organism. Our next set of examples involves signal processing in the VOR.

2.2   Signal Processing in the Vestibulo-Ocular Reflex (VOR)

The function of the vestibulo-ocular reflex (VOR) is to maintain retinal image stability by making eye rotations that counterbalance head rotations (Wilson and Melvill Jones 1979). The VOR is mediated by interneurons, located in the vestibular nuclei of the brainstem, which receive input from vestibular sensory afferent neurons, process that input, and relay the result as a command to the motoneurons of the eye muscles. The vestibular afferents carry signals from hair cells, which are specialized receptor cells located within the semicircular canal vestibular receptors. Through a sensory transduction process occurring within the semicircular canals, the hair cells are activated by head rotational (angular) acceleration. This vestibular sensory signal, carried by semicircular canal afferents, drives the VOR.

In order to operate properly, the VOR must produce eye angular velocities that are equal (but opposite) to head angular velocities over the range of head angular velocities experienced by the organism. Thus, over this range, the VOR produces eye angular velocities that are approximately linearly related to head angular velocities (with a slope approximately equal to −1) (Wilson and Melvill Jones 1979). This linear operation is mediated by sensory afferent neurons, vestibular nucleus neurons, and eye muscle motoneurons whose activities are approximately linearly related to system parameters such as head and/or eye angular velocities over the operational range (Robinson 1981). The approximate linearity of the activities of the neurons mediating the VOR justifies the use of linear neural units in simulating the VOR in this chapter. (We will consider the important role of nonlinearity in VOR processing in Chapter 10.)

The neurons mediating the VOR must take into account not only the magnitude of head rotations but also their dynamics. According to Newton's laws, movement of an object is caused by a force, and force is proportional to acceleration. A force producing a pulse of head angular acceleration to the left, for example, will cause a head angular velocity to the left. To counterbalance this, the VOR will have to produce an eye angular velocity to the right of the same magnitude. Again according to Newton's laws, the head will continue to rotate until it is acted upon by another force. Therefore, in order to work well, the VOR has to maintain its production of eye rotation for some time after the pulse of head angular acceleration.

As indicated above, the semicircular canals, and the vestibular afferents that carry their signals, are activated by head angular acceleration. Due to their physical properties the canals are leaky-integrating angular accelerometers (Wilson and Melvill Jones 1979). Correspondingly, in response to a pulse of head angular acceleration, the vestibular afferents show a sharp initial increase in activation followed by a decaying return to baseline. This pulse response can be described as an exponential decay $e^{-t/\tau}$ (see Math Box 2.1), with a time constant τ of about 5 seconds in primates. Representative neurophysiological data are shown in Figure 2.4. A pulse of whole-body angular acceleration brings head angular velocity (Figure 2.4D) from 0 to 160 degrees/s, and after a duration of about 50 seconds, a pulse of angular deceleration brings head angular velocity back to 0 again. The instantaneous firing rate of a vestibular afferent (Figure 2.4A) abruptly increases in response to the acceleration pulse and then decays with a time constant of about 5 seconds. The afferent, which has a high spontaneous firing rate, shows a similar response in the opposite direction for the deceleration pulse.

Driven by the vestibular canal afferent signal alone, the VOR could continue to produce counterbalancing eye rotations for a few seconds following a

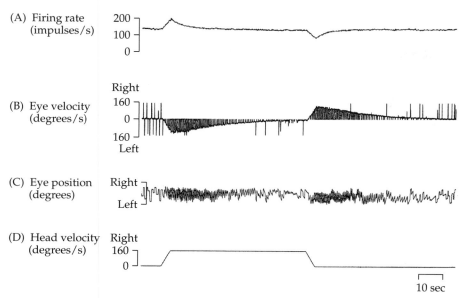

FIGURE 2.4   The response of a semicircular canal primary afferent, and of the overall vestibulo-ocular reflex (VOR), to a step change in head angular velocity (A) The instantaneous firing rate, in impulses/s (spikes/s), of a horizontal semicircular canal primary afferent. (B) The eye angular velocity in degrees/s. (C) The eye angular position in degrees. (D) The head angular velocity in degrees/s. The eye position trace (C) is extremely jagged, due to the fast, resetting eye movements that are made when the VOR carries the eye to an eccentric position in the orbit. The pattern of alternation between the slow, VOR eye movements and the fast, resetting eye movements is known as nystagmus. The velocities of these resetting eye movements are mostly clipped out of the eye velocity trace (B), the envelope of which shows eye velocity due to the VOR. Note that the duration of the VOR response is longer than that of the canal afferent response that drives it. (From Henn 1982.)

pulse of head angular acceleration. However, that amount of counterbalancing is apparently not enough for the primate VOR. Representative VOR data is also shown in Figure 2.4. Head rotation produces a pattern of eye movement, known as nystagmus, in which the smooth, counterbalancing VOR eye rotations that can bring the eye to the edge of the orbit are periodically interrupted by fast, resetting eye movements that return the eye to a more central position in the orbit. The nystagmic pattern is apparent in the eye angular position trace in Figure 2.4C. To analyze the VOR it is more practical to differentiate the position trace, thereby converting it to an eye angular velocity trace (Figure 2.4B). In the eye velocity trace the fast, resetting eye movements appear as sharp spikes, which can be clipped out, and the smooth, counterbalancing VOR eye velocity remains as an envelope.

Examination of the eye angular velocity trace in Figure 2.4B reveals that the response of the VOR to a pulse of head angular acceleration is also characterized by a sharp initial increase in activation, followed by a decaying return to baseline. As for the vestibular canal afferents, the pulse response of the VOR can also be described as an exponential decay, but the time constant of that decay in primates is 20 seconds, four times longer than the decay of the vestibular sensory signal (Wilson and Melvill Jones 1979; Henn 1982).

In contrast to the canal afferents, the pulse responses of the vestibular nucleus neurons, which are the interneurons of the VOR pathway, decay with the same long time constant as the VOR (Figure 2.5). It seems that interactions occurring at the level of the vestibular nuclei in the brainstem have somehow

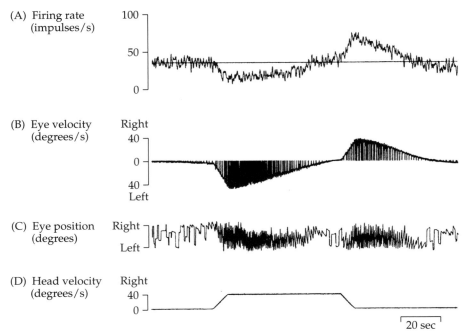

FIGURE 2.5   The response of a vestibular nucleus neuron, and of the overall vestibulo-ocular reflex (VOR), to a step change in head angular velocity (A) The instantaneous firing rate, in impulses/s, of a vestibular nucleus neuron. (B) The eye angular velocity in degrees/s. (C) The eye angular position in degrees (showing a nystagmic pattern). (D) The head angular velocity in degrees/s. As in Figure 2.4, the velocities of the resetting eye movements are clipped out of the eye velocity trace (B), the envelope of which shows eye velocity due to the VOR. Note that the vestibular nucleus neuron response has a sharp onset, but its duration is about the same as that of the VOR. (From Henn 1982.)

prolonged the canal decay time constant from 5 to 20 seconds, but have also retained its sharp initial increase in activation, to produce the VOR. The neural mechanism responsible for this processing has been called velocity storage. Two models have been proposed to account for velocity storage in the VOR (Raphan et al. 1979; Robinson 1981). The models are schematized in Figure 2.6. They are structurally different but functionally equivalent (Anastasio 1993). We will study simplified versions of these models in the following sections.

2.3   The Parallel-Pathway Model of Velocity Storage in the Primate VOR

Raphan and coworkers (1979) proposed a model of the velocity storage mechanism that is composed of two parallel pathways from the vestibular afferents to the motoneurons. One pathway is direct, while the other passes through a leaky integrator. Basically, the direct pathway preserves the sharp, initial increase in afferent activation while the leaky integrator prolongs the response. Their weighted sum exhibits the sharp initial peak and the long decay of the VOR. A simplified version of the parallel-pathway model of the velocity storage mechanism is shown in Figure 2.6A. We will implement the parallel-pathway model by reconfiguring the two-neuron network we studied in the first example.

The configuration of the two-unit network that implements the parallel-pathway model of velocity storage is shown in Figure 2.7. Unit y_1 represents the vestibular nucleus neurons that send their output to the eye muscle

(A) Parallel pathway model

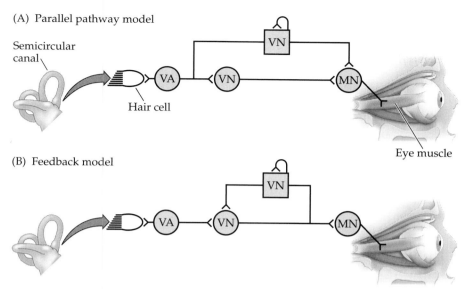

FIGURE 2.6   Two models of velocity storage in the primate vestibulo-ocular reflex (VOR) (A) In the parallel-pathway model, vestibular nucleus neurons (VN) pass the vestibular afferent (VA) signal to the motoneuron (MN) either directly or indirectly through a leaky integrator. (B) In the feedback model, the vestibular nucleus neuron that receives the vestibular afferent signal sends its output to the motoneuron and also feeds back onto itself through a leaky integrator. Leaky integrators are drawn as boxes to distinguish them from the other neural elements drawn as circles. (Note that in our simulations leaky integrators are just like other neural units except that they send excitatory, recurrent connections to themselves. Raphan and Robinson used different methods to model leaky integrators.) (A after Raphan et al. 1979; B after Robinson 1981.)

motoneurons, and unit y_2 represents some of the other vestibular nucleus neurons that mediate the VOR. We could have y_1 itself represent a motoneuron, and receive its input from a vestibular nucleus neuron acting as a simple relay (see Figure 2.6A), but for purposes of comparison with later simulations we have y_1 represent the subset of vestibular nucleus neurons that have response properties like those of motoneurons (Henn 1982). The discrete-time responses of this network are described by Equation 2.2. Script `velocityStoreLeak`, listed in MATLAB Box 2.2, implements this model. For the parallel-pathway model of velocity storage, set the connection weight values at $v_1 = 1$, $v_2 = 0.18$, $w_{11} = 0$, $w_{12} = 0.2$, $w_{21} = 0$, and $w_{22} = 0.95$. This is done straightforwardly using `v1=1, v2=0.18, w11=0, w12=0.2, w21=0,` and `w22=0.95`. The input represents the responses of vestibular semicircular canal afferents to a pulse of head

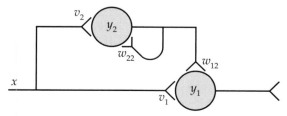

FIGURE 2.7   The two-unit network configured to implement the parallel-pathway model of velocity storage in the primate VOR Input x connects to y_1 and y_2 with weights v_1 and v_2, and unit y_2 connects to unit y_1 and to itself with weights w_{12} and w_{22}, respectively.

MATLAB® BOX 2.2   The script implements the parallel-pathway and positive-feedback models of velocity storage, and the negative-feedback model of velocity leakage.

```
% velocityStoreLeak.m

v1=1; v2=0.18; % set weights from the input
w11=0; w12=0.2; % set feedback weights to unit one
w21=0; w22=0.95; % set feedback weights to unit two

V=[v1;v2]; % compose input weight matrix (vector)
W=[w11 w12;w21 w22]; % compose feedback weight matrix

tEnd=100; % set end time
tVec=0:tEnd; % set time vector
nTs=tEnd+1; % find number of time steps
dkc=0.9; % set input geometric decay constant
x=(dkc).^(tVec); % generate input

y=zeros(2,nTs); % zero the output vector
for t=2:nTs,  % do for each time step
    y(:,t)=W*y(:,t-1) + V*x(t-1); % compute output
end  % end loop
```

angular acceleration. This can be approximated in discrete-time as a geometric decay (see Math Box 2.1). A decay constant of 0.9 makes a nice profile for this example. The input (canal response) is set up using the following MATLAB commands: `tEnd=100`, `tVec=0:tEnd`, `dkc=0.9`, and `x=(dkc).^(tVec)`. The symbols `.^` signify element-wise exponentiation. The result of this last command is a vector (array) x in which each element is the scalar value `dkc` raised to the power of each corresponding element of time vector `tVec`. (The symbol `^` by itself can be used to raise one scalar value to the power of another scalar value, as in command `2^2` which finds the value of 2^2.) The response of the network is computed, exactly as before, using a for-loop, with input $x(t)$ being drawn from the geometric decay in vector time series (array) x. Note that the loop, and the command that computes the response of the network on each time step, is the same in scripts `velocityStoreLeak` and `twoLeakSeries`. As before, the script will zero array y and keep the initial values of units y_1 and y_2 at 0 by starting the loop on time step 2. The results are shown in Figure 2.8.

The input (dot-dashed line) is a geometric decay with decay constant 0.9, as specified. The response of y_2 (dashed line) is a leaky-integrated, sluggish (or roundish) version of the input. It is similar in form to the lopsided bump response of the second leaky integrator in the two leaky-integrator series we studied in the first example (see Figure 2.3). As such, it has a longer duration but a rounded initial response. The response of y_1 (solid line), which represents the vestibular nucleus neurons that send their outputs to the motoneurons, has the sharp initial peak of the vestibular sensory input combined with a longer decay. The motoneurons would use this signal as a command to drive the eye muscles. In that it has both the sharp initial response of the vestibular afferents and the long decay of the VOR, this simple model captures the salient features of the velocity storage mechanism. The function of y_2, which represents some of the other vestibular nucleus neurons, is to leaky integrate

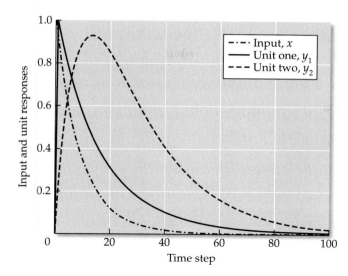

FIGURE 2.8   A simulation of velocity storage in the primate VOR using the parallel-pathway model The input (dot-dashed line, x) is a (geometric) decay that represents the response of vestibular sensory neurons. The response of unit two (dashed line, y_2) is a leaky-integrated version of the input. The response of unit one (solid line, y_1) is the weighted sum of the input and the response of unit two. It has the sharp onset of the input (x) and the long tail (decay) of the response of unit two (y_2).

the sensory input, and thereby "store" it. Unit y_2 adds its stored version to the direct sensory signal x to form the VOR command at y_1. (Note that the contributions of x and y_2 to the response of y_1 are scaled by weights v_1 and w_{12}.) Thus, the storage element itself can be modeled as a leaky integrator.

In the parallel-pathway model, velocity storage arises as the result of positive feedback by a leaky integrator, and we might predict from our model that velocity storage in the real VOR is mediated by positive feedback occurring at the level of the vestibular nuclei. We model a leaky integrator as a single unit that exerts positive feedback directly on itself. Although neurons could in principle directly excite themselves, it is likely that positive feedback in the real VOR involves more complicated patterns of connectivity in neural networks. We will explore more complicated and realistic patterns of positive feedback in Chapter 10, where we will also cite evidence that velocity storage does indeed occur via positive feedback, though not necessarily of the direct sort that we use for single-unit leaky integrators. Our single-unit leaky integrators should be understood as simplifications of actual neural sub-circuits, which nevertheless accomplish the required signal processing function.

Essentially, the "velocity storage mechanism" involves positive feedback, at the level of the vestibular nuclei, of the vestibular semicircular canal sensory afferent signal, and serves roughly as a "memory" for this signal. As explained in the previous section, pulses of head angular acceleration produce enduring head angular velocities, but the vestibular semicircular canals respond transiently to head angular acceleration. Therefore, we can consider the signal being "stored" or "remembered" by the vestibular nuclei as an internal representation of head angular velocity. This representation decays with a time constant of about 20 seconds in primates. This prolonged decay is long enough, because the head angular velocity representation due to a pulse of head angular acceleration does not need to be maintained for very long before the primate experiences another pulse of head angular acceleration.

2.4   The Positive-Feedback Model of Velocity Storage in the Primate VOR

The old saying that "there is more than one way to skin a cat" is as true in neural systems modeling as in life generally. Robinson (1981) proposed a model of velocity storage that is different from Raphan's model. Robinson's model uses positive feedback through a leaky integrator, rather than parallel direct and leaky-integrated pathways, to produce velocity storage. The feedback model of velocity storage is schematized in Figure 2.6B. This model employs a compound form of positive feedback, since the main positive feedback loop includes a leaky integrator, which already has it own, direct positive feedback. We can also implement the positive-feedback model of velocity storage by reconfiguring the two-neuron network we studied in the first example.

The configuration of the two-unit network that implements the positive-feedback model of velocity storage is shown in Figure 2.9. Units y_1 and y_2 represent the vestibular nucleus neurons that mediate the VOR, and y_1 would send its output directly to motoneurons. The discrete-time responses of this network are again described by Equation 2.2. Script `velocityStoreLeak`, listed in MATLAB Box 2.2, implements this model. For the positive-feedback model of velocity storage, set the connection weight values at $v_1 = 1$, $v_2 = 0$, $w_{11} = 0$, $w_{12} = 0.2$, $w_{21} = 0.2$, and $w_{22} = 0.9$. The input, which represents the response of vestibular sensory afferents to a pulse of head acceleration, is approximated as before as a geometric decay with a decay constant of 0.9. The response of the network is computed, exactly as before, using a for-loop, with input $x(t)$ being drawn from the vector time series (array) x. As before, the script will zero array y and keep the initial values of units y_1 and y_2 at 0 by starting the loop on time step 2. The results are shown in Figure 2.10.

The input (dot-dashed line) is a geometric decay with decay constant 0.9, as before. The response of y_2 (dashed line) is a leaky-integrated, sluggish version of the output of y_1, and could be described as a lopsided bump. As such, it has a long duration and a rounded initial response. The response of y_1 (solid line) has the sharp initial peak of the vestibular sensory input combined with a longer decay time. This signal has the characteristics that are required of the VOR motoneuron command. Thus, the positive-feedback model accomplishes essentially the same transformation as the parallel-pathway model, but in a different way.

As in the parallel-pathway model, unit y_2 (dashed line) acts a leaky integrator in the positive-feedback model. Unlike the parallel-pathway model, however, the leaky integrator in the positive-feedback model does not leaky integrate the input directly. Instead it leaky integrates the output of unit y_1 (solid line). Unit y_1 sums the direct sensory input and a leaky-integrated ver-

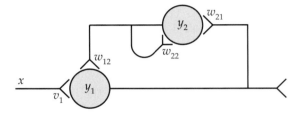

FIGURE 2.9   The two-unit network configured to implement the feedback model of velocity storage in the primate VOR   Input x connects to unit y_1 with weight v_1, unit y_1 connects to y_2 with weight w_{21}, and unit y_2 connects to y_1 and to itself with weights w_{12} and w_{22}, respectively.

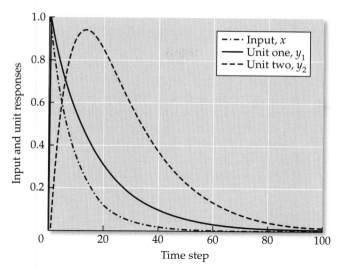

FIGURE 2.10   A simulation of velocity storage in the primate VOR using the positive-feedback model The input (dot-dashed line, x) is a decay that represents the response of vestibular sensory neurons. The response of unit two (dashed line, y_2) is a leaky-integrated version of the response of unit one (y_1). The response of unit one (solid line, y_1) is essentially the weighted sum of the input and the leaky integral of its own response. It has the sharp onset of the input and the long tail (decay) of the response of unit two (y_2).

sion of its own output. This results in a signal with a sharp initial peak and a long decay that can serve as the motoneuron command for the VOR.

The parallel-pathway and positive-feedback models show that there is "more than one way to skin the cat" of velocity storage in the VOR, and it would be reasonable to ask whether one way is better than the other. To answer a cliché with a cliché, the parallel-pathway and positive-feedback models are "six of one and a half-dozen of the other." Both models have the same number of units and the same number of nonzero connections. Both produce neural responses with long decays that qualitatively resemble the actual responses of real vestibular nucleus neurons (see Figure 2.5). Both rely on a leaky integrator to store the vestibular afferent signal, and they both accomplish the same overall velocity-storage transformation. In the last sense they are computationally equivalent (see Anastasio 1993 for a detailed comparison of the parallel-pathway and positive-feedback models of velocity storage in the VOR).

In another sense, though, it can be argued that the feedback model is cleverer, in that it requires less from its leaky integrator. To see this, note that there are really two feedback loops in the feedback model (see Figure 2.9). Unit y_2, which is the leaky integrator, feeds back onto itself directly, but unit y_1 feeds back onto itself indirectly through unit y_2. The combined weight of the recurrent connections needed to produce positive feedback in the feedback model is shared between the leaky-integrator self-connection weight and the weights of the connections between y_1 and y_2. Due to this sharing of the positive-feedback load, the self-connection weight of the leaky-integrator is a bit smaller in the positive-feedback model (0.90) than in the parallel-pathway model (0.95). Thus, the leaky integrator is a bit further from instability (which would occur with a self-connection weight greater than 1) in the positive-feedback than in the parallel-pathway model. It is possible that synapses in real neural networks are subject to small, random fluctuations in strength (which may be involved in learning, see Chapter 7). In the face of random fluctuations in recurrent connection weights that could cause the networks to become unstable, the positive-feedback model would be slightly more robust than the parallel-pathway model, yet both achieve the same amount of time constant lengthening.

We may accept that the parallel-pathway and positive-feedback models are computationally equivalent, but that the positive-feedback model is slightly more robust to random connection weight fluctuations. We still need to ask whether one or the other is a better model of signal processing in the real VOR. We will defer consideration of this important question until Chapter 10, in which we will construct a nonlinear neural network model of velocity storage. For now we will consider a linear model of another form of signal processing in the VOR that is the opposite of velocity storage.

2.5   The Negative-Feedback Model of Velocity Leakage in the Pigeon VOR

While velocity storage is observed in the primate VOR, a phenomenon termed velocity leakage is observed in the pigeon VOR (and perhaps also in the VORs of some other birds). As mentioned previously, the time constants of the vestibular afferent sensory signal and of the VOR in primates are 5 and 20 seconds, respectively (Wilson and Melvill Jones 1979; Henn 1982). In contrast, the time constants of the vestibular sensory signal and of the VOR in pigeons are 10 and 4 seconds, respectively (Anastasio et al. 1985; Anastasio and Correia 1988). Thus, the velocity storage mechanism lengthens the vestibular time constant in primates, but the velocity leakage mechanism shortens it in pigeons (and perhaps also in some other birds). Whereas the velocity storage mechanism has been modeled using positive feedback through a leaky integrator, the velocity leakage mechanism has been modeled using negative feedback through a leaky integrator (Anastasio and Correia 1994).

The configuration of the two-unit network that implements the negative-feedback model of velocity leakage is the same as that which implements the positive-feedback model of velocity storage (see Figure 2.9). As for the positive-feedback model, units y_1 and y_2 represent the vestibular nucleus neurons that mediate the VOR, and y_1 would send its output directly to motoneurons. The discrete-time responses of this network are again described by Equation 2.2. Script `velocityStoreLeak` (see MATLAB Box 2.2) implements this model. For the negative-feedback model of velocity leakage, set the connection weight values as for the positive-feedback model, but make the connection to y_1 from y_2 negative: $v_1 = 1$, $v_2 = 0$, $w_{11} = 0$, $w_{12} = -0.2$, $w_{21} = 0.2$, and $w_{22} = 0.9$. To simulate the longer decay of the vestibular sensory signal in pigeons, increase the decay constant to 0.95 (`dkc=0.95`). As before, the script will zero array y and keep the initial values of units y_1 and y_2 at 0 by starting the loop on time step 2. The response of the network is computed, exactly as before, using a for-loop. Note that the network is updated in exactly the same way for all of the examples we have considered so far in this chapter. The only difference has been the values of the connection weights. The results for velocity leakage are shown in Figure 2.11.

The vestibular input signal $x(t)$, the leaky integrator signal $y_2(t)$, and the motor command $y_1(t)$ have essentially the same form in both the velocity storage and velocity leakage models (compare Figures 2.10 and 2.11). The input, as specified, is a geometric decay, but at a rate slower in the velocity leakage than in the velocity storage model, to reflect the longer decay of vestibular sensory afferent responses in pigeons as compared with primates (dot-dash line). The leaky-integrated output of unit y_2 (dashed line) has a rounded initial response and a long decay. The response of y_1, which represents the command

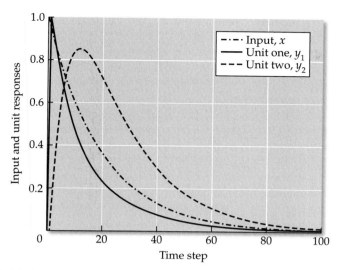

FIGURE 2.11   A simulation of velocity leakage in the pigeon VOR using the negative-feedback model The input (dot-dashed line, x) is a decay that represents the response of pigeon vestibular sensory neurons. The response of unit two (dashed line, y_2) is a leaky-integrated version of the response of unit one (y_1). The response of unit one (solid line, y_1) is essentially the weighted difference between the input and the leaky integral of its own response. It has the sharp onset of the input (x) but it decays faster than the input.

sent to the motoneurons in both models, has a sharply peaked initial response in both cases, as required. However, relative to the vestibular sensory afferent response, the response of y_1 decays faster in the velocity leakage model and slower in the velocity storage model, as required. Thus, the same type of model can simulate both velocity storage and velocity leakage, depending only on the sign of its main feedback pathway (positive or negative, respectively).

In the examples involving velocity storage and leakage, we use the leaky integrator as a system component, which we model as a single unit with a positive self-connection. In several places we have issued the warning that, in the real brain, most neurons probably do not send excitatory, recurrent connections to themselves, but in at least one case they probably do. We will briefly describe this case because it serves to illustrate the potential benefits but also the drawbacks of excitatory self-connections.

The fast, resetting eye movements that occur as part of vestibular nystagmus (see Figures 2.4 and 2.5) are driven by burst commands that are generated by brainstem burst neurons (Strassman et al. 1986). A burst is characterized as a brief period (50–100 ms) of neural discharge at a very high firing rate (up to 1000 action potentials, or spikes, per second). In the brainstem, the burst may be the result of positive feedback produced by excitatory connections from burst neurons onto other burst neurons, and even from the same burst neuron onto itself (Strassman et al. 1986). A model, based on known connections between burst neurons, vestibular nucleus neurons, and other brainstem neural types, has shown how the onsets and offsets of bursts produced by excitatory recurrent connections from burst neurons to themselves could be controlled (Anastasio 1997). An important component of this control is the lack of burst neuron spontaneous activity.

Burst neurons are completely silent (have zero discharge) between bursts, so their self-excitation is engaged only when needed at burst onset. If they were not spontaneously silent, then their excitatory self-connections would cause them to integrate their own spontaneous activity. It is possible that neurons that have excitatory self-connections, and that integrate their own spontaneous activity or that of their inputs, could serve a computationally useful purpose. (We will consider one such possibility in Section 12.4 of Chapter 12.) In most cases, however, it would not be computationally useful to integrate neural background activity. The reason can be appreciated most readily by considering sensory neurons.

Sensory (and other) neurons that provide inputs to real neural systems often do not have a zero baseline. Many neurons have nonzero background activities, and they signal increases or decreases in the quantity they encode as increases or decreases in that background activity. An excellent example of this is provided by the data in Figure 2.4A showing the instantaneous firing rate of a vestibular semicircular canal primary afferent neuron. This sensory neuron has a background firing rate that is well over 100 impulses/s (or spikes/s), and it encodes head rotation in either direction as a symmetrical increase or decrease in this high background firing rate. For vestibular and many other neurons, the signals of interest are the increases and decreases in background activity, not the background activity itself.

A nonzero baseline poses a problem for the simple leaky integrators we have been using in this chapter. Because these simple integrators exert direct positive feedback on themselves, they would integrate the background activity as well as the signal of interest, and this could lead to errors in signal processing. In the next example we consider a solution to this problem. The example involves a model of a neural network known as the integrator of the oculomotor system (also called the oculomotor neural integrator). The solution involves positive feedback that occurs, in part, through other neural units. The solution also relies on the configuration of the network, which has its basis in neuroanatomy.

2.6   Oculomotor Neural Integration via Reciprocal Inhibition

Cannon and coworkers (1983) studied leaky integrators in the context of the eye-movement (i.e., oculomotor) control system. Specifically, they focused on the oculomotor neural integrator, which converts velocity signals into position signals (Robinson 1981). Both signals are needed to control eye movements, and eye-muscle motoneurons carry both components. An example from an early study of eye-muscle motoneurons in the primate (Fuchs and Luschei 1970) is shown in Figure 2.12. The velocity component of the motoneuron command appears as bursts or pauses in spike discharge when eye angular position (smooth trace) changes (and eye angular velocity is nonzero). The position component appears as a constant discharge proportional to eye angular position itself. The oculomotor neural integrator is needed to provide the position component because eye movement commands, such as the fast eye-movement commands from burst neurons or the slow, VOR eye-movement commands from vestibular afferents and vestibular nucleus neurons (see Section 2.2), originate as velocity signals (Robinson 1981). Cannon and coworkers (1983) showed how these velocity signals could be integrated while any background rate (such as that carried by vestibular neurons) would be passed unintegrated to motoneurons.

They noted that inputs to the oculomotor neural integrator that have nonzero background activity (such as vestibular inputs) are provided by two sets of neurons that are bilaterally arranged and encode signals in push–pull. Both sets have approximately equal background activities, and they encode signals by an increase of activity in one set and a decrease in the other set. Cannon

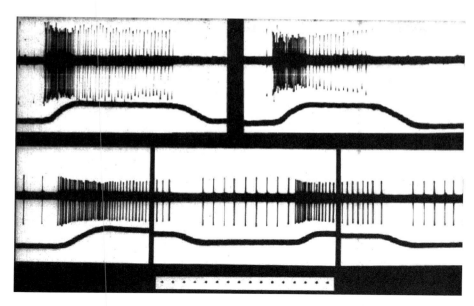

FIGURE 2.12   Activity of two abducens motoneurons in a monkey during horizontal eye movements The activity of motoneuron one is shown in the top row, while that of motoneuron two is shown in the bottom row, during five different eye movements separated in time. Each panel shows motoneuron spike discharge (top trace) and horizontal eye angular position (bottom trace). The discharge rate of the motoneuron encodes both the angular velocity and position of the eye. The velocity component appears as a high-frequency burst of spikes, or as a pause in discharge, for changes in eye angular position (i.e., eye angular velocity) in the "on" (burst) or "off" (pause) directions of eye movement, respectively. The position component appears as steady firing proportional to eye angular position during periods when the eye is not moving. The timing pips (row of dots at bottom) are separated by 20 ms. (From Fuchs and Luschei 1970.)

and coworkers (1983) showed that the push–pull signal of interest, but not the background activity, could be leaky integrated by a pair of neurons that receive oppositely directed inputs (one push, the other pull) and exert positive feedback on themselves, both directly and through reciprocal inhibition of each other. Reciprocal inhibition is a closed-loop (circuit) form of recurrent connectivity that is equivalent to positive feedback, since each unit in the pair exerts positive feedback on itself by inhibiting its inhibitor (inhibition of inhibition is excitation). Neurons that compose the neural integrator are located predominantly in the vestibular nuclei (Robinson 1981). These neurons are in fact bilaterally arranged, with each side receiving oppositely directed inputs, and they reciprocally inhibit each other (Wilson and Melvill Jones 1979). (See Chapter 6 for further details on the neuroanatomy of the vestibulo-oculomotor system.) A schematic of the two-unit version of the model of Cannon and coworkers (1983), which is consistent with this neuroanatomical arrangement, is shown in Figure 2.13.

Equation 2.4 describes the discrete-time responses of the two-unit model of the oculomotor neural integrator:

$$\begin{bmatrix} y_1(t) \\ y_2(t) \end{bmatrix} = \begin{bmatrix} w_{11} & w_{12} \\ w_{21} & w_{22} \end{bmatrix} \begin{bmatrix} y_1(t-1) \\ y_2(t-1) \end{bmatrix} + \begin{bmatrix} v_{11} & v_{12} \\ v_{21} & v_{22} \end{bmatrix} \begin{bmatrix} x_1(t-1) \\ x_2(t-1) \end{bmatrix} \qquad \textbf{2.4}$$

Equation 2.4 differs from Equation 2.2 in that the former has two inputs, x_1 and x_2, whereas the latter has only one, x. Remember that Equation 2.2 described

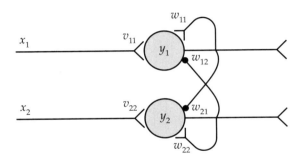

FIGURE 2.13   The two-unit network configured to implement the two-unit model of the oculomotor neural integrator Inputs x_j (j = 1, 2) connect to units y_i (i = 1, 2) with weights v_{ij}, and units y_l (l = 1, 2) connect to units y_k (k = 1, 2) with weights w_{kl}. The Y-shaped and closed-circle endings represent excitatory and inhibitory synaptic connections, respectively.

the two-leak series, as well as the parallel-pathway, positive-feedback, and negative-feedback models of VOR processing that we studied in previous sections of this chapter. Equations 2.2 and 2.4 are both of the general form of Equation 2.3. Because the two-unit integrator has two inputs, its input weight matrix **V** is a square, 2-by-2 matrix (see Equation 2.4). In contrast, for the models with only one input, matrix **V** is a column vector of two elements (see Equation 2.2). The weight matrix **W** of the recurrent connections among the two units is a square 2-by-2 matrix for the two-unit integrator (see Equation 2.4) as for the other networks we have studied so far in this chapter (see Equation 2.2).

Script `twoUnitIntegrator`, listed in MATLAB Box 2.3, will implement the two-unit integrator model. It will evaluate Equation 2.4 on each time step, after first setting up the push–pull inputs $x_1(t)$ and $x_2(t)$. To do this, both inputs are provided with the same background activity, and then the signal of interest is added to one member of the pair and subtracted from the other. Background activity is stored in variable `bg`. Script `twoUnitIntegrator` will produce a push–pull pulse input and store the pair of time series as the two rows of the array x using the following MATLAB commands: `tEnd=1000`, `nTs=tEnd+1`, `x=ones(2,nTs)*bg`, `x(1,101)=x(1,101)+1`, and `x(2,101)=x(2,101)-1`. (Note that each of the two vector time series in x has 1001 elements.) To simulate the oculomotor integrator, set the connection weight values as follows: $v_{11} = 1$, $v_{12} = 0$, $v_{21} = 0$, $v_{22} = 1$, $w_{11} = 0.5$, $w_{12} = -0.499$, $w_{21} = -0.499$, and $w_{22} = 0.5$. The response of the network is computed, as before, using a for-loop, where the only difference is that two inputs, rather than one input, are applied on each time step. Inputs $x_1(t)$ and $x_2(t)$ are drawn from the columns of array x on the previous time step using `x(:,t-1)` in the command `y(:,t)=W*y(:,t-1)+V*x(:,t-1)`, which implements Equation 2.4 in `twoUnitIntegrator`. As before, the output array is defined (and zeroed) using `y=zeros(2,nTs)`, and the initial values of units y_1 and y_2 are kept at 0 by starting the loop on time step 2.

To begin this study of the two-unit integrator, set the background rate to 0 (`bg=0`), and run `twoUnitIntegrator` to observe the response of the network to the push–pull pulse input with a 0 background rate. You will observe that each unit produces a geometric decay, which is a leaky-integrated version of the pulse input, but one unit has a response polarity opposite that of the other. Both units decay toward a baseline of 0. The results show that the two units leaky integrate the input, and respond to push–pull input pulses with push–pull geometric decays.

Now increase the background rate to 10 (`bg=10`) and rerun the simulation. The results are shown in Figure 2.14. The inputs (dot-dashed line) have back-

MATLAB® BOX 2.3   The script implements the two-unit model of the integrator of the oculomotor system.

```
% twoUnitIntegrator.m

bg=0; % set background
v11=1; v12=0; % set weights to unit one from inputs
v21=0; v22=1; % set weights to unit two from inputs
w11=0.5; w12=-0.499; % set feedback weights to unit one
w21=-0.499; w22=0.5; % set feedback weights to unit two

V=[v11 v12;v21 v22]; % compose input weight matrix
W=[w11 w12;w21 w22]; % compose feedback weight matrix

tEnd=1000; % set end time
tVec=0:tEnd; % set time vector
nTs=tEnd+1; % find number of time steps
x=ones(2,nTs)*bg; % set input background
x(1,101)=x(1,101)+1; % set "push" input
x(2,101)=x(2,101)-1; % set "pull" input

y=zeros(2,nTs); % zero the output array
for t=2:nTs, % do for each time step
    y(:,t)=W*y(:,t-1) + V*x(:,t-1); % compute output
end  % end loop

[eVec,eVal]=eig(W); % find eigenvalues and eigenvectors
eVal=diag(eVal); % extract eigenvalues
magEVal=abs(eVal); % find magnitude of eigenvalues
[eVec eVal magEVal] % show eigenvectors, eigenvalues, magnitude
```

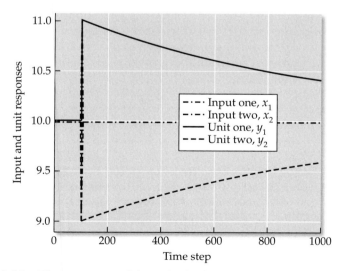

FIGURE 2.14   The responses of the units in the two-unit model of the oculo-motor neural integrator to a push–pull pulse The input pulses (dot-dashed lines) rise ("push," x_1) or fall ("pull," x_2) for a duration of one time step from a nonzero background. The input pulses are just barely discernable behind the unit responses. The units (solid and dashed lines, y_1 and y_2) leaky integrate the push–pull inputs but not their common background.

ground activity of 10, as set. If the network was to leaky integrate this nonzero background, then the states of both units would immediately begin a gradual rise to some new baseline, and this sluggish rise would be maintained for the duration of the simulation. This does not occur. Instead, the states (responses) of both units immediately jump from 0 to about 10 and remain at that level until the time of the push–pull input pulse. When it arrives, the units respond to the push–pull pulse with push–pull geometric decays (solid and dashed lines) as in the previous simulation, except that now they decay toward a baseline near 10 rather than 0. This simulation shows that the push–pull input signal is integrated, but the input background activity is not integrated by the two-unit network model of the oculomotor neural integrator. This behavior is due to the reciprocal inhibitory connections between the units (see analysis later in this section).

The behavior of the two-unit integrator is similar to that observed in integrator networks composed of more than two units (Cannon et al. 1983). The long-duration responses of the units are consistent with the sustained eye position component of the motoneuron command produced by the real neural integrator (see Figure 2.12). We might predict from our simulation that positive feedback via reciprocal inhibition is necessary for integration by the oculomotor neural integrator. Studies in primates confirm this prediction. Lesions of the brainstem midline in monkeys, which disrupt mutually inhibitory connections between the vestibular nuclei on the two sides, produce severe deficits in oculomotor neural integration (Anastasio and Robinson 1991).

The response of the two-unit integrator to the push–pull pulse gives us a good, qualitative view of its dynamic behavior. A more quantitative description is obtained by computing the dynamic modes of the system. The eigenvectors, eigenvalues, and eigenvalue magnitudes are also computed by script `twoUnitIntegrator` and are listed in Table 2.2.

The two-unit integrator has two dynamic modes. Both modes have real, positive eigenvalues less than 1, so the response components due to both modes are stable decays. The dominant mode, which is the one with the larger eigenvalue, has eigenvector $[+0.7071 \; -0.7071]^T$. This is the push–pull pattern in which the responses of the two units change in opposite directions. The eigenvalue of this mode is 0.9990. It governs the rather unleaky decay of the push–pull response. (Note that if the eigenvalue were 1, then the integration would be perfect: no leak, no decay.) The other mode has eigenvector $[+0.7071 \; +0.7071]^T$. This is the pattern in which the responses of both units change in the same direction. The eigenvalue of this mode is 0.0010. It produces integration so leaky that it is essentially no integration at all. It governs the rapid jump of both unit responses from 0 to the constant baseline level they assume

TABLE 2.2   Eigenmode analysis for the two-unit model of the oculomotor neural integrator

Eigenvector	+0.7071	+0.7071
	−0.7071	+0.7071
Eigenvalue	+0.9990	+0.0010
Magnitude	0.9990	0.0010

Eigenvectors, eigenvalues, and eigenvalue magnitude (stability) for each of the two dynamic modes are listed. The signs of the eigenvector elements and eigenvalues are indicated. Magnitudes are always positive.

when their inputs have nonzero background activity. If the eigenvalue of this subdominant mode were larger, then the increase of both unit responses up to the baseline level would be more sluggish and rounded.

The stabilities of the dynamic modes of the two-unit integrator network are determined by the magnitudes of their associated eigenvalues. Both eigenvalues in this case are positive and real, so the magnitude of each eigenvalue is simply equal to the eigenvalue. We already know from the eigenvalues that the two-unit integrator in this case is stable. Yet, with the dominant eigenvalue at 0.9990, the two-unit integrator network with its weights as set is not far from instability. Relatively small changes in the recurrent weights can have dramatic consequences for network dynamics (see Exercise 2.2).

The properties of the dynamic modes of the two-unit integrator network result from the specific values of the recurrent connection weights, including the reciprocally inhibitory weights, in matrix **W**. Thus, the two-unit integrator will integrate push–pull inputs (eigenvalue near 1), which cause the responses of the units to move in opposite directions, but will not integrate the common input background activity (eigenvalue near 0), which causes the responses of the units to move in the same direction. This type of analysis can be applied to integrator network models composed of many more units, provided that all of the units are linear (e.g., Anastasio 1998).

Reciprocal inhibition can do more than just cancel off background activity in push–pull inputs. Reciprocal inhibitory interactions are found throughout the nervous system, especially in the motor system, where they appear to be important for motor coordination. Reciprocal inhibitory interactions are also a prominent feature of many central pattern generator (CPG) neural networks. In the next section we will study simple models of CPGs that will feature both reciprocal inhibition and leaky-integration.

2.7 Simulating the Insect-Flight Central Pattern Generator

Central pattern generators (CPGs) are neural networks that produce oscillatory outputs. They are used to drive repetitive movements such as locomotion (swimming, walking, running, flying, and so on) (Delcomyn 1980). The vertebrate spinal cord contains many CPGs. The most intensively studied invertebrate CPG is that of the stomatogastric ganglion in the lobster, which controls the rhythmic churning movements of its stomach (Elson and Selverston 1992; Marder and Calabrese 1996). A schematic of this CPG, and some data showing the activity of its neurons, is shown in Figure 2.15. It is apparent from the schematic (Figure 2.15A) that many of the neurons in this CPG are connected in reciprocally inhibitory pairs (such as the lateral and medial gastric motoneurons, to take one example). These reciprocally inhibitory interactions may be responsible for coordinating the activity of the neurons in the CPG. As the example in this section will illustrate, reciprocal inhibition is not necessarily responsible for the oscillations.

The first model of a CPG was proposed by Wilson (1961), who studied the flight control CPG in locusts. Wilson found experimentally that the locust flight control CPG converts a constant flight command input into a steady oscillation that drives the beating of the wings. His model took the form of the reciprocal inhibitory network shown in Figure 2.13, with two notable differences. First, the two units y_1 and y_2 both received the same flight command input. This command is either off, or active at some constant level, but the weight of the input was greater to y_1 than to y_2. Second, and more importantly,

FIGURE 2.15   The lobster stomatogastric central pattern generator (A) The known connectivity of the stomatogastric ganglion of the lobster. Connection symbols are: filled circles, chemical (neurotransmitter) inhibition; filled triangles, chemical excitation; open triangles, functional excitation; resistor symbol, electrotonic coupling (via gap junctions, which essentially are membrane pores through which ions flow between two neurons). (B) Spike discharge of stomatogastric neurons. Motoneurons: LG, lateral gastric; MG, medial gastric; LPG, lateral posterior gastric; DG, dorsal gastric; GM, gastric mill; AM, anterior median. Interneuron: INT 1. (From Elson and Selverston 1992.)

(A)

(B)

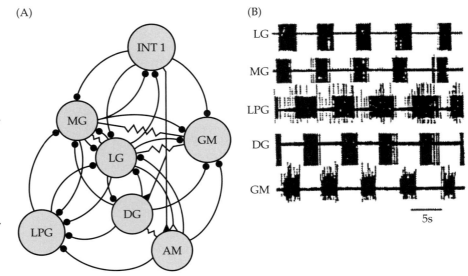

the units y_1 and y_2 had the special property of "fatigue." That is, after unit y_1 or y_2 became active, it would, after a short while, simply "get tired" and shut itself off again through fatigue.

The Wilson CPG works as follows. The flight command input comes on. Unit y_1 is activated more than y_2 and inhibits y_2. After a short while y_1 turns itself off through fatigue. This releases y_2 from inhibition, and allows y_2 to be activated by the constant flight command input and to inhibit y_1. After a short while y_2 turns itself off through fatigue and releases y_1 from inhibition. This allows y_1 to be activated and inhibit y_2, and the process repeats itself.

The property of fatigue was attributed by Wilson to biophysical events occurring within individual neurons of the CPG. We can simulate the same effect using additional leaky-integrator units. This is plausible neurobiologically because real CPGs are composed of many interconnected neurons, and it is realistic to suppose that some of those act as leaky integrators. A simple model for a CPG is shown in Figure 2.16. Note that units y_2 and y_3 also have self connections, but these are not shown for clarity.

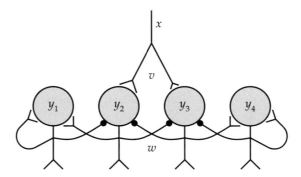

FIGURE 2.16   Wilson's model of the locust-flight central pattern generator (CPG) implemented using leaky integrators Input x connects to units y_i ($i = 1, 2, 3, 4$) with weights v_i, and units y_l ($l = 1, 2, 3, 4$) connect to units y_k ($k = 1, 2, 3, 4$) with weights w_{kl}. For clarity, the self-connections of y_2 and y_3 are not shown, and the individual forward and recurrent weights are not labeled.

In the model in Figure 2.16, units y_2 and y_3 reciprocally inhibit each other. Units y_1 and y_4 are leaky integrators. Unit y_1 leaky integrates the output of y_2 and inhibits y_2, while unit y_4 leaky integrates the output of y_3 and inhibits y_3. As leaky integrators, the responses of y_1 and y_4 are sluggish (they lag the responses of y_2 and y_3), so the effect of their inhibition on y_2 and y_3 takes a while to build up. In this way, units y_1 and y_4 can simulate the "fatigue" postulated by Wilson, but they do so via a network mechanism rather than a cellular, biophysical mechanism.

Equation 2.5 describes the discrete-time responses of the units in the locust flight CPG network:

$$
\begin{bmatrix} y_1(t) \\ y_2(t) \\ y_3(t) \\ y_4(t) \end{bmatrix} = \begin{bmatrix} w_{11} & w_{12} & w_{13} & w_{14} \\ w_{21} & w_{22} & w_{23} & w_{24} \\ w_{31} & w_{32} & w_{33} & w_{34} \\ w_{41} & w_{42} & w_{43} & w_{44} \end{bmatrix} \begin{bmatrix} y_1(t-1) \\ y_2(t-1) \\ y_3(t-1) \\ y_4(t-1) \end{bmatrix} + \begin{bmatrix} v_1 \\ v_2 \\ v_3 \\ v_4 \end{bmatrix} x(t-1) \qquad \textbf{2.5}
$$

Note that Equation 2.5 has the same general form (see Equation 2.3) as all of the other equations we have considered so far in this chapter, but its input weight matrix **V** is a 4-element column vector, while the matrix **W** of the weights of the recurrent connections among the units is a square, 4-by-4 matrix. In this form the response of the CPG network can be computed, as before for the other networks, using a for-loop, in which Equation 2.5 is evaluated on each time step. The script `WilsonCPG`, listed in MATLAB Box 2.4, will do this. As for the networks we studied at the beginning of this chapter, the input to the CPG is a single pulse. The script sets the end time as `tEnd=100`, sets the time vector as `tVec=0:tEnd`, and finds the number of time points as `nTs=tEnd+1`. The script sets `fly=11`, and it then constructs the input $x(t)$ using `x=zeros(1,nTs)` and `x(fly)=1`, which places the input pulse that initiates flight at time 10. To simulate the flight control CPG, set the connection weights as: $v_1 = 0$, $v_2 = 1$, $v_3 = 0$, $v_4 = 0$, $w_{11} = 0.9$, $w_{12} = 0.2$, $w_{13} = 0$, $w_{14} = 0$, $w_{21} = -0.95$, $w_{22} = 0.4$, $w_{23} = -0.5$, $w_{24} = 0$, $w_{31} = 0$, $w_{32} = -0.5$, $w_{33} = 0.4$, $w_{34} = -0.95$, $w_{41} = 0$, $w_{42} = 0$, $w_{43} = 0.2$, and $w_{44} = 0.9$. The script defines (and zeros) the output array using `y=zeros(4,nTs)`. Running `WilsonCPG` simulates the CPG. The input and the responses of units y_2 and y_3 are shown in Figure 2.17.

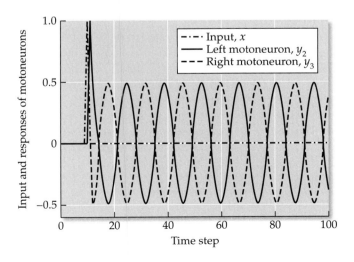

FIGURE 2.17   **The responses of units representing motoneurons in the linear version of Wilson's model of the locust-flight central pattern generator (CPG)** The input (dot-dashed line, x) is a pulse of amplitude 1 and duration one time step. The motoneuron responses (left, y_2; right, y_3) are oscillations at a frequency of about 0.07 cycles per time step. (One full cycle has a period of about 15 time steps.) The oscillations of the motoneurons on the left and right sides of the CPG are one-half cycle out of phase.

MATLAB® BOX 2.4   **The script implements a linear version of Wilson's model of the locust-flight central pattern generator.**

```
% WilsonCPG.m

v1=0; v2=1; v3=0; v4=0; % set input weights
w11=0.9; w12=0.2; w13=0; w14=0; % feedback weights to unit one
w21=-0.95; w22=0.4; w23=-0.5; w24=0; % weights to unit two
w31=0; w32=-0.5; w33=0.4; w34=-0.95; % weights to unit three
w41=0; w42=0; w43=0.2; w44=0.9; % feedback weights to unit four

V=[v1;v2;v3;v4]; % compose input weight matrix (vector)
W=[w11 w12 w13 w14;w21 w22 w23 w24; % compose feedback...
 w31 w32 w33 w34;w41 w42 w43 w44]; % weight matrix

tEnd=100; % set end time
tVec=0:tEnd; % set time vector
nTs=tEnd+1; % find number of time steps
x=zeros(1,nTs); % zero input vector
fly=11; % set time to start flying
x(fly)=1; % set input to one at fly time

y=zeros(4,nTs); % zero output array
for t=2:nTs, % for each time step
    y(:,t)=W*y(:,t-1) + V*x(t-1); % compute output
end % end loop

[eVec,eVal]=eig(W); % find eigenvalues and eigenvectors
eVal=diag(eVal); % extract eigenvalues
magEVal=abs(eVal); % find magnitude of eigenvalues
angEVal=angle(eVal)./(2*pi); % find angles of eigenvalues
[eVec eVal magEVal angEVal] % show eigenmode analysis results
```

The input (dot-dashed line) is a pulse at time 10 that signals the start of flying. The outputs of units y_2 and y_3 show a steady, sinusoidal oscillation. The outputs of units y_1 and y_4 (not shown) also oscillate. Thus, the model simulates the essential behavior of a CPG, which is oscillation. Further, units y_2 and y_3 exhibit oscillations that are one-half cycle out of phase with each other, and so network behavior could be interpreted in terms of the function of a locomotory CPG such as the locust-flight CPG first described by Wilson (1961).

A wing, like any limb, is moved by the coordinated action of antagonistic muscles. These muscles in locust wings are the elevator and depressor muscles. To produce coordinated beating of the wings in a locust, unit y_2 could, say, drive the elevator muscle and unit y_3 could drive the depressor muscle. Because the two oscillations are a half-cycle out-of-phase, y_3 is suppressed when y_2 is activated and vice-versa. When y_2 is activated and y_3 suppressed, the elevator muscle would contract and the depressor muscle would relax, and the wing would rise. During the next half-cycle, when y_2 is suppressed and y_3 activated, the elevator would relax and the depressor contract, and the wing would fall. This cycle would repeat, and coordinated flight would result.

As for the networks we studied in previous sections, the pulse response of the CPG network gives us a qualitative view of its dynamics, but eigenmode analysis gives us a more quantitative description. The eigenvectors, eigenvalues, and eigenvalue magnitudes (stability) of the CPG network model are

TABLE 2.3   Eigenmode analysis for the linear version of Wilson's locust-flight central pattern generator

Eigenvector	+0.0000+j0.2949	+0.0000−j0.2949	+0.4363	+0.1833
	+0.6427−j0.0000	+0.6427+j0.0000	−0.5564	−0.6829
	−0.6427+j0.0000	−0.6427−j0.0000	−0.5564	−0.6829
	−0.0000−j0.2949	−0.0000+j0.2949	+0.4363	+0.1833
Eigenvalue	+0.9000+j0.4359	+0.9000−j0.4359	+0.6449	+0.1551
Magnitude	1.0000	1.0000	0.6449	0.1551
Frequency	0.0718	0.0718	0.0000	0.0000

Eigenvectors, eigenvalues, eigenvalue magnitude (stability), and oscillation frequency (in cycles per time step) for each of the four dynamic modes are listed. The signs of eigenvector elements and eigenvalues are indicated. Magnitudes are always positive. The signs of frequencies are ignored.

computed by script `WilsonCPG` and are listed in Table 2.3. The four-unit CPG model has four dynamic modes; two of these are real and two are complex. For a complex mode the eigenvalue, and each element of the eigenvector, are complex numbers of the form $\mu + j\omega$, where μ is the real part, ω is the imaginary part, and $j = \sqrt{-1}$. Complex modes occur in pairs in which the eigenvalues are complex conjugates ($[\mu + j\omega]$ and $[\mu - j\omega]$ are conjugates), and corresponding elements of the eigenvectors are likewise complex conjugates.

Complex modes produce oscillations, and the frequencies of the oscillations in radians per time step are equal to the angles $\theta = \arctan(\omega / \mu)$ of the complex eigenvalues expressed as vectors in the complex plane. These angles in cycles per time step (where 1 cycle equals 2π radians) are computed in script `WilsonCPG` using `angleEVal=angle(eVal)./(2*pi)` (the symbols `./` signify element-wise division). The angles (frequencies) are also listed in Table 2.3. The complex modes of the CPG model produce its oscillation of about 0.07 cycles per time step. The magnitudes (or absolute values) of complex eigenvalues are equal to the lengths $\sqrt{(\mu^2 + \omega^2)}$ of the eigenvalues expressed as vectors in the complex plane. The MATLAB command `magEVal=abs(eVal)` finds the magnitudes of the real or complex eigenvalues. (Note that a real number is just a complex number with zero imaginary part.) Eigenvalue magnitudes indicate not only the stability of the corresponding dynamic mode, but also indicate the dominance of the mode relative to the other modes in the network. The two complex modes (which form a complex conjugate pair) have magnitude 1, which is larger than the magnitudes of the two real modes (see Table 2.3). Thus, the oscillatory mode dominates the dynamics of the locust-flight CPG model.

Like the purely real eigenvectors considered previously, complex eigenvectors also indicate the pattern of responses among the units in the network, but their complex elements must first be converted to real numbers before they can be related to the actual unit responses they describe (Luenberger 1979). Without entering into the details, we can observe that each element of an eigenvector corresponds to a response component of a unit, so that the first element of each eigenvector corresponds to a response component of unit y_1, the second to y_2, and so on for the other elements and units. Consider eigenvectors 1 and 2 in Table 2.3, which form the complex conjugate eigenvector pair. The second elements of eigenvectors 1 and 2 are both real and positive, and their third elements are both real and negative. This essentially describes the one half-cycle phase difference between the oscillations of units y_2 and y_3, which represent the motoneurons. As noted above, the magnitudes of the eigenvalues associated with the two complex modes (both equal to 1) are larger than those of the other two, real modes. Thus, the dominant modes are the two complex modes. They account for the predominant dynamics of the CPG, which is characterized by oscillations of the two motoneurons at the same frequency that are a half-cycle out of phase with one another.

Complex modes arise from asymmetry in the couplings of the elements of dynamic systems (Luenberger 1979). In our linear networks, complex modes arise from asymmetry in the interconnections between the units. In the CPG network, oscillation occurs not because of the reciprocal inhibitory connections, which are symmetric, but because of the asymmetric coupling between the leaky integrator (y_1 or y_4) and the motoneuron (y_2 or y_3) on each side. To see this we can compare the parameterized versions of the recurrent weight matrices **W** for the two-unit integrator and the CPG.

The recurrent weight matrix **W** that we used for the two-unit integrator model is shown in Equation 2.6:

$$\mathbf{W} = \begin{bmatrix} +0.500 & -0.499 \\ -0.499 & +0.500 \end{bmatrix} \qquad \textbf{2.6}$$

The self-connections, both +0.5 in this network, define the diagonal, about which this matrix is clearly symmetric. The two-unit integrator with this recurrent weight matrix had no complex modes (see Table 2.2). In contrast, the recurrent weight matrix **W** that we used for the CPG model is shown in Equation 2.7:

$$\mathbf{W} = \begin{bmatrix} +0.90 & +0.20 & 0 & 0 \\ -0.95 & +0.40 & -0.50 & 0 \\ 0 & -0.50 & +0.40 & -0.95 \\ 0 & 0 & +0.20 & +0.90 \end{bmatrix} \qquad \textbf{2.7}$$

This matrix is asymmetric, but the asymmetry is not due to the reciprocal inhibitory connections between y_2 and y_3, which are symmetrically –0.50. The asymmetry is due to the connections between the leaky integrator and the motoneuron on each side. Note on the left side that y_1 inhibits y_2 by –0.95, but y_2 excites y_1 by +0.20, and the same asymmetric relationship holds between y_4 and y_3 on the right side. These asymmetries give rise to the complex modes that produce oscillation in the CGP network. Note also that these asymmetries are contained within the 2-by-2 blocks of weights that correspond to each half of the CPG. Indeed, with some weight adjustments, each half of the CPG network is capable of independent oscillation (see Exercise 2.3). Oscillators of this sort, which are formed from asymmetric coupling between neural elements, may be components in many different kinds of oscillatory neural systems.

An asymmetric pattern of connectivity between two neural types may contribute to the production of oscillations in the thalamus. Thalamocortical neurons, which project from the thalamus to the cortex, also send excitatory projections to thalamic interneurons known as reticular neurons. The reticular neurons, in turn, inhibit the thalamocortical neurons (Steriade et al. 1993). In combination with the intrinsic biophysical properties of these neurons, modeling studies suggest that the asymmetric connectivity between thalamocortical and reticular neurons may contribute to the complex oscillations that have been observed in the thalamcortical system (Destexhe and Sejnowski 2003). Asymmetric connectivity between neural types has also been used to simulate vestibular nystagmus, which is the alternation between the slow VOR and fast resetting eye movements that is produced during head rotation (see Section 2.2 and Figures 2.4 and 2.5). In this model the nystagmic pattern is based on an oscillation due to the asymmetric, excitatory–inhibitory connectivity between vestibular nucleus neurons and brainstem burst neurons (Anastasio 1997).

In the CPG model, the symmetric, reciprocal inhibition between the two half-CPG oscillators is not necessary for their oscillation, but it does ensure that their oscillations are out of phase. From this analysis we might predict that the reciprocally inhibitory connections in real CPGs, such as those found in the lobster stomatogastric ganglion (see Figure 2.15), also play a role in the coordination of alternating patterns of rhythmic activity. Oscillation in the model is due to the asymmetric, excitatory–inhibitory connections between the motoneuron and the leaky integrator within each half-CPG. Mixed excitatory and inhibitory interactions between neurons are also observed in real CPGs such as the lobster stomatogastric ganglion (see Figure 2.15), and we might predict that they contribute to the oscillatory behavior of those neural systems.

We found the magnitudes of the eigenvalues associated with the four dynamic modes in the CPG network and used them to determine that the two complex modes were the dominant modes. As explained previously (see also Math Box 2.4), the magnitude (absolute value) of a mode is related to its stability. In linear dynamic systems, the stability of a mode determines whether the response pattern due to that mode will grow, decay, or stay constant. The magnitudes of the modes of the CPG network model are listed in Table 2.3. Note that the magnitudes of the two complex modes have value 1. This means that the complex modes, which produce oscillation in the network, are marginally stable. The consequence is that, once the oscillations are initiated by the input pulse, their amplitudes would persist (remain constant). In order to switch off the oscillations, the states of the units would have to be reset to 0.

The production of a stable oscillation is a straightforward way to use linear units to simulate a CPG. Switching it on with a pulse, and switching it off again with a reset, is a form of control that could occur in the fly. The escape flight of a fly is initiated by a transient visual stimulus (indicating an approaching object) and terminated by a different visual stimulus (indicating approach to a surface) (Holmqvist and Srinivasan 1991). Although it might be appropriate as a model of the fly-flight CPG, the sustained, marginally stable oscillation among linear units produced by our CPG model deviates from Wilson's original model in that the oscillation in the original persisted only as long as the "fly" signal was nonzero. In our linear CPG model the oscillation would begin when the fly signal comes on, but would persist after the fly signal went off again. The form of control in which a CPG oscillates only when a fly signal is active might be better simulated using a network of nonlinear than of linear units.

Linear systems can exhibit rich behaviors, including multiple modes that can grow, decay, and oscillate, and they are amenable to analysis, and for these reasons they can offer insights into the behavior of certain neural systems (e.g., Barreiro et al. 2008). However, nonlinear dynamic systems can exhibit behaviors whose richness completely outstrips that of linear systems. Perhaps for this reason CPGs are usually modeled as nonlinear dynamic systems (Ermentrout and Chow 2002). We will explore specific types of nonlinear systems in later chapters of this book. For present purposes it is enough to point out that a nonlinear version of the CPG model can be made to oscillate only as long as a fly signal is nonzero. Constructing a nonlinear version of the Wilson CPG model is the goal of Exercise 2.4. In Exercise 13.4 (see Chapter 13) we will use the genetic algorithm to set some of the parameters of the nonlinear version of the Wilson CPG model.

Exercises

2.1   We studied the pulse response of two units connected in series, where both units were leaky integrators because they exerted positive feedback on themselves with weights less than 1. Unit 1 leaky integrated the input pulse, while unit 2 leaky integrated the output of unit 1. We observed that the response of unit 2 was a rounded version of the response of unit 1, and could be described as a lopsided bump. What does the response of the 25th leaky integrator in a series look like? Modify script `twoLeakSeries` (listed in MATLAB Box 2.1) to find out. The input matrix **V** will be a column vector of 24 0s preceded by a 1. If n=25, then this input matrix can be set using the command V=[1;zeros(n-1,1)]. The matrix **W** of connections among the units will have their self-connections on the main diagonal, while the connections that link each unit to the next one in the series will be on the next diagonal below it. Set the weight values for the main diagonal (self-connections) using `wmain=ones(1,n)*0.95`, and for the off-diagonal (series connections) using `woff=ones(1,n-1)*0.05`. Then matrix **W** is composed using `W=diag(wmain,0)+diag(woff,-1)`. Note that the feedback weights are all 0.95, while the series connection weights are all 0.05. The responses of units 1 and 2 should be similar to those you observed in the example with two leaky-integrators in series. What do the other 23 look like? How would you describe the pulse response of the 25th leaky integrator?

2.2   Script `twoUnitIntegrator` (listed in MATLAB Box 2.3) implements the two-unit model of the oculomotor neural integrator. In our example, each unit excited itself with a self-connection weight of 0.5, and the two units reciprocally inhibited each other with weights of –0.499. The input was a push–pull pulse, and the push–pull responses of the units were slow decays. What happens if you change the reciprocal weights to –0.5? What happens if you change the reciprocal weights to –0.5001? Can you explain the resulting behavior in each case in terms of the magnitude of the dominant (largest magnitude) eigenvalue?

2.3   Like the original model, our version of Wilson's model of the locust-flight central pattern generator (CPG) has two sides that are interconnected by reciprocal inhibition. We determined, through analysis, that oscillation in our network was not due to the reciprocal inhibitory connections between the two sides, but to the asymmetric excitation and inhibition between the motoneuron unit and the leaky-integrator unit on each side. The analysis indicated that each side should be capable of independent oscillation. Modify script `twoLeakSeries` (listed in MATLAB Box 2.1) to demonstrate this result. Assume that y_1 is the motoneuron and y_2 is the leaky integrator in a half-CPG. For simplicity, have each unit excite itself with a weight of 0.9 (w11=0.9 and w22=0.9). For oscillation, we need the motoneuron to excite the leaky integrator, but we need the leaky integrator to inhibit the motoneuron, so set w21=0.43 and w12=0.44. We want the input to be sent to y_1 but not y_2, so set v1=1 but v2=0. We also want the input to be a pulse, so make sure that tEnd=100, nTs=tEnd+1, x=zeros(1,nTs), start=11, and x(start)=1. We also want the input to be v1=1 but v2=0. What is the result? Can you get a half-CPG to oscillate? What happens if you change the weight values? Can you get an oscillation with decaying or growing amplitude? Can you get oscillations with constant amplitudes at other frequencies? Can you describe aspects of the behavior of the network (e.g., oscillation frequency, stability) on the basis of eigenmode analysis?

2.4   In our linear version of Wilson's model of the locust-flight central pattern generator (CPG), a pulse input initiated an oscillatory response in which there was a half-cycle phase difference between the two sides of the bilateral CPG. Once initiated, this oscillation was sustained. Modify script WilsonCPG (listed in MATLAB Box 2.4) to create a nonlinear version of Wilson's CPG in which an oscillation, with the required phase difference between the two sides, is present when the CPG receives a constant fly command but absent when the fly command is terminated. Use the following commands to set the fly, land, and end times: fly=11, land=351, tEnd=500, and nTs=tEnd+1. Zero the input using x=zeros(1,nTs) and then make the flying/landing command using x(fly:land)=ones(1,land-fly+1). Set the (forward) weights from the inputs as V=[0 12 11.9 0]' and the unit interconnection (recurrent) weights as W=[1 3 0 0; -12 1 -6 0; 0 -6 1 -12; 0 0 3 1]. Define the output array as y=zeros(4,nTs). For each time step, compute the weighted input sum as q=W*y(:,t-1)+V*x(t-1) and then make the unit responses nonlinear using the sigmoidal squashing function, where y(:,t)=1./(1+exp(-q)) (see Chapter 6 for a description of the sigmoidal squashing function). After some initially spluttering (but interesting) activity, the oscillatory pattern should emerge and be sustained as long as the CPG receives the fly command (represented by a constant input of 1). The oscillatory pattern should cease when the fly command is removed (when the input goes back to 0).

References

Anastasio TJ (1993) Modeling vestibulo-ocular reflex dynamics: From classical analysis to neural networks. In: Eeckman FH (ed) *Neural Systems: Analysis and Modeling*. Kluwer Academic Publishers, Norwell, MA.

Anastasio TJ (1997) A burst-feedback model of fast-phase burst generation during nystagmus. *Biological Cybernetics* 76: 139–152.

Anastasio TJ (1998) Nonuniformity in the linear network model of the oculomotor integrator produces approximately fractional-order dynamics and more realistic neuron behavior. *Biological Cybernetics* 79: 377–391.

Anastasio TJ, Correia MJ (1988) A frequency and time domain study of the horizontal and vertical vestibuloocular reflex in the pigeon. *Journal of Neurophysiology* 59: 1143–1161.

Anastasio TJ, Correia MJ (1994) "Velocity leakage" in the pigeon vestibulo-ocular reflex. *Biological Cybernetics* 70: 235–245.

Anastasio TJ, Correia MJ, Perachio AA (1985) Spontaneous and driven responses of semicircular canal primary afferents in the unanesthetized pigeon. *Journal of Neurophysiology* 54: 335–347.

Anastasio TJ, Robinson DA (1991) Failure of the oculomotor neural integrator from a discrete midline lesion between the abducens nuclei in the monkey. *Neuroscience Letters* 127: 82–86.

Barreiro AK, Bronski JC, Anastasio TJ (2009) Bifurcation theory explains waveform variability in a congenital eye movement disorder. *Journal of Computattional Neuroscience* 26: 321–329.

Cannon SC, Robinson DA, Shamma S (1983) A proposed neural network for the integrator of the oculomotor system. *Biological Cybernetics* 49: 127–136.

Dayan P, Abbott LF (2001) *Theoretical Neuroscience: Computational and Mathematical Modeling of Neural Systems*. MIT Press, Cambridge, MA.

Delcomyn F (1980) Neural basis of rhythmic behavior in animals. *Science* 210: 492–498.

Dextexhe A, Sejnowski TJ (2003) Interactions between membrane conductances underlying thalamocortical slow-wave oscillations. *Physiology Review* 83: 1401–1453.

Elson RC, Selverston AI (1992) Mechanisms of gastric rhythm generation in the isolated stomatogastric ganglion of spiny lobsters: Bursting pacemaker potentials, synaptic interactions and muscarinic modulation. *Journal of Neurophysiology* 68: 890–907.

Ermentrout GB, Chow CC (2002) Modeling neural oscillations. *Physiology and Behavior* 77: 629–633.

Fuchs AF, Luschei ES (1970) Firing patterns of abducens neurons of alert monkeys in relationship to horizontal eye movement. *Journal of Neurophysiology* 33: 382–392.

Gallistel CR (1980) *The Organization of Action: A New Synthesis*. Lawrence Erlbaum Associates, Hillsdale, NJ.

Henn V (1982) The correlation between motion sensation, nystagmus, and activity in the vestibular nerve and nuclei. In: Honrubia V, Brazier MAB (eds) *Nystagmus and Vertigo: Clinical Approaches to the Patient with Dizziness*. Academic Press, New York, pp 115–124.

Holmqvist MH, Srinivasan MV (1991) A visually evoked escape response of the housefly. *Journal of Comparative Physiology* 169: 451–459.

Hultquist PF (1988) *Numerical Methods for Engineers and Computer Scientists*. Benjamin/Cummings, Menlo Park, CA.

Luenberger DG (1979) *Introduction to Dynamic Systems: Theory, Models, and Applications*. John Wiley and Sons, New York.

Marder E, Calabrese RL (1996) Principles of rhythmic motor pattern generation. *Physiological Reviews* 76: 687–717.

Purves D, Augustine GJ, Fitzpatrick D, Hall WC, LaMantia A-S, McNamara JO, Williams SM (eds) (2008). *Neuroscience: Fourth Edition*. Sinauer Associates, Sunderland, MA.

Raphan T, Matsuo V, Cohen B (1979) Velocity storage in the vestibuloocular reflex arc (VOR). *Experimental Brain Research* 35: 229–248.

Robinson DA (1981) The use of control systems analysis in the neurophysiology of eye movements. *Annual Review of Neuroscience* 4: 463–503.

Steriade M, McCormick DA, Sennowski TJ (1993) Thalamocortical oscillations in the sleeping and aroused brain. *Science* 262: 679–685.

Strassman A, Highstein SM, McCrea RA (1986) Anatomy and physiology of saccadic burst neurons in the alert squirrel monkey. I. Excitatory burst neurons. *Journal of Comparative Neurology* 249: 337–357.

Wilson DM (1961) The central nervous control of flight in a locust. *Journal of Experimental Biology* 38: 471–490.

Wilson VJ, Melvill Jones G (1979) *Mammalian Vestibular Physiology*. Plenum Press, New York.

3

Forward and Recurrent Lateral Inhibition

Networks with forward and recurrent laterally inhibitory connectivity profiles can shape signals in space and time, and simulate certain forms of sensory and motor processing

Vision is the dominant sensory modality for human beings. Perhaps for that reason, vision has been the most intensively studied of all sensory systems. Although vision is still incompletely understood, research clearly indicates that the brain represents the visual world not as a snap-shot, but as a set of features that it actively extracts from the visual scene. In humans and other vertebrates, processing of the responses of the photoreceptors begins in the retina, which contains at least four layers of other cell types in addition to the photoreceptors (Dowling 1979). The retinal output passes through the lateral geniculate nucleus of the thalamus, and from there enters a hierarchy of cortical areas. The whole process can be described as an extraction from the original photoreceptor input of features of ever increasing complexity (Hubel 1988).

Much of early visual processing involves the separation of essential features, such as edges or spots, from uninformative background such as constant levels or noise. What the brain does with those features ranges from the straightforward to the mysterious. A straightforward example involves the generation of saccade commands by the superior colliculus. In addition to its relay in the lateral geniculate, some of the retinal output also goes to the superior colliculus in the midbrain. Processing in the colliculus appears to extract a localized spot, or target, from noise or from among competing, distracting targets. It then converts the sensory response at that spot into a burst of activity that serves as a command to drive a saccadic eye movement in the direction of the target (Wurtz and Goldberg 1989). We will study a model of target selection by the superior colliculus later in this chapter.

A more mysterious example involves the process that creates the experience of seeing. We will not attempt to solve mysteries such as late vision in this book, but we will attempt to explain the neural mechanisms that underlie the detection of edges in visual scenes, which is the first stage of early vision. The visual representation, as rich as our experience knows it to be, is based on simple features such as edges. Edge detection is as important for other sensory systems as it is for vision (Shepherd 1994). We will study edge detection and related forms of processing in this chapter.

Both target selection and edge detection can be simulated in neural networks that implement laterally inhibitory interactions. Lateral inhibition was arguably the first form of computation by a neural system to be described (Ratliff 1965), and for that reason it may be the most commonly known. As its name implies, lateral inhibition is characterized by inhibition off to the sides of some form of central excitation. Reciprocal inhibition, which we studied in Chapter 2, is a form of lateral inhibition, but in Chapter 2 we limited ourselves to simple networks composed of few units, and all the units had linear input–output (activation) functions. In this chapter we will greatly expand the number of units. The networks we study in this chapter will have two layers, an input layer and an output layer, and each layer will be a one-dimensional array of up to 50 or more units. The spatially extended structure of the networks will allow them to process inputs that can be interpreted as simple images. Input units will project to output units, and output units can project to themselves and to each other, so these networks will be capable of static or dynamic processing. The output units will be linear or nonlinear, and nonlinearity will endow the dynamic, laterally inhibitory networks with critically important capabilities that they would not have if their units were linear. Our explorations in this chapter will combine all of these factors. Specifically, we will study lateral inhibition in spatially extended, two-layered networks of linear or nonlinear units, and will use these networks to process signals spatially and temporally.

As illustrated in Figure 3.1, lateral inhibition takes two basic forms: forward (also called feedforward) and recurrent. In feedforward architectures (Figure 3.1A), lateral inhibition occurs in the projection from input units to output units. In the simplest case of feedforward lateral inhibition, a unit in the input layer makes an excitatory connection to its corresponding unit in the output layer, and makes inhibitory connections with the two nearest neighbors of that output unit. In recurrent architectures (Figure 3.1B), lateral inhibition occurs in the projection of an output unit to other units in the output layer. In the simplest case of recurrent lateral inhibition, an output unit makes inhibitory connections with its two nearest neighbors in the output layer. In general, both feedforward (forward) and recurrent lateral inhibition can involve excitation and inhibition of any number of units. What characterizes lateral inhibition is that excitation occurs over a central core of units, and inhibition occurs over sets of units that flank the central core. We will study both simple and more complex forms of lateral inhibition in this chapter.

(A) **Feedforward lateral inhibition**

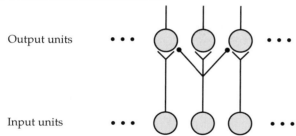

(B) **Recurrent lateral inhibition**

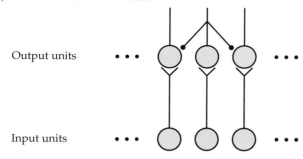

Figure 3.1   The two forms of lateral inhibition in neural networks (A) forward (feedforward) and (B) recurrent lateral inhibition. Y-shaped and dot endings are excitatory and inhibitory, respectively.

Lateral inhibition was first described in the eye of the horseshoe crab (*Limulus*), a photograph of which is shown in Figure 3.2A. Like other invertebrate eyes, the *Limulus* eye is multifaceted. The structures of two facets (ommatidia) are schematized in Figure 3.2B. Each ommatidium contains a retinula cell, which is a visual receptor (photoreceptor), and an eccentric cell. The visual response of each retinula cell is transmitted to the *Limulus* central nervous system by the axon of its associated eccentric cell. Eccentric cells are primary afferent sensory neurons because they are the first neurons in the sensory pathway for the visual modality in *Limulus*.

The action potential firing rate of the eccentric cell from one ommatidium, in response to two types of visual stimuli, is shown in Figure 3.3A. One stimulus is a rectangular light pattern (see Figure 3.2A) that has a higher intensity on one side, and a lower intensity on the other side, of a sharp boundary or edge. The other stimulus is a spot of light, either at the higher or the lower intensity, which is focused on the ommatidium. The activity of the same eccentric cell is

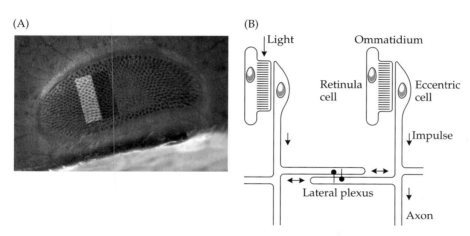

Figure 3.2   Structure of the *Limulus* (horseshoe crab) eye (A) Photograph of a *Limulus* compound eye, showing a visual stimulus pattern consisting of a boundary (edge) between low and high intensities of light. (B) The compound limulus eye is composed of an array of ommatidia. Each ommatidium contains a retinula cell, which transduces light, and an eccentric cell, that is activated by the retinula cell and conducts action potentials into the central nervous system. Eccentric cells in neighboring ommatidia inhibit one another (dots). (A from David McIntyre; B after Shepherd 1994.)

(A)

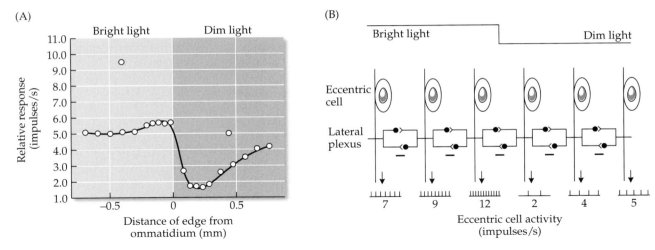

(B)

Figure 3.3 **Edge detection and the organization of the sensory and neural elements in the eye of the *Limulus* (horseshoe crab)** (A) The response of one eccentric cell from the *Limulus* eye. The curvilinear record shows the response of the cell when the light pattern was projected onto the eye with its edge at different positions relative to the location of the ommatidium of the cell. The two isolated dots show the response of the cell to spots of light that are focused on its ommatidium, either at the high or the low intensity. The difference between the two response records reflects the influence of lateral inhibition. (B) The synaptic interaction between the eccentric cells is inhibitory, and this lateral inhibition accounts for the edge detection properties of the *Limulus* eye. (A after Hartline and Ratliff 1959; B after Shepherd 1994.)

recorded in response to either of the two stimuli delivered separately. In one case, the response of the eccentric cell is recorded when the light pattern is presented at different locations on the eye relative to that of the ommatidium, so that the ommatidium is located either in the higher or the lower intensity region of the pattern and at varying distances relative to the edge. In the other case, the focused spot of light at the corresponding intensity is presented by itself. The responses to the light spots or to the light pattern were measured relative to arbitrary controls that differed between the two cases (see Ratliff and Hartline 1959 for methodological details). For this reason, the differences in magnitude between the responses in the two cases are not absolute but are meant to reflect the general observation that the response to a focused light spot is larger than the response to light at the same intensity that covers a wider area. Of particular interest here is the qualitative relationship between the response and light intensity in the two cases. The response (firing rate) of the eccentric cell is proportional to the intensity of the light spot when it is presented by itself (the two unconnected dots in Figure 3.3A). In striking contradistinction, the response to the two-sided, dual-intensity (two-patch) light pattern is largely independent of light intensity, but dependent on the location of the edge relative to the ommatidium (the curvilinear record in Figure 3.3A). This edge dependency is the defining characteristic of the response of the *Limulus* eye to dual-intensity light patterns.

The firing rate of the eccentric cell when the ommatidium is on the higher intensity side of the light pattern is much higher when it is near the edge. Conversely, the firing rate of the eccentric cell when the ommatidium is on the lower intensity side of the light pattern is much lower when it is near the edge. The firing rate of the eccentric cell when the ommatidium is located far from the edge is about the same whether it is in the higher or the lower intensity part of the pattern. Because this effect is observed not when an isolated ommatidium is illuminated by itself, but when many ommatidia are illuminated by the two-patch light pattern, the edge effect is a property not of a single ommatidium but of the entire eye. It seems that the *Limulus* eye as a whole is more responsive to the edges between patches of light of different intensities than to the intensities themselves. This "edge detection" is the result of laterally inhibitory interactions occurring among the eccentric cells in the *Limulus* eye.

The eccentric cells of neighboring ommatidia interact, and the interaction is inhibitory, as shown in Figures 3.2B and 3.3B. Retinula cells are activated little within the low-intensity portion of the light pattern, and the firing rates of their associated eccentric cells are correspondingly low. Retinula cells are activated much more strongly within the high-intensity portion of the light pattern, but their associated eccentric cells also inhibit each other strongly. Consequently, eccentric cell firing rates are about the same whether their associated retinula cells are located within the high-intensity or low-intensity portions of the light pattern. Thus, lateral inhibition explains the general observation that the response to a focused spot of light is larger than the response within a wider patch of light at the same intensity (see Figure 3.3A).

The situation is different at the edge. Eccentric cells on the high-intensity side of the edge are strongly activated by their retinula cells, but are not strongly inhibited by the eccentric cells adjacent to them on the low-intensity side of the edge, so the firing rates are higher for eccentric cells on the high-intensity side of the edge than within the high-intensity portion of the light pattern. Conversely, eccentric cells on the low-intensity side of the edge are not strongly activated by their retinula cells, but they are strongly inhibited by the eccentric cells adjacent to them on the high-intensity side of the edge, so the firing rates are lower for eccentric cells on the low-intensity side of the edge than within the low-intensity portion of the light pattern. Thus, lateral inhibition accounts for the edge-detection capability of the *Limulus* eye. We will simulate this edge detection effect in our first two examples in this chapter.

3.1   Simulating Edge Detection in the Early Visual System of *Limulus*

If we think of the cells in the *Limulus* eye as composing a two-layered neural network, then the retinula and eccentric cells correspond to input and output units, respectively. Because lateral inhibition in the *Limulus* eye occurs between eccentric cells it is, strictly speaking, recurrent lateral inhibition (see Figure 3.1B). Because of these recurrent connections the network of retinula and eccentric cells in the *Limulus* eye is capable both of spatial and temporal signal processing (Ratliff 1965). We will study recurrent lateral inhibition later in this chapter. Here we wish to study the spatial edge-detection effect, and we note that this is a stable-state property of the response of the *Limulus* eye network. We will also study stable states later in this chapter. For now, we note that some stable states, treated as static response patterns, can be approximated by feedforward neural networks. Since this is the case for the edge-detection property we can approximate edge detection in the *Limulus* eye using a feedforward lateral inhibitory network.

We will simulate edge-detection in the *Limulus* eye using a two-layered, feedforward lateral inhibitory network (see Figure 3.1A). The output units will be linear. (Because we specify the activities of the input units, the input unit activation function is not relevant.) Unlike real eccentric cells, which can have only positive firing rates, our linear output units will produce positive and negative responses, so their states will not correspond exactly to firing rates. Our use of linear output units for this example does not change the essential form of the response, but it facilitates the description of network behavior. The responses of the output units in nonlinear versions of this network exhibit the same essential behavior but have only positive values (see Exercise 3.1).

For this feedforward, laterally inhibitory network the first layer of units (inputs) projects to the second layer (outputs) via weighted, feedforward connections. The activity level (or state) of any output unit is just the sum of all its weighted inputs from the input units. If the states of the units are represented as vectors, then the weights connecting the layers can be represented in a matrix. The response, or output of the network (the states of the output units), will simply be the matrix product of the input unit vector and the connectivity matrix: $\mathbf{y} = \mathbf{Vx}$, where $\mathbf{x}$ and $\mathbf{y}$ are input and output (column) vectors and $\mathbf{V}$ is the matrix of the feedforward connection weights. (See Chapter 1 for details on, and numerical examples of, multiplication of a vector by a matrix.)

For our first example, we will construct a network corresponding to the simplest case of feedforward lateral inhibition (see Figure 3.1A). In this case, each unit in the input layer makes an excitatory connection of +2 to its corresponding unit in the output layer, and each input unit makes inhibitory connections of −1 to the two nearest neighbors of that output unit. To take a simple numerical example, consider a feedforward laterally inhibitory network with seven input and seven output units. Assume, for simplicity, that the input and output layers are arranged in circles, so that the first and seventh input units are neighbors, and the first and seventh output units are likewise neighbors. The weight matrix $\mathbf{V}$ is shown in Equation 3.1:

$$\mathbf{V} = \begin{bmatrix} +2 & -1 & 0 & 0 & 0 & 0 & -1 \\ -1 & +2 & -1 & 0 & 0 & 0 & 0 \\ 0 & -1 & +2 & -1 & 0 & 0 & 0 \\ 0 & 0 & -1 & +2 & -1 & 0 & 0 \\ 0 & 0 & 0 & -1 & +2 & -1 & 0 \\ 0 & 0 & 0 & 0 & -1 & +2 & -1 \\ -1 & 0 & 0 & 0 & 0 & -1 & +2 \end{bmatrix} \qquad \textbf{3.1}$$

This weight matrix contains the connection weights in the two-layered, 7-by-7, feedforward laterally inhibitory network. For example, column 2 of $\mathbf{V}$ is $[-1 +2 -1\,0\,0\,0\,0]^T$. It shows the weights from input unit x_2 to each of the seven output units. Specifically, it shows that input unit x_2 excites output unit y_2 with a weight of +2, but inhibits output units y_1 and y_3 with weights of −1 (its connections to all other output units have weights of 0). Thus, the pattern of weights from x_2 is consistent with the simplest feedforward laterally inhibitory connectivity pattern. Column 1 of $\mathbf{V}$, which is $[+2 -1\,0\,0\,0\,0 -1]^T$, illustrates how the circular arrangement of units is managed. Column 1 of $\mathbf{V}$ shows that input unit x_1 excites output unit y_1 with a weight of +2, but inhibits output units y_2 and y_7 with weights of −1. Because output units y_1 and y_7 are neighbors in the circular arrangement, input unit x_1 excites y_1 but inhibits both y_2 and y_7.

We can use this weight matrix $\mathbf{V}$ to find the responses $\mathbf{y}$ of the output units to an input $\mathbf{x}$, which is the column vector $[1\,1\,2\,2\,2\,1\,1]^T$. This input can be interpreted as a spatial visual stimulus pattern in which the central region has a higher intensity than the flanking regions. A one-dimensional array is an admittedly impoverished version of a two-dimensional image or of a three-dimensional scene, but the essential features of edge detection can be adequately and clearly demonstrated with such a simple input. Likewise, a one-dimensional array of neural units seems meager in comparison with essentially two-dimensional neural structures such as the retina, colliculus, and cortex, or with three-dimensional structures such as the vestibular nuclei that we studied in Chapter 2. For simplicity in this book we will restrict our-selves to neural networks having one-dimensional (1D) layers, because they are easier to manage and because their properties are the same as those having two-dimensional (or three-dimensional) arrangements of units.

The equation $\mathbf{V}\mathbf{x} = \mathbf{y}$ in expanded form, for the two-layered, 7-by-7, laterally inhibitory network with feedforward connection weights as described above, is shown in Equation 3.2. Note that Equation 3.2 includes an intermediate step showing the column of weighted input sums to each of the seven output units (the weighted input sums omit the 0s).

$$
\begin{bmatrix}
+2 & -1 & 0 & 0 & 0 & 0 & -1 \\
-1 & +2 & -1 & 0 & 0 & 0 & 0 \\
0 & -1 & +2 & -1 & 0 & 0 & 0 \\
0 & 0 & -1 & +2 & -1 & 0 & 0 \\
0 & 0 & 0 & -1 & +2 & -1 & 0 \\
0 & 0 & 0 & 0 & -1 & +2 & -1 \\
-1 & 0 & 0 & 0 & 0 & -1 & +2
\end{bmatrix}
\begin{bmatrix} 1 \\ 1 \\ 2 \\ 2 \\ 2 \\ 1 \\ 1 \end{bmatrix}
=
\begin{bmatrix}
+2-1-1 \\
-1+2-2 \\
-1+4-2 \\
-2+4-2 \\
-2+4-1 \\
-2+2-1 \\
-1-1+2
\end{bmatrix}
=
\begin{bmatrix} 0 \\ -1 \\ +1 \\ 0 \\ +1 \\ -1 \\ 0 \end{bmatrix}
\qquad \textbf{3.2}
$$

Using the rules for multiplication of a vector by a matrix (as detailed in Math Box 1.2), the responses $\mathbf{y}$ of the output units to the input pattern $\mathbf{x}$ is the col-umn vector $[0\ -1\ +1\ 0\ +1\ -1\ 0]^{\mathrm{T}}$. This response is 0, except at the locations at which the input changes from one intensity level to another. The significance of this type of output response is more easily discerned graphically in a larger network, as we shall see.

In expanded form, the equation describing the responses of the output units in a general n-by-n feedforward, laterally inhibitory network is:

$$
\begin{bmatrix} y_1 \\ y_2 \\ y_3 \\ \vdots \\ y_n \end{bmatrix}
=
\begin{bmatrix}
+2 & -1 & 0 & 0 & 0 & 0 & & -1 \\
-1 & +2 & -1 & 0 & 0 & 0 & \cdots & \\
0 & -1 & +2 & -1 & 0 & 0 & & \\
& & \vdots & & & & \ddots & \\
-1 & \cdots & 0 & 0 & 0 & 0 & -1 & +2
\end{bmatrix}
\begin{bmatrix} x_1 \\ x_2 \\ x_3 \\ \vdots \\ x_n \end{bmatrix}
\qquad \textbf{3.3}
$$

where n is the number of input and output units in the network. We will again assume that the input and output layers are arranged in circles, so that input units x_1 and x_n are neighbors, and so are output units y_1 and y_n. The task in assembling this network consists in constructing its connectivity weight matrix $\mathbf{V}$. Note that each row of the weight matrix contains a shifted version of the pattern $[\ldots\ 0\ -1\ +2\ -1\ 0\ \ldots]$. This is most clearly apparent in rows two and three of the matrix in Equation 3.3. The patterns in the first and last (nth) rows appear to be broken up in the matrix, but in fact they connect the first and nth neighbors in the circular input and output layers of the network, as described above for the 7-by-7 network.

A simple way to construct the matrix in Equation 3.3 is first to set a con-nectivity pattern, or profile, and enter this profile as the rows of the connectiv-ity matrix, after shifting the profile by one element for each successive row. Because weight matrix $\mathbf{V}$ is symmetric (see also Equation 3.1), it could also be constructed using this procedure carried out column-wise. We will use a row-wise procedure because it corresponds more naturally to profiles as we

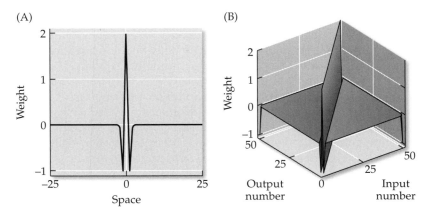

Figure 3.4 A simple, laterally inhibitory connectivity profile (A) and weight matrix constructed from it (B) The profile is shifted to center it relative to the space vector. There are 51 units in the network, which are arranged in a circle, so that units 1 and 51 are neighbors.

would read them on the page. In this chapter we will assemble networks having 51 input and output units, which are extensive by comparison with the small networks we studied in the previous chapter. A connectivity profile with 51 elements that corresponds to the pattern for the matrix in Equation 3.3 can be made with the commands: p=zeros(1,51), p(1)=2, p(2)=-1, and p(51)=-1. This should give you the vector **p** = [+2, –1, 0, 0, 0, ..., –1] with 51 elements in all. Because the units are arranged in a circle, units 1 and 51 are immediate neighbors. A plot of this profile is shown in Figure 3.4A. Note that the original profile has been shifted by 26 elements before plotting, to make its laterally inhibitory structure easier to appreciate.

To make the matrix, you would assign each row of **V** a shifted version of **p** using shiftLam, which is listed in MATLAB® Box 3.1. Note that shiftLam is a function, which is a special type of MATLAB program (m-file) that takes arguments from the command line. The command V=shiftLam(p), with argument p, would make a matrix V with the required connectivity. We use the term "command" liberally. Technically, in computational science a "command" would be of the form help shiftLam. (This particular command will display the comments that describe shiftLam at the beginning of the m-file.) A "function" would be of the form shiftLam(p) and a "statement" would be

MATLAB® BOX 3.1 **This function will make a connectivity matrix by laminating shifted versions of a connectivity profile.**

```
% shiftLam.m
% makes connectivity matrix MX by laminating shifted versions of the
% same row vector rv that contains the desired connectivity profile

function MX = shiftLam(rv) % declare the function

[dum,nUnits] = size(rv); % find the number of units in the network
for i = 1:nUnits % for each unit in the network
   MX(i,:) = rv; % set its row of the weight matrix to the profile
   rv = [rv(nUnits) rv(1:nUnits-1)]; % shift the profile
end % end the loop
```

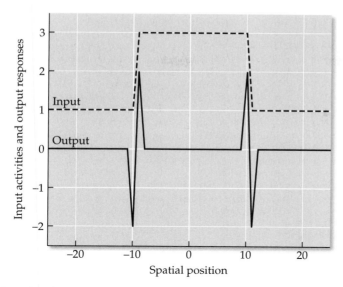

Figure 3.5   Edge detection by a two-layered, feedforward laterally inhibitory network The network connectivity matrix is constructed from the simple laterally inhibitory profile shown in Figure 3.4A. The responses of the output units (solid line) are nonzero at points where the input (dashed line) changes from one level to another.

of the form `V=shiftLam(p)`. For simplicity in this book we will use the term "command" to denote any instruction that can be given to MATLAB, either at the command line or, what is operationally the same thing, from within an m-file (MATLAB program). Thus the "command" `mesh(V)` —technically a function but called a command here—can be used to visualize the resulting connectivity matrix, as shown in Figure 3.4B.

Now that we have assembled the laterally inhibitory network, we can use it to simulate edge detection. Set the input vector (input array) x to correspond to a spatial (1D) light pattern in three sections, the middle section having a higher intensity than the two side sections. This can be done using `x=ones(51,1)` and `x(17:36)=3`. (The command `x(17:36)=3` is shorthand for `x(17:36)=ones(20,1)*3`, a more descriptive form of the kind we used in Chapter 1.) Note that x is a column vector. To find the output response of the network, simply multiply input x by matrix V using `y=V*x`. To visualize the output, you could plot y using `plot(y)`, or you could position the output in the arbitrary "middle" of the simulated space, and of the network, by first making a vector `s=-25:25` and then plotting y against s using `plot(s,y)`. The output of the network to the simulated light pattern is shown in Figure 3.5.

The result of this computation is an output that seems to indicate the points at which the input pattern changes from one intensity level to another. In regions of constant input the activity levels of the output units are 0s. In sharp contradistinction, the activity levels of the output units on the high-intensity and low-intensity sides of the edges are respectively high and low (positive and negative). This pattern of response corresponds qualitatively to that of the *Limulus* eye (see Figure 3.3A). If the input were part of a visual scene, it could be said that the network was detecting the edges in the scene. In this sense the simulation captures the essential characteristics of edge detection in the *Limulus* eye.

In that the network responds not to the intensity level of the input itself but to changes in that level, it seems that the network is computing a derivative of

MATH BOX 3.1   FINITE (DISCRETE) DIFFERENCE APPROXIMATIONS TO CONTINUOUS DERIVATIVES

The derivative of a function $f'(x)$ is defined as in Equation B3.1.1:

$$f'(x) = \lim_{h \to 0} \frac{f(x+h) - f(x)}{h} \qquad \text{B3.1.1}$$

which leads directly to the finite (discrete) difference approximation to the (continuous) first derivative, as shown in Equation B3.1.2:

$$f'(x) \approx \frac{f(x+h) - f(x)}{h} \qquad \text{B3.1.2}$$

where h can be thought of as a sampling interval at which samples of $f(x)$ are taken to compute the finite difference and approximate $f'(x)$. The smaller h is, the better the approximation (Hultquist 1988). In this book we do not sample continuous signals, such as the inputs to neural networks, but do construct discrete versions, and h can be thought of as the temporal resolution with which we construct them (one second per time step, for example). If we are unconcerned about scaling we can simply set h equal to 1. We can consider the value of some "input function" to be the series of values x_j (j=1, 2,..., n). Then the finite difference approximation to the first derivative x_j' of the series x_j is:

$$x_j' \approx x_{j+1} - x_j \qquad \text{B3.1.3}$$

Equation B3.1.3 can be expressed in matrix form as shown in Equation B3.1.4:

$$
\begin{bmatrix} x_1 \\ x_2 \\ x_3 \\ \vdots \\ x_{n-1} \end{bmatrix}'
\approx
\begin{bmatrix}
-1 & +1 & 0 & 0 & 0 & \\
0 & -1 & +1 & 0 & 0 & \cdots \\
0 & 0 & -1 & +1 & 0 & \\
& & \vdots & & & \ddots \\
& \cdots & 0 & 0 & 0 & -1 & +1
\end{bmatrix}
\begin{bmatrix} x_1 \\ x_2 \\ x_3 \\ \vdots \\ x_n \end{bmatrix}
$$

$$\text{B3.1.4}$$

where the approximate first derivative vector **x**′ (with elements x_j') has one element fewer than the vector **x** containing the series x_j. The finite difference approximation to the second derivative of the series of values x_j (j = 1, 2,...,n), shown in Equation B3.1.5, can be derived by applying Equation B3.1.3 recursively:

$$x_j'' \approx x_{j+1} - 2x_j + x_{j-1} \qquad \text{B3.1.5}$$

Equation B3.1.5 can be expressed in matrix form as in Equation B3.1.6:

$$
\begin{bmatrix} x_2 \\ x_3 \\ x_4 \\ \vdots \\ x_{n-1} \end{bmatrix}''
\approx
\begin{bmatrix}
+1 & -2 & +1 & 0 & 0 & 0 & \\
0 & +1 & -2 & +1 & 0 & 0 & \cdots \\
0 & 0 & +1 & -2 & +1 & 0 & \\
& & \vdots & & & & \ddots \\
& \cdots & 0 & 0 & 0 & +1 & -2 & +1
\end{bmatrix}
\begin{bmatrix} x_1 \\ x_2 \\ x_3 \\ \vdots \\ x_n \end{bmatrix}
$$

$$\text{B3.1.6}$$

where the approximate second derivative vector **x″** has two elements fewer than the vector **x** (note that the approximate second derivative vector produced by Equation B3.1.6 starts at x_2 and ends at x_{n-1}). Vector **x** could, for example, be a series of values in time or in space. If the latter, then it might be reasonable to assume that its boundary condition is circular. In that case x_1 and x_n are next to each other, and we could take advantage of the contiguity at the ends to have as many elements in the approximate derivative as in the series **x**. Then the finite difference approximation to the second derivative is shown in Equation B3.1.7:

$$
\begin{bmatrix} x_1 \\ x_2 \\ x_3 \\ \vdots \\ x_n \end{bmatrix}''
\approx
\begin{bmatrix}
-2 & +1 & 0 & 0 & 0 & 0 & & +1 \\
+1 & -2 & +1 & 0 & 0 & 0 & \cdots \\
0 & +1 & -2 & +1 & 0 & 0 & \\
& & \vdots & & & & \ddots \\
+1 & \cdots & 0 & 0 & 0 & 0 & +1 & -2
\end{bmatrix}
\begin{bmatrix} x_1 \\ x_2 \\ x_3 \\ \vdots \\ x_n \end{bmatrix}
$$

$$\text{B3.1.7}$$

The matrix in Equation B3.1.7 is the same as the weight matrix in the first example in this chapter (see Equation 3.3), except that the signs on the elements are reversed to make the neural network laterally *inhibitory*. (The matrix in Equation B3.1.7 is laterally excitatory.) Thus, the lateral inhibitory network in the first example computes the finite difference approximation to the second spatial derivative of its input, with the sign reversed.

its input. In fact, it is. More precisely, the simple laterally inhibitory network with the weight matrix shown in Equation 3.3 computes the finite difference approximation to the second spatial derivative of its input, but with the sign reversed (see Math Box 3.1). The finite difference method can be applied to approximate the derivatives of discrete series of values in time or space. The

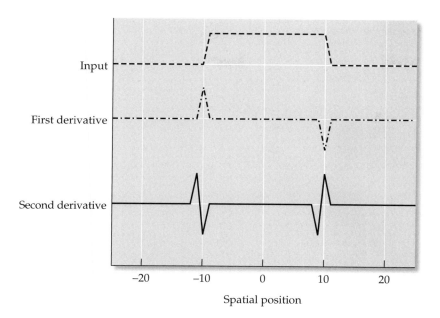

Input

First derivative

Second derivative

$-20 \quad -10 \quad 0 \quad 10 \quad 20$

Spatial position

Figure 3.6 A spatial step (up and down), and its first and second spatial derivatives The first derivative (dot-dashed line) is approximated as the finite difference of the input (dashed line), while the second derivative (solid line) is approximated as the finite difference of the approximate first derivative. (See also Math Box 3.1.) The input and approximate derivatives are vertically separated for clarity.

`diff` command in MATLAB computes the finite difference of vector **x**, with elements x_j $(j = 1, 2, ..., n)$, as $[x_2 - x_1, x_3 - x_2, ..., x_n - x_{n-1}]$. (Note that the resulting difference vector is one element shorter than vector **x**.) Since input vector x is a discrete series of values arrayed in space, the first spatial derivative of x can be approximated using the difference command `fsdx=diff(x)` followed by `fsdx=[fsdx;0]`, which appends a 0 to make difference vector `fsdx` the same length as x. Similarly, the second spatial derivative can be approximated using `ssdx=diff(fsdx)` followed by `ssdx=[ssdx;0]`.

The input and its approximate first and second spatial derivatives are shown in Figure 3.6. Note that the response of the simple laterally inhibitory network (see Figure 3.5, solid line) has the same form as the finite difference approximation to the second spatial derivative (Figure 3.6, solid line), except that it is rotated about the $y = 0$ axis. This is because the connectivity matrix for the simple laterally inhibitory network (see Equation 3.3) is the same as the matrix that computes the finite difference approximation to the second derivative, except the signs of the elements are reversed (see Math Box 3.1). Thus, the transformation being performed by the network is the finite difference approximation to the second spatial derivative, with a rotation about the $y = 0$ axis (sign reversal). This example illustrates that edge detection is essentially differentiation, and specifically double-differentiation, in space.

The computation that we have identified as double-differentiation in space can be considered more generally as a form of spatial filtering. Since we divided our simulated space into discrete steps, the operation performed by our network can also be considered as a form of digital filtering. There are many types of digital filters (Hamming 1998). Our edge detector was constructed using a simple profile for its feedforward, laterally inhibitory connection weights. It filtered its input by "passing" the component of the input that changed rapidly and by "blocking" the component of the input that did not change. Networks constructed using different profiles for their laterally inhibitory connection weights will implement filters having different properties. We will explore some of these in the next section.

A computation similar to that performed by the eye of the *Limulus*, an invertebrate, also occurs in the retinas of vertebrates (Dowling 1979). The structure of the vertebrate retina is shown in Figure 3.7. The visual receptor and gan-

Figure 3.7 Intracellular recordings from neurons in the vertebrate retina The traces beside the cell bodies show the responses of the cells when the receptor cell on the left is stimulated by light (indicated by the bar). Note that some neurons in the vertebrate retina produce action potentials (such as ganglion cell types G_1–G_3, and amacrine cells [A]) but others (such as bipolar cells [B] and horizontal cells [H]) produce only modulations of their resting membrane potentials in response to illumination of the visual receptors. (From Dowling 1979.)

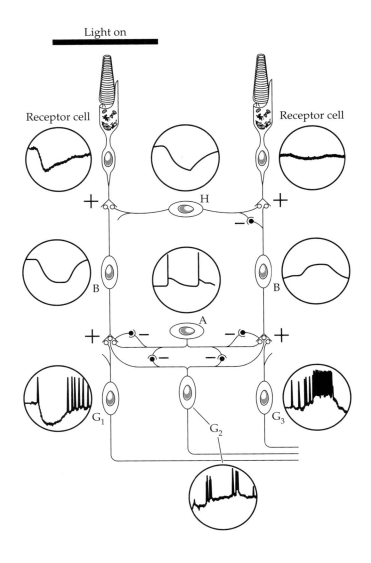

glion cells in the vertebrate retina correspond to the retinula and eccentric cells in the ommatidia of *Limulus* eyes (see Figure 3.2). An important difference between vertebrate retinae and *Limulus* ommatidia is the presence in the former of other cell types that intervene between the photoreceptors and the ganglion cells. Rather than project directly to eccentric cells, as retinula cells do in *Limulus* eyes, the receptor cells in the vertebrate retina project to retinal ganglion cells via bipolar interneurons. The connections from receptor to bipolar cells, and from bipolar to ganglion cells, are excitatory. Lateral inhibition in the vertebrate retina is mediated by horizontal and amacrine cells.

The performance of the vertebrate retina is much more complex than that of the simple, feedforward, laterally inhibitory network we studied in the previous example. Although capable of more complex computations, the vertebrate retina, which has a laterally inhibitory organization analogous to our simple neural network model, would also function as an edge detector. One interesting difference between the vertebrate retina, on the one hand, and both our network model and the *Limulus* eye on the other, is that the visual receptors in the vertebrate retina reverse the sign of their inputs. Without going into the biophysical details, photoreceptors in the vertebrate retina (rods and cones) constantly produce a background activation of bipolar cells, but the receptors, and their activation of bipolar cells, is actually suppressed when the receptors are illuminated. This is the opposite of what happens in the *Limulus* eye, where retinula cells are activated by light and activate eccentric cells when they are illuminated.

The sign reversal that occurs at the photoreceptors in the vertebrate retina is equivalent to a reversal of the signs of the elements in the weight matrix of the laterally inhibitory network. Thus, the vertebrate retina, with sign-reversing receptors and laterally inhibitory connectivity, would compute the actual (not sign-reversed) finite difference approximation to the second spatial derivative of its inputs (see Exercise 3.2). The difference in response polarity of the vertebrate retina compared with the *Limulus* eye is interesting in the context of our example, but probably not of functional significance. It is most likely the edge-detection capability, and not the response polarity, that is the functionally important aspect of lateral inhibition in early visual processing.

The receptors in the vertebrate retina and the ommatidia in the *Limulus* eye are arranged in two dimensions, and it is helpful to conceive of both structures as implementing a mapping between a two-dimensional image of the visual world and the activities of their output neurons (ganglion or eccentric cells). Each output neuron from either structure has a receptive field, which is the region of the visual world in which visual stimuli can activate (or suppress) the neuron. Because of laterally inhibitory interactions that take place in these structures, the receptive fields of the output neurons generally have a center/surround arrangement. An off-center/on-surround receptive field arrangement follows directly from the retinal interactions depicted in Figure 3.7. Due to the complex nature of processing in the vertebrate retina, on-center/off-surround receptive field arrangements are also common (Dowling 1979).

The responses to light of a ganglion cell from the retina of a cat are shown in Figure 3.8. This particular ganglion cell has an on-center/off-surround receptive field, as illustrated in the inset at the upper right of Figure 3.8. Thus, illumination of the center produces activation but illumination of the surround produces suppression of its firing rate. The receptive field illustrated in Figure 3.8 is representative of many visual neurons in the retina and lateral geniculate nucleus. Neurons in other sensory systems, notably somatosensation (touch), also have center/surround receptive fields (Shepherd 1994).

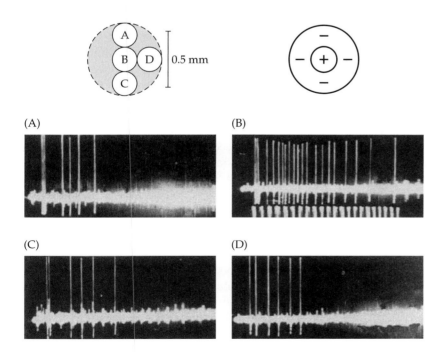

Figure 3.8   Activity of a ganglion cell in the retina of a cat caused by shining a small light spot on different regions of its receptive field The focused light spot was 0.2 mm in diameter. The ganglion cell receptive field is shown in the diagram at the upper left, along with the positions of the light spot (A–D). Stimulation with light at the on-center position B produces high frequency discharge from the ganglion cell that lasts for the duration of the stimulus. Stimulation at the off-center positions A, C, and D cause lower frequency discharge that is not maintained for the duration of the stimulus. (A–D and diagram at upper left from Kuffler 1953.) The diagram at upper right (not part of the original figure from Kuffler 1953) depicts an on-center/off-surround receptive field that is consistent with the data in the rest of the figure.

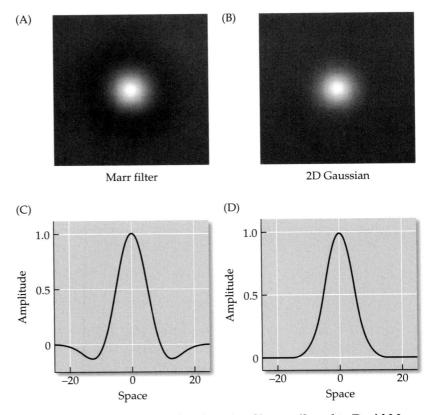

(A)

(B)

Marr filter

2D Gaussian

(C)

(D)

Figure 3.9   Illustration of the edge-detection filter attributed to David Marr
The Marr filter (A) is the Laplacian (the sum of the second spatial derivatives in both
directions) of the two-dimensional Gaussian (B) (see Math Box 3.2). The values for
the plots were computed using Equations B3.2.1 (for B) and B3.2.2 (for A), where the
Gaussian had a variance of 40 in both the x and y directions. The Laplacian (A) has
been scaled and inverted for illustrative purposes. Panels C and D show one-dimensional slices through the centers of the two-dimensional functions, which are shown
in gray scale in panels A and B (white is +1, black is −1).

Various methods have been proposed to mathematically describe the receptive fields of visual (and other) sensory neurons. One such method, which
involves taking the Laplacian of a two-dimensional Gaussian, was proposed
by David Marr (1982). "Gaussian" is a term that can be used to denote any
curve that has the form of a Gaussian probability density function, but is not
necessarily scaled to serve properly as such (see Chapter 9). The Laplacian of a
two-dimensional function is the second partial derivative of the function with
respect to one coordinate, added to the second partial derivative of the same
function with respect to the other coordinate (Math Box 3.2). A "Marr filter"
and the two-dimensional Gaussian from which it is derived are illustrated in
Figure 3.9A and B. The Marr filter has been inverted for purposes of comparison
with other functions in this chapter. One-dimensional slices through the two-
dimensional functions are shown in Figure 3.9C and D. The two-dimensional
Laplacian of a Gaussian (Marr filter; Figure 3.9A) resembles the on-center/off-
surround receptive field of the ganglion cell in Figure 3.8.

In mammals, retinal ganglion cells project from the retina to the lateral geniculate nucleus of the thalamus, and geniculate neurons project, in turn, to neurons in the visual cortex (Hubel 1988). Neurons in the lateral geniculate have
center/surround receptive fields that are similar to those of retinal ganglion
cells, but neurons in visual cortex can have receptive fields that are more ellip-
tical than circular, and their major axes can have a variety of orientations (see

MATH BOX 3.2   THE MARR FILTER

David Marr was a theoretical neuroscientist who contributed many seminal ideas in the area of neural systems modeling. His contributions to modeling of the visual system are among his best known (Marr 1982). Marr maintained that the extraction of edges was an essential part of early visual processing, and proposed that the early visual system employed a spatial filter that resembled a Mexican hat. One way to construct such a filter was to compute the Laplacian of a two-dimensional Gaussian.

The two-dimensional Gaussian function, with variance σ^2 in both the x and y directions, is given in Equation B3.2.1:

$$G(x,y) = \left[1/2\pi\sigma^2\right] \times \exp\left[-\left(x^2 + y^2\right)/2\sigma^2\right]$$ B3.2.1

The Laplacian operator ∇^2 applied to a two-dimensional function is the second partial derivative of the function with respect to coordinate x, added to the second partial derivative of the same function with respect to coordinate y: $(\partial^2/\partial x^2 + \partial^2/\partial y^2)$. Equation B3.2.2 shows the Laplacian of a two-dimensional Gaussian:

$$\nabla^2 G(x,y) = \left[-1/\pi\sigma^4\right] \times \left[1 - \left(x^2 + y^2\right)/2\sigma^2\right] \times \exp\left[-\left(x^2 + y^2\right)/2\sigma^2\right]$$ B3.2.2

The Laplacian of a Gaussian (Marr filter) is illustrated in Figure 3.9. For a Gaussian with equal variance in both the x and y directions, the Laplacian resembles the circular center-surround receptive fields of retinal ganglion cells (see Figure 3.8) and of lateral geniculate nucleus neurons. Marr pointed out that there are many ways to create filters in the shape of a Mexican hat, including the difference of Gaussians (DOG) that we use, for simplicity, in the examples in this chapter (see main text).

also Chapters 5 and 8). The Gabor function has been proposed as a mathematical description for this type of receptive field (Daugman 1985). Essentially, the spatial Gabor function is a two-dimensional sinusoidal wave, of some particular orientation, multiplied point-for-point by a two-dimensional Gaussian (Math Box 3.3). A spatial Gabor function, and its two-dimensional sinusoidal and Gaussian components, are shown in Figure 3.10A–C. One-dimensional slices through these two-dimensional functions are shown in Figure 3.10D–F.

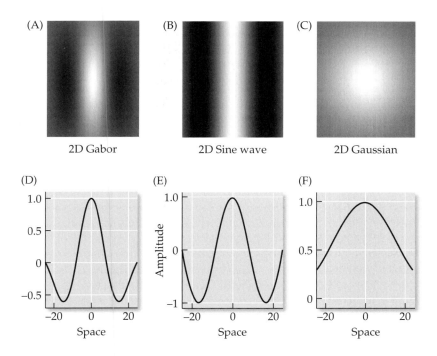

(A) 2D Gabor   (B) 2D Sine wave   (C) 2D Gaussian

(D) (E) Amplitude (F)   Space   Space   Space

Figure 3.10   Illustration of the approximate, two-dimensional Gabor function Basically, the approximate 2D Gabor function (A) is a 2D sine wave (B) multiplied point-for-point by a 2D Gaussian (C) (see Math Box 3.3). The values for the plots were computed using Equation B3.3.4 where the sine wave had a frequency of 0.18 radians per space unit and a phase of $\pi/2$, and the Gaussian had a variance of 500 in both the x and y directions. The Gabor function (A) has been scaled for illlustrative purposes. Panels D, E, and F show one-dimensional slices through the centers of the two-dimensional functions, which are shown in gray scale in panels A, B, and C (white is +1, black is −1).

MATH BOX 3.3   ONE- AND TWO-DIMENSIONAL GABOR FUNCTIONS

The two-dimensional Gabor function is a widely used formalism for describing the receptive fields of visual (and other sensory) neurons, and it is expressed mathematically in a variety of different ways. This very rough summary is adapted from Stork and Wilson (1990).

For temporal signal $f(\hat{t})$, where $\hat{t}$ is continuous time (we use t for discrete time in this book), observers face a trade-off in which they would need a narrow temporal window to determine precisely the timing of signal transients, but would need a wide temporal window to determine precisely the frequencies of signal components. The frequency components of temporal signal $f(\hat{t})$ are found by the Fourier transform $F(\omega_t)$, as shown in Equation B3.3.1:

$$F(\omega_t) = \int_{-\infty}^{\infty} f(\hat{t}) \exp(-j\omega_t \hat{t}) d\hat{t} \qquad \text{B3.3.1}$$

where ω_t is temporal frequency and j is $\sqrt{-1}$ (Oppenheim et al. 1983). Note that the temporal Fourier transform is the integral of the product of the temporal signal $f(\hat{t})$ and the complex wave $\exp(-j\omega\hat{t})$ [where $\exp(-j\omega\hat{t}) = \cos(\omega\hat{t}) - j\sin(\omega\hat{t})$], so the value of the Fourier transform is a complex number. Equation B3.3.2 gives the (un-normalized) one-dimensional temporal Gabor function (Gabor 1946; Daugman 1985; Stork and Wilson 1990):

$$B(\hat{t}) \propto \exp\left[-(\hat{t})^2/\sigma^2\right] \times \exp(-j\omega_t \hat{t}) \qquad \text{B3.3.2}$$

which is a Gaussian-modulated complex wave, where σ and ω_t are arbitrary constants that correspond roughly to the standard deviation of the Gaussian and the temporal frequency of the complex wave, respectively. Observers that apply the temporal Gabor function (see Equation B3.3.2) to temporal signals achieve the optimal balance between precisely determining the timing of transients and the temporal frequencies of components.

The Gabor function was generalized to two-dimensions and applied in describing the spatial receptive fields of visual neurons by Daugman (1985). The (un-normalized) two-dimensional (2D) Gabor function for spatial coordinates x and y is given in Equation B3.3.3:

$$B(x,y) = \exp\left[-\left(x^2/\sigma_x^2 + y^2/\sigma_y^2\right)\right] \times \exp\left[-j\left(\omega_x x + \omega_y y\right)\right] \qquad \text{B3.3.3}$$

where the σ and ω terms can be roughly thought of as the standard deviations of Gaussians and the frequencies of complex waves, respectively (see Daugman 1985 for details). Observers that apply the spatial Gabor function (see Equation B3.3.3) to images achieve the optimal balance between precisely determining the locations of features and the spatial frequencies of components. Equation B3.3.3 can be approximated as Equation B3.3.4:

$$B(x,y) = \exp\left[-\left(x^2/\sigma_x^2 + y^2/\sigma_y^2\right)\right] \times A\sin\left(\omega_s x + \theta\right) \qquad \text{B3.3.4}$$

where σ_x and σ_y are the standard deviations of a 2D Gaussian that is modulated by a sinusoidal wave with amplitude A, spatial frequency ω_s, and phase θ and is oriented along the x dimension (the sinusoid could have any orientation). The approximate 2D Gabor function (see Equation B3.3.4) specifies a real-valued function that resembles the receptive fields of many visual neurons. The approximate 2D Gabor function is illustrated in Figure 3.10. While the complex-valued 2D Gabor function (see Equation B3.3.3) would optimally balance the ability to determine the spatial locations and spatial frequencies of visual stimuli, the real-valued, approximate 2D Gabor function (see Equation B3.3.4) would not (Stork and Wilson 1990). However, the approximate form is useful descriptively.

The Gabor function was proposed for functional as well as descriptive purposes. Daugman (1985) argued that the two-dimensional Gabor function provides the optimal compromise between determining the spatial locations of features in a visual scene and the spatial frequency components of the scene (see MathBox 3.3). Subsequently, computer models that constructed representations of real visual scenes, which both maximized information but minimized activity, produced elements with receptive fields that resembled Gabor functions (see Chapter 8). The Gabor function continues to provide an effective mathematical description of the receptive fields of sensory neurons, especially in the visual system (e.g., Malone et al. 2007). However, for both descriptive and functional reasons, the Gabor function is not necessarily always the best model of sensory receptive fields (Stork and Wilson 1990). For most purposes a simpler receptive field description, also proposed by Marr (1982), which consists of a difference of two-dimensional Gaussians, is sufficient. For simplicity in this book, we study neural networks in which layers of units are arranged in one-dimensional arrays only. The examples in the next section explore the properties of one-dimensional difference-of-Gaussians connectivity profiles in feedforward lateral inhibitory networks.

3.2 Simulating Center/Surround Receptive Fields Using the Difference of Gaussians

In simplest terms, the one-dimensional Gaussian is the familiar bell-shaped curve. Over a series x of numbers from $-n$ to $+n$ including 0, the Gaussian function is simply $f(x) = \exp[-(x^2 / 2\sigma^2)]$, where the variance σ^2 determines the width of the bell-shaped curve. (The function $\exp[x]$ is equivalent to e^x where e is the base of the natural logarithms.) The difference-of-Gaussians (DOG) is a common connectivity pattern in use in neural systems modeling. In two-dimensions it can resemble a Mexican hat, and the pattern sometimes also takes that name. It is easily constructed as a Gaussian with a larger variance that is scaled down and subtracted from a Gaussian with a smaller variance. In one-dimension the DOG resembles both the Laplacian of the Gaussian (see Figure 3.9C) and the Gabor function (see Figure 3.10D).

The function gaussPro, listed in MATLAB Box 3.2, will make discrete, one-dimensional Gaussian profiles that can be used in the construction of one-dimensional DOGs. Function gaussPro issues the command gd=exp((s/sd).^2*(-0.5)), where s is a series of numbers (typically from $-n$ to $+n$ including 0), and sd is the standard deviation σ, which is the square root of the variance σ^2. For computational purposes it is convenient to specify the relative widths of the Gaussians using the standard deviation (SD) rather than the variance. For the argument of the Gaussian function we can use the s vector constructed above as s=-25:25, which represents space, and is just a series of 51 equally spaced points from −25 to +25.

A discrete Gaussian with a standard deviation of 0.75 can be constructed using g=gaussPro(s,0.75). If we make another Gaussian d with an SD of 1.5 using d=gaussPro(s,1.5), we can scale it by half and construct a nice DOG profile p using p=g-(0.5*d). To make the DOG profile, the broader Gaussian (the one with the larger SD) is being scaled down and subtracted from the narrower Gaussian (the one with the smaller SD). This DOG profile, which could be described as a very narrow Mexican hat, is shown in Figure 3.11A. It is similar to the simple laterally inhibitory profile we used in the

MATLAB® BOX 3.2 **This function will make a Gaussian connectivity profile.**

```
% gaussPro.m
% this function computes a discrete Gaussian curve, where s is a row
% vector of values and sd is the standard deviation of the Gaussian

function gd = gauss(s,sd) % declare the function

gd = exp((s/sd) .^ 2 * (-0.5)); % compute the Gaussian curve
```

Figure 3.11   A narrow difference-of-Gaussians laterally inhibitory connectivity profile (A) and weight matrix constructed from it (B) The profile in (A) was constructed by subtracting a Gaussian with a standard deviation (SD) of 1.5 and amplitude 0.5 from another Gaussian with an SD of 0.75 and amplitude 1. The 51 output units are arranged in a circle, so that units 1 and 51 are neighbors.

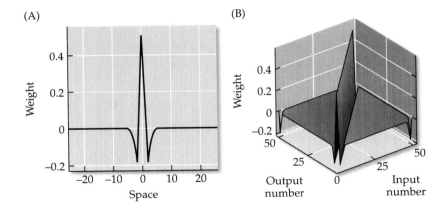

previous example, but instead of exciting only one output unit and inhibiting only its two nearest neighbors, this narrow DOG profile excites a few output units in a central core and inhibits a few output units on the two flanks of this core.

This DOG profile can be incorporated into matrix **V** as before, using `V=shiftLam(p)`, but for convenience in interpreting the results we will rotate it first so that inputs and outputs are aligned: `p=[p(26:51) p(1:25)]`. The resulting connectivity matrix is shown in Figure 3.11B. The response to the spatial light pattern x (a step up and down in intensity) of the feedforward, laterally inhibitory network with this DOG as its connectivity-matrix weight profile can be computed, as before, by matrix multiplication: `y=V*x`. The results are shown in Figure 3.12.

The output appears as a smoother version of the sign-reversed second spatial derivative that was observed for the output in the previous example. This makes sense, because the DOG from which the connectivity matrix in this example is constructed is a smoother version of the sharp profile used in the previous example. The output of the feedforward laterally inhibitory network with the DOG profile in this example resembles a bit more closely the responses of eccentric cells in the *Limulus* eye (see Figure 3.3A).

Feedforward laterally inhibitory networks with DOG connectivity profiles have also been used to model the responses of secondary neurons

Figure 3.12   Responses of the units in a two-layered, feedforword laterally inhibitory network The connectivity matrix is constructed from the narrow difference-of-Gaussians profile shown in Figure 3.11A. The responses of the output units (solid line) are nonzero near points at which the input changes from one level to another.

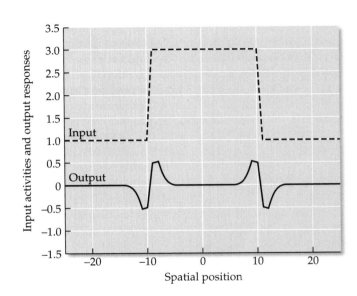

in the lateral-line sensory system of fish (Coombs et al. 1998). The lateral line is a sensory organ found in all aquatic vertebrates. In some fish it can be seen, unaided, as a line running down their flanks. Small pockets are arrayed at intervals along the line, and water flowing into the pockets is sensed by specialized sensory cells that activate the primary lateral-line afferents (Shepherd 1994). The responses of secondary lateral-line neurons can be simulated using a two-layered, feedforward network in which the input units, representing the linear array of primary lateral-line afferents, project to the output units, representing the secondary neurons, according to a DOG profile. Our one-dimensional, laterally inhibitory neural network provides an especially apt model of the lateral-line system, which is also arranged in one-dimension.

Whatever their connectivity profiles, laterally inhibitory networks act as spatial filters, and different profiles will block or pass different components of the input. To illustrate this we will construct two more DOGs with different widths and compare the responses of networks incorporating them on a spatial filtering task. We already have a network constructed from a narrow DOG, and we can rename its weight matrix `VN=V` to distinguish it from the others. Make a medium-width DOG by subtracting a Gaussian with SD 3 and scale factor (amplitude) 0.5, from a Gaussian with SD 1.5 and amplitude 1 using `s=-25:25`, `g=gaussPro(s,1.5)`, `d=gaussPro(s,3)`, and `p=g-(0.5*d)`. Then make the connectivity matrix using `p=[p(26:51) p(1:25)]` followed by `VM=shiftLam(p)`. Use the same procedure to make a wide DOG by subtracting a Gaussian with SD 6 and amplitude 0.5 from a Gaussian with SD 3 and amplitude 1, and construct matrix `VW` from it. The medium and wide DOG profiles and weight matrices are shown in Figure 3.13. The wide DOG (Figure 3.13C) looks more like a Mexican hat than the narrower versions.

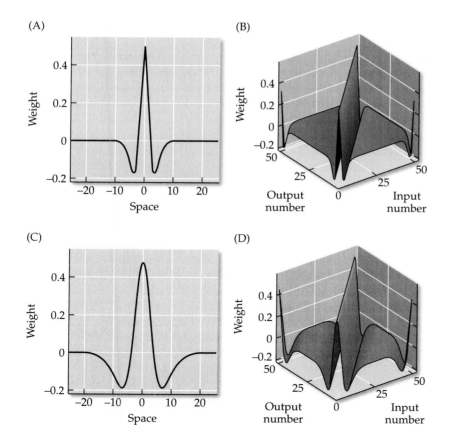

(A)

(B)

(C)

(D)

Figure 3.13   Medium and wide difference-of-Gaussians laterally inhibitory connectivity profiles (A and C) and weight matrices constructed from them (B and D) The medium DOG profile in (A) was constructed by subtracting a Gaussian with SD 3 and amplitude 0.5 from another Gaussian with SD 1.5 and amplitude 1. The wide DOG profile in (C) was constructed by subtracting a Gaussian with SD 6 and amplitude 0.5 from another Gaussian with SD 3 and amplitude 1. The output units are arranged in a circle.

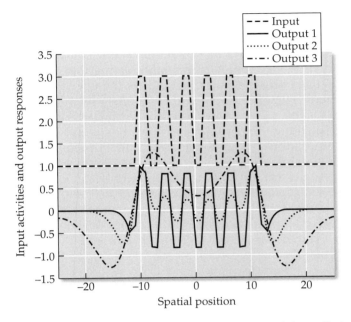

Figure 3.14 Spatial filtering properties of feedforward, laterally inhibitory networks with connectivity profiles consisting of differences-of-Gaussians with different widths The spatial input (dashed line) is a series of pulses. The networks have connectivity matrices constructed from the differences-of-Gaussians shown in Figures 3.11A (solid line), 3.13A, (dotted line), and 3.13C (dot-dash line).

To explore the spatial filtering properties of these DOGs we will construct a more complex light pattern as an input. Construct a "spiky" input using `x=ones(51,1)` and `x([16,17,20,21,24,25,28,29,32,33,36,37])=3`. This input is a series of 6 pulses, each 2 space units wide, with a base at 1 and a top at 3. The outputs to this new, spiky input, of the networks with weight matrices incorporating each of the three DOG profiles we generated above can be found by multiplying each matrix by the input vector using `yn=VN*x`, `ym=VM*x`, and `yw=VW*x`. We can compare the input and the outputs using `plot(s,x,s,yn,s,ym,s,yw)`. The results, shown in Figure 3.14, illustrate the spatial filtering properties of these three laterally inhibitory networks.

As the standard deviations of the Gaussians in each DOG profile increase, the networks made from them become less able to follow the high spatial frequency components of the input (see Figure 3.14, dashed line). The output of the network incorporating the narrowest DOG (solid line) follows well the high spatial frequency, spiky components of the input. The output of the network incorporating the widest DOG (dot-dashed line) seems mushy, but it does indicate the mean amplitude (or zero-frequency component) of the signal, which is higher in the spiky region than on either side of it. Note that the output that follows the spiky signal best has lost this mean signal component. Thus, the different networks act as distinct spatial filters that would provide useful and complementary information regarding the input. The outputs of an ensemble of filters could constitute the representation of the visual scene by the early visual system (Marr 1982). While real neurons in the visual system can be thought of as implementing spatial filters, they would more accurately be characterized as detectors of features such as the position of stationary items, the speed and direction of moving items, and the orientation and extent of edges (e.g., Marr 1982; Hubel 1988). Various aspects of feature-detection in sensory systems will be touched on in later chapters in this book.

3.3 Simulating Activity Bubbles and Stable Pattern Formation

Feedforward (forward) laterally inhibitory networks are quite powerful spatial processors but, to get temporal processing, recurrent (feedback) connections are needed. Recurrent connections between units can occur from a subsequent layer to a previous layer, or between units in the same layer, or both. Networks can employ recurrent laterally inhibitory connections between the units in the output layer, as well as feedforward laterally inhibitory connections from the input to the output layer. As for forward connection weights, recurrent connection weights are held in a matrix. The states of the output units in such a recurrent network will then be a function both of forward and recurrent connections.

It is necessary to represent (discrete) time in recurrent networks, because the states of the output units on time step t are functions of the states of the input and output units on time step $t - 1$. This temporal relationship can be expressed by Equation 3.4:

$$\mathbf{y}(t) = \varphi\left(\beta \mathbf{W}\mathbf{y}(t-1) + \mathbf{V}\mathbf{x}(t-1)\right) \qquad \textbf{3.4}$$

where $\mathbf{x}$ and $\mathbf{y}$ are the input and output state vectors, and $\mathbf{V}$ and $\mathbf{W}$ are the feedforward and recurrent connection weight matrices, respectively. Note that Equation 3.4 is equivalent to Equations 1.7 and 2.3, except for the function $\varphi(\cdot)$ and parameter β. To explain the roles of $\varphi(\cdot)$ and β it is helpful to express Equation 3.4 alternatively as in Equation 3.5:

$$y_i(t) = \varphi\left(q_i(t)\right) = \varphi\left(\sum_l \beta w_{il} y_l(t-1) + \sum_j v_{ij} x_j(t-1)\right) \qquad \textbf{3.5}$$

where $i = j = l = 1, ..., n$. The term $q_i(t)$ is the weighted sum of all the inputs to unit y_i, from the input units x_j and the other output units y_l, at the previous time step $(t - 1)$. According to the convention established in Chapter 1, v_{ij} is the weight of the connection to output unit y_i from input unit x_j, while w_{il} is the weight of the connection to output unit y_i from output unit y_l. Note that the summation ($\Sigma\cdot$) terms in Equation 3.5 are equivalent to the matrix terms in Equation 3.4. (For a brief note on summation notation see Math Box 3.4.) In Equations 3.4 and 3.5, $\varphi(\cdot)$ is a nonlinear function meant to represent the neurobiological limits on neural firing rate. It operates on the weighted input sum $q_i(t)$ and ensures that the elements y_i of $\mathbf{y}$ are bounded inclusively between 0 and a saturation level S as described in Equation 3.6:

$$y_i(t) = \varphi\left(q_i(t)\right) = \begin{cases} S, & q_i(t) > S \\ q_i(t), & 0 \le q_i(t) \le S \\ 0, & q_i(t) < 0 \end{cases} \qquad \textbf{3.6}$$

When the recurrent connectivity profile (making up matrix $\mathbf{W}$) is a DOG having both positive and negative values, the recurrent connections form both positive and negative feedback loops. The result of this for network dynamics is that some output units can be driven to the saturation limit S while other units are driven to zero. In networks described by Equations 3.4–3.6, the overall strength of the feedback is controlled by the value of parameter β. The network is said to "relax" into an activity pattern that is specific for a given input. Because time in the network is discrete, the equations describing relaxation in the network (see Equations 3.4–3.6) can be solved iteratively. We will use a recurrent laterally inhibitory network to simulate the formation of activity bubbles. The example in this section is adapted from Haykin (1999).

MATH BOX 3.4 SUMMATION NOTATION

The finite series $y = x_1 + x_2 + \cdots + x_n$ would be expressed using summation notation as in Equation B3.4.1:

$$y = \sum_{j=1}^{n} x_j \qquad \text{B3.4.1}$$

If we define our indices (e.g., $j = 1, \ldots, n$), and/or it is understood that we sum over all possible values of the variables in the summation, then we can express Equation B3.4.1 alternatively as in Equation B3.4.2:

$$y = \sum_j x_j \qquad \text{B3.4.2}$$

In some cases it is convenient to use summation notation rather than vector notation. For example, suppose we have a single, linear unit y that receives inputs over weights v_j from input units x_j ($j = 1, \ldots, n$). Suppose further that the v_j and x_j are the elements of column vectors $\mathbf{v}$ and $\mathbf{x}$,

respectively. Then Equation B3.4.3 shows the equivalence between vector notation and summation notation:

$$y = \mathbf{v}^{\mathrm{T}}\mathbf{x} = v_1 x_1 + v_2 x_2 + \cdots + v_n x_n = \sum_j v_j x_j \qquad \text{B3.4.3}$$

where superscript T is the transpose operator and $\mathbf{v}^{\mathrm{T}}\mathbf{x}$ is the inner (dot) product (see Math Box 1.2). If y_i ($i = 1, \ldots, m$) is a linear unit in a network that receives input over weights v_{ij} from input units x_j ($j = 1, \ldots, n$) then its response in summation notation can be expressed as in Equation B3.4.4:

$$y_i = \sum_j v_{ij} x_j \qquad \text{B3.4.4}$$

We use a time dependent form of Equation B3.4.4 in Equation 3.5 of the main text. We will use summation notation in many contexts throughout this book.

We will construct a recurrent laterally inhibitory network of the same dimensions as the feedforward networks we constructed in the previous sections, having two layers of 51 units each. To make things simple, set the forward weight matrix $\mathbf{V}$ to be the identity matrix: `V=eye(51)`. To make things interesting, make the recurrent weight profile a DOG. Subtract a Gaussian with SD 15 and amplitude 0.3 from a Gaussian with SD 3 and amplitude 1 using `s=-25:25, g=gaussPro(s,3), d=gaussPro(s,15)`, and `p=g-(0.3*d)`. Now the recurrent weight matrix $\mathbf{W}$ can be made after first rotating the weight profile using `p=[p(26:51) p(1:25)]` and `W=shiftLam(p)`. This DOG profile and the recurrent connectivity weight matrix constructed from it are shown in Figure 3.15.

Make an input vector that is the positive half-cycle of a sinusoid with an amplitude of 2: `x=2*sin(pi*(0:50)./50)'`. (Note the apostrophe makes x a column vector.) The response of the network to this input can be found by computing and re-computing its response iteratively. The script `winnersTakeAll`, listed in MATLAB Box 3.3, will do this. Set the cutoff to 0 (`cut=0` in `winnersTakeAll`), the saturation level to 10 (`sat=10`), and the number of iterations to 20 (`nTs=20`). Note that `winnersTakeAll` is a script, rather than a function, and some of its parameters must already be set at the command line and available in the MATLAB workspace for it to run prop-

(A)

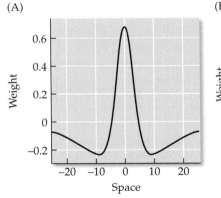

(B)

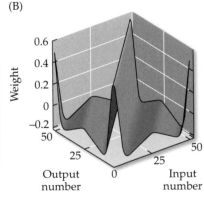

Figure 3.15 A wide difference-of-Gaussians laterally inhibitory connectivity profile (A) and weight matrix constructed from it (B) The profile in (A) was constructed by subtracting a Gaussian with SD 15 and amplitude 0.3 from another Gaussian with SD 3 and amplitude 1. Output units are arranged in a circle.

MATLAB® BOX 3.3   This script implements the winners-take-all network that has recurrent, lateral inhibitory and central excitatory connections and nonlinear units.

```
% winnersTakeAll.m
% forward weight matrix V and recurrent weight matrix W
% must already be available in the workspace

nTs=20; % set number of iterations
rate=1; % set the rate parameter
cut=0; % set the cutoff level (usually zero)
sat=10; % set the saturation level (usually ten)
[nUnits,dum]= size(W); % find number of output units
y=zeros(nUnits,nTs); % zero the output y array

for t = 2:nTs % for each time step
    y(:,t) = rate*W*y(:,t-1) + V*x; % update y
    y(:,t) = max(y(:,t),cut); % impose the cutoff
    y(:,t) = min(y(:,t),sat); % impose the saturation
end % end the t loop
```

erly. For script winnersTakeAll, the required parameters are the forward and recurrent weight matrices V and W that we have already made. Script winnersTakeAll will first find the number of output units ([nUnits, dum] = size(W)) and then define (and zero) the output unit state array (y=zeros(nUnits,nTs)). Note that y has one row for each unit and one column for each iteration (time step). The script updates the states of the units in y using y(:,t)=rate*W*y(:,t-1)+V*x. Note that the input x is not explicitly a function of time in winnersTakeAll. It is a static image that is presented at the input to the network and remains there over the course of the simulation. (In Chapter 2 both the inputs and the outputs were functions of time.) The cutoff and saturation limits in winnersTakeAll are implemented using y(:,t)=max(y(:,t),cut) and y(:,t)=min(y(:,t),sat).

For our first run of this simulation, set the rate parameter β to 0.1 (rate=0.1) in script winnersTakeAll. Of course, when parameters are set within the script the m-file must be resaved in order for them to be expressed when the script is run. The advantage of setting certain parameters outside the script is that they can be changed directly from the command line without having to resave the script. When run, the script winnersTakeAll will compute the output y resulting from input x as the recurrent network relaxes for nTs time steps. To run the script, simply issue its filename, without the .m extension, at the command line: winnersTakeAll. Following the run you can plot the output responses over one another using plot(y) or see them separated at each time step using mesh(y). The results for $\beta = 0.1$ are shown (using command plot (y)) in Figure 3.16A. For our second run, set the rate to 1: rate=1 (resave the script after you make this parameter change). The results for $\beta = 1.0$ are shown in Figure 3.16B.

The parameter β scales the weights in recurrent weight matrix **W** (see Equations 3.4 and 3.5; β is left inside the summation in Equation 3.5 to emphasize its weight-scaling role). With β set at 0.1 (Figure 3.16A) the recurrent weights are weak, and the output changes little from the input, which is the first half-cycle of a sinusoid. However, with β set at 1.0 (Figure 3.16B) the recurrent weights are at full strength, and the output reaches the point where some states have been driven to the saturation limit of 10 while the rest have been driven to

Figure 3.16   Responses of output units to a sinusoid-half-cycle input in a recurrent, nonlinear laterally inhibitory network The recurrent connectivity matrix is constructed from the difference-of-Gaussians profile shown in Figure 3.15A. Each curve shows the responses of all 51 output units on one time step. An activity bubble fails to form with a rate value of 0.1 (A), but forms nicely with a rate value of 1.0 (B).

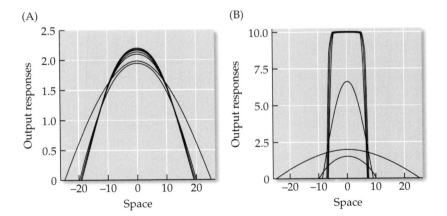

the cut-off of 0. With the recurrent weights at full strength, an activity bubble forms in the network that is centered on the peak of the input sinusoidal half-cycle. Once formed, the activity bubble would persist for all subsequent time steps. Specifically, our activity bubble formed within nTs=20 time steps, and it would persist if we iterated the network for another 20, or for another 200, or for an infinity of additional time steps. Thus, the activity bubble is a stable state of this recurrent laterally inhibitory network, and it can form because the units in the network are nonlinear.

A linear network would have only one stable state, and that would be the network state in which all units have activations of 0. Nonlinearity is required to achieve stable states in which some (possibly all) of the units have nonzero activations. As explained in Chapter 2, some neural systems require that their constituent neurons operate approximately linearly over the operational range of the system of which they are a part. The activity-bubble network is an example in which the nonlinearity of the units is essential for the operation of the overall neural system.

Our activity bubble has arisen in a network that we characterize as laterally inhibitory, but it would not form without the excitation at the center of its recurrent connectivity profile. An activity bubble is an example of a stable-state activity pattern that can form in a neural system provided it has two essential attributes: positive feedback and nonlinearity. In our activity-bubble network, the positive feedback is provided by the local excitation at the central core of the recurrent connectivity profile, and the nonlinearity is provided by the cut-off and saturation limits on neural unit activity. The laterally inhibitory connections of the network, which are essential for the selective properties that we will study in the next section, are not required for stable-state pattern formation. In fact, networks having only positive feedback (recurrent excitatory connections) and nonlinearity (unit activity limits) can form stable-state patterns that play useful computational roles. We will consider the activity-bubble network further in this chapter, and will study nonlinear neural units and networks in many contexts throughout the rest of this book.

An activity-bubble network is a special case of a winners-take-all network. In a winners-take-all network, the output relaxes to a pattern (stable state) in which some units are fully active while the rest are silent. In an activity-bubble network, the winners are neighbors in the network. The winners-take-all paradigm is useful for many purposes and it is possible that something like winners-take-all processing occurs in many regions of the brain. In the next section of this chapter we will use a winners-take-all network to retrieve a weak signal from noise. We will suggest this process may be similar to that which occurs in a brain structure known as the superior colliculus, as it creates an activity bubble in a sub-region of its structure that corresponds to the location in space of the target of the next saccadic eye movement.

3.4   Separating Signals from Noise and Modeling Target Selection in the Superior Colliculus

A weak signal is one that is difficult to distinguish from background noise, and much of sensory processing involves separating signals from noise. The signal-to-noise ratio is the ratio of the amplitude of a signal to the amplitude of the noise in which it is embedded. If the signal of interest is a pulse, or some other feature that is circumscribed in space, then a winners-take-all network can amplify the signal by creating an activity bubble at the location of the signal. Because the activity of the units in the bubble, representing the signal, would be maximal, and the activity of the units outside the bubble, representing the noise, would be 0, an activity-bubble winners-take-all network can essentially increase the signal-to-noise ratio to infinity. In so doing, the activity-bubble network essentially retrieves the signal from the noise.

To construct an input that has a pulse-like signal imbedded in noise, first generate a signal that is simply a vector of 0s with three contiguous 1s in the middle: `signal=zeros(51,1)` and `signal(25:27)=1`. Then corrupt this signal with noise to make the input vector: `noise=rand(51,1)` and `x=signal+noise`. Note that `rand` draws a random deviate from a uniform distribution between 0 and 1, and `rand(51,1)` creates a column vector of 51 such deviates. We can use the same recurrent weight matrix `W` that we used in the previous section, and we can use the script `winnersTakeAll` to create our activity bubble. Set the forward weight matrix as before: `V=eye(51)`. Check to ensure that the internal parameters are set as: `nTs=20`, `cut=0`, `sat=10`, and `rate=1`. (This check assumes that you have been experimenting with the parameters on your own! There is no need to resave the m-file if you have not changed the internal parameters from their values for the previous simulation.) Now run `winnersTakeAll`. Following the run you can again plot the output responses over one another using `plot(y)` or see them separated at each time step using `mesh(y)`. The results are shown (using `plot(y)`) in Figure 3.17.

(A)

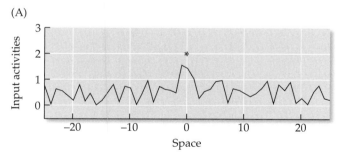

(B)

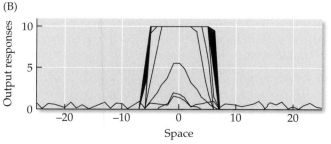

Figure 3.17   Responses of the output units in a winners-take-all, recurrent laterally inhibitory network   The recurrent connectivity matrix is constructed from the difference-of-Gaussians profile shown in Figure 3.15A. The input (A) is a pulse, three space units wide, that is embedded in noise (the center of the pulse is marked with an asterisk). The response of the output units (B) is an activity bubble centered on the input pulse.

The network successfully retrieves the signal from the noise, and re-running the simulation many times, each time with a different noise profile, will demonstrate that the activity-bubble network does this reliably (not shown). The network forms an activity bubble that is centered at the location of the pulse. In this example the pulse is always located at the center of the simulated space s, but the network could form an activity bubble that is centered on any location (see Exercise 3.3). Because each activity bubble is a stable state of the network, the activity-bubble winners-take-all network has multiple stable states. Thus, the activity-bubble example demonstrates another important property of nonlinear, recurrent neural networks: not only can they reach stable states in which some of the units have nonzero activation levels, but they can have multiple such stable states. We will re-examine this important property in later chapters (specifically Chapters 4 and 10).

The retrieval of a signal from noise that we studied in the previous example can also be thought of as the selection of one signal from potentially many others. Such a selection process may occur in a region of the midbrain known as the superior colliculus. The colliculus is an essentially two-dimensional structure that is topographically organized (Wurtz and Goldberg 1989). It implements a sensorimotor transformation in which it localizes the sources of stimuli in the environment, and seems to select one from among them as the target of a fast (saccadic) eye movement that brings the fovea (the region of the retina with the highest receptor density) in line with that target.

The activity of a neuron in the superior colliculus of a monkey during a saccade-to-target task is shown in Figure 3.18. In this task the monkey is presented with one or more potential target lights, and makes a saccade to the

Figure 3.18 The activity of a superior colliculus neuron during a saccade-to-target task In this task one or more potential target lights appear and the monkey makes a saccade to the light that dims. For these results the target (that dims) is in the receptive/movement field of the neuron. Each trial is divided into two phases: pre-selection and selection. The three columns represent activity at the following times: left, all potential target lights come on (indicated by black in the array diagram); middle, the intended target light dims (indicated by gray); right, the saccade command is generated. The saccade command results in eye movement (Eye). Each panel shows the average action potential firing rate over five trials. The number of potential targets increases progressively: A, one; B, two; C, four; D, eight. The initial sensory response (left column) decreases as the number of potential targets increases, but the burst of activity forming the saccadic motor command (right column) is independent of the number of potential targets. (From Basso and Wurtz 1998.)

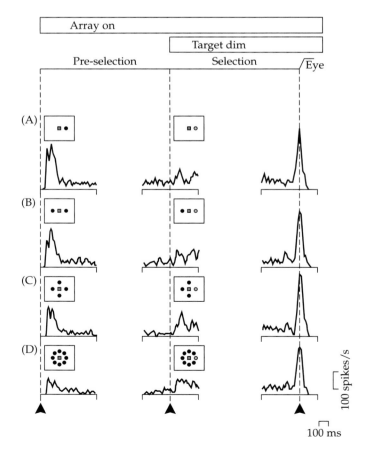

light that dims. Like many neurons in the superior colliculus, this neuron has both sensory and motor related activity, and it has both a receptive and a movement field. The neuron responds to visual stimuli presented in its receptive field, and generates commands for saccades that bring the fovea into register with its movement field. The receptive and movement fields of collicular neurons are generally coextensive. Because the neuron has sensory related activity, it responds to a target light that appears in its receptive field (left column of Figure 3.18). Because it has motor related activity, it also generates a burst that commands a saccade that aligns the fovea with this target (right column). That burst can be thought of as an activity bubble.

Clues concerning the neural processing that occurs in the superior colliculus are provided by data on the activity of collicular neurons when more than one potential target light is presented. Collicular neurons are generally described as having on-center receptive fields with no surround (Wurtz and Goldberg 1989), but experimental evidence is suggestive of laterally inhibitory interactions. For example, Basso and Wurtz (1998), in experiments using monkeys trained to make saccades to visual targets, showed that the sizes of the bursts generated by collicular neurons for saccades into their movement fields are independent of the number of potential targets. In striking contradistinction, the sensory related activity of collicular neurons decreases as the number of target lights presented outside their receptive fields increases (see Figure 3.18). These results are consistent with the idea that saccade targets are selected, and that saccade commands are generated, by a winners-take-all competition that takes place within the superior colliculus.

We can use the winners-take-all network to simulate some of the salient features of the data in Figure 3.18. We can use exactly the same network we used in the activity-bubble and signal-from-noise examples. (That will enable us to use the same recurrent weight matrix W that we constructed in the previous section.) However, we will need two new input signals, one with a single target and another with an intended target and several distracters. To make the single target input, zero an array x1 and place a pulse at the center, three spaces wide, with an amplitude of 2 using x1=zeros(51,1) and x1(25:27)=2. To make the target with distracters, set an array x7 the same as x1 using x7=x1, but add several distracter pulses of amplitude 1 that flank the intended target using x7([7:9,13:15,19:21,31:33,37:39,43:45]) =1. To make the results of this simulation easier to interpret we will present the inputs without noise.

Set the forward weight matrtix as V=eye(51), and make sure the internal parameters for script winnersTakeAll are set as before: nTs=20, cut=0, sat=10, and rate=1. Now we can run the script on each of the inputs and save the output. To find the response to the first input (single target by itself), set x=x1, run script winnersTakeAll, and save the output as y1=y. To find the response to the second input (target with distracters), set x=x7, run script winnersTakeAll, and save the output as y7=y. In both cases the network will retrieve, or select, the intended target and, after the 20 time steps, will form an activity bubble at its location. The responses on all time steps in each case can be plotted using plot(y1) and plot(y7). The activity bubbles in each case can be plotted using plot(y1(:,20)) and plot(y7(:,20)). Because we start the for-loop in winnersTakeAll on time step 2 (see MATLAB Box 3.3), we can consider the response of the network on time step 3 to be the initial response, because this is the first time point at which the effects of the recurrent connections are expressed. The initial responses for each case can be plotted using plot(y1(:,3)) and plot(y7(:,3)). The inputs are plotted using plot(x1) and plot(x7). A comparison of the two cases (single

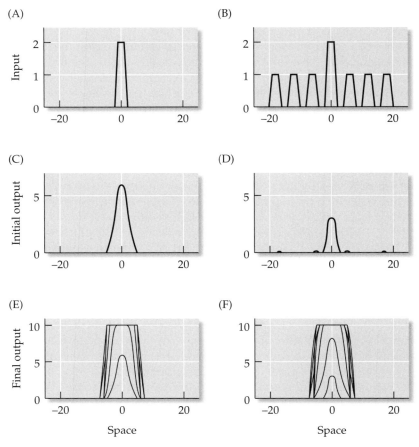

Figure 3.19   Simulating the selection of a saccade target as it might occur in the superior colliculus using a winners-take-all recurrent, laterally inhibitory neural network Each visible target is simulated as a pulse, three space units wide. The input in (A) consists of a single target of amplitude 2 presented at the central location. The input in (B) consists of a target of amplitude 2 presented at the central location that is flanked on either side by three distracter targets of amplitude 1. The initial response of the network is taken to be that which occurs on time step 3, because the recurrent connections first affect the output responses at that time. Note that the initial output responses to the central target are much larger in (C) (without distracters) than in (D) (with distracters), demonstrating that the presence of distracters greatly reduces the initial response to the target. The output responses at subsequent times ultimately achieve the same height in (F) (with distracters) as in (E) (without distracters), demonstrating that the winners-take-all network produces the same size activity bubble at the location of the largest initial response, regardless of its size.

target by itself or target with distracters) reveals an important effect of the competitive interactions in winners-take-all networks.

The results of the colliculus-selection simulation are plotted in Figure 3.19. Note that the initial response at the target location (Figure 3.19C) to the single target presented by itself (Figure 3.19A) is much larger than the initial response (Figure 3.19D) to the same intended target when it is flanked by distracters (Figure 3.19B). Competition from the distracters reduces the initial response at the intended target location in the recurrent, laterally inhibitory network. The reduction in intended target response due to distracters in the model agrees well with the data. The left column in Figure 3.18 clearly shows that the response of a real superior colliculus neuron to a target presented in its receptive field is decreased by distracters presented outside its receptive field. Our modeling results could lead us to hypothesize that the initial response reduction due to distracters results from laterally inhibitory interactions occurring in the real superior colliculus. Electrophysiological evidence supports this hypothesis (Munoz and Istvan 1998).

In our simulation the intended target is indicated by its amplitude, and the delay between input presentation and activity-bubble formation is due only to the dynamics of the winners-take-all mechanism. In the experiment whose results are depicted in Figure 3.18, the intended target is distinguished from the distracters by dimming it, and that occurs after the distracter array (including the intended target) is presented fully lit. The experimental protocol requires the monkey to suppress the generation of any saccade command until the dimming signal that identifies the target. The activity level of the neuron decreases during the interval between distracter-array presentation and target identification (Figure 3.18 between the left and middle columns), but target dimming actually causes the activity level of the neuron to increase (Figure 3.18, middle column), which leads to burst formation (Figure 3.18, right column). Saccade command suppression, and the increased activation due to target dimming, are probably caused by inputs to the superior colliculus from saccade-related regions of the basal ganglia and cortex, such as the substantia nigra and frontal eye fields (Wurtz and Goldberg 1989). Clearly, the neural system that produces the results shown in Figure 3.18 is much more complicated than the recurrent, laterally inhibitory neural network that we use to form activity bubbles. Yet in the model as in the real monkey, a burst of activity is generated at the location on the colliculus corresponding to the location of the intended target, and the amplitude of this burst is the same regardless of the size of the initial response that gave rise to it. This is shown for the model in Figure 3.19 E and F, and for the real colliculus in the right column of Figure 3.18. The data are consistent with the idea that the colliculus generates a saccade command through a mechanism analogous to activity-bubble formation. It is possible that the superior colliculus implements a winners-take-all interaction as part of the decision-making process by which it chooses the target of the next saccade.

The agreement between the model and the data leads us to speculate that a winners-take-all interaction could mediate collicular processes that include response modulation due to distracters, competition between and selection from among multiple possible targets, and generation of bursts that serve as commands for saccades that align the fovea with the selected target. The reduction in the sensory responses of collicular neurons to stimuli presented inside their receptive fields, due to other stimuli presented outside their receptive fields, could result from the competitive component of a winners-take-all interaction (brought about through recurrent laterally inhibitory connections). The fixed size of the burst associated with saccades into the movement fields of collicular neurons, which is the same no matter what array of stimuli triggered it, could result from neural firing-rate saturation and the cooperative component of a winners-take-all interaction (brought about through central excitatory recurrent connections). The activity-bubble network we studied in this section separated a signal from noise or distracters, and produced a burst of activity of the same size regardless of the size of the signal of interest or the spatial distribution of the overall input. This recurrent, laterally inhibitory network could serve as a simple model of the processing that occurs in structures such as the superior colliculus.

Follow up studies suggest that the extent of lateral inhibition in the superior colliculus may be limited. McPeek and Keller (2002) showed that neurons in the superior colliculus can respond to sensory stimuli presented in their receptive fields even as burst commands are being generated for saccades to non-coextensive movement fields. Limitations in lateral inhibition would allow for a softer form of competition and could make winners-take-all mechanisms more flexible. McPeek and Keller (2002) suggest that the ability of some collicular neurons to respond to sensory stimuli while others are engaged in the generation of saccade commands could enable the superior colliculus to make sequences of target-driven saccades with shorter inter-saccadic intervals. A possible consequence of limiting lateral inhibition for activity-bubble networks is the topic of Exercise 3.4.

Exercises

3.1   In the first example of lateral inhibition we set up a feedforward lateral inhibitory network that had a simple weight profile in which each input unit excited its corresponding output unit with a connection of weight +2, but inhibited the nearest neighbors of that output unit with connections of weight −1. We constructed this profile using commands `p=zeros(1,51)`, `p(1)=2`, `p(2)=−1`, and `p(51)=−1`. We then constructed the weight matrix using `V=shiftLam(p)` (function `shiftLam` is listed in MATLAB Box 3.1). We studied the output of this network to an input that represented a light pattern in space, constructed using `x=ones(51,1)` and `x(17:36)=3`. Double the amplitude of the profile (`p=p*2`), reconstruct the weight matrix, and find the response to the input pattern (`y=V*x`). Has increasing the absolute values of the weights changed the essential form of the response? Now make the output units nonlinear using the squashing function (see Chapter 6). This is done by first computing the weighted input sum `q` using `q=V*x` and then squashing it to find `y` using `y=1./(1+exp(−q))`. How has the nonlinearity changed the response? Does it change its essential form?

3.2   Again consider the first lateral inhibitory network we studied, that had a simple connectivity profile in which each input unit excited its corresponding output unit with a weight of +2, but inhibited the nearest neighbors of that output unit with weights of −1. The response of this network to a spatial step input could be described as a second spatial derivative with its sign reversed. Reverse the polarity of the connectivity profile using `p=zeros(1,51)`, `p(1)=−2`, `p(2)=1`, and `p(51)=1`. (If you already have the original profile `p` from the previous exercise you can reverse its polarity simply using `p=−p`). Then reconstruct the weight matrix using `V=shiftLam(p)`. Set up the same spatial step input that you used in the previous exercise, which was constructed using `x=ones(51,1)` and `x(17:36)=3`, and retest the feedforward lateral inhibitory network using `y=V*x`. How would you characterize its response now?

3.3   We constructed a winners-take-all, recurrent lateral inhibitory network using the difference-of-Gaussians connectivity profile made by subtracting a Gaussian with SD 15 and amplitude 0.3 from another Gaussian with SD 3 and amplitude 1 (see Figure 3.15A). We did this using `s=−25:25`, `g=gaussPro(s,3)`, `d=gaussPro(s,15)`, `p=g−(0.3*d)`, `p=[p(26:51) p(1:25)]`, and `W=shiftLam(p)`. We found that this winners-take-all network was able to separate a pulse signal from noise by forming an activity bubble that was centered on the location of the pulse. In the example we set the input pulse at the center of the input array. See if the network will form activity bubbles over input pulses at other locations. First, zero the signal as before using `signal=zeros(51,1)`, but then place the pulse at other locations using, for example, `signal(17:19)=1` or `signal(37:39)=1`. Make some noise and add it to each signal to make the input: `noise=rand(51,1)` and `x=signal+noise`. Then set the feedforrward weight matrix using `V=eye(51)`. Ensure in `winnersTakeAll` that its internal parameters are set as follows: `nTs=20`, `rate=1`, `cut=0`, and `sat=10`. Then run script `winnersTakeAll`. Is the winners-take-all network able to form activity bubbles at other locations? An activity bubble, once it is fully formed, will remain on all subsequent time steps. Thus, a fully formed activity bubble is a stable state of a nonlinear, recurrent, lateral inhibitory network with an excitatory central core. What do your findings in this exercise tell you about the number of stable states possessed by this type of network?

3.4   Again consider the winners-take-all activity-bubble network, but this time return the pulse to its original location (`signal=zeros(51,1)`, `signal(25:27)=1`, `noise=rand(51,1)`, and `x=signal+noise`). Use Gaussians with the same SDs in constructing the difference-of-Gaussians connectivity profile, but this time reduce the amplitude of the Gaussian with the larger SD. Specifically, construct the difference-of-Gaussians by subtracting a Gaussian with SD 15 and amplitude 0.1 (rather than 0.3) from another Gaussian with SD 3 and amplitude 1. What happens to the performance of the network? Does it reach a stable state? If so, then how would you characterize it? Is the network able to retrieve the signal from the noise? What does this tell you about the sensitivity of the network to the values of the connection weights? We will revisit this issue in Chapter 13, where we will use the genetic algorithm to find a difference-of-Gaussians profile for activity-bubble networks.

References

Basso MA, Wurtz RH (1998) Modulation of neuronal activity in superior colliculus by changes in target probability. *Journal of Neuroscience* 18: 7519–7534.

Coombs S, Mogdans J, Halstead M, Montgomery J (1998) Transformation of peripheral inputs by the first-order lateral line brainstem nucleus. *Journal of Comparative Physiology A* 182: 609–626.

Daugman JG (1985) Uncertainty relation for resolution in space, spatial frequency, and orientation optimized by two-dimensional visual cortical filters. *Journal of the Optical Society of America* A2: 1160–1169.

Dowling JE (1979) Information processing in local circuits: The vertebrate retina as a model system. In: Schmitt FO, Worden FG (eds) *The Neurosciences: Fourth Study Program*. MIT Press, Cambridge, MA, pp 163–182.

Gabor D (1946) Theory of communication. *Journal of Instrumentation and Electrical Engineering* 93: 429–457.

Hamming RW (1998) *Digital Filters*. Dover, Ontario, Canada.

Haykin S (1999) *Neural Networks: A Comprehensive Foundation. Second Edition.* Prentice Hall, Upper Saddle River, NJ.

Hubel DH (1988) *Eye, Brain, and Vision*. Scientific American Library, WH Freeman, New York.

Hultquist PF (1988) *Numerical Methods for Engineers and Computer Scientists*. Benjamin/Cummings, Menlo Park, CA.

Kuffler SW (1953) Discharge patterns and functional organization of mammalian retina. *Journal of Neurophysiology* 16: 37–68.

Malone BJ, Kumar VR, Ringach DL (2007) Dynamics of receptive field size in primary visual cortex. *Journal of Neurophysiology* 97: 407–414.

Marr D (1982) *Vision*. WH Freeman, San Francisco.

McPeek RM, Keller EL (2002) Superior colliculus activity related to concurrent processing of saccade goals in a visual search task. *Journal of Neurophysiology* 87: 1805–1815.

Munoz DP, Istvan PJ (1998) Lateral inhibitory interactions in the intermediate layers of the monkey superior colliculus. *Journal of Neurophysiology* 79: 1193–1209.

Oppenheim AV, Willsky AS, Young IT (1983) *Signals and Systems*. Prentice Hall, Englewood Cliffs, NJ.

Ratliff F (1965) *Mach Bands: Quantitative Studies on Neural Networks in the Retina*. Holden-Day, San Francisco.

Ratliff F, Hartline HK (1959) The responses of *Limulus* optic nerve fibers to patterns of illumination on the receptor mosaic. *Journal of General Physiology* 42: 1241–1255.

Shepherd GM (1994) *Neurobiology, Third Edition*. Oxford University Press, New York, pp 239–242.

Stork DG, Wilson HR (1990) Do Gabor functions provide appropriate descriptions of visual cortical receptive fields? *Journal of the Optical Society of America A* 7: 1362–1373.

Wurtz RH, Goldberg ME (1989) *The Neurobiology of Saccadic Eye Movements*. Elsevier, Amsterdam.

4

Covariation Learning and Auto-Associative Memory

Networks with recurrent connection weights that reflect the covariation between pattern elements can dynamically recall patterns and simulate certain forms of memory

We know from common experience that we can form detailed memories of items and events with only one exposure. I can recall a detailed mental image of my neighbor building a snowman for his daughter this morning. With hints from my own family, I could recall many other detailed images of our neighborhood on the first snowy morning of the year. With time, most of those images will probably fade from memory, or get confused with other memories, but the fact remains that I was able to retain, for many hours, detailed memories of items and events to which I had only one exposure.

Many of the characteristics of single-exposure memory can be simulated using recurrent networks of nonlinear neural units. If we represent an item or event as a specific pattern of activity over the set of units, and if the recurrent connection weights reflect the covariation between the various elements of the pattern, then the units in the network can express that pattern and dynamically return to it if they are given a "hint" in the form of a partial, weak, or slightly corrupted pattern. Just like real memory, these recurrent networks can produce errors in memory recall, and they have a limited capacity, but they can learn to store patterns with one exposure. The recurrent structure and learning mode of these artificial networks resemble real neural networks in the hippocampus (Rolls and Kesner 2006; Rolls 2007), which is a brain region known to be critical for forming detailed memories from single exposures (Squire 1992; Smith and Mizumori 2006). Our goal in this chapter is to explore covariation learning and memory in these recurrent neural networks, and discuss their similarities with the hippocampus.

The only form of learning we have studied so far in this book has been habituation (see Chapter 1). Habituation is a decrease in the weight of a synaptic connection that occurs each time its pre-synaptic neuron is activated. While habituation can be considered as the simplest form of learning, covariation learning can be considered as the next simplest because it is a type, or a generalization, of Hebbian learning. Donald Hebb (1949) postulated that the weight of the connection between two neurons is increased if the neurons are both active at the same time. A colloquial way of stating Hebb's rule, and the easiest way to remember it, is that "neurons that fire together wire together." Many theorists have applied Hebb's rule, and variations on it, in developing neural models of storage and retrieval of memories. David Marr (1971) showed how application of Hebb's rule to a set of interconnected neurons could "store" a memory pattern that later could be "recalled."

Marr's idea is illustrated in Figure 4.1. Assume initially that all of the neurons are interconnected, but only very weakly. If some set of neurons is active at the same time (Figure 4.1A, filled circles) then, by Hebbian learning, the connections between them become stronger (Figure 4.1B). Later, if a partial pattern is presented to the neurons (Figure 4.1C), the mutually excitatory connections between them produce pattern completion, and the original pattern of neural activity is reinstated (Figure 4.1D). This example illustrates how a memory item can be represented as pattern of activity over a network of neurons. It also shows how the neural network can be trained using Hebb's rule to store the pattern as a set of interconnection weights, and how the memory can later be recalled by reinstating the complete pattern given only a "hint" (partial pattern).

FIGURE 4.1 Marr's model of memory storage and recall in archicortex (basically, the hippocampus) (A) A pattern of active neurons (filled circles) corresponds to a potential memory item. (B) The synapses of the connections between the active neurons are strengthened according to Hebb's postulate ("Neurons that fire together wire together"). (C) Following learning, a part of the remembered pattern is presented. (D) The full pattern is restored due to the mutual excitation of the neurons. Pattern completion corresponds to memory recall. (After Marr 1971.)

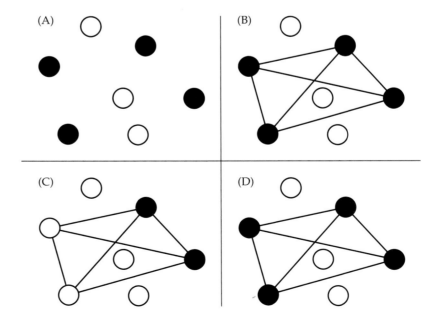

A network such as Marr's memory network is often called a content addressable memory, because a stored pattern can be accessed by a partial version of it. A network such as Marr's is also called an auto-associator neural network, because it learns to associate the various elements of the same memory pattern with each other. In the example in Figure 4.1, all of the active units forming the memory pattern developed excitatory connections with each other. Just as importantly, the active units did not develop excitatory connections with the inactive units. The configuration of the excitatory weights is critical to memory recall in this network.

Perusal of Figure 4.1 might lead you to wonder whether the memory network would benefit if the active units developed inhibitory connections with the inactive units. This might keep inactive those units that should be inactive for a particular memory pattern. Contemplation of Figure 4.1 might also lead you to wonder whether such a network of units could learn to accurately recall more than one pattern. As we will see, auto-associator neural networks of the type schematized in Figure 4.1 can indeed store and recall multiple patterns, and inhibitory connections can indeed improve performance, especially when multiple and overlapping patterns are involved. Learning to develop inhibitory connections between active pre-synaptic units and inactive post-synaptic units requires an extension of Hebb's original postulate. Other extensions of Hebb's rule are also possible, and all of them can be considered as subtypes of covariation learning.

Covariation learning is a method for training neural networks in which changes to the weights of the connections between units depend on the covariation between their pre-synaptic and post-synaptic activities. Specifically, two units will have a positive or a negative covariation over some set of activations if their states are more often the same or different, respectively. What we mean by "covariation" is a relaxed form of true covariance. A more precise definition of covariation, stated in terms of covariance, is given in Math Box 4.1.

In this chapter we will consider covariation learning in the context of networks of binary units, the states of which can only be 0 or 1. For binary units, a simple form of covariation learning would stipulate that the weight of the connection from a pre-synaptic to a post-synaptic unit should be increased each time both units have the same state, and decreased each time the two units have different states. We will also consider learning rules that can be characterized as subtypes of the covariation rule but are more neurobiologically plausible. In that all of these update rules involve only the activity pre-synaptic and post-synaptic to the connection weight being modified, all of them can be referred to as "Hebbian" learning rules. In this chapter will use Hebbian learning to train recurrent neural networks to auto-associate patterns.

In general, an auto-associator is any neural network that learns to associate patterns with themselves. Auto-associative neural networks can have various architectures, and can be purely feedforward rather than recurrent. They can be trained using various methods, including but not limited to Hebbian rules. Conversely, recurrent neural networks can be trained to perform functions other than auto-association using rules other than Hebbian. We will study some of these variations in later chapters. In this chapter we will focus on auto-associator networks of nonlinear neural units that have recurrent architectures and are trained using Hebbian rules, because this class of network lends itself most readily as a model of the real memory network in the hippocampus.

The most important property of recurrent networks of nonlinear units trained using Hebbian rules is that they have multiple stable states. The activity-bubble networks we studied in Chapter 3 provide a different example of nonlinear recurrent networks that have multiple stable states (see especially

MATH BOX 4.1   COVARIATION AND ITS RELATIONSHIP WITH COVARIANCE

We use the term "covariation" as an un-normalized measure of the degree to which two units have the same state (positive covariation) or different states (negative covariation) over a set of activations. It is best understood by comparison with true covariance.

The arithmetic mean of a set of numbers p_l ($l = 1,\ldots, n$) is given in Equation B4.1.1:

$$\bar{p} = \frac{1}{n}\sum_{l=1}^{n} p_l \qquad \text{B4.1.1}$$

and the variance (assuming that n is the complete set and not just a sample) is computed using Equation B4.1.2:

$$\sigma_{\mathrm{P}}^2 = \frac{1}{n}\sum_{l=1}^{n} (p_l - \bar{p})^2 \qquad \text{B4.1.2}$$

The covariance between two, paired sets of numbers p_l and q_l ($l = 1,\ldots, n$) is shown in Equation B4.1.3:

$$\sigma_{\mathrm{P,q}}^2 = \frac{1}{n}\sum_{l=1}^{n} (p_l - \bar{p})(q_l - \bar{q}) \qquad \text{B4.1.3}$$

If $\mathbf{p}_l$ ($l = 1,\ldots, n$) are a set of n vectors (row vectors in this case), then the mean vector is described by Equation B4.1.4:

$$\bar{\mathbf{p}} = \frac{1}{n}\sum_{l=1}^{n} \mathbf{p}_l \qquad \text{B4.1.4}$$

Every element of $\bar{\mathbf{p}}$ is the mean of the corresponding element of the $\mathbf{p}_l$. Now we can find the variance of every individual element of the $\mathbf{p}_l$, and we can also find the covariance between the elements of the $\mathbf{p}_l$, as shown in Equation B4.1.5 using the outer product (see Math Box 4.2):

$$\Omega = \frac{1}{n}\sum_{l=1}^{n} (\mathbf{p}_l - \bar{\mathbf{p}})^{\mathrm{T}}(\mathbf{p}_l - \bar{\mathbf{p}}) \qquad \text{B4.1.5}$$

where Ω is the covariance matrix (because the vectors are row vectors their difference is also a row vector, but the transpose of their difference is a column vector). The variances of each element of the $\mathbf{p}_l$ are the diagonal elements of Ω, while the covariances between the elements of the $\mathbf{p}_l$ are the off-diagonal elements of Ω. What we call the "covariation" is shown in Equation B4.1.6:

$$\mathbf{W} = \sum_{l=1}^{n} (2\mathbf{p}_l - 1)^{\mathrm{T}}(2\mathbf{p}_l - 1) \qquad \text{B4.1.6}$$

where the $\mathbf{p}_l$ are binary pattern (row) vectors, and the $(2\mathbf{p}_l - 1)$ vectors would have +1 and −1 elements in place of 1 and 0 elements, respectively. Equation B4.1.6 is equivalent to the outer-product version of the Hopfield rule (see Section 4.1). Thus, we can call the Hopfield rule the "covariation" rule. For the special case where every binary element of the $\mathbf{p}_l$ has probability 0.5 of being a 1, so that every element of $\bar{\mathbf{p}}$ is 0.5, then dividing each element of $\mathbf{W}$ by $4n$ would convert $\mathbf{W}$ into a true covariance matrix.

Using Equation B4.1.6 as it is, the signs of the elements of $\mathbf{W}$ indicate positive or negative covariance, but their absolute values can grow as the number n of pattern vectors increases. Various methods exist for constraining or normalizing connection weights adapted using the Hopfield rule and other Hebbian rules (e.g., Miller and MacKay 1994), but they would not change the essential behavior of the recurrent auto-associative networks that we study in this book, so we use the Hopfield rule and the other Hebbian rules in their original and simplest forms.

Exercise 3.3). The units in activity-bubble networks have their activities non-linearly bounded between cut-off and saturation levels, and the recurrent connection weights between the units have Mexican-hat profiles characterized by excitatory centers and inhibitory surrounds. When primed with an input, an activity bubble forms at the location of the largest initial response. This occurs as the excitatory recurrent connections drive units within the bubble into saturation, and the inhibitory recurrent connections drive the units outside the bubble into cut-off. The dynamics can be characterized as winners-take-all, since the units in the bubble take their highest activity (saturation) while those outside the bubble take their lowest activity (cut-off). An activity bubble is a stable state of the network, which will persist indefinitely. The network has multiple stable states because it can form an activity bubble centered on any location.

A recurrent network of nonlinear units trained on a pattern using a Hebbian learning rule can also function as a winners-take-all network. In this case the winners are not confined to a bubble but can be arranged over the output according to the specific, learned pattern. Provided that certain conditions are met, these recurrent auto-associator networks can have multiple stable states

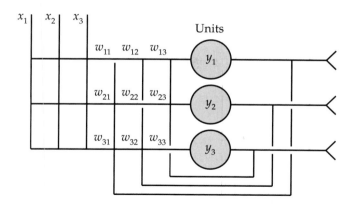

FIGURE 4.2   A model of three neurons, each receiving three inputs and each feeding back on each other (but not on themselves) The weights of the recurrent (feedback) connections are designated as w_{ij}, where y_i and y_j ($i = 1,2,3$ and $j = 1,2,3$) are the post-synaptic and pre-synaptic units, respectively. Note that $w_{11} = w_{22} = w_{33} = 0$.

corresponding to multiple learned patterns, and when primed with an input, their dynamics will bring them to the stable state corresponding to the learned pattern closest to the input. In such networks, whether activity bubble or auto-associator, the multiple stable states can be referred to as "attractors," and the networks themselves can be referred to as "attractor networks."

Auto-associative attractor networks, which must be composed of nonlinear units, can be composed of units having continuous, sigmoidal activation functions (Hopfield 1984), or even of spiking neural units (Buhmann and Schulten 1986). For simplicity in this chapter we will limit ourselves to networks composed of binary units that can take only one of two states (1 or 0). Networks of binary units are the easiest to implement yet possess all of the important properties of networks composed of more complicated units (Hopfield 1984). With this background, we can precisely define the subject of our study in this chapter as auto-associative attractor networks that are composed of binary neural units and are trained using Hebbian learning rules.

David Marr's memory network (see Figure 4.1), with which we began our discussion, essentially is a recurrent network in which each unit connects to every other unit but not to itself. Inputs from outside the network serve only to initialize the states of the units, as with a training pattern, or with an incomplete pattern that prompts recall of the complete pattern. Another way to visualize this type of network is shown in Figure 4.2. In this network, w_{ij} ($i = 1,2,3$ and $j = 1,2,3$) is the weight to post-synaptic unit y_i from pre-synaptic unit y_j, according to the convention established in Chapter 1. The inputs (x_1, x_2, and x_3) only initialize the states of the units (y_1, y_2, and y_3). In this chapter we will use Hebbian rules to study auto-association in neural networks with the general architecture of the network shown in Figure 4.2.

4.1   The Four Hebbian Learning Rules for Neural Networks

Hebbian rules are local, in that they depend only on the activity of neurons pre- and post-synaptic to any particular synapse (i.e., connection). The locality of Hebbian rules lends them neurobiological plausibility. The original rule proposed by Hebb specified an increase in synaptic strength whenever pre- and post-synaptic neurons were active together. The classic Hebb rule has received strong experimental support (e.g., Bliss and Lømo 1973; Neves et al. 2008). The classic Hebb rule provides no mechanism for inhibition, but other Hebbian rules with inhibition have also been proposed (Willshaw and Dayan 1990; Dayan and Wilshaw 1991). In addition to the original Hebb increase, the post-synaptic rule specifies a decrease in synaptic strength if the post-synaptic neuron is active when the pre-synaptic neuron is not, and vice-versa for the pre-synaptic rule. Both of these rules have received experimental support (post-synaptic, Stent 1973, Singer 1985; pre-synaptic, Stanton and Sejnowski 1989; see also Neves et al. 2008). The covariation rule proposed by Hopfield (1982) incorporates all three of the above mechanisms, with the addition of a specified increase in synaptic strength if pre- and post-synaptic neurons are *inactive* together. This last mechanism is not (so far) supported by experimental evidence. Thus, of the four Hebbian rules, the Hopfield covariation rule is considered the least plausible neurobiologically. We will consider this issue in more detail in Section 4.7 in the context of models of the hippocampus.

The four Hebbian rules are presented together in Table 4.1, where the absolute values of all specified increases and decreases are equal to 1. The unit states are binary (0 or 1). The rules can be implemented using the following four formulae (shown in Equations 4.1–4.4):

Hebb $$\Delta w_{ij} = (y_i)(y_j) \tag{4.1}$$

Post-synaptic $$\Delta w_{ij} = (y_i)(2y_j - 1) \tag{4.2}$$

Pre-synaptic $$\Delta w_{ij} = (2y_i - 1)(y_j) \tag{4.3}$$

Hopfield $$\Delta w_{ij} = (2y_i - 1)(2y_j - 1) \tag{4.4}$$

In these formulae y_i is the activity of the post-synaptic unit, y_j is the activity of the pre-synaptic unit, and Δw_{ij} is the change to the weight of the connection to y_i from y_j as specified by each rule. Because the units are binary their activities can only be 1 or 0. Thus, when the post- and pre-synaptic units are both active at 1, the product of their activities $(y_i)(y_j)$ is 1, and Hebb's rule (see Equation 4.1) specifies a weight change Δw_{ij} of +1. Terms of the form $(2y - 1)$ take value +1 or −1 when y is 1 or 0, respectively. Thus, when the post- and pre-synaptic units are both active at 1, each of the other three rules (see Equations 4.2–4.4) also specify a weight change Δw_{ij} of +1 (see Table 4.1).

The classic Hebb rule (see Equation 4.1) will specify a nonzero weight change only when both the pre-synaptic and post-synaptic units are active. The post-synaptic rule will specify a nonzero weight change only when the post-synaptic unit is active, and it specifies a weight change of $\Delta w_{ij} = -1$

TABLE 4.1   The four Hebbian learning rules: Hebb, post-synaptic, pre-synaptic, and Hopfield (covariation)

Unit activations	Post-synaptic	1	1	0	0
	Pre-synaptic	1	0	1	0
Weight updates	Hebb	+1	0	0	0
	Post-synaptic	+1	−1	0	0
	Pre-synaptic	+1	0	−1	0
	Hopfield	+1	−1	−1	+1

when the post-synaptic unit is active but the pre-synaptic unit is inactive. Conversely, the pre-synaptic rule will specify a nonzero weight change only when the pre-synaptic unit is active, and it specifies a weight change of Δw_{ij} = −1 when the pre-synaptic unit is active but the post-synaptic unit is inactive. The Hopfield (covariation) rule specifies a nonzero weight change in all cases. It specifies a weight change of Δw_{ij} = −1 when the post-synaptic unit is active but the pre-synaptic unit is inactive, and vice-versa. In addition, the Hopfield rule specifies a weight change of Δw_{ij} = +1 when both the post- and pre-synaptic units are inactive (see Table 4.1).

Unlike all the other learning methods we will consider in this book, covariation learning is not iterative. As emphasized in the preamble, this form of learning requires only a single exposure to each pattern. The weight changes due to each pattern are summed over all patterns. The weight values for the four Hebbian rules, in which the weight changes are summed over all patterns, are given in the following formulae (shown in Equations 4.5–4.8):

Hebb
$$w_{ij} = \sum_{l} \left(y_i^l\right)\left(y_j^l\right)$$
4.5

Post-synaptic
$$w_{ij} = \sum_{l} \left(y_j^l\right)\left(2y_j^l - 1\right)$$
4.6

Pre-synaptic
$$w_{ij} = \sum_{l} \left(2y_j^l - 1\right)\left(y_j^l\right)$$
4.7

Hopfield
$$w_{ij} = \sum_{l} \left(2y_j^l - 1\right)\left(2y_j^l - 1\right)$$
4.8

The binary unit activities, or states y, which are indexed with i or j ($i = 1, \ldots, d$ and $j = 1, \ldots, d$), are the elements of state vector $\mathbf{y}$ that has dimension d (where d is the number of units in the network). Vector $\mathbf{y}$ differs for each binary training pattern $\mathbf{p}_l$ ($l = 1, \ldots n$ where n is the number of training patterns). The training patterns $\mathbf{p}_l$ also have dimension d (i.e., the $\mathbf{p}_l$ correspond element-for-element with $\mathbf{y}$). These equations show that, for recurrent auto-associative neural networks, the recurrent weight matrix can be computed directly from the patterns that we want the network to store.

The application of these formulae can be illustrated with simple numerical examples. We wish to train the network in Figure 4.2, which has units y_1, y_2, and y_3, to auto-associate two patterns: $\mathbf{p}_1 = [1\ 1\ 0]$ and $\mathbf{p}_2 = [0\ 0\ 1]$. To do this we use one of the Hebbian rules to compute weight changes of the form Δw_{ij}^l where i and j are the indices of the post- and pre-synaptic units and l is the pattern index. First, we will use the classic Hebb rule (see Equation 4.5) to compute the value of w_{12}, which is the weight of the connection to unit y_1 from unit y_2. For pattern $\mathbf{p}_1$ we note that $y_1 = 1$ and $y_2 = 1$, so the weight change due to pattern $\mathbf{p}_1$ is $\Delta w_{12}^1 = (y_1)(y_2) = (1)(1) = 1$. For pattern $\mathbf{p}_2$ we note that $y_1 = 0$ and $y_2 = 0$, so the weight change due to pattern $\mathbf{p}_2$ is $\Delta w_{12}^2 = (y_1)(y_2) = (0)(0) = 0$. The value of w_{12} is the sum of the weight changes due to both patterns: $w_{12} = \Delta w_{12}^1 + \Delta w_{12}^2 = 1 + 0 = 1$.

Next we will use the Hopfield rule (see Equation 4.8) to compute the value of w_{12} given patterns $\mathbf{p}_1 = [1\ 1\ 0]$ and $\mathbf{p}_2 = [0\ 0\ 1]$. The computation using the Hopfield rule is essentially the same as that using the Hebb rule except that, due to terms of the form $(2y - 1)$, activities of 0 are changed to −1 (activities of 1 stay +1). Thus, for pattern $\mathbf{p}_1$, we note that $y_1 = 1$ and $y_2 = 1$, so the weight change due to pattern $\mathbf{p}_1$ is $\Delta w_{12}^1 = (2y_1 - 1)(2y_2 - 1) = (1)(1) = 1$, as for the Hebb

MATLAB® BOX 4.1 **This script implements three different methods to make connection weight matrices for recurrent auto-associative networks using the Hebb, post-synaptic, pre-synaptic, and Hopfield (covariation) rules.**

```
% autoConnectivity.m
% this script makes the Hebb (HB), post-synaptic (PO),
% pre-synaptic (PR), and Hopfield (HP) auto-associator
% connectivity matrices using pattern matrix P; pattern
% matrix P must already be available in the workspace

[nPat,nUnits] = size(P); % find numbers of patterns and units
HB = zeros(nUnits); PO = zeros(nUnits); % define and zero HB and PO
PR = zeros(nUnits); HP = zeros(nUnits); % define and zero PR and HP

% this method implements the summation for each connection in turn
for i=1:nUnits % for each unit as the post-synaptic unit
    for j=1:nUnits % for each unit as the pre-synaptic unit
        for l=1:nPat % for each pattern (loop variable is letter l)
            HBDW=P(l,i) * P(l,j); % compute Hebbian update
            PODW=P(l,i) * (2*P(l,j) -1); % compute post-synaptic update
            PRDW=(2*P(l,i) -1) * P(l,j); % compute pre-synaptic update
            HPDW=(2*P(l,i) -1) * (2*P(l,j) -1); % compute Hopfield update
            HB(i,j) = HB(i,j) + HBDW; % update Hebb connection
            PO(i,j) = PO(i,j) + PODW; % update post-synaptic connection
            PR(i,j) = PR(i,j) + PRDW; % update pre-synaptic connection
            HP(i,j) = HP(i,j) + HPDW; % update Hopfield connection
        end % end pattern loop
    end % end pre-synaptic unit loop
end % end post-synaptic unit loop

% this method implements outer product summation pattern-by-pattern
% for l=1:nPat, % for each pattern (loop variable is letter l)
%     HBDW=P(l,:)' * P(l,:); % compute entire Hebb matrix update
%     PODW=P(l,:)' * (2*P(l,:) -1); % compute post-synaptic update
%     PRDW=(2*P(l,:)' -1) * P(l,:); % compute pre-synaptic update
%     HPDW=(2*P(l,:)' -1) * (2*P(l,:) -1); % compute Hopfield update
%     HB = HB + HBDW; % update entire Hebbian matrix
%     PO = PO + PODW; % update entire post-synaptic matrix
%     PR = PR + PRDW; % update entire pre-synaptic matrix
%     HP = HP + HPDW; % update entire Hopfield matrix
% end % end pattern loop

% this method implements matrix multiplication over all patterns
% HB=P' * P; % compute Hebbian matrix
% PO=P' * (2*P -1); % compute post-synaptic matrix
% PR=(2*P' -1) * P; % compute pre-synaptic matrix
% HP=(2*P' -1) * (2*P -1); % compute Hopfield matrix

MSK = (ones(nUnits) - eye(nUnits)); % construct the masking matrix
HB = HB .* MSK; % zero self-connections in Hebbian matrix
PO = PO .* MSK; % zero self-connections in post-synaptic matrix
PR = PR .* MSK; % zero self-connections in pre-synaptic matrix
HP = HP .* MSK; % zero self-connections in Hopfield matrix
```

rule. For pattern $\mathbf{p}_2$, we note that $y_1 = 0$ and $y_2 = 0$, so the weight change due to pattern $\mathbf{p}_2$ using the Hopfield rule is $\Delta w_{12}^2 = (2y_1 - 1)(2y_2 - 1) = (-1)(-1) = 1$. As for the Hebb rule, the value of w_{12} using the Hopfield rule is the sum of the weight changes due to both patterns: $w_{12} = \Delta w_{12}^1 + \Delta w_{12}^2 = 1 + 1 = 2$. The values of the other weights are computed similarly. This method of using all of the patterns to compute the value of each connection weight in turn is implemented using three nested for-loops in script `autoConnectivity`, listed in MATLAB® Box 4.1. The values for all of the weights, computed using the Hopfield rule on patterns $\mathbf{p}_1$ and $\mathbf{p}_2$, are shown in Table 4.2, where the final weight matrix is shown on the right-hand side of the equation in the last panel. Note that the value corresponding to w_{12} is +2.

The connection weights in Table 4.2 were not computed one at a time but were computed using the method of outer products. This procedure applies naturally to auto-associative networks. In fully recurrent networks, such as the auto-associative networks we study in this chapter (see also Figure 4.2), each unit is both pre-synaptic and post-synaptic to every other unit. During training, the activity determined by each element of any pattern is both pre-synaptic and post-synaptic to that determined by every other element. Thus, in computing the weight updates due to a pattern we need to compute the products associated with every possible pair of pre-synaptic and post-synaptic activities for that pattern. This array of products can be computed using the outer product procedure, which is summarized in Math Box 4.2. The outer product of two vectors, where the first vector is a column and the second a row, is a matrix of the products of all pairs of elements of the two vectors.

TABLE 4.2   Computing the connection weights for a three-unit, recurrent network using the Hopfield rule

Step 1: Compute outer product for $\mathbf{p}_1$

$$\left(2\mathbf{p}_1^T - 1\right)\left(2\mathbf{p}_1 - 1\right) = \begin{bmatrix} +1 \\ +1 \\ -1 \end{bmatrix}\begin{bmatrix} +1 & +1 & -1 \end{bmatrix} = \begin{bmatrix} +1 & +1 & -1 \\ +1 & +1 & -1 \\ -1 & -1 & +1 \end{bmatrix}$$

Step 2: Compute outer product for $\mathbf{p}_2$

$$\left(2\mathbf{p}_2^T - 1\right)\left(2\mathbf{p}_2 - 1\right) = \begin{bmatrix} -1 \\ -1 \\ +1 \end{bmatrix}\begin{bmatrix} -1 & -1 & +1 \end{bmatrix} = \begin{bmatrix} +1 & +1 & -1 \\ +1 & +1 & -1 \\ -1 & -1 & +1 \end{bmatrix}$$

Step 3: Sum the outer products

$$\begin{bmatrix} +1 & +1 & -1 \\ +1 & +1 & -1 \\ -1 & -1 & +1 \end{bmatrix} + \begin{bmatrix} +1 & +1 & -1 \\ +1 & +1 & -1 \\ -1 & -1 & +1 \end{bmatrix} = \begin{bmatrix} +2 & +2 & -2 \\ +2 & +2 & -2 \\ -2 & -2 & +2 \end{bmatrix}$$

Step 4: Zero the diagonal (∘ denotes element-wise multiplication)

$$\begin{bmatrix} +2 & +2 & -2 \\ +2 & +2 & -2 \\ -2 & -2 & +2 \end{bmatrix} \circ \begin{bmatrix} 0 & 1 & 1 \\ 1 & 0 & 1 \\ 1 & 1 & 0 \end{bmatrix} = \begin{bmatrix} 0 & +2 & -2 \\ +2 & 0 & -2 \\ -2 & -2 & 0 \end{bmatrix}$$

The Hopfield (covariation) rule is applied via the method of outer products to two patterns: $\mathbf{p}_1 = [1\ 1\ 0]$ and $\mathbf{p}_2 = [0\ 0\ 1]$. Note that, in this book, pattern vectors $\mathbf{p}_i$ are expressed as rows, so that the $\mathbf{p}_i^T$ are columns.

MATH BOX 4.2   THE OUTER PRODUCT OF TWO VECTORS

The outer product between two vectors is in some sense the opposite of the inner (or dot) product (see Math Box 1.2). Whereas the inner product of two vectors is a scalar (a single number), the outer product of two vectors is a matrix (Noble and Daniel 1988). Specifically, the inner product is the sum of the products of the corresponding elements of the two vectors, but the outer product is the matrix of products of all pairs of elements of the two vectors. Unlike the inner product, the outer product can be computed between two vectors that do not have the same dimension (i.e., the same number of elements). Both the inner and outer products are computed by matrix multiplication according the rule "across the row and down the column" (see Math Box 1.2), so for both, one vector must be a row and the other a column. The inner and outer products differ in the order of the row and column. For the inner product the row vector is first, but for the outer product the column vector is first. For example, the outer product between $[a\ b\ c]^T$ and $[x\ y]$ is described by Equation B4.2.1:

$$\begin{bmatrix} a \\ b \\ c \end{bmatrix} \begin{bmatrix} x & y \end{bmatrix} = \begin{bmatrix} ax & ay \\ bx & by \\ cx & cy \end{bmatrix} \qquad \text{B4.2.1}$$

Note that in finding the pairs of elements to multiply, we moved across each one-element row of the column vector and down each one-element column of the row vector. The resulting matrix has row number equal to the dimension of the first (column) vector and column number equal to the dimension of the second (row) vector. Again unlike the inner product, the result of the outer product operation depends on the order of the vectors. For example, the outer product between $[x\ y]^T$ and $[a\ b\ c]$ is:

$$\begin{bmatrix} x \\ y \end{bmatrix} \begin{bmatrix} a & b & c \end{bmatrix} = \begin{bmatrix} xa & xb & xc \\ ya & yb & yc \end{bmatrix} \qquad \text{B4.2.2}$$

The outer product of two vectors of the same dimension is a square matrix.

Computing the outer product between a given pattern vector expressed as a column, and the same pattern vector expressed as a row, gives the array of products that constitute the weight updates due to that pattern. The outer products for all patterns are then summed to find the weight values for the whole set of patterns.

Table 4.2 illustrates the outer product method for computing weight values using the Hopfield rule on patterns $\mathbf{p}_1 = [1\ 1\ 0]$ and $\mathbf{p}_2 = [0\ 0\ 1]$. For the Hopfield rule the binary pattern vectors, with elements of 1 or 0, are first converted to pattern vectors with elements of +1 or –1 using terms of the form $(2\mathbf{p} - 1)$. Note in the expression $(2\mathbf{p} - 1)$ that each element in $\mathbf{p}$ is first multiplied by 2 and then has the value 1 subtracted from it. The outer product is computed as the converted vector expressed as a column multiplied by the same converted vector expressed as a row. As shown in Step 1 of Table 4.2, the outer product of the converted vector for pattern $\mathbf{p}_1$ is computed as $(2\mathbf{p}_1^T - 1)(2\mathbf{p}_1 - 1)$, where T is the transpose operator that converts a row to a column (or vice-versa). The transpose operator is used here to convert pattern vectors, which we express as rows by convention in this book, into column vectors. The same procedure applies for $\mathbf{p}_2$ (Step 2). The two outer products are then summed to get the weight values (Step 3). Because self-connections are not allowed in Hopfield networks, the diagonal of the weight matrix is set to 0 through element-by-element multiplication by another matrix in which all diagonal elements are 0 and in which all off-diagonal elements are 1 (Step 4). The reasons for disallowing diagonal connectivity matrix elements (which correspond to unit self-connection weights) will be explained later in this section.

The sum of outer products we compute in order to determine the network connection weights using the Hopfield rule (see Equation 4.8) can be thought of as the "covariation matrix" for the unit activations, given the set of patterns on which they are trained. As explained in more detail in Math Box 4.1, the covariation matrix is different from a true covariance matrix in two specific ways. First, for a covariance matrix, the individual outer products are computed not directly from the unit activations but from the differences between the activation of each unit and its mean activation. Second, for a covariance matrix, the sum of the outer products is divided by the number of outer products in the sum. Under certain circumstances the covariation matrix computed using the Hopfield rule (see Equation 4.8) can easily be converted to a true covariance matrix (see Math Box 4.1), but using the true covariance matrix in place of the covariation matrix would not change the dynamic behavior of the networks we wish to study. Also, the covariation (Hopfield) matrix is more easily compared with the other Hebbian matrices we will study in this chapter.

The numerical example illustrates how the covariation matrix stores the covariations in activity among the units in the network, as determined by the patterns we want the network to store. Again consider patterns $\mathbf{p}_1 = [1\ 1\ 0]$ and $\mathbf{p}_2 = [0\ 0\ 1]$. These patterns are different, but in both patterns the desired activities of y_1 and y_2 are the same, and in both patterns the desired activities of y_1 and y_2 are different from those of y_3. Thus, units y_1 and y_2 have a positive covariation with each other, while y_1 and y_2 both have a negative covariation with y_3. This is apparent in the covariation matrix on the right-hand side of the equation in Step 4 of Table 4.2.

The computations in Table 4.2 also illustrate the fact that the variation (as opposed to covariation) of the activity of a unit with itself is always positive. (Note the positive diagonal on the right-hand side of the equation in Step 3 of Table 4.2.) Thus, the variations (as opposed to covariations) of the unit activities indicate nothing about the associations of the elements of the patterns with each other that the network needs to store. Because they contribute nothing, and because their removal simplifies the analysis of the dynamics of the Hopfield network (to be described in the next section), the diagonal of the Hopfield weight matrix is set to 0 (see Haykin 1999).

To recap, the outer product procedure for the Hopfield rule consists in summing outer products of the form $(2\mathbf{p}_l^T - 1)(2\mathbf{p}_l - 1)$ for all patterns indexed by l, where $\mathbf{p}_l$ is a pattern vector and $\mathbf{p}_l^T$ is its transpose. The same outer product procedure that we used for the Hopfield rule can also be used for the other Hebbian rules by restricting the conversion from binary (1 and 0) to +1 and −1. For the three other rules the outer products are computed as: Hebb $\mathbf{p}_l^T\mathbf{p}_l$, post-synaptic $\mathbf{p}_l^T(2\mathbf{p}_l - 1)$, and pre-synaptic $(2\mathbf{p}_l^T - 1)\mathbf{p}_l$. Script `autoConnectivity` uses the outer product method to compute the weights for the classic Hebb, post-synaptic, pre-synaptic, and Hopfield rules using a single loop.

The outer product method will become useful later in this chapter when we make hetero-associative updates due to two different pattern vectors (see Section 4.6). The outer product method is also useful for conceptually working up to the full matrix computation of the connectivity weights of recurrent, auto-associative networks. If $\mathbf{P}$ is the matrix of patterns, where each pattern constitutes a row of $\mathbf{P}$, then the matrix forms of the four rules are: Hebb $\mathbf{P}^T\mathbf{P}$, post-synaptic $\mathbf{P}^T(2\mathbf{P} - 1)$, pre-synaptic $(2\mathbf{P}^T - 1)\mathbf{P}$, and Hopfield $(2\mathbf{P}^T - 1)(2\mathbf{P} - 1)$. Note that $\mathbf{P}^T$ is the transpose of matrix $\mathbf{P}$, so the columns of $\mathbf{P}^T$ are the rows of $\mathbf{P}$. For the $(2\mathbf{P} - 1)$ terms, all elements of $\mathbf{P}$ are first multiplied by 2 and then have 1 subtracted from them [and similarly for the $(2\mathbf{P}^T - 1)$ terms]. Then the matrix forms of each of the four rules are computed via matrix multiplication, which is summarized in Math Box 4.3.

These matrix operations are equivalent to the outer product method shown in Table 4.2, and to the weight-by-weight computations shown in Equations 4.5 through 4.8. Script `autoConnectivity` also uses the matrix method to compute the weights for the classic Hebb, post-synaptic, presynaptic, and Hopfield rules. Note that the outer product and matrix methods are commented-out in MATLAB Box 4.1. You will need to comment-out the commands for the other methods, and uncomment the commands for the method you wish to use in order for the script to operate properly. The script removes the diagonals from all of the weight matrices computed using any method.

MATH BOX 4.3 MATRIX MULTIPLICATION: ACROSS THE ROW AND DOWN THE COLUMN

The rule for multiplying two matrices is the same as the rule for multiplying two vectors, or multiplying a matrix and a vector (see Math Box 1.2). The rule is "across the row and down the column" (Noble and Daniel 1988). While the inner (or dot) product of two vectors is a scalar, and the product of a matrix and a vector is another vector, the product of two matrices is another matrix. Two matrices can be multiplied provided they are conformable (i.e., the number of columns of the first matrix to be multiplied must equal the number of rows of the second), in which case the resulting product matrix has as many rows as the first matrix to be multiplied and as many columns as the second. Note that two square matrices having the same dimensions can be multiplied in either order but, because matrix multiplication is not commutative in general, the resulting product matrices will not necessarily be the same.

The elements of the product matrix are sums of products of pairs of elements of the matrices to be multiplied. The rule "across the row and down the column" determines which pairs of elements are multiplied and summed. This is illustrated in Equation B4.3.1:

$$\begin{bmatrix} a & b & c \\ d & e & f \\ g & h & i \\ j & k & l \end{bmatrix} \begin{bmatrix} u & x \\ v & y \\ w & z \end{bmatrix} = \begin{bmatrix} au+bv+cw & ax+by+cz \\ du+ev+fw & dx+ey+fz \\ gu+hv+iw & gx+hy+iz \\ ju+kv+lw & jx+ky+lz \end{bmatrix} \qquad \text{B4.3.1}$$

In finding the pairs of elements to be multiplied we moved across each row of the first matrix and down each column of the second. The result is another matrix having as many rows as the first matrix to be multiplied and as many columns as the second.

We can compare and contrast the Hebb, post-synaptic, pre-synaptic, and Hopfield connectivity weight matrices after first using script `autoConnectivity` to compute them for the following set of two patterns (as shown in Equation 4.9):

$$\mathbf{P} = \begin{bmatrix} 1 & 1 & 1 & 1 & 0 & 0 & 0 & 0 & 0 & 0 \\ 0 & 0 & 0 & 0 & 0 & 0 & 1 & 1 & 1 & 1 \end{bmatrix} \qquad \textbf{4.9}$$

This set of two patterns can be loaded into the MATLAB workspace using the command `P=[1 1 1 1 0 0 0 0 0 0; 0 0 0 0 0 0 1 1 1 1]`. Note that each pattern vector (row of P) has ten elements. Therefore, a network would need ten units to represent and auto-associate these patterns. The command `autoConnectivity` will generate weight matrices of the correct dimensions directly from the training patterns. Using any of the three methods (weight-by-weight, outer product, or matrix) the script `autoConnectivity` computes the weight values and stores them in matrix variables HB for Hebb, PO for post-synaptic, PR for pre-synaptic, and HP for the Hopfield matrix.

The four connectivity matrices computed for the two patterns in Equation 4.9 are shown in Table 4.3. Their dimensions are all 10-by-10, which are the correct dimensions for recurrent networks of ten units. The Hebb, post-synaptic, pre-synaptic, and Hopfield auto-association matrices are similar in that they all have a 0 diagonal (which is set to 0 by `autoConnectivity` to disallow unit self-connections). Other similarities and differences in the Hebb, post-synaptic, pre-synaptic, and Hopfield matrices are apparent. The Hebb and Hopfield matrices are symmetric. The pre-synaptic and post-synaptic matrices are asymmetric, but they are each other's transpose. The Hebb matrix lacks negative connections, which are present in the other three matrices. Also, the Hebb matrix is the sparsest because its rule is the most restrictive. Connections in the Hopfield matrix are stronger. Some of these characteristics

COVARIATION LEARNING AND AUTO-ASSOCIATIVE MEMORY **109**

TABLE 4.3 **Recurrent auto-associator weight matrices constructed using each of the four Hebbian rules**

Hebb										Post-synaptic									
0	+1	+1	+1	0	0	0	0	0	0	0	+1	+1	+1	−1	−1	−1	−1	−1	−1
+1	0	+1	+1	0	0	0	0	0	0	+1	0	+1	+1	−1	−1	−1	−1	−1	−1
+1	+1	0	+1	0	0	0	0	0	0	+1	+1	0	+1	−1	−1	−1	−1	−1	−1
+1	+1	+1	0	0	0	0	0	0	0	+1	+1	+1	0	−1	−1	−1	−1	−1	−1
0	0	0	0	0	0	0	0	0	0	0	0	0	0	0	0	0	0	0	0
0	0	0	0	0	0	0	0	0	0	0	0	0	0	0	0	0	0	0	0
0	0	0	0	0	0	0	+1	+1	+1	−1	−1	−1	−1	−1	−1	0	+1	+1	+1
0	0	0	0	0	0	+1	0	+1	+1	−1	−1	−1	−1	−1	−1	+1	0	+1	+1
0	0	0	0	0	0	+1	+1	0	+1	−1	−1	−1	−1	−1	−1	+1	+1	0	+1
0	0	0	0	0	0	+1	+1	+1	0	−1	−1	−1	−1	−1	−1	+1	+1	+1	0

Pre-synaptic										Hopfield (covariation)									
0	+1	+1	+1	0	0	−1	−1	−1	−1	0	+2	+2	+2	0	0	−2	−2	−2	−2
+1	0	+1	+1	0	0	−1	−1	−1	−1	+2	0	+2	+2	0	0	−2	−2	−2	−2
+1	+1	0	+1	0	0	−1	−1	−1	−1	+2	+2	0	+2	0	0	−2	−2	−2	−2
+1	+1	+1	0	0	0	−1	−1	−1	−1	+2	+2	+2	0	0	0	−2	−2	−2	−2
−1	−1	−1	−1	0	0	−1	−1	−1	−1	0	0	0	0	0	+2	0	0	0	0
−1	−1	−1	−1	0	0	−1	−1	−1	−1	0	0	0	0	+2	0	0	0	0	0
−1	−1	−1	−1	0	0	0	+1	+1	+1	−2	−2	−2	−2	0	0	0	+2	+2	+2
−1	−1	−1	−1	0	0	+1	0	+1	+1	−2	−2	−2	−2	0	0	+2	0	+2	+2
−1	−1	−1	−1	0	0	+1	+1	0	+1	−2	−2	−2	−2	0	0	+2	+2	0	+2
−1	−1	−1	−1	0	0	+1	+1	+1	0	−2	−2	−2	−2	0	0	+2	+2	+2	0

The Hebb, post-synaptic, pre-synaptic, and Hopfield rules are listed in Table 4.1. The connectivity matrices are constructed from the patterns in Equation 4.9. The Hebb and Hopfield matrices are symmetric. The post-synaptic and pre-synaptic matrices are not symmetric but they are each other's transpose.

will have functional consequences, which we will explore in the following sections. Many of the examples in this chapter, particularly those involving performance comparisons between auto-associative neural networks trained using the four different Hebbian rules, take their inspiration from Orchard and Phillips (1991).

4.2 Simulating Memory Recall Using Recurrent Auto-Associator Networks

Once the connectivity weights are trained, using one of the rules detailed in the previous section, recurrent networks can be used as pattern auto-associators. They can, for example, recall a pattern when the states of the units are initialized with some partial or corrupted version of it. Thus, recurrent auto-associators can act as content addressable memories, and can serve as models for certain types of neurobiological memory. As mentioned in the preamble, and discussed in detail in Section 4.7, recurrent auto-associative neural networks are often used to model part of the hippocampus, which is a brain region closely linked to memory formation and recall. The mechanism by which recurrent auto-associative networks recall patterns is intrinsic to their dynamics. The use of these dynamic neural systems as content addressable memories is one of the most beautiful and elegant modeling paradigms in all of computational neuroscience.

Recurrent neural networks are dynamic systems that process signals in time. The recurrent auto-associator networks we will consider in this chapter consist of one layer of neural units that are all interconnected, except that self-connections are disallowed (see Figure 4.2). The units are nonlinear, with binary states that can take values only of 0 or 1. Any state of the neural network intended as a stored memory state will be represented by some pattern of 0s and 1s over the units.

Recurrence and nonlinearity lie at the heart of auto-associative network behavior. Recurrence allows desired states to emerge via dynamic interactions between the units. Nonlinearity prevents the network from becoming unstable, and instead encourages the network to settle into a stable state. Provided that certain conditions are satisfied, an auto-associative network will settle, or relax, from any initial state into a stable state, also known as an attractor. If the initial state is a partial pattern, and the stable state is a stored memory pattern, then upon reaching the stable state the attractor network can be said to have "recalled" the pattern.

We previously studied both linear and nonlinear recurrent neural networks in Chapters 1 through 3. In those networks the external input, expressed as vector $\mathbf{x}$, was present over the entire time course of the simulation. For the auto-associative networks we will study in this chapter, the input is used only to present complete patterns to the network during training, or to initialize the states of the units with partial, weak, or corrupt patterns for recall. Because the input is not present throughout the simulation, we will describe the dynamics of recurrent auto-associative networks without external inputs. The input to each unit in the recurrent network will arrive only from the other units in the network. The sums of the weighted inputs to the units in a recurrent, auto-associative network, from the other units in the network, can therefore be computed as shown in Equation 4.10:

$$\mathbf{q}(t) = \mathbf{W}\mathbf{y}(t-1) \qquad\qquad \textbf{4.10}$$

where t is discrete time, $\mathbf{W}$ is the matrix of the recurrent connection weights between the units, $\mathbf{y}$ is the vector of unit states (activations), and $\mathbf{q}$ is the vector of sums of the weighted inputs to each unit. The nonlinear activation function of each unit can be described as in Equation 4.11:

$$y_i(t) = \begin{cases} 1, & q_i(t) > \theta \\ 0, & q_i(t) \le \theta \end{cases} \qquad\qquad \textbf{4.11}$$

The threshold θ is set to 0 in the examples in this chapter. The state update described by Equations 4.10 and 4.11 is synchronous, in that each unit y_i in $\mathbf{y}$ updates its state at the same time. For asynchronous updates each unit computes its weighted input sum individually and in random order according to:

$$q_i(t) = \mathbf{W}_{\text{row } i}\ \mathbf{y}(t-1) = \sum_{j \ne i} w_{ij} y_j(t-1) \qquad\qquad \textbf{4.12}$$

where $\mathbf{W}_{\text{row } i}$ is the ith row of $\mathbf{W}$. The unit being updated then thresholds its weighted input sum according to the nonlinear function in Equation 4.11. We will explore both synchronous and asynchronous updates in the examples which follow.

The reason that recurrent networks of threshold units, with connection weights $\mathbf{W}$ trained using the covariation rule, can operate as content addressable memories was shown through analysis by Hopfield (1982). By analogy with certain physical systems, Hopfield defined the "energy" E of the network as shown in Equation 4.13:

$$E = -\frac{1}{2}\sum_{i}\sum_{j\neq i} w_{ij}y_i y_j \qquad\qquad \textbf{4.13}$$

Hopfield then used Equation 4.13 to derive the change in energy of the network, due to the change in state of a unit, based on the following conditions. First, self-connections are disallowed, so that the recurrent connectivity matrix **W** has a 0 diagonal ($w_{ii} = 0$). Second, the weight matrix **W** must be symmetric ($w_{ij} = w_{ji}$). Third, the state updates must be asynchronous, so that the units can only update their states one at a time and in random order.

These conditions can be satisfied for the Hopfield auto-associator. Because the self-connection weights (diagonal elements of **W**) trained using the Hopfield rule are just the variations of the pattern elements with themselves, they contribute nothing toward associating the various elements of the patterns with each other, so they can be set to 0 without affecting the auto-associative properties of the network. The off-diagonal elements of matrix **W** are constrained to be symmetric if the weights are trained using the Hopfield (covariation) rule. Finally, there is no restriction on the order of unit state updates, which can be made one at a time using Equations 4.11 and 4.12 (in reverse order). With these conditions satisfied the change in energy of the network due to a change in the state of any unit y_i is described in Equation 4.14:

$$\Delta E = -\Delta y_i \sum_{j\neq i} w_{ij}y_j \qquad\qquad \textbf{4.14}$$

Equation 4.14 shows that the Hopfield recurrent auto-associative network is stable in that its energy can only decrease or remain at 0. Table 4.4 evaluates Equation 4.14 (for threshold θ of 0) and shows that the change in energy is either 0 or decreasing under all possible circumstances. Further analysis (Amit 1989) shows that the Hopfield network can have many different stable states (stable attractors). Thus, from whatever state in which a Hopfield network finds itself (such as a partial pattern) the energy of the network will decrease until the network settles into a stable state (such as a stored memory pattern).

The stable states of the Hopfield network are best thought of as the corners of a d-dimensional hypercube, where d equals the number of elements in the pattern vectors to be stored as unit state vectors in the network. The vector **y** (with elements y_i, $i = 1,..., d$) describes the state of the Hopfield network (see Equations 4.11 and 4.12) as a point that "bounces" from one corner to another of the hypercube until it finds the "lowest energy" corner. Because a hypercube is difficult to visualize, an abstraction is provided in Figure 4.3 that reduces the dimensionality of the state vector from d to 1, but gives at least an intuitive view of the movement of the state of a Hopfield network from a higher to a lower energy.

Essentially the same behavior attributable to Hopfield networks composed of binary (discrete) units can be attributed to Hopfield networks composed of sigmoidal (continuous) units. The sigmoid is an s-shaped curve that provides a simple but continuous model of the cut-off and saturation properties of real neurons (see Chapter 6). Hopfield

TABLE 4.4   The "energy" of a Hopfield network always decreases or stays zero

Old y_i	$\sum_{j\neq i} w_{ij}y_j$	New y_i	Δy_i	$\Delta E = -\Delta y_i \sum_{j\neq i} w_{ij}y_j$
0	Positive	1	+1	Negative
0	Negative	0	0	Zero
1	Positive	1	0	Zero
1	Negative	0	−1	Negative

The five columns represent, in order, the value of any unit y_i before it is updated (Old y_i), the sign of its weighted input sum (see also Equations 4.11 and 4.12), the value of y_i after thresholding its input sum at 0 (New y_i), the change in unit activity (Δy_i), and the change in network energy (ΔE). The values in the first four columns exhaust all the possibilities, and determine the value of the expression for the change in energy in the last column.

MATH BOX 4.4   LIAPUNOV FUNCTIONS

The dynamics of linear systems can be described explicitly. We considered the dynamics of linear (and discrete) systems in Math Box 2.4. Nonlinear systems are capable of much richer behavior than linear systems. For example, a nonlinear system can have multiple stable states, where each region Φ of the state space has its own stable state vector $\tilde{\mathbf{y}}$. Explicit descriptions of nonlinear system dynamics are rarely available, but implicit methods can be used to infer their behavior. The most common method for inferring the behavior of a nonlinear system involves the Liapunov function, which is a function of the state vector that summarizes the entire system and also conforms with certain conditions (Luenberger 1979).

Consider the system $\mathbf{y}(t) = f(\mathbf{y}(t-1))$, where $\mathbf{y}$ is the state vector, t is discrete time, and $f(\mathbf{y})$ is a nonlinear function.

Define a summarizing function $L(\mathbf{y})$ for this system. If at any time $t-1$ the state of the system is $\mathbf{y}$, then at time t the state will be $f(\mathbf{y})$, and the values of the summarizing function will be $L(\mathbf{y})$ and $L(f(\mathbf{y}))$, respectively. Then the change in the summarizing function is $\Delta L(\mathbf{y}) = L(f(\mathbf{y})) - L(\mathbf{y})$.

Function $L(\mathbf{y})$ is a Liapunov function if $L(\mathbf{y})$ has a unique minimum (stable state $\tilde{\mathbf{y}}$) with respect to all other points in Φ, and if $\Delta L(\mathbf{y}) \equiv L(f(\mathbf{y})) - L(\mathbf{y}) \leq 0$ for all $\mathbf{y}$ in region Φ of the state space (see Luenberger (1979) for further conditions and a fuller discussion of this concept). Thus, the value of $L(\mathbf{y})$ can only decrease until stable point $\tilde{\mathbf{y}}$ in region Φ is reached. Note that the nonlinear system $\mathbf{y}(t) = f(\mathbf{y}(t-1))$ may have many different stable states, but $L(\mathbf{y})$ is a Liapunov function for a given region of its state space only if that region has only one minimum (stable state).

(1984) established this correspondence by deriving an "energy" equation for networks of sigmoidal units that is analogous to Equation 4.13 for networks of binary units. In the larger context of dynamic systems theory, these equations are Liapunov functions (Haykin 1999). Liapunov functions are used to infer the behavior of dynamic systems and are especially useful for nonlinear systems (see Math Box 4.4).

The classic example of a Liapunov function describes the energy of an unforced mechanical system with friction, which always decreases from some initial state until the system is at rest. It could be visualized as a marble that is not initially located at the bottom of a bowl. The marble may move up and down the sides of the bowl, but its energy (potential plus kinetic) continues to decrease, due to friction between the marble and bowl, until the marble comes to rest at the bottom of the bowl. A nonlinear system such as a recurrent, auto-associative neural network will have many stable states, and can be visualized as a set of many adjacent bowls whose edges have been deformed and welded together (Figure 4.3 can be thought of as the side view of a vertical cut through such a set of adjacent, welded bowls). While Hopfield's analysis specifically concerns networks trained using the covariation rule, Cohen and Grossberg (1983) earlier showed, also using Liapunov functions, that many different types of recurrent neural networks could be stable.

All of the Hebbian rules we presented in Section 4.1 can be used to set the matrix $\mathbf{W}$ of the connection weights of a recurrent neural network. Depending on the number and properties of the patterns to be stored, all of the Hebbian rules can thereby train networks to act as content addressable memories. We will demonstrate this ability using the networks we already trained in the previous section on the two patterns given in Equation 4.9. For these patterns, correct recall can be achieved using synchronous updates. We will begin by using synchronous updates because they are easier to implement and they yield more reproducible results, which will aid our comparison of the networks trained using the different rules. We will switch to asynchronous updates in a later section.

We will first show that the training patterns are stable states of each of the networks. To do this, we will initialize each network with the first training pattern and synchronously update the network for ten time steps. Note

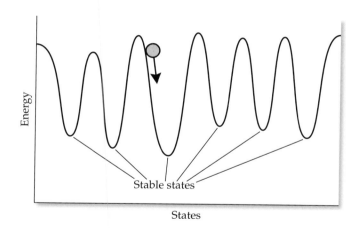

FIGURE 4.3   An abstraction providing an intuitive illustration of the multiplicity of stable states (attractors) of a Hopfield network The stable states can be thought of as "energy minima," and the state of the network "moves" from a high-energy to a low-energy region of the state space. The abstraction essentially reduces the dimensionality of the network unit state vector from d to 1, where d is the number of units in the network.

that every unit is updated on each synchronous time step. Since there are 10 units in each network, 10 synchronous updates are equivalent to 100 individual unit updates. The function synchUp, listed in MATLAB Box 4.2, will compute synchronous updates of recurrent networks by implementing Equations 4.10 and 4.11. To initialize the network with the first pattern, set yInitial=P(1,:)'. Note that the half-quote converts the pattern row vector into a unit state column vector. Then 10 synchronous updates of the Hebb network can be carried out using the function call (which we also call a command) YHB=synchUp(yInitial,HB,10), where HB is the classic Hebb connectivity matrix we computed in the previous section, and it corresponds to matrix **W** in Equation 4.10. Matrix variable YHB is an array in which each column corresponds to a unit and each row corresponds to an update. Thus, YHB is arranged in rows, like the pattern array, but each row of YHB shows the states of the units in the network on each time step.

The array YHB showing the initial state vector (as the first row) and the state vector following each of ten synchronous updates (rows two through eleven) is shown in numeric form in Table 4.5. Note that the initial state [1 1 1 1 0 0 0 0

MATLAB® BOX 4.2   This function computes synchronous updates of recurrent auto-associative networks. The entire state vector is updated on each time step.

```
% synchUp.m
% yIinitial is the initial state (column) vector, W is
% the connectivity matrix, nTs is the number of time steps,
% and Y is an array to hold state vector y through time

function Y = synchUp(yInitial,W,nTs) % declare the function

[dum,nUnits]=size(W); % find the number of units in the network
Y=zeros(nTs,nUnits); % zero the output Y array
y=yInitial; % initialize the state of y to yInitial
for t=1:nTs % for each time step
    q = W*y; % synchronously update y
    y = q>0; % impose the threshold nonlinearity
    Y(t,:)=y'; % save this state y to the output array Y
end % end the synchronous update loop
Y=[yInitial';Y]; % place yInitial as the first row of Y
```

TABLE 4.5   Showing that a training pattern can be a stable state of a recurrent auto-associator network trained using the Hebb rule

1	1	1	1	0	0	0	0	0	0
1	1	1	1	0	0	0	0	0	0
1	1	1	1	0	0	0	0	0	0
1	1	1	1	0	0	0	0	0	0
1	1	1	1	0	0	0	0	0	0
1	1	1	1	0	0	0	0	0	0
1	1	1	1	0	0	0	0	0	0
1	1	1	1	0	0	0	0	0	0
1	1	1	1	0	0	0	0	0	0
1	1	1	1	0	0	0	0	0	0
1	1	1	1	0	0	0	0	0	0

The network was trained on the non-overlapping patterns in Equation 4.9. The 10-unit network has a 10-element state vector. The network undergoes 10 synchronous updates. The initial state vector is shown at the top row, and each subsequent row shows the state vector following each successive synchronous update.

0 0], which is the first training pattern, is maintained over all ten synchronous updates. This shows that the first training pattern is a stable state of the auto-associative network trained using the classic Hebb rule.

Since it is tedious to look at output pattern arrays in numeric form, we can convert the array to an image using the `image` command in MATLAB. Start by finding the dimensions of the array to be converted to an image using `[r,c]=size(YHB)`. The `size` command will find that array YHB has ten columns c, corresponding to the ten units, and has eleven rows r, where the first row corresponds to the initial state and the next ten rows correspond to the ten synchronous updates. The image array is three-dimensional, and each pixel in the image is associated with three numbers that determine the color of the pixel. Define the image hold matrix using `YHBim=zeros(r,c,3)`. For black-and-white images, each of the three color numbers has the same value, so to make a black-and-white image of YHB use the three commands: `YHBim(:,:,1)=YHB`, `YHBim(:,:,2)=YHB`, and `YHBim(:,:,3)=YHB`. Now the image can be generated using the command `image(YHBim)`.

The image, with the initial state at the top and subsequent states moving successively downward, is shown in Figure 4.4A. In the image, white and black correspond to 1 and 0, respectively. (Intermediate values would show up in shades of gray.) The image (see Figure 4.4A), like the numerical array (see Table 4.5) shows that the first training pattern, which is [1 1 1 1 0 0 0 0 0 0], is a stable state of the network trained using the classic Hebb rule. Similar computations show that the first training pattern is also a stable state for the post-synaptic, pre-synaptic, and Hopfield networks (not shown). Thus, the first training pattern has been stored as a stable memory pattern in each of the four networks.

The same approach can be used to test whether the second training pattern (see Equation 4.9) is also a stable state of the auto-associator trained using the classic Hebb rule. This time, set the initial state to the second pattern using `yInitial=P(2,:)'`. Ten synchronous updates of this network can be carried out as before using the command `YHB=synchUp(yInitial,HB,10)`. The result is shown in Figure 4.4B. The pattern [0 0 0 0 0 0 1 1 1 1], which is the second training pattern, is a stable state of the auto-associator trained using the classic Hebb rule. Similar computations show that the second training pat-

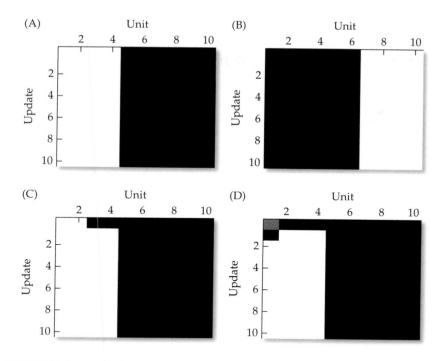

FIGURE 4.4   Stable states, pattern completion, and pattern amplification in auto-associators   Each panel is a pictorial visualization of the state vector of a recurrent auto-associator neural network having 10 units and trained using the Hebb rule. The units are arrayed horizontally, and state vector updates are arrayed vertically. The initial state vector is shown at the top, and the state vectors following each of 10 synchronous updates are shown progressively moving downward in each plot. Each network was trained on the two patterns shown in Equation 4.9. (A) The initial state **y** = [1 1 1 1 0 0 0 0 0 0] is a stable state for the Hebb network. Plot A is a pictorial representation of the data shown in Table 4.5, where 1 is white and 0 is black. (Values between 1 and 0 would show up proportionately as levels of gray.) (B) The initial state **y** = [0 0 0 0 0 0 1 1 1 1] is also a stable state of the Hebb network. (C) The Hebb network reaches the stable state **y** = [1 1 1 1 0 0 0 0 0 0] (also shown in A) from the incomplete state **y** = [1 1 0 0 0 0 0 0 0 0]. (D) The Hebb network reaches the same stable state **y** = [1 1 1 1 0 0 0 0 0 0] from the weak and incomplete state **y** = [0.1 0 0 0 0 0 0 0 0 0]. The performances of auto-associator networks trained on the same patterns (see Equation 4.9) using the post-synaptic, pre-synaptic, and Hopfield rules are the same as shown here for the Hebb auto-associator.

tern is likewise a stable state for the post-synaptic, pre-synaptic, and Hopfield networks (not shown). Thus, the second training pattern has also been stored as a stable memory pattern in each of the four networks.

Now that we have established that both training patterns have successfully been stored as stable states of the four auto-associators, we can use them to recall patterns given hints in the form of incomplete patterns. Set the initial state to an incomplete version of the first pattern using `yInitial=[1 1 0 0 0 0 0 0 0 0]'`. Then update the Hebb auto-associator 10 times from this initial state using `YHB=synchUp(yInitial,HB,10)`. The result is shown in Figure 4.4C. The classic Hebb auto-associator was able to complete the pattern by settling to the stable state [1 1 1 1 0 0 0 0 0 0], which corresponds to the first training pattern. The Hebb recurrent neural network auto-associator was able to "recall" the first pattern.

Now set the initial state to an incomplete and weak version of the first pattern using `yInitial=[0.1 0 0 0 0 0 0 0 0 0]'` and update the Hebb auto-associator 10 times using `YHB=synchUp(yInitial,HB,10)`.

The result is shown in Figure 4.4D. The Hebb auto-associator was able both to amplify and complete the pattern by settling to the stable state [1 1 1 1 0 0 0 0 0 0], which corresponds to the first training pattern. Similar computations show that all four auto-associators have the same pattern completion and amplification abilities for both the first and second patterns (not shown). Thus, all four auto-associators are able to "recall" the training patterns given "hints" or "reminders" in the form of weak and incomplete patterns. The ability of all four networks to amplify and complete patterns is due to their recurrent connections, which allow parts of the pattern to reinforce the whole pattern.

4.3 Recalling Distinct Memories Using Negative Connections in Auto-Associators

While recall from a weak hint is difficult, we know from our own experience that recall from an ambiguous hint, one that could correspond to more than one memory, is even more difficult. The same is the case for "recall" in recurrent auto-associative neural networks. To see this, set the initial state to a corrupted version of the first training pattern using `yInitial=[1 1 1 1 0 0 0 0 0 1]′`. This initial state is a combination of the first pattern and a small part of the second pattern (see Equation 4.9). Now update the Hebb auto-associator 10 times starting from this corrupted initial state using `YHB=synchUp(yInitial,HB,10)`. The result is shown in Figure 4.5A. The Hebb auto-associator settles to a state that does not correspond to either of the two training patterns. Such stable states are called spurious states. The spurious state reached by the Hebb auto-associator in Figure 4.5A is a mixture of the first and second training patterns. The spurious states that can arise in recurrent auto-associative neural networks include mixture states, as well as reversed states, which are the reverse of training patterns, and other types of states that are not related in any clear way to the training patterns (Amit 1989; Haykin 1999). By settling to a spuri-

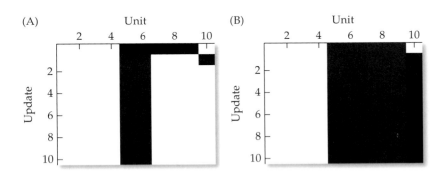

FIGURE 4.5   Negative connections can separate non-overlapping patterns in auto-associators Each panel is a pictorial visualization of the state vector of a recurrent auto-associator neural network having 10 units. The graphic conventions are as in Figure 4.4. The networks were trained on the two patterns shown in Equation 4.9. In both panels the auto-associator networks take the initial state **y** = [1 1 1 1 0 0 0 0 0 1], which is a corrupted version of the first training pattern **y** = [1 1 1 1 0 0 0 0 0]. The networks undergo 10 synchronous updates. (A) An auto-associator trained using the Hebb rule reaches the spurious stable state **y** = [1 1 1 1 0 0 1 1 1 1] from this initial state. (B) An auto-associator trained with the post-synaptic rule reaches the stable state corresponding to the first training pattern **y** = [1 1 1 1 0 0 0 0 0 0]. Recurrent auto-associators trained using the pre-synaptic and Hopfield rules (not shown) also reach a stable state corresponding to the first training pattern when initialized with the same corrupted version of it (**y** = [1 1 1 1 0 0 0 0 0 1]).

ous state the Hebb auto-associator fails to reproduce the first pattern from an ambiguous version of it.

The fact that the Hebb auto-associator failed to disambiguate the corrupted pattern does not mean that the other three auto-associator networks will also fail at this task. Reinitialize the state to the same corrupted version of the first training pattern using `yInitial=[1 1 1 1 0 0 0 0 0 1]'`, and update the post-synaptic auto-associator 10 times starting from this corrupted initial state using `YPO=synchUp(yInitial, PO, 10)`. (In this command matrix `PO` corresponds to matrix **W**.) The result is shown in Figure 4.5B. Unlike the Hebb auto-associator, the post-synaptic auto-associator settles to a state that does correspond to first training pattern. Similar computations (not shown) demonstrate that the pre-synaptic and Hopfield networks can also produce the first training pattern from the corrupted version. The other three auto-associators succeed where the Hebb auto-associator failed.

The reason the Hebb network fails in this task is that the initial pattern, which was a corrupted version of the first training pattern, had elements of both the first and second training patterns in it. The Hebb network completed both patterns and stabilized in a spurious state that combined both patterns (see Figure 4.5A). It was unable to let elements of the first pattern suppress elements of the second. The post-synaptic auto-associative network is able to suppress elements of the second pattern using elements of the first (see Figure 4.5B). It can do so because it has negative (inhibitory) as well as positive (excitatory) recurrent connections (see Table 4.3). The pre-synaptic and Hopfield networks, which also have negative recurrent connections, are also able to suppress elements of the second pattern using elements of the first (not shown). The post-synaptic, pre-synaptic, and Hopfield networks are able to take an initial state that is composed mostly of one pattern, but partly of another, and produce the correct pattern. This ability can be called pattern separation or pattern differentiation. This example demonstrates that post-synaptic, pre-synaptic, and Hopfield recurrent auto-associative neural networks are more powerful than those trained using the classic Hebb rule on these patterns.

The first set of training patterns (see Equation 4.9) were relatively easy to recall because they were non-overlapping. Overlapping patterns present additional challenges for auto-associative neural networks. To explore the behavior of auto-associators on a set of overlapping patterns, we will retrain all four networks on the two patterns shown in Equation 4.15:

$$\mathbf{P} = \begin{bmatrix} 1 & 1 & 1 & 1 & 1 & 0 & 0 & 0 & 0 & 0 \\ 1 & 0 & 1 & 0 & 1 & 0 & 1 & 0 & 1 & 0 \end{bmatrix} \qquad \textbf{4.15}$$

These patterns can be entered into the MATLAB workspace using `P=[1 1 1 1 1 0 0 0 0 0; 1 0 1 0 1 0 1 0 1 0]`, and recurrent auto-associator networks with connectivity matrices **W** trained using each of the four rules can be generated using the script `autoConnectivity`. Now set the initial state to the first training pattern using `yInitial=P(1,:)'`, and update the Hebb auto-associator network 10 times from this initial state using `YHB=synchUp(yInitial, HB, 10)`. The result is shown in Figure 4.6A. The first training pattern is not a stable state of the Hebb network. The Hebb network has settled from an initial state corresponding to the first training pattern to a spurious state that is a mixture of the first and second training patterns. The Hebb network settles to this same spurious state starting from an initial state corresponding to the second training pattern (not shown). Similar computations demonstrate that the post-synaptic network also settles to this spurious mixture state starting from initial states corresponding either to the first or the second training pattern (not shown). The Hebb and post-synaptic networks both fail in this task.

FIGURE 4.6 Negative connections can separate overlapping patterns in auto-associators Each panel is a pictorial visualization of the state vector of a recurrent auto-associator neural network having 10 units. The graphic conventions are as in Figure 4.4. The networks were trained on the two patterns shown in Equation 4.15. In both panels the auto-associator networks take the initial state **y** = [1 1 1 1 1 0 0 0 0 0], which corresponds to the first training pattern (see Equation 4.15). The auto-associator networks undergo 10 synchronous updates. (A) An auto-associator trained using the Hebb rule reaches the spurious stable state **y** = [1 1 1 1 1 0 1 0 1 0] from this initial state. An auto-associator trained using the post-synaptic rule (not shown) reaches this same, spurious stable state. (B) The first training pattern **y** = [1 1 1 1 1 0 0 0 0 0], taken as the initial state, is a stable state for an auto-associator trained using the pre-synaptic rule. The first training pattern is also a stable state for an auto-associator trained using the Hopfield rule (not shown).

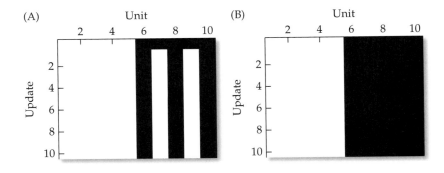

The fact that the Hebb and post-synaptic auto-associators fail to differentiate the overlapping patterns in Equation 4.15 does not imply that the pre-synaptic and Hopfield networks will also fail. To examine the behavior of the pre-synaptic network on this task, set the initial state to the first training pattern using `yInitial=P(1,:)'`, and update the pre-synaptic auto-associator 10 times from this initial state using `YPR=synchUp(yInitial,PR,10)`. (Now PR corresponds to **W**.) The result is shown in Figure 4.6B. The second training pattern is a stable state of the pre-synaptic auto-associator. Similar computations demonstrate that both the first and second training patterns are stable states of both the pre-synaptic and the Hopfield recurrent auto-associators. The pre-synaptic and Hopfield networks have succeeded in a pattern differentiation task where the Hebb and post-synaptic networks have failed.

The inability of the Hebb network to differentiate these overlapping patterns is related to its lack of inhibitory connections. The post-synaptic network fails to differentiate these patterns because the post-synaptic rule produces no weight update in cases where the pre-synaptic unit is 1 but the post-synaptic unit should be 0. The pre-synaptic rule does produce weight updates in that case, because it allows the network to learn to use a pre-synaptic unit to inhibit a post-synaptic unit. This sometimes allows networks trained using the pre-synaptic rule to separate partly overlapping patterns. However, if the patterns overlap too much, or if there are too many patterns, then the ability of a pre-synaptic network to differentiate them degrades as well. The Hopfield network is also able to separate these patterns and, in general, it is the most robust in terms of differentiating overlapping patterns. We will take a deeper look into these issues in Section 4.7.

4.4 Synchronous versus Asynchronous Updating in Recurrent Auto-Associators

The examples in Sections 4.2 and 4.3 demonstrated some of the strengths and weaknesses of recurrent auto-associative networks trained using the four Hebbian learning rules. Because recurrent auto-associative networks trained using the Hopfield rule were the most robust, we will study Hopfield networks in this and the next two sections. The proof (in Section 4.2) that the Hopfield network will always settle to a stable state depended on three conditions: first, that unit self-connection weights are 0; second, that the matrix of unit interconnection weights is symmetric; and third, that the units update asynchronously. The first condition is met by zeroing the diagonal of the weight matrix following training using the Hopfield rule, and the second condition is met by the nature of the Hopfield (covariation) rule itself. We have violated the third condition so far in this chapter, but we did this intentionally because synchronous updates are easier to implement and they are deterministic, which provided a reproducibility that facilitated the performance comparison we made of the networks trained using the four different learning rules. The goal of the examples in this section is to illustrate the problem with synchronous updates and to show how this problem is avoided by asynchronous updates.

To begin, we will train a Hopfield network on the set of two patterns shown in Equation 4.16:

$$\mathbf{P} = \begin{bmatrix} 1 & 0 & 1 & 0 & 1 & 0 & 1 & 0 & 1 & 0 \\ 1 & 0 & 0 & 1 & 1 & 1 & 1 & 0 & 0 & 1 \end{bmatrix} \qquad \textbf{4.16}$$

These patterns can be entered into the MATLAB workspace using `P=[1 0 1 0 1 0 1 0 1 0; 1 0 0 1 1 1 1 0 0 1]`, and a recurrent auto-associator network with connectivity matrix trained according to the Hopfield rule can be generated using the script `autoConnectivity`. Now set the initial state to the pattern `yInitial=[0 0 1 0 1 0 1 0 1 0]'`, which is an incomplete version of the first training pattern, and synchronously update the Hopfield network 10 times from this initial state using the command `YHP=synchUp(yInitial,HP,10)`. (Now HP corresponds to **W**.) The result is shown in Figure 4.7A. The network settles to a stable state that corre-

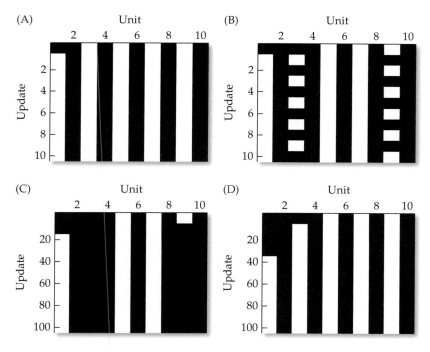

FIGURE 4.7 Synchronous versus asynchronous updating in auto-associators Each panel is a pictorial visualization of the state vector of a recurrent auto-associator network having 10 units. The graphic conventions are as in Figure 4.4. The network was trained on the two patterns shown in Equation 4.16 using the Hopfield rule. (A) The network takes the initial state **y** = [0 0 1 0 1 0 1 0 1 0]. It is synchronously updated 10 times and reaches the stable state **y** = [1 0 1 0 1 0 1 0 1 0], which corresponds to the first training pattern (see Equation 4.16). (B) The network takes the initial state **y** = [0 0 0 0 1 0 1 0 1 0]. It is synchronously updated 10 times but never reaches a stable state. Instead, it alternates between state **y** = [1 0 1 0 1 0 1 0 0 0] and **y** = [1 0 0 0 1 0 1 0 1 0]. (C) The network again takes the initial state **y** = [0 0 0 0 1 0 1 0 1 0], but now it is asynchronously updated 100 times. (A single unit chosen at random is updated on each asynchronous update; the state vector is shown on every tenth update.) The network reaches a stable state but it is a spurious state. (D) The network again takes the initial state **y** = [0 0 0 0 1 0 1 0 1 0] and is asynchronously updated 100 times. The network again reaches a stable state, but this time the stable state corresponds to the first training pattern.

MATLAB® BOX 4.3   This function computes asynchronous updates of recurrent auto-associative networks. The state of only one unit, chosen at random, is updated on each time step.

```
% AsynchUp.m
% yIinitial is the initial state (column) vector, W is the
% connectivity matrix, nTs is number of time steps (a multiple
% of ten) and array Y holds state vector y through time

function Y = AsynchUp(yInitial,W,nTs) % declare the function

[dum,nUnits]=size(W); % find the number of units in the network
Y=zeros(nTs/10,nUnits); % zero the output Y array
y=yInitial; % initialize the state of y to yInitial
for t=1:nTs % for each time step
    rIndx=ceil(rand*nUnits); % randomly choose a state in y to update
    q=W(rIndx,:)*y; % update the selected state in y
    y(rIndx)=q>0; % impose the threshold nonlinearity
    if rem(t,10)==0, Y(t/10,:)=y'; end, % at intervals save to Y array
end % end the asynchronous update loop
Y=[yInitial';Y]; % place yInitial as the first row of Y
```

sponds to the first training pattern. The network has succeeded in completing the first training pattern using synchronous updates.

Now set the initial state to the pattern yInitial=[0 0 0 0 1 0 1 0 1 0]', which is an even more incomplete version of the first training pattern, and synchronously update the Hopfield network 10 times from this initial state using YHP=synchUp(yInitial,HP,10). The result is shown in Figure 4.7B. In this case the Hopfield network does not settle to a stable state. Instead, it oscillates between two states, neither of which bears a clear relationship with the training patterns. This interesting but faulty behavior results from the use of synchronous updating. The discrete Hopfield network, composed of binary units, is guaranteed to reach a stable state only if it is updated asynchronously (see Section 4.2).

The script AsynchUp, listed in MATLAB Box 4.3, will produce asynchronous updates of recurrent auto-associator networks. This script implements Equations 4.11 and 4.12 (in reverse order). As these equations specify, the state of only one unit is updated on each asynchronous update. Because there are ten units in this network, ten asynchronous updates are equivalent to one synchronous update, since all ten units are updated on every synchronous update. This equivalence is approximate. Because units are chosen for asynchronous update at random, individual units will probably not be updated the same number of times using equivalent numbers of asynchronous as compared with synchronous updates. In script AsynchUp, the index of the unit to be updated is chosen at random on each time step using rIndx=ceil(rand*nUnits), in which variable nUnits is the number of units in the network. The script saves the state vector in array Y every ten updates.

Set the initial state to the same incomplete pattern that produced oscillation with synchronous updates using yInitial=[0 0 0 0 1 0 1 0 1 0]'. Then, to make a valid comparison with the synchronous results, asynchronously update the Hopfield network 100 times from this initial state using YHP=AsynchUp(yInitial,HP,100). The result is shown in Figure 4.7C. Using asynchronous updates the network reaches a stable state, but in this case it is a spurious state, which is not related in any clear way to the training patterns. This result is not unexpected. When the required conditions are met, the Hopfield network is guaranteed to reach a stable state, but that state can be a spurious state as well as a desired, trained memory state.

Due to the stochasticity (randomness) inherent in the asynchronous update procedure, the same network can reach different stable states from the same initial state. For this reason, the results produced on different asynchronous simulations can differ from one another, and it is necessary to run the simulation several times to get a feel for the behavior of the network. We can reinitialize the network with the same incomplete pattern that produced oscillatory behavior using synchronous updates (see Figure 4.7B), and reached a spurious stable state using asynchronous updates (see Figure 4.7C), by repeating the command `yInitial=[0 0 0 0 1 0 1 0 1 0]'`. (Note that it is not necessary to reset `yInitial` if you have not changed it since the last simulation.) We then update the Hopfield network 100 times from this initial state by again using `YHP=AsynchUp(yInitial,HP,100)`. The result is shown in Figure 4.7D. Using asynchronous updates the network again reaches a stable state, but in this case it is the state corresponding to the first training pattern. The Hopfield network using asynchronous updates has succeeded in completing this pattern.

Computationally, asynchronous updates are clearly to be preferred over synchronous updates, and we might be led to wonder if there is any neurobiological significance to this modeling result. Neurobiologically, asynchronous updates seem the more plausible. Synchronous updating would require that all the neurons in a network operate in lock step, and this seems unrealistic. However, synchronous updates can produce oscillation because the units composing our Hopfield network are binary. Hopfield networks composed of sigmoidal units will not oscillate even if updated synchronously (Hopfield 1984). Sigmoidal units are more like real neurons, and we will make extensive use of them in later chapters. We use binary units in this chapter because Hopfield networks composed of them have the same essential features (i.e., multiple stable states) as Hopfield networks composed of sigmoidal units (Hopfield 1984), but the binary networks are easier to analyze and explain. These considerations indicate that the oscillation observed in our binary Hopfield network when we updated it synchronously, and the elimination of that oscillation when we updated it asynchronously, is more of computational than of neurobiological significance.

4.5 Graceful Degradation and Simulated Forgetting

Not only are recurrent auto-associative neural networks elegant as nonlinear dynamic systems, but they also seem to capture some of the features of neurobiological memory. We have seen how auto-associators can "remember" certain patterns and "recall" them from partial or corrupted versions of those patterns. Another way in which auto-associative networks resemble neurobiological memory is in their fault tolerance. Auto-associators can still recall patterns correctly, or nearly so, even when some of their connection weights are destroyed. We will explore the robustness of recurrent auto-associators in this section.

To do a fair test of robustness we will not want to train our networks beyond their capacity. The capacity of a Hopfield network, expressed in terms of the number of patterns it can store and correctly recall, is about 15% of the number of units in the network (Hopfield 1982; Amit 1989). The networks we have studied so far in this chapter had ten units but were trained on two patterns. This number of patterns probably exceeded their capacity, but this may have helped us demonstrate their weaknesses as well as their strengths. To test robustness we will train a Hopfield network right at its capacity. We will also restrict ourselves to asynchronous updates.

First, generate a set of 3 binary random patterns, each 20 elements long, in which each element has a 50% chance (probability 0.5) of being a 1. This can be done using the command `P=double(rand(3,20)>0.5)`. (Note that `double` converts the logical data type to the double precision data type so that the values in P can be used in double-precision computations.) Next train a Hopfield network on these patterns using script `autoConnectivity` (which will make a connectivity matrix for an auto-associative network having 20 units). We will first verify that the intact network can amplify the training patterns. Set the initial state to the first training pattern at half strength using `yInitial=0.5*P(1,:)'`, and asynchronously update the Hopfield network 100 times using `YHP=AsynchUp(yInitial,HP,100)`. The result is shown in Figure 4.8A. The Hopfield network reaches a stable state that corresponds to the first training pattern, as expected. Note that we generated a set of random

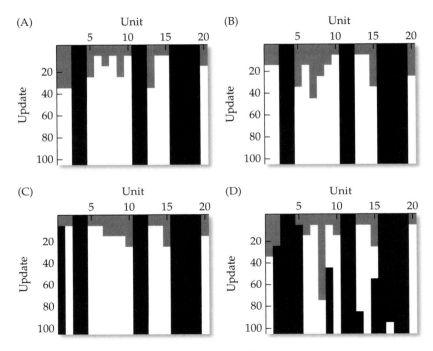

FIGURE 4.8 Graceful degradation of recall in auto-associators Each panel is a pictorial visualization of the state vector of a recurrent auto-associator neural network having 20 units. The graphic conventions are as in Figure 4.4 (where 1 is white and 0 is black, and values between 1 and 0 show up proportionately as levels of gray). The network was trained on three binary random patterns using the Hopfield rule. In each panel the network takes an initial state corresponding to the first training pattern at half strength (the pattern vector is multiplied by 0.5) and is asynchronously updated 100 times. (A) The network reaches the stable state corresponding to the first training pattern. (B) The connectivity matrix is "lesioned" through element-by-element multiplication by a "lesioning" matrix having 25% 0s and 75% 1s at randomly determined locations. The lesioned network also reaches the stable state corresponding to the first training pattern. (C) The already lesioned connectivity matrix is again lesioned with a fresh (re-randomized) lesioning matrix and asynchronously updated 100 times. It reaches a stable state that is close to, but different from, the first training pattern. (D) The already twice lesioned connectivity matrix is again lesioned with a fresh (re-randomized) lesioning matrix and asynchronously updated 100 times. It does not reach a stable state.

training patterns for this example, so the pattern you observe when you run this simulation will be different from the one shown in Figure 4.8A.

To simulate neurological damage we will "lesion" the connectivity matrix. To do this we will generate a "shotgun" lesioning matrix, of the same size as the Hopfield connectivity matrix, in which each element has probability 0.25 of taking value 0 and probability 0.75 of taking value 1. This can be done using `[dum,nUnits]=size(HP)` (where `dum` is an unused placeholder variable) and `shotgun=rand(nUnits)>0.25`. The connectivity matrix can be "lesioned" by element-wise multiplication of the connectivity and the shotgun matrices: `HP=HP.*shotgun`, where (`.*`) corresponds to element-by-element multiplication. This command should eliminate (set to 0) about 25% of the weights in the Hopfield network weight matrix. (Note that many of the weights will already be 0.) To see the effects of the lesion we will again set the initial state to the first training pattern at half strength using `yInitial=0.5*P(1,:)'`. (This step is unnecessary if you have not changed `yInitial` since the last simulation.) Then we will update the lesioned Hopfield network 100 times starting from this initial state using `YHP=AsynchUp(yInitial,HP,100)`. The result is shown in Figure 4.8B. The Hopfield network again reaches a stable state that corresponds to the first training pattern. Thus, the lesion in this case did not affect the pattern amplification ability of the Hopfield network. This recurrent auto-associative network is robust to damage.

To further damage the network we will lesion it a second time by first generating a new shotgun matrix using `shotgun=rand(nUnits)>0.25` and then lesioning the network using `HP=HP.*shotgun`. Again (if necessary) set the initial state to the first training pattern at half strength using `yInitial=0.5*P(1,:)'` and update the Hopfield network 100 times using `YHP=AsynchUp(yInitial,HP,100)`. The result is shown in Figure 4.8C. The Hopfield network again reaches a stable state. This state is not exactly the same as the first training pattern but it is close to it. This demonstrates graceful degradation. Rather than abruptly failing, the performance gradually worsens as the connections are gradually removed. Graceful degradation is another aspect of the robustness of recurrent auto-associative networks.

It is important to point out again here that the randomness of the patterns in this example, the stochasticity inherent in asynchronous updates, and the randomness involved in the lesioning procedure will cause the results to vary considerably from simulation to simulation. For this reason it is necessary to generate several random pattern sets and run the simulation several times to get a feel for network behavior. The results on any give run are unlikely to resemble those shown in Figure 4.8. The results in the figure are meant as representative of the types of network behavior observed.

We will lesion the Hopfield connectivity matrix a third time using `shotgun=rand(nUnits)>0.25` and `HP=HP.*shotgun`. Again (if necessary) set the initial state to the first training pattern at half strength using `yInitial=0.5*P(1,:)'` and update the Hopfield network 100 times using `YHP=AsynchUp(yInitial,HP,100)`. The result is shown in Figure 4.8D. Even though the updates are asynchronous, the Hopfield network does not seem to reach a stable state in this case. This may be due to asymmetry that has been introduced into the connectivity matrix by the lesioning process. Remember that an important condition for stability of the Hopfield network is weight matrix symmetry (see Section 4.2). Our shotgun matrices had 0s at random locations, and they were generally asymmetric. Thus, the lesions they inflicted not only eliminated weights from the connectivity matrix, but they also made it asymmetric. It is possible that matrix asymmetry is preventing the network from reaching a stable state. This last simulation demonstrates that there is a limit to the amount of damage a Hopfield network can sustain and still produce correct, or nearly correct, pattern amplification or completion.

4.6   Simulating Storage and Recall of a Sequence of Patterns

The last simulation of the previous section suggested that the introduction of asymmetry into the connectivity matrix of a Hopfield, recurrent auto-associative neural network could prevent it from reaching a stable state. Although asymmetry might appear detrimental to the performance of a Hopfield network, in some contexts it might be beneficial. Real neurobiological memory often involves more than just reaching a stable state. It sometimes requires recall of a sequence of states. While reaching a stable state might be the equivalent of recalling a word from a partial word (like reaching "HAPPY" from "APPY"), recalling a sequence might be the equivalent of recalling a whole phrase (such as "HAPPY BIRTHDAY TO YOU!"). Hopfield (1982) suggested that networks could be trained to move in sequence from one state to another if their connectivity matrices had a symmetric component, due to the sum of the covariation of each pattern with itself, and an asymmetric component, due to the sum of the covariation of each pattern with the next one in the sequence. Such covariation matrices can be generated from a set of patterns using script `AsimConnectivity`, which is listed in MATLAB Box 4.4. This script uses the matrix method to generate the symmetric component of the connectivity matrix, and the outer product method to generate the asymmetric component.

We will demonstrate movement over a sequence of states by a Hopfield network having 50 units. The network is trained on 3 patterns generated using the following commands: `P=zeros(3,50)`, `P(1,[1:2:49])=1`, `P(2,[1:5 11:15 21:25 31:35 41:45])=1`, and `P(3,[2:2:50])=1`. The first pattern has value 1 for every odd element and 0 for every even element. The third

MATLAB® BOX 4.4   **This script makes asymmetric Hopfield connection weight matrices for sequence recall in recurrent auto-associative neural networks.**

```
% AsimConnectivity.m
% this script makes an asymmetric Hopfield matrix (HP);
% pattern matrix P must already be available in the workspace

a=2; % set size of asymmetric modulation
[nPat,nUnits] = size(P); % find numbers of patterns and units

HP = zeros(nUnits); % zero the Hopfield connectivity matrix
HP=(2*P' -1) * (2*P -1); % compute Hopfield auto-covariation matrix
for l=1:nPat-1, % for each pair of successive patterns
    HPDW=(2*P(l+1,:)' -1) * (2*P(l,:) -1); % compute asymmetric update
    HP = HP + a*HPDW; % update entire Hopfield connectivity matrix
end % end pattern loop

MSK = (ones(nUnits) - eye(nUnits)); % construct the masking matrix
HP = HP .* MSK; % zero self-connections in Hopfield matrix
```

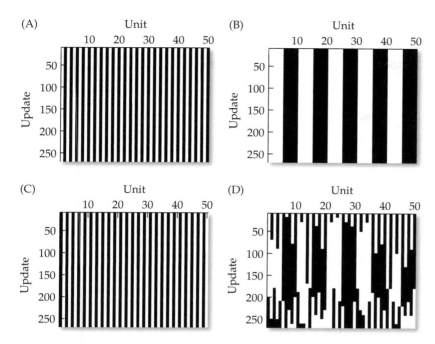

FIGURE 4.9   Sequence recall in an auto-associator Each panel is a pictorial visualization of the state vector of a recurrent auto-associator neural network having 50 units. The graphic conventions are as in Figure 4.4. The network was trained on three, binary patterns using the Hopfield rule. For the results in panels A, B, and C, the network has the symmetric connection weight matrix that is the sum of the covariation of each pattern with itself. For the results in panel D the network has the symmetric weight matrix to which is added a scaled, asymmetric matrix due to the sum of the covariations of each pattern with the next one in the sequence. Each panel shows the state of the network as it is asynchronously updated 250 times. (A) The network with symmetric connections takes an initial state corresponding to the first training pattern and stays in that state. (B) The network with symmetric connections is initialized with the second training pattern and stays in that state. (C) The network with symmetric connections is initialized with the third training pattern and stays in that state. (D) The network with added asymmetric connections is initialized with the first pattern and moves from a state corresponding to the first pattern to a state corresponding to the second pattern, and then to a state corresponding to the third pattern.

pattern has the opposite (value 0 for every odd element and 1 for every even element). The second pattern alternates between 1s and 0s every five elements. We will first verify that each of these training patterns could be a stable state of a purely auto-associative Hopfield network (symmetric connections only). To do this we will use the three patterns as before to generate a symmetric Hopfield connectivity (weight) matrix using the script `autoConnectivity` (see MATLAB Box 4.1). Then we will initialize the network with the first training pattern using `yInitial=P(1,:)'` and asynchronously update it 250 times using `YHP=AsynchUp(yInitial,HP,250)`. The result is shown in Figure 4.9A. This procedure is repeated for the second and third patterns, and the results are shown in Figure 4.9B and C, respectively. All three training patterns are stable states of the symmetric Hopfield network. This is expected since three patterns are well within the capacity of a 50-unit Hopfield network.

To demonstrate movement over a sequence of patterns we add to the symmetric connectivity matrix an asymmetric component computed as the sum of the covariation of each pattern with the next one in the sequence. Actually, the whole procedure can be carried out using `AsimConnectivity` (see MATLAB Box 4.4). Note that the asymmetric component is scaled by a factor of 2 before adding it to the symmetric component. We initialize the network with the first training pattern and asynchronously update it 250 times using `yInitial=P(1,:)'` and `YHP=AsynchUp(yInitial,HP,250)`. The result is shown in Figure 4.9D. The network clearly moves from the first training pattern to the second, and from the second to the third. Note that none of the patterns are stable states, yet the network stays in the first state for a while and then moves on to the second, and stays in the second state for a while and then moves on to the third. The asymmetric, recurrent Hopfield network is used as the starting point for models of sequence learning and sequence production in the hippocampus (e.g., Rolls and Kesner 2006). In the last section we take a closer look at the correspondence between Hopfield networks and the structural and functional properties of the hippocampus.

4.7   Hebbian Learning, Recurrent Auto-Association, and Models of Hippocampus

The hippocampus is a part of the forebrain that is heavily connected with other forebrain regions and is essential for the formation and retrieval of certain types of memories (Squire 1992). The structure and connectivity of the hippocampus is diagrammed in Figure 4.10. The hippocampus is subdivided into three regions: the dentate gyrus, in which the principle neurons are called granule cells, and areas CA3 and CA1, in which the principle neurons are called pyramidal cells. (The principle neurons in a brain region are generally larger than the other neurons, such as interneurons, and provide the main output from the region.) Distinct fiber tracts connect the three hippocampal regions. Granule cells in the dentate gyrus project as mossy fibers to pyramidal cells in CA3, and pyramidal cells in CA3 project to pyramidal cells in CA1 over Schaffer collaterals. (Neuroanatomically, a collateral is just a branch of an axonal projection.) One of the most notable features of hippocampal circuitry is that CA3 pyramidal cells also send collaterals to each other. These recurrent connections strongly resemble the recurrent connections in Hopfield and other recurrent auto-associative neural networks. This has led many researchers to search for parallels between recurrent auto-associative networks (or attractor networks) and the hippocampus (for reviews see: Rolls 1989; Rolls and Kesner 2006).

Another notable feature of the hippocampus is that the percentage of active neurons within it is low compared with other regions of the forebrain, even those that provide direct input to the hippocampus and receive direct output from it. Figure 4.11 shows schematically the volume of neural connections (roughly the number of neuronal axons) linking regions inside and outside the hippocampus to each other and, in the case of CA3, to itself. The diagram indicates that the volume of connections is considerably higher inside than outside the hippocampus. Figure 4.12 shows that the percentage of active neurons is considerably lower inside the hippocampus than in forebrain regions immediately outside it, including the entorhinal cortex, which provides input to the hippocampus, and the subiculum, which receives output from the hippocampus. These findings indicate that active neurons in the hippocampus are sparse, and imply that activity patterns that represent memories in the hippocampus would be composed of few active neurons arranged among many inactive neurons. The sparseness of active neurons in hippocampus has important implications for models of hippocampus that are based on recurrent auto-associative neural networks.

Theoretical work by Willshaw and Dayan has shown that the capacity of recurrent auto-associative neural networks increases as the density of the patterns decreases (Willshaw and Dayan 1990; Dayan and Willshaw 1991). Thus,

(A)

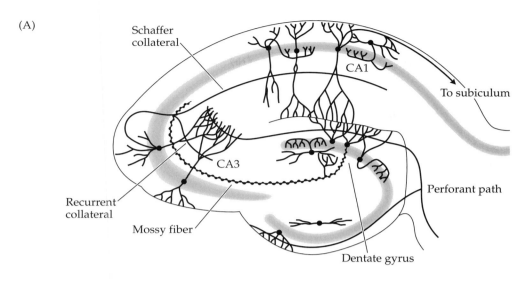

(B)

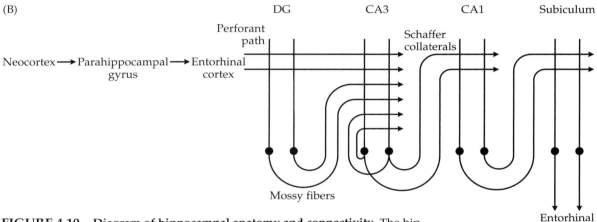

FIGURE 4.10   Diagram of hippocampal anatomy and connectivity The hippocampus is subdivided into the dentate gyrus (DG) and regions CA3 and CA1. The entorhinal cortex provides the input to the hippocampus (via the perforant path), and the subiculum receives the output from the hippocampus. (A and B) Perforant path inputs contact granule cells in the dentate gyrus and pyramidal cells in CA3. The dentate gyrus granule cells send mossy fibers to CA3 pyramidal cells. The CA3 cells also project heavily to themselves via recurrent collaterals (branched connections). The CA3 pyramidal cells project via Schaffer collaterals to CA1 pyramidal cells, and the CA1 cells project out to the subiculum. (B) Schematic representation of hippocampal connectivity, also showing interaction with neocortex, which is involved in long-term memory formation (see Chapter 14). Neocortex projects to hippocampus via parahippocampal gyrus and entorhinal cortex, and hippocampus projects back to neocortex via subiculum, entorhinal cortex, and parahippocampal gyrus. Note recurrent connections in CA3. (After Rolls 1989.)

a recurrent neural network can store and recall more patterns correctly if the patterns are sparse. A sparse binary pattern, for example, would be characterized by few 1s arranged among many 0s. Theoretical work also shows that the covariation rule produces recurrent auto-associative neural networks with the highest capacity, but that the size of the weight update should depend both on the density of the patterns and on the specific combination of pre-synaptic and post-synaptic activity at the connection being updated (Willshaw and Dayan 1990; Dayan and Willshaw 1991). Recall that the four post-synaptic/pre-synaptic activity combinations for binary units are (1, 1), (1, 0), (0, 1), and

FIGURE 4.11   Diagram illustrating the volume of connections between brain regions within and outside the hippocampus   The hippocampal regions include the dentate gyrus, CA3, and CA1. Connections to the hippocampus (via the perforant path) and within the hippocampus (via the Schaffer collaterals, recurrent collaterals, and mossy fibers) are broad and diffuse (broad white arrows). Regions outside the hippocampus that are involved in long-term memory formation (see Chapter 14) include the entorhinal cortex (which provides input to the hippocampus), the subiculum (which receives output from the hippocampus), the parahippocampal gyrus, and the neocortex. Connections to subiculum, and between the cortical areas, are dense and narrow (thin black arrows). (After O'Reilly and McClelland 1994.)

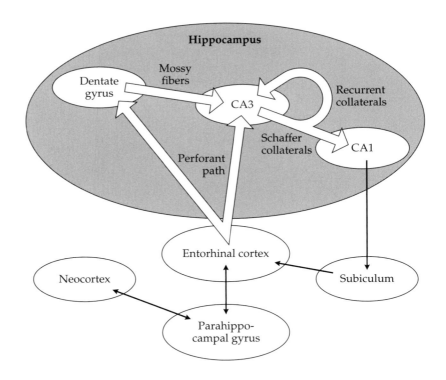

(0, 0). The covariation (Hopfield) rule stipulates connection weight increases for (1, 1) and (0, 0) and weight decreases for (1, 0) and (0, 1) (see Table 4.1). The theory confirms what we observed for covariation learning in Section 4.3, that weight increases for (1, 1) and (0, 0) and weight decreases for (1, 0) and (0, 1) all contribute toward the ability of a recurrent neural network to recall and separate patterns. But the theory goes beyond that and tells us that the amount of weight change that is optimal for recall should differ for the various post-synaptic/pre-synaptic activity combinations and should depend on the density of the patterns.

Consider a dense set of binary patterns in which each element as a 50% chance of being a 1, so that the mean activity over all elements in all patterns is 0.5. Note that such patterns would require probabilities of activation of 0.5 in the units that represent them. For Hopfield networks, the theory essentially tells us that the positive weights due to positive covariation, and the negative weights due to negative covariation, will balance out and produce optimal

FIGURE 4.12   **Activity levels in brain regions within and immediately outside the hippocampus**   The percentage of active neurons is relatively low in all of these regions (less than 10%). However, the percentage of active neurons in entorhinal cortex (EC), which provides input to the hippocampus, and in subiculum (Sub), which receives output from the hippocampus, is notably higher than the percentage of active neurons within the hippocampus itself (dentate gyrus (DG), CA3, and CA1). (After O'Reilly and McClelland 1994.)

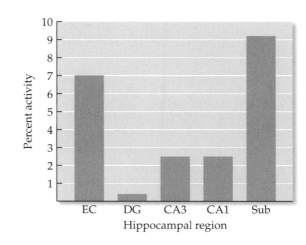

TABLE 4.6 Optimal auto-associative covariation learning rules

Unit activations				
Post-synaptic	1	1	0	0
Pre-synaptic	1	0	1	0
Weight updates				
Optimal	$(1-p_d)^2$	$-p_d(1-p_d)$	$-p_d(1-p_d)$	p_d^2
$p_d = 0.5$	+0.25	−0.25	−0.25	+0.25
$p_d = 0.1$	+0.81	−0.09	−0.09	+0.01
$p_d = 0.01$	+0.98	−0.01	−0.01	+0.0001

Listed are the optimal covariation rule formulas and weight-change values for three different probabilities p_d (pattern density probabilities) with which each element in the binary training patterns takes value 1.

Source: After Willshaw and Dayan 1990.

pattern recall and separation for these dense patterns. Now consider a sparse set of binary patterns in which each element only has a 1% chance of being a 1, so that the mean activity over all elements (and network units) in all patterns is 0.01. With such sparse activity the need for negative weights to separate overlapping patterns is less critical, while the positive weights that develop due to the overwhelming occurrence of the (0, 0) activity pattern are actually damaging to recall because they will tend to activate units that should be inactive in sparse patterns. Thus the optimal weight change for each activity combination should be a function of the mean activity of the units, which is the same as the probability that any unit (and likewise any pattern element) is active for a given set of patterns.

Willshaw and Dayan (1990) found the theoretically optimal weight updates for the covariation rule, which are shown in Table 4.6. The numerical values of the updates are computed for patterns of different densities, where the value of p_d signifies the probability (pattern density probability) with which each element of each binary pattern takes value 1. For $p_d = 0.5$ the optimal covariation rule is a scaled version of the Hopfield rule shown in Table 4.1. As the pattern density probability decreases to $p_d = 0.1$ and to $p_d = 0.01$, meaning that the patterns become progressively sparser, the optimal rule resembles more and more the classic Hebb rule. These theoretical results suggest that the Hebb rule should outperform the Hopfield rule for sparse patterns, which is the opposite of what we observed in Section 4.3 using dense patterns. We can confirm this suggestion (see also Exercises 4.2 and 4.3).

We will use asynchronous updates for this example. We will begin with a variation on the synchronous simulation from Section 4.3 using asynchronous updates. Use command P=[1 1 1 1 1 0 0 0 0 0; 1 0 1 0 1 0 1 0 1 0], to enter patterns consistent with Equation 4.15 into the MATLAB workspace. Note that the elements in these dense patterns are active at 50%, or with probability 0.5. Use script autoConnectivity (see MATLAB Box 4.1) to generate weight matrices from these patterns for Hebb (matrix HB) and Hopfield (matrix HP) recurrent auto-associator networks. Set the initial state to an incomplete and corrupted version of the first dense training pattern using yInitial=[1 1 1 1 0 0 0 0 0 1]′, and asynchronously update the Hebb network 100 times from this initial state using YHB=AsynchUp(yInitial,HB,100). Do the same for the Hopfield network using YHP=AsynchUp(yInitial,HP,100). The results are shown in Figure 4.13.

As we observed in Section 4.3 using synchronous updates, the Hebb network using asynchronous updates also fails to recall the first dense training

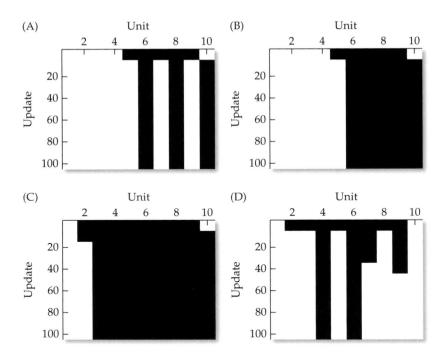

FIGURE 4.13 **Recall in auto-associators depends on pattern density** Each panel is a pictorial visualization of the state vector of a Hebb or Hopfield recurrent auto-associator network having 10 units. The graphic conventions are as in Figure 4.4. The networks in A and B were trained on the two dense patterns shown in Equation 4.15, and both networks take the initial state **y** = [1 1 1 1 0 0 0 0 0 1], which is an incomplete, corrupted version of the first dense training pattern (see Equation 4.15). The networks in C and D were trained on the two sparse patterns shown in Equation 4.17, and both networks take the initial state **y** = [1 0 0 0 0 0 0 0 0 1], which is an incomplete, corrupted version of the first sparse training pattern (see Equation 4.17). All networks undergo 100 asynchronous updates. (A) The network trained with the Hebb rule on the dense patterns reaches the spurious stable state **y** = [1 1 1 1 1 0 1 0 1 0]. (B) The network trained with the Hopfield rule on the dense patterns successfully recalls the first dense training pattern **y** = [1 1 1 1 1 0 0 0 0 0]. (C) The network trained with the Hebb rule on the sparse patterns successfully recalls the first sparse training pattern **y** = [1 1 0 0 0 0 0 0 0 0]. (D) The network trained with the Hopfield rule on the sparse patterns reaches the spurious stable state **y** = [1 1 1 0 1 0 1 1 1 1]. The results show that the Hopfield rule outperforms the Hebb rule for dense patterns, but Hebb outperforms Hopfield for sparse patterns.

pattern from an incomplete and corrupted version of it, and instead settles to a spurious state that is a combination of the first and second training patterns (Figure 4.13A). In contrast, the Hopfield network successfully recalls the pattern using asynchronous updates (Figure 4.13B). As we observed in Section 4.3 and observe again here, the Hopfield network was able to separate the dense, overlapping patterns but the Hebb network was not. This situation is reversed using sparse patterns.

To confirm this we will train both a Hebb and a Hopfield network on the following set of two patterns shown in Equation 4.17:

$$\mathbf{P} = \begin{bmatrix} 1 & 1 & 0 & 0 & 0 & 0 & 0 & 0 & 0 & 0 \\ 0 & 0 & 0 & 1 & 0 & 1 & 0 & 0 & 0 & 0 \end{bmatrix} \qquad \textbf{4.17}$$

Note that the elements in these sparse patterns are active at 20%, or with probability 0.2. This probability is small enough that the Hebb rule outperforms the Hopfield rule, as we shall see. Use P=[1 1 0 0 0 0 0 0 0 0; 0 0 0 1 0 1 0 0 0 0] to enter patterns consistent with Equation 4.17 into the MATLAB workspace, and use autoConnectivity to generate weight matrices from these patterns for Hebb (matrix HB) and Hopfield (matrix HP) networks, as before. Set the initial state to an incomplete and corrupted version of the first sparse training pattern using yInitial=[1 0 0 0 0 0 0 0 0 1]' and asynchronously update the Hebb network 100 times from this initial state using YHB=AsynchUp(yInitial,HB,100). Do the same for the Hopfield network using YHP=AsynchUp(yInitial,HP,100). This time the Hebb network correctly recalls the first training pattern (Figure 4.13C), while the Hopfield network settles to a spurious state that is the reverse of the second training pattern (Figure 4.13D). Note that, due to the randomness inherent in asynchronous updates, the results you obtain will differ from run to run, but will generally be consistent with the results presented in Figure 4.13. Intertrial variability would be avoided using synchronous updates but, interestingly, synchronous updates cause both networks to oscillate in this task. In any case, the simulation demonstrates that the Hebb rule outperforms the Hopfield rule when patterns are sparse.

The interplay between theoretical and experimental results concerning sparseness provides support for the hypothesis that the hippocampus, specifically the CA3 region, functions as a recurrent auto-associative neural network. Theoretical work shows that recurrent auto-associative neural networks are more capacious for sparse patterns (Willshaw and Dayan 1990). Experimental work indicates that activity in the hippocampus is indeed sparse (see Figures 4.11 and 4.12). Theoretical work also shows that the optimal rule approaches the classic Hebb rule for very sparse patterns (see Table 4.6). Experimental work provides convincing evidence for the Hebb rule as the rule underlying synaptic plasticity in the hippocampus (Bliss and Lømo 1973; Neves et al. 2008). This confluence of theoretical and experimental work is augmented by more recent observations supporting the hypothesis that the CA3 region of hippocampus functions as a recurrent auto-associative (attractor) network (Rolls 2007). Evidence includes the findings that CA3 can undergo one-trial (i.e., single-exposure, non-iterative) learning and is capable of pattern completion, and that CA3 may also be involved in the recall of sequences.

Like all of the models in this book, models of hippocampus based on recurrent auto-associative neural networks are hypotheses that must be evaluated through experiment. At this stage, further experimental validation is required before auto-association in recurrent neural networks can be accepted as a theory for hippocampal function. For now, recurrent auto-associative neural networks can be appreciated as among the most beautiful and elegant paradigms in all of computational neuroscience, and may yet provide real insight into the function of brain systems involved in memory, including the hippocampus.

Exercises

4.1   Recurrent auto-associator neural networks trained on a certain pattern can be used to recall that pattern by reaching the corresponding stable state from an initial state corresponding to an incomplete pattern. These auto-associators can be used in a similar way to amplify signals and reduce noise, provided that the signals correspond to stable states of the network. To see this, train a recurrent auto-associator using the Hopfield rule on the following patterns shown in Equation E4.1:

$$P = \begin{bmatrix} 1 & 1 & 1 & 1 & 1 & 0 & 0 & 0 & 0 & 0 \\ 0 & 0 & 0 & 0 & 0 & 1 & 1 & 1 & 1 & 1 \end{bmatrix} \qquad \text{E4.1}$$

This set of two patterns can be loaded into the MATLAB workspace using the command `P=[1 1 1 1 1 0 0 0 0 0; 0 0 0 0 0 1 1 1 1 1]`. The script `autoConnectivity` (see MATLAB Box 4.1) can accomplish the required training, and it will store the weights of the Hopfield network in matrix `HP`. Then set the initial state of the network to `yInitial=[0.4 0.3 0.5 0.3 0.4 0.2 0.1 0.1 0.2 0.1]'` and asynchronously update the network 100 times. This can be done using the command `AsynchUp(yInitial,HP,100)`. Without a semicolon following the command the resulting state array `Y` will by displayed on the monitor. You might want to run this several times. What happens?

4.2 A recurrent auto-associator neural network trained using the Hopfield rule has a capacity, in terms of the number of patterns it can correctly recall, of about 15% of the number of units in the network. To see this, generate a set of 5 binary patterns, each having 20 elements, where each element takes value 1 with probability 0.5. This can be done using `Phld=double(0.5>rand(5,20))`, where `double` ensures that the 1 and 0 pattern elements can be used as real (double precision) numbers in calculations. Train a 20-unit Hopfield network on the first pattern `P=Phld(1,:)` (using `autoConnectivity`), then initialize it with that pattern at half strength (`yInitial=0.5*Phld(1,:)'`) and asynchronously update the network 100 times (`AsynchUp(yInitial,HP,100)`). Does the network correctly recall the pattern? Repeat the entire process (retraining and retesting) with two (`P=Phld(1:2,:)`), three (`P=Phld(1:3,:)`), four (`P=Phld(1:4,:)`), and then all five patterns (`P=Phld`). Each time, test the network on all of the patterns used to train it. How many patterns can it correctly recall?

4.3 The capacity of a recurrent auto-associator network depends both on the rule used train the network and on the density/sparseness of the patterns. In Exercise 4.2 we tested the capacity of a 20-unit network by training it using the Hopfield rule on increasing numbers of patterns and seeing how many the network could correctly recall. The patterns were binary, and each element had probability 0.5 of being a 1. Repeat Exercise 4.2, but set up the binary patterns so that each element has probability 0.1 of being a 1. What is the capacity of the Hopfield network for these sparser patterns? Does the Hopfield network have a higher capacity for the sparse (probability 0.1) or the dense (probability 0.5) patterns? Now use the Hebb rule to train the network on the sparse or dense patterns and test its capacity with increasing numbers of patterns. Does the Hebb network have a higher capacity for the sparse or the dense patterns?

4.4 Hopfield networks with asymmetric weight matrices are not guaranteed to reach stable states and may pass from one stable state to another. Train a 50-unit Hopfield network on 3 binary patterns constructed using commands: `P=zeros(3,50)`, `P(1, [1:2:49])=1`, `P=(2, [1:5 11:15 21:25 31:35 41:45])=1`, and `P=(3, [2:2:50])=1`. Train the network symmetrically on the covariations of each pattern with itself, and also asymmetrically on the covariation between the first and second, and the second and third patterns. This is done automatically using `AsimConnectivity` (see MATLAB Box 4.4). Then initialize the network with the first pattern and asynchronously update it 750 times: `yInitial=P(1,:)'` and `AsynchUp(yInitial,HP,750)`. Does the state of the network cycle from pattern to pattern? Does it cycle through a pattern that is not a training pattern? How would you characterize that spurious pattern?

References

Amit DJ (1989) *Modeling Brain Function: The World of Attractor Neural Networks.* Cambridge University Press, New York.

Bliss TVP, Lømo T (1973) Long-lasting potentiation of synaptic transmission in the dentate area of the anaesthetized rabbit following stimulation of the perforant path. *Journal of Physiology* (London) 232: 331–356.

Buhmann J, Schulten K (1986) Associative recognition and storage in a model network of physiological neurons. *Biological Cybernetics* 54: 319–335.

Cohen MA, Grossberg S (1983) Absolute stability of global pattern formation and parallel memory storage by competitive neural networks. *IEEE Transactions on Systems, Man, and Cybernetics* SMC-13: 815–826.

Dayan P, Willshaw DJ (1991) Optimizing synaptic learning rules in linear associative memories. *Biological Cybernetics* 65: 253–265.

Haykin S (1999) *Neural Networks: A Comprehensive Foundation.* Prentice Hall, Upper Saddle River, N J, pp 680–709.

Hebb DO (1949) *The Organization of Behavior: A Neuropsychological Theory.* Wiley, New York.

Hopfield JJ (1982) Neural networks and physical systems with emergent collective computational abilities. *Proceedings of the National Academy of Sciences* 79: 2554–2558.

Hopfield JJ (1984) Neurons with graded response have collective computational properties like those of two-state neurons. *Proceedings of the National Academy of Sciences* 81: 3088–3092.

Luenberger DG (1979) *Introduction to Dynamic Systems: Theory, Models, and Applications.* John Wiley and Sons, New York.

Marr D (1971) Simple memory: A theory for archicortex. *Philosophical Transactions of the Royal Society* (London) B 262: 23–81.

Miller KD, MacKay DJC (1994) The role of constraints in Hebbian learning. *Neural Computation* 6: 100–126.

Neves, G, Cooke SF, Bliss TVP (2008) Synaptic plasticity, memory and the hippocampus: A neural network approach to causality. *Nature Reviews Neuroscience* 9: 65–75.

Noble B, Daniel JW (1988) *Applied Linear Algebra, Third Edition*. Prentice Hall, Englewood Cliffs, NJ.

Orchard GA, Phillips WA (1991) *Neural Computation: A Beginners Guide*. Lawrence Erlbaum, East Sussex, pp 37–55.

O'Reilly RC, McClelland JL (1994) Hippocampal conjunctive encoding, storage, and recall: Avoiding a trade-off. *Hippocampus* 4: 661–682.

Rolls ET (1989) Functions of neuronal networks in the hippocampus and neocortex in memory. In: Byrne JH, Berry WO (eds) *Neural Models of Plasticity: Experimental and Theoretical Approaches*. Academic Press, San Diego, pp 240–265.

Rolls ET (2007) An attractor network in the hippocampus: Theory and neurophysiology. *Learning and Memory* 14: 714–731.

Rolls ET, Kesner RP (2006) A computational theory of hippocampal function, and empirical tests of the theory. *Progress in Neurobiology* 79: 1–48.

Singer W (1985) Activity-dependent self-organization of synaptic connections as a substrate of learning. In: Changeux JP, Konishi M (eds) *The Neural and Molecular Bases of Learning*. Wiley, New York, pp 301–335.

Squire LR (1992) Memory and the hippocampus: A synthesis from findings with rats, monkeys, and humans. *Psychological Review* 99: 195–231.

Smith DM, Mizumori SJ (2006) Hippocampal place cells, context, and episodic memory. *Hippocampus* 16: 716–729.

Stanton P, Sejnowski TJ (1989) Associative long-term depression in the hippocampus: Induction of synaptic plasticity by Hebbian covariance. *Nature* 339: 215–218.

Stent GS (1973) A physiological mechanism for Hebb's postulate of learning. *Proceedings of the National Academy of Sciences* 70: 997–1001.

Willshaw DJ, Dayan P (1990) Optimal plasticity in matrix memories: What goes up must come down. *Neural Computation* 2: 85–93.

5

Unsupervised Learning and Distributed Representations

Unsupervised learning algorithms, given only a set of input patterns, can train neural networks to form distributed representations of those patterns that resemble brain maps

Although objectively the same entity, the face you see at one moment has a different configuration from the same face you see after it turns a moment later. Extending this example to all objects and all sensory modalities convinces us that the world presents to the brain an unlimited number of sensory input patterns. In order for the brain to make computations that have functional relevance in the world it must first represent these highly variable input patterns. How the brain manages to create a sufficiently rich representation of the world has been a central question in neuroscience. In this chapter we will explore mechanisms by which the brain may learn to represent sensory input configurations efficiently.

The human brain has on the order of 10^{11} neurons. The monkey brain has maybe one-tenth as many, and other animals have fewer still, but the fact remains that brains in general contain a lot of neurons. A brain could represent the world by assigning individual neurons to individual input configurations, but that would not be the most efficient use of its neuronal resources. Instead, the brain appears to develop neurons that are most responsive to particular input patterns, but can also respond, though less intensely, to similar input patterns. Then a particular input is encoded by a whole population of neurons, each one responding according to the similarity between the current input configuration and its preferred configuration. In this way even a relatively small population of neurons can represent many different input patterns. This type of efficient encoding, in which an input configuration is represented by the activity of many neurons, is known as a distributed representation (Hinton et al. 1986).

A beautiful example of this is provided by "face cells," which have been discovered in the lower (inferior) part of the temporal cortex in monkeys (Desimone et al. 1984). These neurons are specialists for monkey faces seen at particular orientations (such as from the front or in profile). A face cell will respond, by increasing its firing rate, when presented with an image of a monkey face at its preferred orientation (Figure 5.1). Importantly, it will also respond, though progressively less intensely, for images that differ more and more from the preferred facial image of the cell. Thus, a face cell is a "specialist" in that it has a preferred stimulus configuration, but it is also "broadly tuned" in that it will also respond (although less intensely) to non-preferred stimuli that are similar to its preferred stimulus. Putting both notions together, we could describe a face cell as a "broadly tuned specialist," and describe its response as proportional to the similarity between the actual and the preferred stimulus configuration of the cell.

Because all the neurons in the face area of the monkey inferotemporal cortex can be characterized as broadly tuned specialists, the representation in this region for any particular face is encoded by the whole population of cells, each one responding according to the similarity between the face currently in view and its own preferred face. One important aspect of this representation is that it does not require a specialist for every possible type of face. In the simplest case, a particular face that is intermediate between the preferred faces of two face cells would be encoded by both cells responding at intermediate levels. Another aspect of this kind of representation is that a cell with the same preferred face as another face cell contributes nothing to the expressive power of the representation. These ideas can be extended to the whole population, which achieves its greatest expressive power when every cell is a specialist for its own unique, preferred face. By appropriately tuning the preferred faces of the available cells, the population could produce distinct representations for the many faces it encounters. Another interesting (and possibly important) aspect of the representation of faces in the monkey inferotemporal cortex is that the region is organized as a map, in which neurons with similar preferred faces are located near each other on the cortex (Wang et al. 1996). Many other types of neurons can be characterized as broadly tuned specialists, and many other brain regions are organized as maps (Knudsen et al. 1987).

In this chapter we will study adaptive mechanisms that can train each output unit in a two-layered neural network to become a broadly tuned specialist for its own, unique input configuration. These adaptive mechanisms are neural network learning algorithms, and they accomplish their goal by training individual units to respond preferentially to input patterns that share distinct sets of common features (Haykin 1999). The algorithms are "unsupervised" in the sense that they receive no guidance concerning the nature of the output representation that they generate (in contrast to supervised and reinforcement paradigms, as described in Chapters 6 and 7).

Competitive learning represents unsupervised learning in its most basic form (Rumelhart and Zipser 1986). A competitive algorithm trains the input–output connection weights in two-layered neural networks so that each output

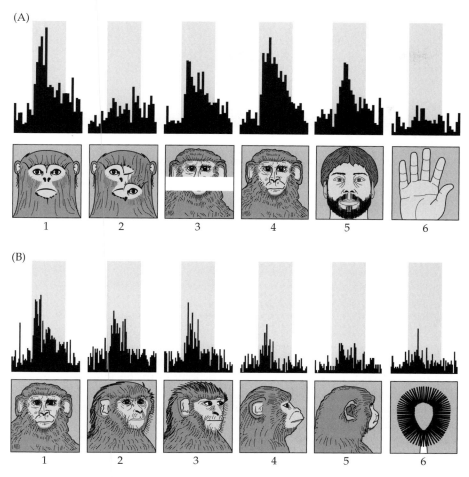

FIGURE 5.1   Reponses of a "face cell" recorded in the inferior part of the temporal cortex of a monkey Neural responses are shown as histograms where each bar is proportional to the number of action potential discharges falling within each time bin. (A) This particular face cell is specialized for faces seen from the front. It prefers whole faces of monkeys but will also respond to partial (but not scrambled) monkey faces, or to bearded human faces, seen from the front. (B) This face cell also responds, but progressively less intensely, to faces rotated away from the frontal view. Thus, this face cell is a "broadly tuned specialist" in that it responds best for a face of a specific type (monkey) and of a specific orientation (frontal) but will also respond, though progressively less intensely, to stimuli that differ more and more from its preferred stimulus. (After Desimone et al. 1984.)

unit becomes specialized for its own unique, preferred input configuration (pattern). Self-organizing map (SOM) algorithms (Kohonen 1982, 1997) add cooperation to competition, and train the connection weights so that output units that have similar preferred input patterns will actually be close together in the output layer, thereby forming a "map" of the features over the network. The simulated maps formed by the SOM often resemble real brain maps. The algorithms are neurobiologically plausible, especially considering that all they need is exposure to the input. Much of the development of the real nervous system is known to occur through exposure to the sensory environment (Knudsen et al. 1987). We will explore both forms of unsupervised learning, competitive and SOM, in detail in this chapter.

Notions such as input configuration (or input pattern), and the similarity between an input pattern and a preferred pattern, can be formalized in terms of feature vectors and feature spaces. A very simple (and slightly whimsical) example is illustrated in Table 5.1. Along the top of the table are listed seven attributes of various animals (fur, barks, meows, fins, gills, feathers, and wings). Along the left edge of Table 5.1 are listed five specific types of animals (dog, cat, fish, bird, and bat). The rows of the table are the feature vectors that describe each animal. The "dog" feature vector is [1 1 0 0 0 0 0], because the dog has fur and it barks, but it does not meow, nor does it have fins, gills, feathers, or wings. The "cat" feature vector [1 0 1 0 0 0 0] is the same as the "dog" feature vector except at two places, indicating that the cat does not bark but does meow. The "fish" feature vector [0 0 0 1 1 0 0] and the "bird" feature

TABLE 5.1   Using animals to illustrate the concepts of feature vector and feature space

	Fur	Barks	Meows	Fins	Gills	Feathers	Wings
Dog	1	1	0	0	0	0	0
Cat	1	0	1	0	0	0	0
Fish	0	0	0	1	1	0	0
Bird	0	0	0	0	0	1	1
Bat	1	0	0	0	0	0	1

An item, such as an animal, can be described as a set of elements in a feature vector. Items that have overlapping feature vectors are "neighbors" in that their vectors are closer to each other than to non-overlapping vectors in feature space. Elements of feature vectors need not be binary.

vector [0 0 0 0 0 1 1], in contrast, share features neither with the "dog" nor the "cat" vectors, nor with each other. Interestingly, the "bat" feature vector [1 0 0 0 0 0 1] shares one feature with both "dog" and "cat" (fur) and shares one other feature with "bird" (wings), but none with "fish." (Note that feature vectors need not be binary in general.)

These "animal" feature vectors are located in a seven-dimensional feature space, with one dimension for each feature. Of course, the complete description of an animal would require a tremendously long feature vector. Seven features are enough to illustrate the principles involved, but still, a seven-dimensional vector space is very hard (probably impossible) to visualize. Fortunately, similarity among vectors is easy to determine. Regardless of the dimension of the feature space, feature vectors that overlap (i.e., share non-zero elements in common) point in similar directions in that space (Noble and Daniel 1988). Thus, the "dog" and "cat" feature vectors are "neighbors" because they fall in the same vector cluster in feature space. The "fish" and "bird" vectors are neighbors neither of each other nor of "dog" and "cat." The "bat" vector points in a direction between the "dog–cat" cluster (of two vectors) and the "bird" vector.

Input patterns in unsupervised learning can be thought of as feature vectors. We could use competitive learning to train a two-layered network with seven input units, one for each feature, and five output units, one for each animal, on the five feature vectors in Table 5.1. The result would be that each output unit would learn to specialize for its own unique feature vector, or "animal." Thus, one output unit would be specialized for "dog," one for "cat," and so on for the other animals, but the locations of the units in the output layer would be independent of their preferred input patterns (feature vectors). When trained using the SOM, output units that specialize for input patterns that are neighbors in feature space will also be neighbors the network, thereby forming a map of the features over the network. Following SOM training on the "animal" patterns, output units that prefer the "dog" and "cat" patterns would be neighbors, and "bat" units would be located between "dog–cat" and "bird" units, but the locations of "fish" units would not depend on the locations of units preferring the other "animal" patterns. We will use competitive learning to demonstrate the basic operation of unsupervised algorithms, and will then use the SOM to simulate the formation of some well-known brain maps.

Unlike covariation learning (see Chapter 4), in which weight training requires only one exposure to each pattern to be learned, unsupervised learning is an iterative process. As such, input patterns must be presented repeatedly to the network, and small weight adjustments are made on each training iteration. (Note that most neural network learning algorithms are iterative, and all of the algorithms we will consider in this and later chapters in this book are iterative.)

Input units   Output units

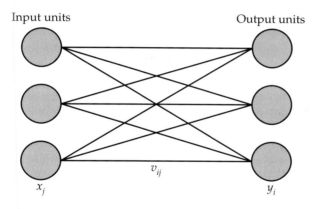

v_{ij}

x_j y_i

FIGURE 5.2 **A generic, two-layered neural network** The x_j are input units, the y_i are output units, and the v_{ij} are the weights of the connections from input to output units. The index ranges are $j = 1, ..., n_x$ and $i = 1, ..., n_y$, where n_x and n_y are the numbers of input and output units, respectively.

As mentioned above, unsupervised learning algorithms are generally used to train neural networks having two layers, one input and one output (Figure 5.2), where input units x_j (in input state vector **x**) project to output units y_i (in output state vector **y**) over weights v_{ij} (in matrix **V**). The number of input units n_x ($j = 1, ..., n_x$) can be different from the number of output units n_y ($i = 1, ..., n_y$). The responses of the output units y_i in networks trained using unsupervised learning are most easily interpreted if the output units are linear. (We will use only linear output units in this chapter, but certain types of nonlinear units, such as sigmoidal units, could also be used in networks that undergo unsupervised training.) The input–output connection weights **V** are positive (i.e., excitatory), and are randomized before learning begins.

Competitive learning is known as such because the output units compete for preferred input patterns (Rumelhart and Zipser 1986). In the simplest case, this competition involves choosing the output unit with the largest response to a given input pattern (the "winner"). The algorithm then specifies that the connection weights to the winning output unit from all input units should be adjusted so that the winner will be *even more* sensitive to this input pattern and those like it. The algorithm also specifies that the winner should become *less* sensitive to unlike patterns, leaving other output units to win the competitions for those. This training process is repeated each time an input pattern is chosen from the pool at random, presented to the network, the winning output unit is determined, and its weights from the inputs are adjusted. After many iterations, competitive learning causes the output units to specialize so that each one responds best to a distinct feature vector (input pattern).

The SOM algorithm is an elaboration of competitive learning. It stipulates not only that the winning output unit, but also its neighbors, should undergo weight adjustments. In this case, the network becomes organized so that output units that are near to each other in the network respond to input patterns that are near in feature space. Thus, SOM training leads to map formation. We can consider competitive learning as a special case of the SOM in which the training neighborhood consists only of the winning output unit.

Kohonen (1982, 1997) expressed the three steps in the SOM algorithm as shown in Equations 5.1–5.3:

$$\mathbf{y} = \mathbf{V}\mathbf{x} \qquad\qquad \textbf{5.1}$$

$$y_m = \max_i \{y_i\} \qquad\qquad \textbf{5.2}$$

$$\mathbf{V}_{\text{row } h}(c+1) = \frac{\mathbf{V}_{\text{row } h}(c) + a\,\mathbf{x}^{\mathrm{T}}(c)}{\left\|\mathbf{V}_{\text{row } h}(c) + a\,\mathbf{x}^{\mathrm{T}}(c)\right\|_2} \qquad\qquad \textbf{5.3}$$

where input vector $\mathbf{x}$ has elements x_j ($j = 1, ..., n_x$) and output vector $\mathbf{y}$ has elements y_i ($i = 1, ..., n_y$). Equation 5.1 simply expresses that the output unit response vector $\mathbf{y}$ is the product of connection weight matrix $\mathbf{V}$ and input vector $\mathbf{x}$. Equation 5.2 embodies the output unit competition most simply, by finding the output unit with the maximal response (element y_m), where m equals the index i of the winning output unit. On each update cycle c, Equation 5.3 trains the input weights to all output units y_h, where h is the subset of indices i of the output units to be trained. The subset of indices in h includes index m of the winner y_m and the indices of any of its specified neighbors (so h indexes the training neighborhood).

Essentially, the SOM weight update involves adding a scaled version of the input vector to the weight vector of the winning output unit, and to the input weight vectors of the other output units in the training neighborhood. The vector of input weights to a unit y_h is the hth row of weight matrix $\mathbf{V}$ ($\mathbf{V}_{\text{row } h}$ is row h of the connectivity matrix $\mathbf{V}$). Because input vector $\mathbf{x}$ is a column, we must transpose it before we can add it to row vector $\mathbf{V}_{\text{row } h}$. (Note that $\mathbf{x}^T$ is the transpose of $\mathbf{x}$, where superscript T is the transpose operator.) Before adding it to the weights in $\mathbf{V}_{\text{row } h}$ the transposed input vector $\mathbf{x}^T$ is scaled by learning rate a. (The learning rate a can be decremented as learning proceeds to improve the process; see Haykin 1999.) The vector sum $\mathbf{V}_{\text{row } h} + a\mathbf{x}^T$ is then normalized by dividing it by its two-norm $\| \mathbf{V}_{\text{row } h} + a\mathbf{x}^T \|_2$. (The two-norm, or Euclidean norm, is explained in Math Box 5.1.) Because the inputs and weights are non-negative in SOM learning, the weight updates are also non-negative, so normalization is needed to prevent the connection weights from growing without bound. Connection weight normalization also ensures specialization (see numerical example below). Unsupervised learning is accomplished by repeating the steps specified in Equations 5.1–5.3 for some number of training cycles. The procedure is the same for competitive as for SOM training, but for the former only the winner is trained on any iteration ($h = m$), while for the latter all of the output units in a training neighborhood encompassing the winner are trained.

The Kohonen SOM algorithm (expressed in simplest terms in Equations 5.1–5.3) is plausible neurobiologically. Equation 5.1 approximates synaptic integration as the computation by a neural unit of its weighted input sum (see Chapter 1). Equation 5.2 finds the output unit with the largest response, which determines the center of the training neighborhood. SOMs are sometimes implemented using recurrent, Mexican-hat connections between the output units. This arrangement results in activity-bubble formation that can find a winning set of output units through its intrinsic dynamics. There is good evidence that certain brain structures are also capable of forming activity bubbles (see Chapter 3). Here we will use the simpler method of simply choosing as the winner the output unit with the largest response to a given input pattern, and designating neighbors as needed. Equation 5.3 actually updates the weights. This learning mechanism is essentially Hebbian, since the synapses (connection weights) to active post-synaptic neurons (the winning output unit and its neighbors) are modified in proportion to pre-synaptic (input unit) activity (see Chapter 4 for a discussion of Hebbian learning mechanisms). The body of evidence that Hebbian forms of synaptic plasticity actually occur in the real nervous system is large and growing (Caporale and Dan 2008). The update equation involves normalization that essentially keeps constant the total amount of synaptic input to a neural unit. Homeostatic mechanisms appear to play the same role in real neurons (Turrigiano 1999; Shah and Crair 2008).

The following numerical example illustrates unsupervised learning in the purely competitive case, in which only the winning output unit is trained. Consider a two-layered network having four input units and two output units.

MATH BOX 5.1　VECTOR NORMS, NORMALIZATION, AND INNER PRODUCTS REVISITED

A vector norm provides some measure of the "size" of a vector (Noble and Daniel 1988). The three most common vector norms are shown in Equations B5.1.1–B5.1.3:

$$\|\mathbf{x}\|_1 = |x_1| + |x_2| + \cdots + |x_n| \qquad \text{B5.1.1}$$

$$\|\mathbf{x}\|_2 = \left(|x_1|^2 + |x_2|^2 + \cdots + |x_n|^2 \right)^{1/2} \qquad \text{B5.1.2}$$

$$\|\mathbf{x}\|_\infty = \max_j |x_j| \qquad \text{B5.1.3}$$

where $\|\mathbf{x}\|_1$, $\|\mathbf{x}\|_2$, and $\|\mathbf{x}\|_\infty$ are the one-, two-, and infinity-norms, respectively, and the absolute value $|x_j|$ of any element x_j ($j = 1, \ldots, n$) is used in all definitions for consistency, even in terms of the form $|x_j|^2$ where taking the absolute value is not necessary. The two-norm (Equation B5.1.2) is the Euclidian, or geometric, length of a vector. It is found using the Pythagorean theorem, as in Equation B5.1.2 or, equivalently, by finding the square root of the inner (or dot) product of the vector with itself (see Math Box 1.2 for a description of the inner product). Division of a vector by its two-norm will "normalize" the vector and make its length 1. Thus, after the vector has been normalized, the inner product of the vector with itself is 1. The inner product of two normalized vectors also equals the cosine of the angle between them. Thus, when two vectors point in the same direction, their inner product following normalization equals +1. When they point in opposite directions it equals –1, and when they point in orthogonal directions (i.e., they are at right angles to each other) it equals 0.

Connectivity matrix $\mathbf{V}$ for this network has two rows (one row for each output unit), and four columns (one column for each input unit), so that each row of $\mathbf{V}$ holds the weights to one output unit from all input units. Assume for the current weight values (from update c) that the first row of $\mathbf{V}$ is $\mathbf{V}_{row1}(c) = [0\ 0.7071\ 0\ 0.7071]$ and the second row of $\mathbf{V}$ is $\mathbf{V}_{row2}(c) = [0.5\ 0.5\ 0.5\ 0.5]$. Note that both of these weight vectors have been normalized, so that their lengths (Euclidian or two-norms) are equal to 1 (see Math Box 5.1). We wish to train the network on two input patterns (row vectors) that have the same dimension as the input vector: $\mathbf{p}_1 = [1\ 0\ 0\ 0]$ and $\mathbf{p}_2 = [0\ 1\ 0\ 0]$. (To keep track of the pattern vectors $\mathbf{p}_l$, and corresponding input vectors $\mathbf{x}_l$, we subscript them with $l = 1, \ldots, n_p$, where n_p equals the number of training patterns.)

We present input pattern 1, $\mathbf{x}_1 = \mathbf{p}_1^T = [1\ 0\ 0\ 0]^T$, and find the response of the output units to this input (see Equation 5.1) to be $\mathbf{y} = \mathbf{V}\mathbf{x}_1 = [0\ 0.5]^T$. The unit with the maximal response, or the winning output unit, is unit 2, so $m = 2$ (see Equation 5.2). We update the weight vector of output unit 2 by first adding to it a scaled version of the input vector (see Equation 5.3). If the learning rate is 1 ($a = 1$), then $\mathbf{V}_{row2}(c) + a\mathbf{x}_1^T = [0.5\ 0.5\ 0.5\ 0.5] + [1\ 0\ 0\ 0] = [1.5\ 0.5\ 0.5\ 0.5]$. The two-norm is $\|\mathbf{V}_{row2}(c) + a\mathbf{x}_1^T\|_2 = \|[1.5\ 0.5\ 0.5\ 0.5]\|_2 = 1.73$. Dividing the updated weight vector by its two-norm gives the normalized, updated weight vector for update $c + 1$ as $\mathbf{V}_{row2}(c + 1) = [0.87\ 0.29\ 0.29\ 0.29]$. The weight matrices before and after the update in this simple, numerical example are shown in Table 5.2.

TABLE 5.2　Weight matrices before and after a single, unsupervised weight update for the simple, numerical example

Before update	After update
$\mathbf{V}(c) = \begin{bmatrix} 0 & 0.7071 & 0 & 0.7071 \\ 0.5 & 0.5 & 0.5 & 0.5 \end{bmatrix}$	$\mathbf{V}(c+1) = \begin{bmatrix} 0 & 0.7071 & 0 & 0.7071 \\ 0.87 & 0.29 & 0.29 & 0.29 \end{bmatrix}$

The updated weight vector ($\mathbf{V}_{\text{row2}}(c + 1) = [0.87\ 0.29\ 0.29\ 0.29]$) is closer to input pattern vector 1 ($\mathbf{x}_1 = \mathbf{p}_1^T = [1\ 0\ 0\ 0]^T$) than the weight vector before the update ($\mathbf{V}_{\text{row2}}(c) = [0.5\ 0.5\ 0.5\ 0.5]$). Thus, the unsupervised learning algorithm has moved the weight vector for output unit 2 closer to this input vector in vector space. Because the response of output unit 2 is the inner (or dot) product of its weight vector and the input pattern vector (see Math Box 5.1), moving its weight vector closer to input pattern 1 ($\mathbf{p}_1$) makes output unit 2 more sensitive to input pattern 1 than it was before the update. This can be seen by comparing the inner products of the weight ($\mathbf{V}_{\text{row2}}$) and input ($\mathbf{x}_1 = \mathbf{p}_1^T$) vectors before ($c$) and after ($c + 1$) the update: $\mathbf{V}_{\text{row2}}(c)\ \mathbf{x}_1 = 0.5 < 0.87 = \mathbf{V}_{\text{row2}}$ ($c + 1$) $\mathbf{x}_1$. Because of weight normalization, making output unit 2 more sensitive to input pattern 1 ($\mathbf{x}_1 = \mathbf{p}_1^T = [1\ 0\ 0\ 0]^T$) necessarily makes it less sensitive to other patterns, such as input pattern 2 ($\mathbf{x}_2 = \mathbf{p}_2^T = [0\ 1\ 0\ 0]^T$). This can be seen by comparing the inner products of the weight ($\mathbf{V}_{\text{row2}}$) and input pattern 2 ($\mathbf{x}_2 = \mathbf{p}_2^T$) vectors before ($c$) and after ($c + 1$) the update: $\mathbf{V}_{\text{row2}}(c)\ \mathbf{x}_2 = 0.5 > 0.29 = \mathbf{V}_{\text{row2}}(c + 1)\ \mathbf{x}_2$. Compared with output unit 2, output unit 1 has an even stronger response to input pattern 2, after the update of the output unit 2 weight vector by input pattern 1 (compare $\mathbf{V}_{\text{row1}}(c)\ \mathbf{x}_2 = 0.7071$, $\mathbf{V}_{\text{row2}}(c)\ \mathbf{x}_2 = 0.5$, and $\mathbf{V}_{\text{row2}}(c + 1)\ \mathbf{x}_2 = 0.29$). Repeated iterations (cycles) of unsupervised training on these two patterns would cause output unit 1 to specialize for $\mathbf{x}_2 = \mathbf{p}_2^T = [0\ 1\ 0\ 0]^T$ and cause output unit 2 to specialize for $\mathbf{x}_1 = \mathbf{p}_1^T = [1\ 0\ 0\ 0]^T$. The specialization of output units for specific input patterns lies at the heart of unsupervised learning.

The computations specified by Equations 5.1–5.3, and illustrated in the numerical example, are implemented by script `KohonenSOM`, which is listed in MATLAB® Box 5.1. We will use `KohonenSOM` to train networks using simple (competitive) unsupervised learning, in which only the winner is trained, and progress to full SOM strategies in which feature maps of various types are formed.

5.1   Learning through Competition to Specialize for Specific Inputs

The ability of unsupervised learning to cause output units to specialize for specific input patterns can be demonstrated by using it to train a three-input, three-output (3-by-3) network to represent the three basis vectors in R^3. (R stands for the real numbers, and R^3 is the space that contains all vectors that have three real elements.) These basis vectors are shown as input patterns in Table 5.3A. They can be entered into the MATLAB workspace for use by script `KohonenSOM` using the command `InPat=[1 0 0;0 1 0;0 0 1]`. The script will determine the number of input patterns `nPat`, and the number of input units `nIn` required to represent those patterns, by finding the

---

TABLE 5.3   Input (A) and output (B) of a two-layered, 3-by-3 network following SOM training on the basis vectors of three-space (R^3)

(A) Input patterns			(B) Output patterns after SOM training		
1	0	0	1	0	0
0	1	0	0	0	1
0	0	1	0	1	0

MATLAB® BOX 5.1   This script implements the Kohonen self-organizing map (SOM) algorithm.

```
% KohonenSOM.m
% pattern array InPat must already be available in the workspace

nOut=3; % set the number of output units
a=1; % set the learning rate
dec=1; % set the learning rate decrement
nHood=0; % set the neighborhood size
nIts=100; % set the number of iterations
[nPat,nIn]=size(InPat); % find number of patterns and of input units
V=rand(nOut,nIn); % set initially random connectivity matrix
for c=1:nIts, % for each learning iteration
    pIndx=ceil(rand*nPat); % choose an input pattern at random
    x=InPat(pIndx,:)'; % set input vector x to chosen pattern
    y=V*x; % compute output to chosen input pattern
    [winVal winIndx]=max(y); % find the index of the winning output
    fn=winIndx-nHood; % find first neighbor in training neighborhood
    ln=winIndx+nHood; % find last neighbor in training neighborhood
    if fn < 1, fn=1; end, % keep first neighbor in bounds
    if ln > nOut, ln=nOut; end, % keep last neighbor in bounds
    for h=fn:ln, % for all units in training neighborhood
        hld=V(h,:)+a*x'; % apply Kohonen update
        V(h,:)=hld/norm(hld); % normalize new weight vector
        a=a*(dec); % decrement the learning rate
    end, % end neighbor training loop
end; % end learning loop
Out=(V*InPat')'; % find the output for all input patterns
```

numbers of rows and columns, respectively, of the input pattern array (here 3 each) using the `size` command. The required number of output units must be specified in the script by setting `nOut=3`. The script will generate an initial connectivity matrix `V` with uniformly distributed, positive random numbers using `V=rand(nOut,nIn)`. For purely competitive learning, in which only the winning output unit is trained on each iteration, the neighborhood size should be 0, so set `nHood=0`. For this simple problem we can set the learning rate to 1 using `a=1`, and we need not decrement the learning rate during training, so we can set `dec=1`. We will train for 100 iterations, so set `nIts=100`.

Each iteration begins by choosing one of the input patterns at random using `pIndx=ceil(rand*nPat)`. The variable `pIndx` is then used as an index into the input pattern array. Thus, `x=InPat(pIndx,:)'` will extract the whole row of `InPat` corresponding to input pattern `pIndx`, convert it to a column, and then set input vector `x` equal to it. (Recall that the apostrophe stands for the transpose in MATLAB.) The response of the output units to the input can be computed using `y=V*x`. The winning output unit is found using `[winVal winIndx]=max(y)`, where `winIndx` is the index of the winning output unit. Because we train only the winner in this example, the only output unit in the training neighborhood `h` is the winning output unit. Update of the weight vector `V(h,:)` of the winner begins by transposing the input vector, scaling it by the learning rate, and adding it to the weight vector using `hld=V(h,:)+a*x'`, where `hld` is an intermediate variable. Normalization using `V(h,:)=hld/norm(hld)` completes the weight vector update.

Following `nIts` training iterations, the output of the network to all the input patterns is computed in one step using `Out=(V*InPat')'`. In this command the input pattern array is transposed using `InPat'`, so that all of the patterns are arranged as columns, and matrix multiplication (see Math Box 4.3) of weight matrix `V` and the transposed input pattern matrix (`V*InPat'`) produces another matrix where the output vectors for each input pattern are arranged as columns. Transposition of that matrix produces output array `Out` where the output patterns are arranged as rows to facilitate their comparison with the input patterns. (Recall that input patterns are expressed as row vectors in this book.)

The output patterns following training on the set of input patterns corresponding to the basis vectors in R^3 are shown in Table 5.3B. Each column of numbers in Table 5.3A or B corresponds to a different input or output unit, respectively. Each row in Table 5.3A contains a different input pattern, while each row in Table 5.3B contains the output pattern produced by the trained network in response to the corresponding input pattern. For example, for input pattern [1 0 0], input units 1, 2, and 3 take values 1, 0, and 0, respectively. The output pattern for this input is also [1 0 0], meaning that output units 1, 2, and 3 produce responses of 1, 0, and 0 to input pattern 1. Thus, output unit 1 has become specialized for input pattern 1. Similarly, Table 5.3 shows that output unit 2 has become specialized for input pattern 3, and output unit 3 has become specialized for input pattern 2.

Examination of the connectivity matrix for the network after training (Table 5.4) reveals the basis of the selectivity of each output unit. (In this very simple case, in which the input patterns are just the basis vectors in R^3, the three output unit responses are the same as their weight vectors, but this is not the case in general.) Because there are as many output units as input patterns, the result of the competitive learning procedure is that each output unit weight vector aligns with a different one of the input pattern vectors. Consequently, each output unit becomes specialized for a different one of the input patterns. Specifically, the weight vectors for output units 1, 2, and 3 have become aligned with input pattern vectors 1, 3, and 2, respectively. In this case the spatial arrangement of the output units with regard to their preferred input pattern is arbitrary. Different runs of the simulation will produce different arrangements, which depend on the values in the random initial connectivity matrix and on the random order of presentation of the input patterns.

In this 3-by-3 network trained without neighbors, no map forms at the output on any run, but failure of map formation is not due only to lack of neighbor training. The three basis vectors in R^3 are mutually orthogonal, meaning that they are all at 90 degrees to one another. Because all the input pattern vectors are mutually orthogonal (and mutually non-overlapping), they are all equally distant from each other in vector space. Even if output units neighbor-

TABLE 5.4   Weight matrix for a two-layered, 3-by-3 network following SOM training on the basis vectors of R^3

	From input unit		
To output unit	**1**	**2**	**3**
1	1	0	0
2	0	0	1
3	0	1	0

ing the winner were trained, the input patterns in this example would provide no neighborhood relationships for them to represent.

In the simple example just considered there were as many output units as input patterns, but unsupervised learning is often used in contexts in which there are many more input patterns than output units. In the extreme the input patterns can vary continuously so there are infinitely many of them. Obviously, in such contexts it is impossible for every input pattern to have an output unit that is specialized for it. Instead, unsupervised learning in such contexts causes individual output units to become specialized for whole clusters of input pattern vectors. These networks can be thought of as vector quantizers, in the sense that they represent a large, and potentially infinite, number of input pattern vectors using a finite set of specialized output unit weight vectors (Haykin 1999). In the next example we will explore this clustering idea using the same 3-by-3 network, but we will use more than three input patterns.

5.2 Training Few Output Neurons to Represent Many Input Patterns

Strictly speaking, vector quantization involves the representation of a continuously varying, infinite number of input vectors using a finite set of output vectors that, in our examples, are the output unit weight vectors of two-layered neural networks. In this section we will consider a much smaller version of the general problem. We will increase the input pattern set of the last example by adding six more vectors that, together with the R^3 basis vectors, will form three clusters of vectors around the basis vectors. The set of nine input patterns is shown in Table 5.5A. They can be entered using `InPat=[5 0 0;4 1 0;3 1 1;0 5 0;0 4 1;1 3 1;0 0 5;0 1 4;1 1 3]`. To facilitate the interpretation of the results, we will normalize each input pattern vector by dividing it by its two-norm before we use the patterns to train the network. For example, for the first input pattern, normalization is accomplished using `InPat(1,:)=InPat(1,:)/norm(InPat(1,:))`. The normalized input patterns are shown in Table 5.5B.

The connectivity matrix of the 3-by-3 network is re-randomized and the network is trained on these patterns using `KohonenSOM` with the same settings as for the previous example (with `nOut=3`, `a=1`, `dec=1`, `nHood=0`, and

TABLE 5.5 **Input (A) and output (C) of a two-layered, 3-by-3 network following SOM training on the three vector clusters in R^3**

(A) Input patterns			(B) Normalized inputs			(C) Outputs after SOM		
5	0	0	1.00	0.00	0.00	0.00	0.26	0.96
4	1	0	0.97	0.24	0.00	0.24	0.32	0.99
3	1	1	0.90	0.30	0.30	0.34	0.60	0.98
0	5	0	0.00	1.00	0.00	0.99	0.29	0.26
0	4	1	0.00	0.97	0.24	0.99	0.51	0.27
1	3	1	0.30	0.90	0.30	0.93	0.62	0.55
0	0	5	0.00	0.00	1.00	0.12	0.92	0.10
0	1	4	0.00	0.24	0.97	0.36	0.96	0.16
1	1	3	0.30	0.30	0.90	0.41	0.99	0.46

Normalized input patterns are shown in B. The values in A and C are shown pictorially in Figure 5.3A and B, respectively.

MATLAB® BOX 5.2   **This script can be used to visualize SOM output responses to sets of input patterns as black-and-white images.**

```
% SOMoutImage.m
% KohonenSOM.m must be run first

inImage=zeros(nPat,nIn,3); % define 3D input image array
outImage=zeros(nPat,nOut,3); % define 3D output image array
inImage(:,:,1)=InPat; % for black-and-white, set each
inImage(:,:,2)=InPat; % dimension of the input image array
inImage(:,:,3)=InPat; % to the same intensity value
hld=Out; % place the output array in a hold array
hld=hld-min(min(hld)); % subtract the minimum value
hld=hld./max(max(hld)); % scale by the new maximal value
outImage(:,:,1)=hld; % for black-and-white, set each
outImage(:,:,2)=hld; % dimension of the output image array
outImage(:,:,3)=hld; % to the same intensity value
subplot(121) % open a subplot
image(inImage) % image the input pattern array
set(gca,'fontsize',14) % set the font size
xlabel('input unit number') % add an x-axis label
ylabel('input pattern number') % add a y-axis label
text(0,0.4,'A','fontsize',14) % label panel A
subplot(122) % open another subplot
image(outImage) % image the output array
set(gca,'fontsize',14) % set the font size
xlabel('output unit number') % add an x-axis label
ylabel('input pattern number') % add a y-axis label
text(0,0.4,'B','fontsize',14) % label panel B
```

nIts=100). The output unit responses following training are shown in Table 5.5C, in which each column corresponds to an output unit, and each row corresponds to the responses of the three output units to each input pattern. Scanning down each column of the output response array shows that output unit 1 has its strongest responses for input patterns 4, 5, and 6. Similarly, output 2 prefers input patterns 7 through 9, while output 3 prefers input patterns 1 through 3. Thus, each output unit has become specialized for its own cluster of input pattern vectors.

To aid visualization, the input pattern and output response arrays can be viewed as images, in which the value of input or output activity is coded on a gray-level scale from black to white for activity levels from 0 to 1. This can be done using script SOMoutImage, listed in MATLAB Box 5.2. The image, shown in Figure 5.3, has the same format as Table 5.5. Thus, each column of Figure 5.3A corresponds to an input unit, and each column of Figure 5.3B corresponds to an output unit. The rows correspond to the input unit patterns (see Figure 5.3A) or to the output unit responses to those input patterns (see Figure 5.3B). The image shows that when input 1 is most active (the whitest pixels in column 1 of Figure 5.3A are for rows 1 through 3), then output 3 is most active (the whitest pixels in rows 1 through 3 in Figure 5.3B are for column 3). Thus, output unit 3 receives its strongest connection from input unit 1. Similarly, output unit 2 receives its strongest connection from input unit 3, and output unit 1 receives its strongest connection from input unit 2.

As in the previous example, examination of the connectivity matrix (Table 5.6) for the network after training on the vector clusters reveals the basis

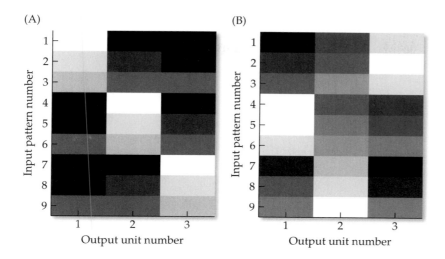

FIGURE 5.3   Competitive learning results in specialization The input (A) and output (B) patterns are viewed as images in which each row represents a pattern and each column represents the activity level of an input (A) or output (B) unit in the 3-by-3 network. Activity level is encoded as brightness; the brighter the pixel the higher the activity level. The input patterns represent vector clusters in R^3. Competitive learning causes the units in the network to specialize for distinct pattern vector clusters: output unit 1 prefers input patterns 4 through 6 (cluster 2), output unit 2 prefers patterns 7 through 9 (cluster 3), and output unit 3 prefers input patterns 1 through 3 (cluster 1). The input and output response values are given numerically in Table 5.5B and C.

for the selectivity of each output unit. The weight matrix confirms what we observed in Figure 5.3 (and Table 5.5). Output unit 1 receives its strongest connection from input unit 2, output 2 from input 3, and output 3 from input 1. The response of each output unit is the inner (or dot) product of the input pattern vector and its weight vector. As such, the output unit will respond strongly or weakly to input pattern vectors that are more nearly aligned with, or more nearly orthogonal to, its weight vector, respectively (see Math Box 5.1). Thus, each output unit will respond strongly to any of the three input pattern vectors from its own cluster, but weakly (if at all) to any input pattern vectors from other clusters.

For the linear units we use in this chapter, the response of an output unit to any input pattern is simply the inner product of the input vector and the vector of weights to that output unit from the input units (see Math Box 1.2). The inner product of two normalized vectors is equal to the cosine of the angle between them (see Math Box 5.1). When the input pattern vectors and weight vectors are normalized, the response of an output unit is equal to the cosine of the angle between the input vector and its weight vector. As such, the units in these networks not only respond well to their preferred input but also respond, to a lesser extent, to inputs that are similar to their preferred input. This is also true for many real neurons, and for this reason their "broad tuning" is sometimes referred to as "cosine tuning." If the input pattern and weight vectors are not normalized, then the output unit response (i.e., the inner product between the input pattern vector and the weight vector) is not equal but is proportional to the cosine between them. Thus, units that compute the weighted sum of their inputs are inherently cosine tuned.

TABLE 5.6   Weight matrix of a two-layered, 3-by-3 network following SOM training on the three vector clusters in R^3

To output unit	From input unit		
	1	2	3
1	0.28	0.91	0.29
2	0.01	0.05	0.99
3	0.99	0.00	0.17

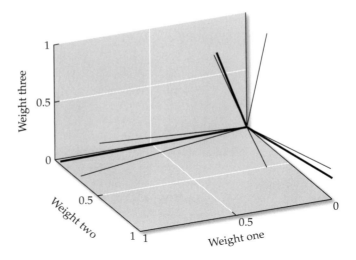

The relationship between the input pattern vectors and the weight vectors can also be visualized using a three-dimensional plot (Figure 5.4). The input pattern vectors (lighter lines) form three separate clusters in R^3. One member of each cluster is a basis vector, while the two other members of each cluster fall nearby. Thus, the three vector clusters are roughly orthogonal to each other. Following training, each output unit weight vector (heavy lines) falls within a different one of the input pattern clusters. Thus, each weight vector represents its whole cluster of input pattern vectors, and each output unit has become specialized for a different input pattern cluster. Again, because of cosine (broad) tuning, each output unit will respond strongly to an input pattern vector from its own cluster, but weakly (if at all) to patterns from the other, roughly orthogonal clusters.

In this particular run, output units 1, 2, and 3 become specialized for input vector clusters 2, 3, and 1, respectively, but any arrangement of the three output units with regard to input pattern preference is possible. Without training neighbors, the spatial arrangement of the output units with regard to input pattern preference depends only on the values in the random initial connectivity matrix, and on the random order of presentation of input pattern vectors during training. However, the input pattern vectors within each cluster are obviously neighbors in vector space. In a network with more than three output units, it should be possible to form at least a fractured map of these patterns, in which output units that prefer inputs from the same input pattern cluster are neighbors in the map (see Exercise 5.1). The next example explores map formation explicitly.

5.3   Simulating the Formation of Brain Maps using Cooperative Mechanisms

Map-like representations abound in the brain (Knudsen et al. 1987). The best known example is the homunculus (little man) map found in the primary somatosensory cortex (Figure 5.5). Neurons in the primary somatosensory cortex respond to touch inputs that originate from touch receptors in the skin. The homunculus in the primary somatosensory cortex nicely illustrates the main characteristic of brain maps, which is that neurons that respond to inputs that are near each other in feature space are located near each other in the map. In the primary somatosensory cortex, neurons that are neighbors respond to

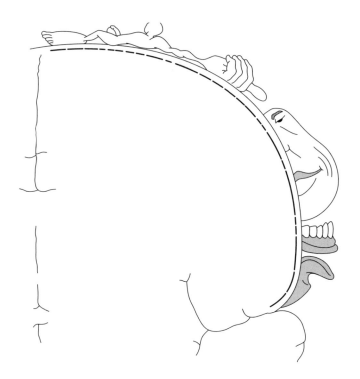

FIGURE 5.5 A slightly updated view of the homunculus in the human somatosensory cortex The original homunculus was described by Penfield and Rasmussen (1950) from direct electrical stimulation of the brains of alert human patients. The mouth (inside) and tongue representations are located below that of the chin. (After Kell et al. 2005.)

touch at neighboring regions on the body surface. Thus, neurons in the primary somatosensory cortex that respond to touch of the hand are near those that respond to touch of the wrist, which are near those that respond to touch of the arm, and so on.

The somatosensory homunculus illustrates two further characteristics of brain maps. First, the homunculus map is fractured, in that a continuous and smooth mapping is interrupted in places, after which another continuous and smooth mapping ensues. An example of a fracture in the homunculus occurs between the representations for the fingers and the forehead (see Figure 5.5). Second, the map is distorted, in that regions of the skin surface that are more densely packed with touch receptors, and which therefore send more frequent input into the brain, occupy more space in the neural representation. An example of distortion can be observed by comparing the sizes of the representations of the mouth and the torso. These and other features of brain maps are captured by the SOM algorithm, as we shall see in the examples to follow.

Formation by unsupervised learning of a map at the output layer of a neural network requires that two conditions be satisfied. First, the input pattern vectors must be non-orthogonal. That is, the input patterns cannot all be equally distant from each other in pattern (feature-vector) space. Instead, some input pattern vectors must be closer than others in vector space so that neighbor relationships exist among the patterns. Second, the unsupervised learning procedure must include cooperative as well as competitive mechanisms. Specifically, training on each input pattern must occur not only for the output unit that wins the competition for that input pattern, but also for the neighbors of the winning output unit. In the first example we used competitive learning to train output units to become specialized for the three basis vectors in R^3. Because these vectors are mutually orthogonal, no map for their representation could form even if cooperative mechanisms (specifically, neighbor training) were employed. To demonstrate map formation in this example, we will use a non-orthogonal input pattern set in which the neighbor relationships between the input patterns will be obvious from their overlap.

TABLE 5.7   Input (A) and output (B) of a two-layered, 11-by-3
network following SOM training on the diagonal-
bar patterns

(A) Input patterns	(B) Output patterns after SOM training		
1 1 1 1 0 0 0 0 0 0 0	0.38	0.00	1.53
0 1 1 1 1 0 0 0 0 0 0	0.92	0.00	1.99
0 0 1 1 1 1 0 0 0 0 0	1.45	0.00	1.50
0 0 0 1 1 1 1 0 0 0 0	1.95	0.05	0.99
0 0 0 0 1 1 1 1 0 0 0	1.75	0.57	0.49
0 0 0 0 0 1 1 1 1 0 0	1.22	1.08	0.00
0 0 0 0 0 0 1 1 1 1 0	0.68	1.59	0.00
0 0 0 0 0 0 0 1 1 1 1	0.17	1.99	0.00

The values in A and B are shown pictorially in Figure 5.6A and B, respectively.

These input patterns are listed in Table 5.7A. Each binary input pattern
(row) vector consists of a set of four contiguous 1s amidst seven 0s. Each successive input pattern overlaps the previous pattern in three places, and each
input pattern vector overlaps at least three other vectors in at least one place.
There is a clear neighborhood relationship among these input pattern vectors,
and this relationship could be represented spatially in a map according to the
locations of the output units with regard to their input pattern preferences.
This pattern set was first suggested by Orchard and Phillips (1991), and the
example in this section is an adaptation of their work.

We will begin our exploration of map formation by training a network
having only three output units on these patterns. To specify 3 output units
set nOut=3 in script KohonenSOM, as before. The input patterns are entered
using InPat=[1 1 1 1 0 0 0 0 0 0 0;0 1 1 1 1 0 0 0 0 0 0],
where only the first and second patterns are shown; the whole pattern set is
entered by extending this command, with semicolons separating each pattern. Eleven input units are required to represent these eleven-dimensional
patterns. Because it would be difficult (if not impossible) to visualize these
patterns as vectors, we can instead regard the whole set as a coarse, black-and-
white image (Figure 5.6A). As such, there is no need to normalize the patterns.
In the order in which they are listed and displayed, the input patterns form a
diagonal-bar arrangement that extends from the upper left to the lower right
of the coarse image.

Training on the diagonal-bar patterns is more effective if it occurs over
many iterations and if the learning rate decrements on each iteration, so set
nIts=1000 and dec=0.999 in script KohonenSOM. We begin using competitive learning (i.e., only the winner is trained, not its neighbors), so set
nHood=0. Then command KohonenSOM will construct a network having
eleven inputs and three outputs, randomize its connectivity matrix, train it
on the diagonal-bar patterns, and determine the output unit responses to all
of the input patterns after training. The output responses after one run are
listed in Table 5.7B and shown as an image in Figure 5.6B.

Figure 5.6B illustrates how the three output units represent the eight input
patterns that form the diagonal-bar. Output unit 1 prefers input patterns from
the middle of the bar, output 2 from the bottom right, and output 3 from the
top left of the bar. Because no neighbors are trained, any arrangement of the
three output units with regard to input pattern preference is possible and
depends only on the values in the random initial connectivity matrix and the
random order of input pattern presentation. Other runs would produce dif-

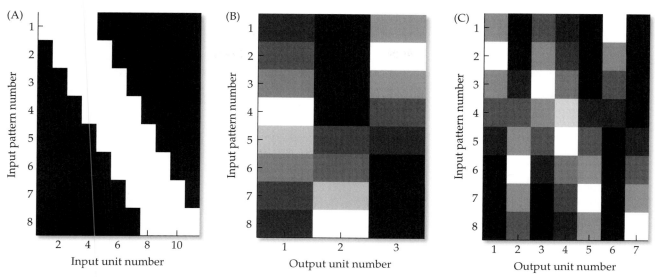

FIGURE 5.6   Specialization without map formation using purely competitive learning The networks providing data for this figure were trained on the diagonal bar patterns using competitive learning only (i.e., there was no cooperative neighbor training). (A) The eight, 11-element diagonal-bar patterns consist of a series of four 1s in a row of 0s that shifts by one place for each subsequent input pattern. (B) In a trained 11-by-3 network, output unit 1 prefers input pattern 4, output 2 prefers input pattern 8, and output 3 prefers input pattern 2. Each unit also responds well for nearby patterns. Thus, the output units specialize for different "regions" of the "bar" image: output 1 prefers the middle set of patterns (middle of the bar), output 2 prefers the bottom set (lower right of the bar), and output 3 prefers the top set of patterns (upper left of the bar). The input and output unit response values are given numerically in Table 5.7. (C) In a trained 11-by-7 network, output unit 1 prefers input pattern 2, output 2 prefers input pattern 6, output 3 prefers input pattern 3, and so on. The output units in the larger network also specialize, but output units that respond to similar input patterns are not neighbors, indicating that no map forms.

ferent output response arrangements, but in all cases the output units group (quantize) the inputs into three clusters: upper-left, middle, and lower-right regions of the bar. Obviously, the simple learning procedure being used here does not "see" a bar having three distinct regions. Instead, it simply groups the vectors together on the basis of their closeness in the eleven-dimensional vector space that contains the input vectors. We can interpret these patterns as "nearby regions of a bar" but, to the learning algorithm and the resulting trained network, they are simply vectors that happen to be close together in vector (feature) space.

To demonstrate map formation we will increase the number of output units and observe the effects of training with and without neighbors. To begin, we set nOut=7 in script KohonenSOM, but keep all of the other settings the same, including the neighborhood size of 0 (nHood=0). The responses of the seven output units are shown as an image in Figure 5.6C. The output units are located randomly with respect to their input pattern preferences. For example, the input pattern preferences of output units 1 and 2 tend toward the upper left (pattern 2) and the lower right (pattern 6), respectively. There appears to be no consistent spatial relationship between the locations of any of the output units in the network and their preferred features. Again, since no neighbors are trained, any arrangement of output units with regard to input pattern preference is possible. The spatial arrangement of the outputs changes dramatically when cooperative mechanisms are employed.

FIGURE 5.7 Specialization and map formation using combined competitive and cooperative learning All of the 11-by-7 networks providing data for this figure were trained on the diagonal bar patterns using the self-organizing map (SOM) algorithm (i.e., competitive learning combined with cooperative neighbor training). (A) The diagonal bar input patterns are as described in Figure 5.6. In SOM training, the competitive component causes the output units to specialize, while the cooperative component causes output units that are neighbors to prefer similar input patterns, thereby forming a map. Due to the initially random connection weights, and the random order of pattern presentation, the configuration of the resulting maps will differ between simulations. In the network in (B), the order of pattern preference of the output units matches the order of the input patterns, but this is not always the case. In the network in (C), the order of pattern preference of the output units is opposite to the order of the input patterns. In the network in (D) the map is fractured, such that a smooth progression of output preference from the middle to the top left of the bar is interrupted, after which another smooth progression of output preference continues from the bottom right to the middle of the bar.

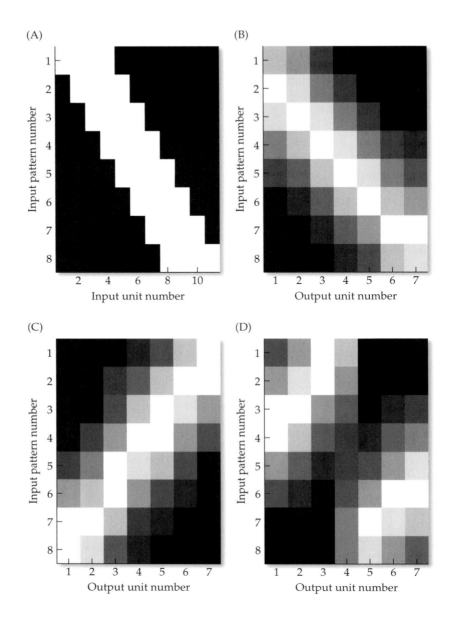

To observe the effects of neighbor training (cooperation) we retrain the network (i.e., rerun `KohonenSOM`), but first set `nHood=1`. This will implement SOM training. Specifically, setting `nHood=1` will cause the winner and its one nearest neighbor on either side to undergo training on each cycle. Script `KohonenSOM` will use the neighborhood size and the index of the winner to find the first neighbor `fn` and the last neighbor `ln` that define the boundaries of the training neighborhood `h` on each cycle. The output responses that result from training with one nearest neighbor on either side are shown as an image in Figure 5.7B (the input pattern image shown in Figure 5.6A is shown again in Figure 5.7A for reference). An output map has clearly formed. Output units that are neighbors in the output array prefer similar (overlapping) input patterns. Training with neighbors will usually produce an orderly arrangement of the output units with regard to input pattern preference. In this case (see Figure 5.7B) the output map has the same orientation as the input pattern array (see Figure 5.7A), but this will not be the case in general. Figure 5.7C shows the results of another run in which the orientation of the map is the reverse of the input pattern array. Figure

5.7D shows a fractured map, in which output units 1 through 3 represent the middle through the top left of the bar, while output units 5 through 7 represent the bottom right through the middle of the bar. Many other map configurations are possible, but SOM training, which is cooperative as well as competitive, will generally produce a map-like output arrangement.

The diagonal-bar SOM simulations capture some of the essential features of map-like representations in the brain. The main feature of neural maps is that output units that are neighbors in the network respond to similar input patterns. The maps can have various orientations, and they can be continuous or fractured. In a fractured map, continuous mapping regions are separated by sharp breaks, as in the somatosensory homunculus (see Figure 5.5). The type of map that forms depends on many factors, including the initial state of the connectivity matrix and the size of the training neighborhood, but increasing the neighborhood size does not necessarily improve the map. As we will discuss in detail in Chapter 8, an important function of a neural representation, whether or not it forms a map, is to represent its inputs as "fully" as possible. We will define "fully" more precisely in Chapter 8, but for now we can state that a good representation is one in which each unit becomes specialized for its own preferred input pattern, and no input patterns are left unrepresented. If the training neighborhood is too large, maps can form in which nearby output units have the *same* preferred input pattern, and in which some input patterns activate no output units (see Exercise 5.2). It is likely that the initial state of the connectivity matrix, and the extent of cooperative mechanisms, are factors that also play an important role in the activity-dependent mechanisms that shape maps in the actual nervous system (Rauthazer and Cline 2004).

5.4   Modeling the Formation of Tonotopic Maps in the Auditory System

While the somatosensory homunculus may be the most famous brain map, it is by no means the only map-like sensory representation in the brain. Auditory input is also represented in map-like arrangements in many brain regions, including parts of the auditory cortex and the cochlear nuclei (Spirou et al. 1993). Many neurons in the auditory system are most sensitive to sound at their preferred or "central" frequency, and many auditory brain structures are arranged tonotopically, in that neurons that neighbor each other in the structure have central frequencies that are neighbors on the frequency spectrum. A tonotopic map in the cochlear nucleus of the cat is diagrammed in Figure 5.8.

The goal of the example in this section is to simulate the formation of the tonotopic map in the cochlear nucleus using the SOM algorithm. Located in the brainstem of mammals, the cochlear nucleus contains the secondary auditory neurons that receive input from cochlear afferents, which are the primary afferents of the auditory system. The cochlear afferents transmit auditory signals from the cochlea, which is the snail-shaped, peripheral auditory receptor in mammals. (Other vertebrates have auditory receptors that are not snail-shaped; see Purves et al. 2004 for details.) We will simulate the formation of the tonotopic map in the mammalian cochlear nucleus by using the SOM to train a two-layered, 20-by-10 neural network, in which the 20 input units represent the cochlear afferents and the 10 output units represent the neurons in the cochlear nucleus. The first step is to set up the input, which will be a simplification of the sensory input received by the cochlear nucleus from cochlear afferents.

Cochlear afferents are most sensitive to sound at their central frequency but, like many neurons throughout the auditory system, they are broadly tuned, so

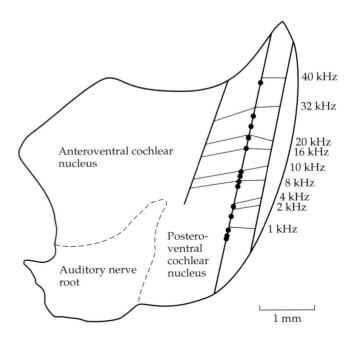

FIGURE 5.8 Map of isofrequency bands within the dorsal cochlear nucleus of the cat Neurons in each band are most sensitive to sound at their "central" frequency (in kilohertz [kHz], or thousands of cycles per second), which is indicated to the right of each band. The locations of the bands were determined by finding the central frequencies of neurons encountered along three microelectrode passes (heavy lines mark the electrode tracks; dots mark the locations of the responses of single neurons recorded along the middle track). The isofrequency bands are tonotopically ordered (i.e., arranged in order of frequency). (From Spirou et al. 1993.)

they also respond to sounds at other frequencies. We discussed broad tuning in the context of output units in Section 5.2. To properly represent the cochlear afferents we must make the input units broadly tuned. There are many ways to model the broad tuning of individual cochlear afferents for the purposes of simulating tonotopic map formation. Some examples are shown in Figure 5.9. The only requirement is that the input as a whole produces different but overlapping patterns for simulated sounds at nearby frequencies. This requirement is satisfied by having broadly tuned input units that differ from one another in their central frequencies. The tuning curve we will use in this example is the back-to-back exponential (solid curve), but any of the curves illustrated in Figure 5.9 would suit the purposes of the simulation.

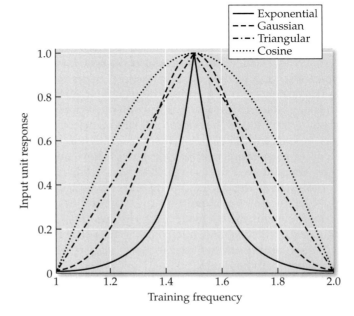

FIGURE 5.9 Types of input unit tuning curves Any one of these could be used to train the tonotopic SOM. The training frequencies are simply scalars in the range from 1 to 2. The back-to-back exponential tuning curve (solid curve) is used in the tonotopic map example. Other broad input tuning curves that would also produce SOM output maps are the Gaussian (dashed), triangular (dot-dashed), and cosine (dotted).

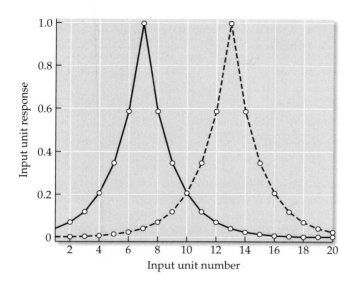

FIGURE 5.10   The responses of a tonotopically ordered set of broadly tuned input units The figure shows the responses of each of the 20 simulated auditory input units (circles) for sounds at training frequencies of 1.3 (solid curve) and 1.6 (dashed curve). Each input unit has the same back-to-back exponential tuning curve (see Figure 5.9). Note that the curve describing the responses of all the input units at a single frequency (this figure) has the same form as the responses of a single input unit over the range of frequencies (see Figure 5.9). Because of the broad tuning of the input units, the input pattern vectors (the elements of which are the responses of the input units) for these two training frequencies overlap. This is illustrated by the overlap of the curves (solid or dashed) describing the responses of all the input units at the two frequencies.

The input pattern vectors for the tonotopic map simulation have as their 20 elements the responses to sound, at any training frequency, of the set of 20 input units. Figure 5.10 illustrates how the broad tuning of individual input units will produce patterns of responses over the input array for nearby frequencies that are distinct but overlapping. Note that when all of the input units have the same tuning curve, the curve describing the responses of all the input units at a single frequency (see Figure 5.10) will have the same form as the response of an individual input unit over the range of frequencies (see Figure 5.9). The result is that the input patterns for nearby frequencies are distinct but overlapping (see Figure 5.10). Thus, the input pattern vectors for nearby frequencies would point in similar directions in vector space. Note here that sound frequency, a single quantity, or a single "dimension" of a sound stimulus, is being encoded by many (in this case 20) input units, which represent a 20-dimensional vector space in the mathematical sense. We will discuss issues of dimensionality in Section 5.5. Here we show that broad tuning of input units can lead to map formation at the output using the SOM algorithm

The script `tonotopicSOM`, listed in MATLAB Box 5.3, implements training of the tonotopic SOM. In the script, the `nIn=20` model cochlear afferents respond to sound frequencies, represented simply as scalars, in an arbitrary range from 1 to 2. Each input unit (model cochlear afferent) is assigned a different central frequency `cf` in this range using `cf=linspace(1,2,nIn)`. Its response to a sound at its central frequency is 1, and its response falls off exponentially for sounds at lower and higher frequencies. The following MATLAB command is used to calculate the input vector x given the vector `cf` of 20 equally spaced central frequencies: `x=exp(-abs(cf-tf)*qf)`. In this command `tf` is a scalar representing a training (or testing) frequency and `qf` can be thought of as a "quality factor," in that the larger it is the tighter the tuning. (In audio engineering, high quality is associated with tight tuning.) The SOM is trained as before, except that instead of drawing the input patterns from an array, the training frequency `tf` is chosen at random from the range and input vector x is generated afresh on each iteration.

The network trained using `tonotopicSOM` is set up to have 10 output units (`nOut=10`). The quality factor is set at 3 (`qf=3`). To make a map we need cooperative training, so set `nHood=1`. For SOM learning set `a=2`, `dec=0.99`, and `nIts=500`. Following training the script will test the network at equally spaced frequencies (held in vector `tfVec`) and store the output responses for

MATLAB® BOX 5.3 This script uses the Kohonen SOM algorithm to simulate the formation of a tonotopic map.

```
% tonotopicSOM.m

nIn=20; % set the number of input units
nOut=10; % set the number of output units
a=2; % set the learning rate
dec=0.99; % set the learning rate decrement
nHood=1; % set the neighborhood size
nIts=500; % set the number of iterations
qf=3; % set the quality factor

cf=linspace(1,2,nIn); % set evenly spaced central frequencies
% cf=[linspace(1.0,1.385,7) linspace(1.45,1.55,6)... % alternate
% linspace(1.615,2.0,7)]; % set of cf's with expanded midrange
V=rand(nOut,nIn); % set initially random connectivity matrix
for c=1:nIts, % for each learning iteration
    tf=rand+1; % choose a test frequency at random
    x=exp(-abs(cf-tf)*qf); % compute the input pattern for tf
    y=V*x'; % compute output to chosen input pattern
    [winVal winIndx]=max(y); % find the index of the winning output
    fn=winIndx-nHood; % find first neighbor in training neighborhood
    ln=winIndx+nHood; % find last neighbor in training neighborhood
    if fn < 1, fn=1; end, % keep first neighbor in bounds
    if ln > 10, ln=nOut; end, % keep last neighbor in bounds
    for h=fn:ln, % for all units in training neighborhood
        hld=V(h,:)+a*x; % apply Kohonen update
        V(h,:)=hld/norm(hld); % normalize new weight vector
        a=a*(dec); % decrement the learning rate
    end, % end neighbor training loop
end; % end learning loop

Out=zeros(10); % define an output array
tfVec=linspace(1,2,10); % set test frequencies
for f=1:10, % for each test frequency
    x=exp(-abs(cf-tfVec(f))*qf); % compute the input
    Out(f,:)=(V*x')'; % compute the output
end; % end test loop
```

each input pattern in array Out. Using plot(tfVec,Out), the responses of each of the ten output units at all of the test frequencies are plotted as overlain curves (Figure 5.11A). Note that the output units have become selective for specific (central) frequencies, but their responses are even more broadly tuned than are those of the inputs, meaning that the output units would respond even more strongly than the inputs to frequencies that are near but not equal to their central frequencies.

Using mesh(1:10,tfVec,Out), the output responses are laid out both as a function of test frequency and their position in the linear output array (Figure 5.11B). The contour plot shows that output units that are neighbors in the array respond to sounds that are neighbors on the frequency spectrum, thereby forming a tonotopic map. As in previous examples, the specific configuration of the map will differ from simulation to simulation, but in general the output units will show some ordering in the array according to their central frequencies.

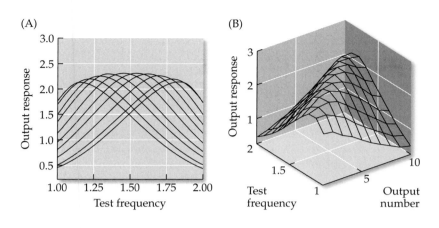

FIGURE 5.11 **Responses of the output units in a 20-by-10 network trained using the SOM to form a tonotopic map** The 20, broadly tuned input units provide a distributed encoding of the frequency of simulated sounds (as shown for two frequencies within the range in Figure 5.10). The responses of each of the 10 output units to this input at every test frequency are plotted in two-dimensions with overlain curves (A), one for each output unit, or with curves that are spread out in a three-dimensional contour plot (B).

The nature of a map-like distributed representation is nicely illustrated by the responses of the output units in the tonotopic map (see Figure 5.11A). A midrange test frequency of 1.6, for example, would most strongly activate output unit 6. It would also activate output units 5 and 7, but less strongly, and activate output units 4 and 8, but less strongly still, and so on for the other units. The output units in our tonotopic map model are so broadly tuned that any frequency in the range would activate all of the output units, but to different levels. Each frequency in the range would be encoded by a unique pattern of activity over the population of output units. Thus, the distributed tonotopic representation, over a population of broadly tuned specialists, could represent every frequency in the range.

The efficiency of a distributed representation via broadly tuned specialists can be appreciated by comparing it with a representation based on very narrowly tuned specialists. Continuing with the auditory network as a specific example, imagine that each of the ten output units was specialized for its own unique central frequency, but that it could respond only to sound at that frequency. Then the network could encode any one of those ten frequencies but no others. Frequencies falling between the preferred (central) frequencies of the very-narrowly-tuned output units would not be represented. This limitation would be made even worse if two or more of the output units had the same preferred frequency, or if any of the output units were simply unresponsive and produced no output at all for any of the inputs.

This comparison illustrates that an output representation is most efficient when the units are broadly tuned specialists, and when all of the output units participate in the representation but none have the same preferred input pattern (Hinton et al. 1986). However, this comparison does not explain why many sensory representations in the brain are organized as maps. Nor does it explain what functional consequences a map formed through SOM training might have. A population of broadly-tuned specialists could represent input patterns just as efficiently and effectively if they were not organized as a map. A consideration of the three essential characteristics of an efficient distributed representation, and how it comes about through SOM training, can shed some light on this issue.

First, an efficient distributed representation should be composed of broadly tuned output units. An output unit that computes the weighted sum of its inputs naturally provides broad (or cosine) tuning, because the weighted input sum is the same as the inner (dot) product between the input vector and the weight vector, and the inner product is proportional to the cosine of the angle between those two vectors (see Section 5.2 and Math Box 5.1). The weight vectors are trained by the SOM to locate themselves within clusters of input pattern vectors. Thus, each output unit would be broadly tuned to the input patterns in the cluster represented by its weight vector.

The second essential characteristic of an efficient distributed representation is that each of the output units should have its own, unique preferred input pattern. The competitive component of SOM training forces this specialization among the output units (see Section 5.1). Third, all of the available output units should participate in the representation. It is the cooperative component of SOM training that forces all of the output units to work together to represent the input patterns. When the input patterns overlap, then the cooperative component of the SOM will bring about map formation. However, the essential role of the cooperative component may be to engage all of the output units in the task of learning to efficiently represent the input patterns. Map formation per se may be incidental. We will consider this important issue in greater depth in Chapter 8. For our next example in this chapter we will continue to explore map formation, but will switch from the auditory to the visual system. Specifically, we will consider the representation of multiple attributes, or dimensions, of visual stimuli by the visual cortex.

5.5 Simulating the Development of Orientation Selectivity in Visual Cortex

The idea of dimension is central to neural network learning algorithms in general and to the SOM in particular. We can think of the SOM as an algorithm that "maps" an input of one dimension into an output of a potentially different dimension. Mathematically, the dimension of a space is the number of coordinates needed to locate a point in that space. In the abstract and whimsical "animal" example that we discussed in the preamble, each of the animals (dog, cat, fish, bird, and bat) could be located in a seven-dimensional space, where the seven dimensions were: fur, barks, meows, fins, gills, feathers, and wings. Various input configurations, characterized according to the simple presence or absence of each of these features, could be described using seven-dimensional, binary feature vectors that could be represented by seven input units. This seven-dimensional input could be mapped by the SOM into an output of arbitrary dimension. If the output had five dimensions (five output units), then each output unit could become a specialist for each animal, and we might expect that the "dog" and "cat" output units would be neighbors. If the output had only three units then, depending on factors including the initially random connectivity matrix and the random order of training pattern presentations, the first output unit might become a specialist for dog and cat, the second for bird and bat, and the third for fish. In both cases, the SOM would have accomplished a dimensionality reduction, from a seven-dimensional input down to a five- or three-dimensional output.

The SOM is often used in the context of dimensionality reduction, in which input patterns of dimension n_x (the input pattern vectors have n_x elements corresponding to n_x input units) are mapped onto a set $n_y < n_x$ of output units. The tonotopic map simulation involved a mapping from a broadly tuned input representation to a broadly tuned output representation of a lower dimension. It offers another example of dimensionality reduction by the SOM, because the input vector of $n_x = 20$ elements (or input units) is mapped onto a set of only $n_y = 10$ output units. Here n_x and n_y are the dimensions of the vector spaces that contain the feature (input) and output vectors, respectively.

There is another important respect in which dimensionality reduction applies to brain maps. This involves dimensionality in the sense of measurable quantities and the anatomical arrangements of units, independent from dimensionality in the mathematical sense of input and output vector spaces. In terms of stimulus attributes, a single measurable quantity, such as sound frequency, can be represented by any number of broadly tuned neurons, and the number of attributes and the number of neurons that encode them are independent. For example, a set of n_x input units could represent one dimension (attribute) of a stimulus in a vector space of n_x dimensions.

In terms of anatomical arrangement, a set of units in a linear array is arranged in one-dimension, because each unit can be located using a one-dimensional vector (a scalar, see Chapter 1). Similarly, a set of units in a square or rectangular array would be arranged in two-dimensions, because each unit could be located using a two-dimensional vector (in terms of x-y coordinates, for example). The dimensionality of the array, as an arrangement of units, is independent from the number of units in the array. Thus, a linear array of n_x input units can encode a feature space of n_x dimensions, but it is arranged in one dimension. Similarly, a rectangular or square array of n_y output units can represent sensory input configurations in an output vector space of n_y dimensions, but it is arranged in two dimensions. Dimensionality with respect to stimulus attributes and anatomical arrangements of neurons has interesting implications for brain maps.

For some brain maps, a single quantity is mapped onto a one-dimensional array of neurons. The tonotopic map in the cochlear nucleus is an example of a one-to-one dimensional mapping, in which the single quantity of sound frequency is mapped onto an essentially linear array of neurons (see Figure 5.8). For other brain maps, two stimulus attributes are mapped onto a two-dimensional array of neurons. The sensory homunculus is an example of a two-to-two dimensional mapping, in which the two spatial coordinates of the body surface are mapped onto the essentially rectangular array of neurons in the primary somatosensory cortex (see Figure 5.5). The situation is more complicated when the number of stimulus attributes exceeds the number of dimensions in which the neurons that encode them are arranged.

Many brain maps occur essentially on two-dimensional arrays (arrangements) of neurons (such as the "sheet" of cortical columns; see Section 5.6), but they sometimes represent more than two dimensions of input attributes (features). The best known example involves the primary visual (striate) cortex. This structure is organized retinotopically, meaning that nearby neurons in striate cortex respond to visual stimuli that activate nearby regions of the retina. The two-dimensions of the retinal representation (describable using two-dimensional feature vectors containing the x-y coordinates of the images of stimuli on the retina) are laid out as a map on the two-dimensional sheet (array) of striate cortex (Hubel 1988). But the striate cortex also represents other attributes associated with visual input, such as the orientations of elongated stimuli. The representation of orientation is also map-like, in the sense that neighboring neurons (or cortical columns) in striate cortex have similar preferred orientations. This third feature dimension (attribute) of orientation specificity is "squeezed" into the underlying two-dimensional retinotopic arrangement and distorts it. The interplay of the retinotopic and orientation features produces a characteristic map structure.

This structure was first explored computationally by van der Malsburg (1973). He modeled the input to the striate cortex using a two-dimensional array of units that represented a patch of retina. Simulated stimuli were bars of light in nine different orientations that activated the input units on which they fell. Thus, the retinal patch encoded the elongated, and variously orientated, visual stimuli according to the arrangement of the units in the input array that

FIGURE 5.12 **The two-dimensional input pattern arrays used in the original model of self-organization in the primary visual (striate) cortex** Each input pattern represents the responses of the units in a patch of model retina to an elongated stimulus of a different orientation. (From von der Malsburg 1973.)

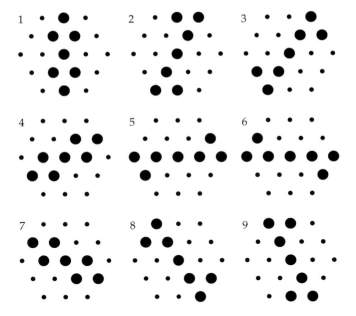

were active (Figure 5.12). Van der Malsburg modeled the striate cortex itself as a larger, two-dimensional array of output units. Each unit in the input array projected to every unit in the output array. The orientations of the simulated stimuli were chosen randomly on each training iteration. Van der Malsburg used an unsupervised algorithm (a progenitor of the Kohonen SOM) to train the network on input patterns that varied in orientation, and tested the trained network to determine the orientation preferences of the output units. Many output units in the trained network became selective for orientation. The orientation preferences of these output units changed smoothly, and swirled around other output units that were orientationally unspecific (Figure 5.13). This configuration became known as the "orientation pinwheel" structure. Its existence was later confirmed experimentally.

The work of van der Malsburg (1973) was extended using the Kohonen algorithm to create models of striate cortex that represented not only orientation, but also location and ocular dominance (i.e., the eye, left or right, from which a striate cortical neuron receives its predominant input). These maps were shown to correspond well with the actual structure of striate cortex (Obermayer et al. 1990; Obermayer and Blasdel 1993). Specifically, the output units were arranged in ocular dominance stripes (appearing roughly like zebra stripes in the model as in the brain). They were also arranged in patches in which the output units had the same location specificity. The location-specific patches were arranged roughly retinotopically, but the location map was distorted by the orientation map, which exhibited a pinwheel structure similar to that originally demonstrated by van der Malsburg.

We will undertake a simplified version of the striate cortex simulation in which input patterns, representing images of bars of light of different orientations, are encoded by a two-dimensional array of input units and are compressed by the SOM into a one-dimensional array of output units. The four two-dimensional input pattern arrays are shown in Table 5.8. Each pattern array can be entered as a matrix. The first pattern array can be entered as `P1=[1 1 0 0 0;1 1 0 0 0;0 0 1 0 0;0 0 0 1 1;0 0 0 1 1]`, and similarly for the other two-dimensional pattern arrays. To use the MATLAB script `KohonenSOM` to train a network on these patterns, these two-dimen-

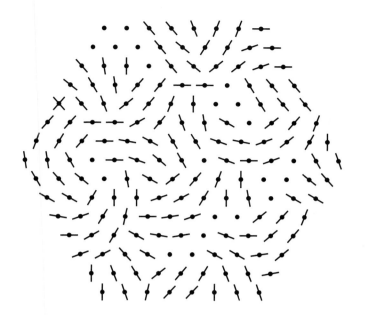

FIGURE 5.13   The preferred orientations of output units in a model of the striate cortex following training using the self-organization algorithm of von der Malsburg Units that are near each other in the two-dimensional array have similar preferred orientations. The orientation preferences of the units change progressively and swirl around orientationally unselective units, forming a repeating pinwheel structure. (From von der Malsburg 1973.)

sional 5-by-5 pattern arrays would have to be converted into the 1-by-25 rows of input pattern matrix InPat. This can be done by first defining the matrix using InPat=zeros(4,25), and then converting each two-dimensional pattern array into its own row of InPat. The command that accomplishes this for pattern 1 is InPat(1,:)=reshape(P1,1,25). The commands for the other pattern arrays are similar.

For simplicity in this book we restrict ourselves to networks having one-dimensional layers (linear arrays of units), but networks having two-dimensional layers (square or rectangular arrays) could be treated using the same algorithms after the two-dimensional layers are reshaped into one-dimensional arrays. The reshape command, used here for input pattern arrays, could also be used to convert two-dimensional arrays of unit states into one-dimensional arrays. We consider only networks having one-dimensional layers because they are easier to manage computationally, but they exhibit all of the properties we wish to study (this issue is also discussed in Chapter 3).

The two-dimensional pattern arrays, reshaped into the rows of the input pattern matrix, are shown in Table 5.9. Now the input patterns can be considered either as two-dimensional images (arrays) or as pattern (feature) vectors (rows of the input pattern matrix). Note that the patterns as image arrays are arranged in two-dimensions, but they correspond to feature vectors that have 25 dimensions. All four input pattern vectors share the same middle element,

TABLE 5.8   Orientation selectivity input patterns, arranged as two-dimensional arrays (images)

1	2	3	4
1 1 0 0 0	0 1 1 1 0	0 0 0 1 1	0 0 0 0 0
1 1 0 0 0	0 0 1 0 0	0 0 0 1 1	1 0 0 0 1
0 0 1 0 0	0 0 1 0 0	0 0 1 0 0	1 1 1 1 1
0 0 0 1 1	0 0 1 0 0	1 1 0 0 0	1 0 0 0 1
0 0 0 1 1	0 1 1 1 0	1 1 0 0 0	0 0 0 0 0

TABLE 5.9 Orientation selectivity input patterns, arranged as feature vectors

1	1	0	0	0	0	1	1	0	0	0	0	0	1	0	0	0	0	0	1	1	0	0	0	1	1
0	1	1	1	0	0	0	1	0	0	0	0	1	0	0	0	0	1	0	0	0	1	1	1	0	
0	0	0	1	1	0	0	0	1	1	0	0	1	0	0	1	1	0	0	0	1	1	0	0	0	
0	0	0	0	0	1	0	0	0	1	1	1	1	1	1	1	1	0	0	0	1	0	0	0	0	0

The corresponding input patterns arranged as two-dimensional arrays are shown in Table 5.8.

so all the pattern vectors overlap in one place. Patterns encoding nearby orientations, when viewed as two-dimensional images, have corresponding pattern vectors that overlap in two additional places. Patterns encoding orthogonal orientations, when viewed as two-dimensional images, have corresponding pattern vectors that have no overlap beyond the one place they all share. Thus, some patterns are nearer than others in vector space, and these neighbor relationships can be represented in a simulated map. To produce the map, script KohonenSOM is set to train the winner among seven output units (nOut=7), along with the one nearest neighbor on either side of the winner (nHood=1), with a learning rate of one and no decrement (a=1 and dec=1) for 100 iterations (nIts=100). The responses of the seven output units to each input pattern following training on a typical run are shown in Table 5.10, in which each row corresponds to one of the four patterns and each column corresponds to a different output unit.

Each output unit develops a preferred orientation, which may correspond to one of the input orientations or to an orientation that is intermediate between two input orientations. Indicated below each column is the number of the pattern (or pattern combination) to which the corresponding output unit has become the most responsive, and below that is drawn a line illustrating the approximate, preferred orientation of each unit. The orientation selectivity of the output units progresses continuously with their position in the network (linear output unit array). This map forms because the feature vectors representing the pattern arrays (images) are closer to some than to others in vector (feature) space, and these neighborhood relationships are represented in the SOM because neighbors are trained along with winners. Various map configurations,

TABLE 5.10 Orientation selectivity of output units arranged in a linear array following SOM training

Input patterns	Output patterns after SOM training						
1	1.00	0.84	0.33	0.86	1.00	2.42	3.00
2	3.00	2.52	1.00	0.77	0.3	0.81	1.00
3	1.00	2.37	3.00	2.31	1.00	0.83	0.33
4	0.33	0.79	1.00	2.57	3.00	2.48	1.00
Best pattern	2	2–3	3	3–4	4	4–1	1
	|	/	/	╱	—	╲	\

The elongated-bar input patterns are arranged as image arrays in Table 5.8 and as feature vectors in Table 5.9.

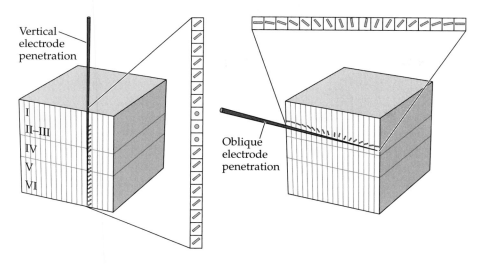

FIGURE 5.14   Orientation selectivity and columnar organization in the primary visual cortex The visual (and most other) regions of cortex are composed of six layers of neurons. Inputs to the cortex arrive at layer IV. The cortex is also organized into functional columns. In the primary visual (striate) cortex, all of the neurons in the same functional column are selective for elongated visual stimuli (such as bars of light) of the same orientation (except for neurons in the input layer IV, which are orientationally unselective). An electrode inserted perpendicularly with respect to the surface of the striate cortex, which only encounters neurons in one functional column, would record responses all having the same orientation selectivity (except in layer IV). The experiments by Hubel and Wiesel (1974), which originally established the orderly progression of orientation selectivity in striate cortex, were made using electrodes inserted obliquely with respect to the surface of the striate cortex that encountered neurons in a series of adjacent cortical columns. (From Purves et al. 2004.)

including fractured continua, can also occur, but with overlapping input patterns and neighbor training, strong spatial structure will emerge in the SOM.

The simulation in this section illustrates how individual neurons in visual cortex could become specialized for specific orientations, and how a map could form in which neurons with similar orientation specificity would be located near each other in the map. In the simulation, orientation selectivity progresses smoothly from unit to unit along the linear output array, and this is analogous to the smooth progression of orientation specificity observed in striate cortex. In fact, the orderly progression in orientation selectivity that develops in our linear array of output units resembles that observed in the original experiments on striate cortex of Hubel and Wiesel (1974). They recorded the responses to oriented light-bars of neurons that were encountered along oblique electrode passes into striate cortex that ran in a straight line through a sequence of adjacent cortical columns (Figure 5.14). Of course, the one-dimensional output array we used could not reproduce the orientation pinwheels that develop in a two-dimensional array of output units, but our simple SOM simulation using a linear array captures the essential feature of the orientation map without the added complexity of two-dimensional input and output layers. The learning algorithm proposed by van der Malsburg (1973) was a bit more complicated than the SOM (Kohonen 1982, 1997) but, as described above, the SOM algorithm is also capable of training two-dimensional arrays of output units to form orientation pinwheels (Obermayer et al. 1990; Obermayer and Blasdel 1993). Other work using the Kohonen SOM algorithm suggests that a pinwheel structure may exist in a different, non-cortical brain region. We briefly review this example in the next section.

5.6 Modeling a Possible Multisensory Map in the Superior Colliculus

The models of map formation in the striate cortex (van der Malsburg 1973; Obermayer et al. 1990; Obermayer and Blasdel 1993) instantiate the hypothesis that orientation pinwheels develop because activity-dependent, unsupervised learning mechanisms cause neighboring neurons in the two-dimensional, striate cortical array to prefer nearby two-dimensional retinotopic locations, but also to prefer similar stimulus orientations. In order for the model of the two-dimensional striate cortical array to represent the two-dimensions of retinotopy plus the additional dimension of stimulus orientation, the SOM has to "squeeze" orientation into the retinotopic map. Orientation pinwheels, and retinotopic map distortion, result. An analogous model suggests that a pinwheel arrangement might occur in a topographically organized, two-dimensional but non-cortical array that must also squeeze in a third stimulus attribute. The structure is the superior colliculus, and the third stimulus attribute is selectivity for combinations of sensory input modalities.

Located in the midbrain, the superior colliculus is a layered structure, and its deep layers receive inputs of multiple sensory modalities, including visual, auditory, and somatosensory (Stein and Meredith 1993). The various inputs are represented topographically, but the maps of each modality are not separate. Instead, individual neurons in the colliculus can receive inputs of multiple modalities, and all the possible modality combinations are found among them (Stein and Meredith 1993). A model based on the SOM suggests that modality selectivity may be represented in a pinwheel organization within the deep layers of the superior colliculus.

The input to the model is represented by three, square, 20-by-20 arrays of input units, one array for each stimulus modality (visual V, auditory A, and somatosensory S). Each input array is topographically organized, such that input units that are neighbors in the array respond best to stimuli from neighboring regions of the environment (Figure 5.15A). Individual input units are broadly tuned, and have tuning curves that are two-dimensional versions of the one-dimensional Gaussian tuning curve shown in Figure 5.9.

The colliculus is modeled as a square, 20-by-20 array of output units. The matrix of the weights of the connections from inputs to outputs is randomized and the network is trained using a version of the Kohonen SOM algorithm that is similar to `KohonenSOM` (see MATLAB Box 5.1). A notable difference is that the output training neighborhood in the colliculus model is a two-dimensional Gaussian with a variance that decreases as learning proceeds. This implementation of the neighborhood function improves the performance of the SOM algorithm (Kohonen 1997; Haykin 1999).

On each training cycle a stimulus location and sensory modality combination are chosen at random. For example, a visual-auditory stimulus at coordinates (5, 5) would activate input units according to a two-dimensional Gaussian profile centered at coordinates (5, 5) in the visual and auditory input arrays. No input units in the somatosensory array would be activated. Training using the SOM causes the output units to become selective both for stimulus location and modality combination. A topographic map of location forms at the output, but this map is distorted (Figure 5.15B) because the output units also represent modality selectivity. The percentages of units that become specialized for each modality combination can be manipulated by adjusting

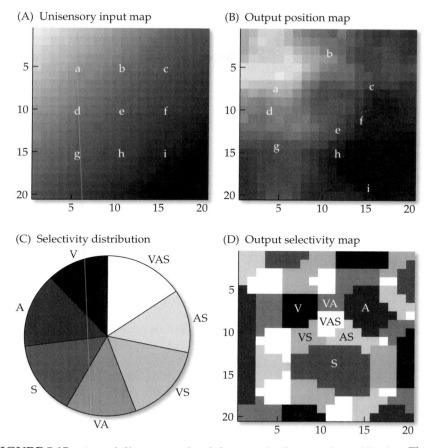

FIGURE 5.15   A modality map as it might occur in the superior colliculus The map is the output layer of a two-layered SOM neural network. The multisensory output layer and the three unisensory input layers are modeled as two-dimensional 20-by-20 square arrays of units. Each unisensory input array has the same topographic organization, which is illustrated in (A) using shading (from white in the upper left to black in the lower right). Following training, the output map has a distorted representation of topography, as illustrated in (B) using shading. Topography distortion in the output map (B) is also indicated by the irregular spacing of the units that respond best to inputs from the reference locations (labeled a–i), which are regularly spaced in the input maps (A). The topography of the output map is distorted because it also represents modality selectivity. The seven modality selectivities are: visual V, auditory A, somatosensory S, visual-auditory VA, visual-somatosensory VS, auditory-somatosensory AS, and visual-auditory-somatosensory VAS. To facilitate illustration, the percentages of the seven modality selectivities (C) are roughly equal in this simulation. (D) The output selectivity map has a repeating modality pinwheel structure that is analogous to the orientation pinwheels of striate cortex.

the relative numbers of inputs of different modality combinations that are presented to the network. To aid visual interpretation of the resulting map, the numbers of inputs of different modality combinations are set so that the percentages of output units that become specialized for each modality combination are roughly equal (Figure 5.15C).

The main feature of the map is that output units with the same modality selectivity form clusters, and that the selectivities of unisensory (V, A, or S) and bisensory (VA, VS, or AS) clusters change smoothly as they swirl around trisensory (VAS) clusters, thus forming pinwheels (Figure 5.15D). The smooth change in selectivity in swirling around the pinwheel is manifested as an alternation between unisensory and bisensory clusters. If we choose an arbitrary beginning for, and swirling direction around, the pinwheel, then the smooth change would be V, VA, A, AS, S, and VS. The trisensory output units (VAS), found in clusters around which the unisensory and bisensory clusters swirl, can be considered as unselective for modality because they respond to inputs of all modalities. In this sense the trisensory output units are analogous to the orientationally unselective output units that form the "pin" in the center of the orientation pinwheels in the striate cortex model (the dots without lines through them in Figure 5.13).

The multisensory map model (see Figure 5.15D) stands as a prediction that pinwheels of modality selectivity should exist in the superior colliculus. Validating this prediction would establish that the pinwheel organization, observed so far only in visual cortex, can also occur in a non-cortical structure. Although the prediction is straightforward, testing it is problematic. Since the colliculus is a deep structure, optically imaging its actual organization, as was done for striate cortex (Obermayer and Blasdel 1993), is not possible. As illustrated in Figure 5.14, the observations that originally established the orderly progression of orientation selectivity in striate cortex were made by noting the order with which neurons of various orientation specificities were encountered along long, oblique recording-electrode trajectories through the striate cortex (Hubel and Wiesel 1974). The multisensory map model can be used to derive predictions about the order in which neurons of the various modality selectivities should be encountered along oblique recording-electrode trajectories through the deep layers of the superior colliculus. Although such recordings can be made experimentally, interpreting the results would be difficult.

In the striate cortex experiment the electrodes passed through cortical columns (Hubel and Wiesel 1974; Hubel 1988). Cortical columns are microstructures that form functional subsystems, with input, processing, and output stages (Purvis et al. 2004). In striate cortex, all the neurons in a column (except those at the input stage) have the same orientation specificity (see Figure 5.14). Experimentally, it was feasible to determine the orientation specificity of a column with a recording electrode, because within a column most of the neurons, including their cell bodies and processes (axons and dendrites) have the same orientation selectivity. In contrast, the superior colliculus does not have a columnar organization. An electrode passing through the colliculus will record not only from cell bodies, but also from axons and dendrites that can have modality selectivities very different from the cell bodies they are located near. The model predicts a pinwheel organization for clusters of cell bodies, but not for axons and dendrites, which could come from all over the superior colliculus. Because it is difficult to distinguish cell bodies from neural processes using electrode recording, encounters with axons and dendrites will obscure any map structure due to the arrangement of the cell bodies. Current experimental techniques may not provide resolution adequate to test predictions from the multisensory map model of the superior colliculus.

Although in some ways technically challenging, the superior colliculus (and the optic tectum, its non-mammalian homolog) is neurobiologically advantageous as a subject for models of brain map formation (Rauthazer and Cline 2004). Findings on map formation following manipulations (such as lesioning) of the optic tectum are generally consistent with mechanisms like those simulated by the SOM algorithm (Fraser and Perkel 1990). However, further experimentation is required to determine what roles, if any, competition, cooperation, Hebbian plasticity, and synaptic homeostasis actually play in the formation of real brain maps (Miller 1994). As emphasized at the beginning of this book, models are hypotheses that need to be verified experimentally. As the example of the multisensory map model illustrates, the definitive experiments are not always so easy to do.

Exercises

5.1   In training a network with three input units and three output units on the three vector clusters in R^3, using the nine input pattern vectors in Table 5.5, the network was trained using KohonenSOM (see MATLAB Box 5.1) without training neighbors (i.e., nHood=0, so only the winning output unit was trained on any learning cycle), and no map formed. Clearly, the input pattern vectors in each cluster are neighbors in vector space, so a fractured map at the output layer could potentially form. Can you change the structure of the network, and change the learning procedure, to get a fractured map of the clusters in R^3 to form? (Think in terms of numbers of output units nOut and nonzero training neighborhood size nHood.)

5.2   In training SOM networks with 11 input units and 7 output units using the diagonal-bar patterns (as in Table 5.7A), we used neighborhood sizes of 0 or 1. No map formed with neighborhood size 0. With neighborhood size 1, maps formed such that output units that are neighbors in the output array prefer similar input patterns. While some neighboring output units preferred the same input pattern, all of the output units had their own unique selectivity to the set of input patterns. Again set the number of output units to 7 (nOut=7) and retrain using the diagonal-bar patterns with neighborhood sizes greater than 1. The effects of larger neighborhood sizes will be more apparent with the decrement set to 1 (dec=1 in script KohonenSOM). Describe the output map and the responses of the output units when the network is trained with a neighborhood size of 5 (nHood=5). Does a map form? Do each of the output units have their own unique preferred input patterns? Would a SOM trained with 5 neighbors on each side be as good at representing the various inputs as a SOM trained with 1 neighbor on each side?

5.3   In training the SOM model of a tonotopic auditory representation using tonotopicSOM (see MATLAB Box 5.3), the central frequencies of the input units were equally spaced. In some creatures, such as echo-locating bats that emit calls over a narrow frequency range, many auditory afferents are specialized for inputs over that specific range. Set the central frequencies of the input units so that relatively more of them are tuned for frequencies over the middle of the frequency range using the command cf=[linspace(1.0,1.385,7) linspace(1.45,1.55,6) linspace(1.615,2.0,7)]. This command is already available in tonotopicSOM, and to use it you need only uncomment it. Retrain the network on this input arrangement using tonotopicSOM (you should run the script several times to get a nice map). How does this unequal spacing of input central frequencies change the map? Is the frequency range uniformly represented by the output units after training, or are more output units devoted to the midrange? Are the all the output units equally broadly tuned, or are some more tightly tuned to midrange frequencies? Would this make sense behaviorally?

5.4 In training SOM networks with seven output units on the orientation selectivity pattern arrays (see Table 5.8) and neighborhood size one, we found that output units that were neighbors in the output array had similar orientation specificities (see Table 5.10). The orientation selectivity patterns can be considered either as crude "image" arrays in two spatial dimensions or as feature vectors in 25 dimensions. As images they can be considered "nearby" each other if the angle between them is 45 degrees, and "orthogonal" if it is 90 degrees. We saw in Table 5.9 that orientation selectivity patterns, which were nearby as image arrays, overlapped in three places when reformatted as feature vectors. Examine the sparser orientation pattern arrays in Table E5.1, after reformatting them as feature vectors. In how many places do the sparser orientation selectivity patterns that are nearby as image arrays overlap as feature vectors? Do nearby pattern images overlap more than orthogonal pattern images when reformatted as vectors? Now retrain the network using `KohonenSOM` on the sparser orientation patterns with neighborhood size 1 (`nHood=1`), are retest the trained network to determine the output unit orientation specificities as before. Does a map form? Should a map form?

TABLE E5.1   Sparser orientation selectivity input pattern arrays for use in Exercise 5.4

1	2	3	4
1 0 0 0 0	0 0 1 0 0	0 0 0 0 1	0 0 0 0 0
0 1 0 0 0	0 0 1 0 0	0 0 0 1 0	0 0 0 0 0
0 0 1 0 0	0 0 1 0 0	0 0 1 0 0	1 1 1 1 1
0 0 0 1 0	0 0 1 0 0	0 1 0 0 0	0 0 0 0 0
0 0 0 0 1	0 0 1 0 0	1 0 0 0 0	0 0 0 0 0

References

Caporale N, Dan Y (2008) Spike timing-dependent plasticity: A Hebbian learning rule. *Annual Review of Neuroscience* 31: 25–46.

Desimone RT, Albright D, Gross CG, Bruce C (1984) Stimulus-selective properties of inferior temporal neurons in the macaque. *Journal of Neuroscience* 4: 2051–2062.

Fraser SE, Perkel DH (1990) Competitive and positional cues in the patterning of nerve connections. *Journal of Neurobiology* 21: 51–72.

Haykin S (1999) *Neural Networks: A Comprehensive Foundation, Second Edition.* Prentice Hall, Upper Saddle River, NJ, pp 443–483.

Hinton GE, McClelland JL, Rumelhart DE (1986) Distributed representations. In: Rumelhart DE, McClelland JL, PDP Research Group (eds) *Parallel distributed processing: Explorations in the microstructure of cognition, vol 1: foundations.* MIT Press, Cambridge, MA, pp 77–109.

Hubel DH (1988) *Eye, Brain, and Vision.* Scientific American Library, WH Freeman, New York.

Hubel DH, Wiesel TN (1974) Sequence regularity and geometry of orientation columns in the monkey striate cortex. *Journal of Comparative Neurology* 158: 267–293.

Kell CA, von Kriegstein K, Rösler A, Kleinschmidt A, Laufs H (2005) The sensory cortical representation of the human penis: Revisiting somatotopy in the male homunculus. *Journal of Neuroscience* 25: 5984–5987.

Kohonen T (1982) Self-organized formation of topologically correct feature maps. *Biological Cybernetics* 43: 59–69.

Kohonen T (1997) *Self-Organizing Maps, Second Edition*. Springer-Verlag, Berlin.

Knudsen EI, du Lac S, Esterly SD (1987) Computational maps in the brain. *Annual Review of Neuroscience* 10: 41–65.

Miller KD (1994) Models of activity-dependent neural development. *Progress in Brain Research* 102: 303–318.

Noble B, Daniel JW (1988) *Applied Linear Algebra, Third Edition*, Prentice Hall, Englewood Cliffs, NJ.

Obermayer K, Ritter H, Schulten K (1990) A principle for the formation of the spatial structure of cortical feature maps. *Proceedings of the National Academy of Science* 87: 8345–8349.

Obermayer K, Blasdel (1993) Geometry of orientation and ocular dominance columns in monkey striate cortex. *Journal of Neuroscience* 13: 4114–4129.

Orchard GA, Phillips WA (1991) *Neural Computation: A Beginner's Guide*. Lawrence Erlbaum, London, pp 63–91.

Penfield W, Rasmussen T (1950) *The Cerebral Cortex of Man*. Macmillan, New York.

Purves D, Augustine GJ, Fitzpatrick D, Hall WC, LaMantia A-S, McNamara JO, Williams SM (eds) (2004) *Neuroscience: Third Edition*. Sinauer, Sunderland, MA.

Rauthazer ES, Cline HT (2004) Insights into activity-dependent map formation from the retinotectal system: A middle-of-the-brain perspective. *Journal of Neurobiology* 59: 134–146.

Rumelhart DE, Zipser D (1986) Feature discovery by competitive learning. In: Rumelhart DE, McClelland JL, PDP Research Group (eds) *Parallel distributed processing: explorations in the microstructure of cognition, vol 1: foundations*. MIT Press, Cambridge, MA, pp 151–193.

Shah RD, Crair MC (2008) Mechanisms of response homeostasis during retinocollicular map formation. *Journal of Physiology* 586: 4363–4369.

Spirou GA, May BJ, Wright DD, Ryugo DK (1993) Frequency organization of the dorsal cochlear nucleus in cats. *Journal of Comparative Neurology* 329: 36–52.

Stein BE, Meredith MA (1993) *The Merging of the Senses*. MIT Press, Cambridge, MA.

Turrigiano GG (1999) Homeostatic plasticity in neuronal networks: The more things change, the more they stay the same. *Trends in Neuroscience* 22: 221–227.

von der Malsburg CH (1973) Self-organization of orientation sensitive cells in the striate cortex. *Kybernetik* 14: 85–100.

Wang G, Tanaka K, Tanifuji M (1996) Optical imaging of functional organization in the monkey inferotemporal cortex. *Science* 272: 1665–1668.

6

Supervised Learning and Non-Uniform Representations

Supervised learning algorithms can train neural networks to associate patterns and simulate the non-uniform distributed representations found in many brain regions

Two factors determine the properties of a real neural system. The first is the function that the neural system performs. The second is the process by which it acquired that function. While evolution and development count heavily in determining the properties of real neural systems, much of the function of the brain is acquired through learning. No human, for example, is born speaking a language, but each one must learn it, and the representation for language in the brain depends on certain variables including which language is learned, for how long, and whether or not it is the mother tongue (e.g., Hull and Vaid 2007).

Full language learning has so far eluded simulation, but aspects of it have been modeled using neural networks. These networks have input units, output units, and one or more layers of units that intervene between the input and output layers. They are trained using neural network learning algorithms on tasks that require the production of a correct output in response to an input. The algorithm compares the correct output with the actual output to determine network error, which it then uses to adjust network connection weights so as to minimize error and thereby correctly learn the task. Neural network learning algorithms that have this mode of operation are known as supervised algorithms, and what they implement is known as error-driven learning.

Multilayered neural network models trained using supervised learning algorithms have an uncanny, almost eerie ability to reproduce aspects of language learning such as word pronunciation (Sejnowski and Rosenberg 1987) or semantic category formation (McClelland and Rogers 2003). They do this by developing "internal representations," which are the collective response properties of units in the layers that intervene between the input and output layers. These internal units develop responses for combinations of input features that could not be learned via covariational or unsupervised mechanisms (see Chapters 4 and 5). Although the internal representations that develop in these language-learning networks are consistent with phenomena on the cognitive level, the responses of the units do not have clear counterparts on the neurophysiological level in real brains. A closer correspondence is achieved by multilayered neural networks trained using supervised learning to simulate simpler, sensorimotor tasks. These networks develop internal representations characterized by units that combine input features idiosyncratically, and the diversity of their responses resembles that observed neurophysiologically among real neurons. Such representations are known as non-uniform distributed representations. In this chapter we will demonstrate the power of supervised learning through comparison with covariation learning, and will use supervised learning algorithms to construct non-uniform distributed representations that resemble those observed in real neural systems.

Supervised learning algorithms can train neural networks to associate specific input patterns with specific desired output patterns. The desired output patterns are generally different from the input patterns, so the trained networks function as pattern associators. Unsupervised learning algorithms (see Chapter 5) cannot be used to train pattern associating networks. Hebbian learning algorithms (see Chapter 4), which are used mainly to train autoassociative networks, can also be used to train pattern associating networks, but they have limitations as we shall see.

Recall that the four Hebbian rules are the classic Hebb rule, the pre-synaptic rule, the post-synaptic rule, and the covariation (Hopfield) rule (see Chapter 4). Hebbian learning algorithms compute weight updates on the basis of pre-synaptic and post-synaptic activity only. In contrast, supervised learning algorithms compute weight updates on the basis of pre-synaptic activity and post-synaptic *error*, which is some measure of the difference between the desired and the actual output of a network. Supervised learning algorithms are more flexible and powerful as trainers of pattern associators.

The delta rule and back-propagation algorithms are the two most commonly used forms of supervised, error-driven learning. The delta rule is used for two-layered networks, because it can only train the weights of connections onto output units for which a desired output is known, and for which an explicit error can be computed. In contrast, back-propagation can be used to train networks with one or more layers of units that intervene between the input and the output layers, because back-propagation can determine the contribution to network error of units in layers that precede the output layer (Rumelhart et al. 1986). Because their activities are neither specified (as are the inputs) nor observed (as are the outputs), the units in intervening layers of multilayered networks are called "hidden" units. The properties of the hidden units in neural network models often provide insight into the organization of real neural systems.

Network error, which is a function of the difference between the desired and actual outputs of a network, is easy to determine. The challenge in deriving the back-propagation learning algorithm was in determining the contribution that the hidden units make to network error. The solution involved generating signals related to output unit error and propagating them backward to the hidden units, in the direction opposite to that in which the hidden units project to the output units. This feature casts some doubt on the neurobiological validity of back-propagation. While Hebbian rules receive strong support from neurophysiological studies that demonstrate synaptic weight changes associated with pre-synaptic and post-synaptic activity (see Chapter 4), there is no direct evidence that error signals propagate backward down axons. This has led to a search for alternatives to back-propagation. In the next chapter we will consider reinforcement learning algorithms that do not require backward propagation of signals but can train networks on some of the same tasks as back-propagation. Although reinforcement learning is less efficient than back-propagation, it is more plausible neurobiologically (see Chapter 7).

Of course, back-propagation is not the only way that error-driven learning could occur in the brain. Neurobiologically plausible mechanisms have been proposed by which neural projections from higher levels to lower levels, which abound in the brain (see Chapter 12), could carry error signals and mediate supervised learning (Zipser and Rumelhart 1990; O'Reilly 1996). Perhaps the best way to conceive of back-propagation is as a tool that very efficiently accomplishes a form of learning that may actually occur in the brain via different mechanisms. There is ample evidence of feedback, error-driven processes in operation in the brain. You use one of yours whenever you keep your car on the road. Neural feedback (servo) mechanisms range from high-level processes such as driving a car, down to the muscle-spindle stretch reflexes that regulate muscle tension (Gallistel 1980). These are feedback, error-driven mechanisms that regulate neural activity rather than synaptic strength, but it is conceivable that feedback, error-driven processes could also be used by the brain to regulate synapses.

Back-propagation can be thought of as a pervasive form of feedback in which every synapse in a neural network can regulate the value of its weight according to error. Networks trained using back-propagation can learn a wide variety of tasks in an equally wide variety of ways, and they can produce desired outputs that require learning complicated relationships among their inputs. Considering the power of error-driven learning, it would be surprising to find that the brain did not employ something similar. In any case, we will use back-propagation not as a model of actual learning but as a tool to construct neural network models that accomplish sensorimotor tasks, and in so doing simulate the response properties of real neurons. We will begin by demonstrating the power of back-propagation by comparing its capabilities with those of some Hebbian rules and the delta rule. Sections 6.1, 6.3, and 6.4 are adapted from McClelland and Rumelhart (1989) and Orchard and Philips (1991).

6.1 Using the Classic Hebb Rule to Learn a Simple Labeled Line Response

Hebbian pattern associators are similar to Hebbian auto-associators, except that the former have two layers instead of just one, and the connections are feedforward rather than recurrent. (All of the networks we will study in the chapter will be feedforward.) A generic, two-layered pattern associator neural network is shown in Figure 6.1. Units x_j in the input layer project to units y_i in the output layer over connections with weights v_{ij}. (Note that i and j index

FIGURE 6.1 **A generic, two-layered feedforward neural network** Input units x_j project to output units y_i over connections with weights v_{ij} ($j = 1, \ldots, n_x$ and $i = 1, \ldots, n_y$, where n_x and n_y are the numbers of input and output units, respectively.)

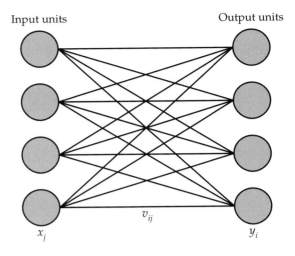

the output and input units, respectively, and $i = 1, \ldots, n_y$ while $j = 1, \ldots, n_x$ where n_x and n_y are the numbers of input and output units, respectively.) Hebbian pattern associators are trained according to the same rules as Hebbian auto-associators (see Chapter 4), except that in a pattern associator the pre-synaptic and post-synaptic units are in different layers. Equation 6.1 specifies the weight values using the classic Hebb rule to train a pattern associator:

$$v_{ij} = \sum_l y_i^l x_j^l \tag{6.1}$$

The post-synaptic units y_i are in the output layer, while the pre-synaptic units x_j are in the input layer. Any pattern l links a specific input unit activity pattern to a specific output unit activity pattern.

To illustrate pattern association by the Hebb rule, we will use the Hebb rule to train a network having four input units and one output unit on the four input and desired output patterns shown in Table 6.1. These patterns can be interpreted in the context of a simple labeled-line arrangement. For example, we could imagine that the output drives an escape response, which is elicited for noxious stimuli that come over input lines one and two, but not for neutral stimuli that come over input lines three and four. Note that the four patterns are non-overlapping. This makes them especially easy to learn.

To train weights v_{ij} using the classic Hebb rule, we initialize them all to 0, and then compute each weight as the sum over the weight adjustments for all four patterns (see Equation 6.1). Consider weight v_{11}, which connects input x_1

TABLE 6.1 **Learning the non-overlapping (labeled-line) patterns using the Hebb rule**

Input patterns				Desired output patterns	Actual output patterns
1	0	0	0	1	1
0	1	0	0	1	1
0	0	1	0	0	0
0	0	0	1	0	0

The input, desired output, and actual output following training are listed for a two-layered, feedforward network of binary threshold units. The network has four input units and one output unit.

to the single output y_1. For the first pattern, the desired output for y_1 is 1 and the activity specified for input unit x_1 is 1. The product of this post-synaptic and pre-synaptic activity is 1, so the adjustment to weight v_{11} due to the first pattern is 1 (see Equation 6.1). For the second pattern, the desired output for y_1 is again 1, but the activity specified for input unit x_1 is now 0. The product of this post-synaptic and pre-synaptic activity is 0, so the adjustment to weight v_{11} due to the second pattern is 0. The desired output for y_1 is 0 for both the third and fourth patterns so, regardless of the specified input activity, the weight updates for these patterns would be 0. The value of weight v_{11} specified by Hebb rule training, which is the sum of the weight changes over all four of the non-overlapping (labeled-line) patterns (see Table 6.1), is therefore equal to 1. The values of the other weights are computed similarly.

This method for computing the weight updates in a pattern associator using the classic Hebb rule is implemented by script `HebbPatAssoc`, which is listed in MATLAB® Box 6.1. To use this script, the input and desired output patterns would first need to be entered into the MATLAB workspace. The input and desired output patterns for the non-overlapping set given in Table 6.1 could be entered as rows into arrays `InPat` and `DesOut` using `InPat=` `[1 0 0 0;0 1 0 0;0 0 1 0;0 0 0 1]` and `DesOut=[1;1;0;0]`. (Since there is only one output unit in this example, `DesOut` has only one element per row, so it is really just a column vector in this case.) Script `HebbPatAssoc` uses these pattern arrays and the `size` command to find the number of patterns (`nPat`), and also the numbers of input (`nIn`) and output (`nOut`) units. It then defines the weight matrix `V` (just a row vector in this case), initializes all elements to 0, and computes the values for each weight according to the classic Hebb rule as outlined above (see Equation 6.1).

MATLAB® BOX 6.1   This script trains two-layered networks of binary units to associate patterns using the Hebb rule.

```
% HebbPatAssoc.m
% input InPat and desired output DesOut patterns
% must be supplied in workspace

[nPat,nIn]=size(InPat); % find numbers of patterns and inputs
[nPat,nOut]=size(DesOut); % find numbers of patterns and outputs
V=zeros(nOut,nIn); % initialize connectivity matrix V to all zeros
for i=1:nOut, % for each output unit
    for j=1:nIn, % for each input unit
        for l=1:nPat, % for each pattern (letter l indexes patterns)
            x=InPat(l,j); % set input x to input pattern
            y=DesOut(l,i); % set output y to desired output
            deltaV=y*x; % compute Hebb weight update
            V(i,j)=V(i,j)+deltaV; % apply weight update
        end % end pattern loop
    end % end input unit loop
end % end output unit loop

Out=zeros(nPat,nOut); % define array to hold output responses
for l=1:nPat, % for each pattern (letter l indexes patterns)
    x=InPat(l,:)'; % set input x to input pattern l
    q=V*x; % find the weighted input sum q
    y=q>0; % threshold the weighted input sum to find y
    Out(l,:)=y'; % set row l of array Out to output y
end % end pattern loop
```

TABLE 6.2 **Weight matrix after Hebb rule training on the non-overlapping (labeled-line) patterns**

To output unit	From input unit			
	1	**2**	**3**	**4**
1	1	1	0	0

Script `HebbPatAssoc` computes the weights using the nested-loop method (see Chapter 4). Specifically, it takes one weight `V(i,j)` at a time (the two outer loops) and computes its value over all the patterns (the inner loop). Thus, for each pattern `l=1:nPat`, the script sets `x=InPat(l,j)` and `y=DesOut(l,i)`. It computes the Hebb weight change due to each pattern as `deltaV=y*x` and updates the weight using `V(i,j)=V(i,j)+deltaV`. The weight values computed using the Hebb rule on the non-overlapping (labeled-line) patterns of Table 6.1 are shown in Table 6.2. Note that the weight values are either positive (excitatory) or 0. Because the activities (states) of the units in the network are non-negative (binary in this case) the classic Hebb rule cannot produce negative (inhibitory) connection weights

The output unit responses y_i of our Hebb pattern associator networks are binary, as were those of the auto-associative networks we studied in Chapter 4. Their responses are computed by first finding the weighted input sum q_i and then applying a threshold of 0, as shown in Equations 6.2 and 6.3:

$$q_i = \sum_j v_{ij} x_j \tag{6.2}$$

$$y_i = \begin{cases} 1, & q_i > 0 \\ 0, & q_i \leq 0 \end{cases} \tag{6.3}$$

Equation 6.2 is equivalent to $\mathbf{q} = \mathbf{V}\mathbf{x}$, where $\mathbf{q}$ is the vector of weighted input sums, $\mathbf{x}$ is the input vector, and $\mathbf{V}$ is the weight matrix.

After it trains the network, script `HebbPatAssoc` finds the actual output for each input pattern. It again does this in a loop, one pattern at a time, and stores the results in array `Out`. (Since there is only one output unit in this example, `Out` is just a column vector.) For each pattern `l=1:nPat`, the script sets the input (column) vector as `x=InPat(l,:)'`. It then implements Equations 6.2 and 6.3 in matrix and vector form using `q=V*x` followed by `y=q>0`, and sets the corresponding row (element in this case) of `Out` as `Out(l,:)=y'`. The actual outputs of the network trained on the non-overlapping input patterns are also shown in Table 6.1. The classic Hebb rule is able to train the network to correctly produce the desired output for each of the non-overlapping input patterns. Thus, the Hebb rule can successfully train a two-layered network on the labeled-line task.

The weight values and actual outputs are computed using loops in script `HebbPatAssoc` to facilitate explanation, and to show the correspondence between the MATLAB code and Equations 6.1–6.3. They can both be computed more efficiently using matrices. The weight values can be computed in one step using the command `V=DesOut'*InPat`. Computation of the weighted input sums and their conversion to binary can be accomplished in one step using `Out=(V*InPat')'>0`. The transpositions in this command cause the actual output patterns for each input pattern to be arrayed as the rows of `Out`. This facilitates comparison with the desired output. (Input and desired output pattern vectors are expressed as rows in this book.)

TABLE 6.3   Failure to learn the sparse-overlapping (simple contingency) patterns using the Hebb rule

Input patterns				Desired output patterns	Actual output patterns
1	0	0	0	1	1
1	1	0	0	1	1
1	0	1	0	0	1
0	0	0	1	0	0

The input, desired output, and actual output following training are listed for a two-layered, feedforward network of binary threshold units. The network has four input units and one output unit.

The classic Hebb rule was capable of training a pattern associator network on the set of non-overlapping input patterns, but this rule can fail on overlapping patterns. To illustrate this we train the network using the classic Hebb rule on the input and desired output patterns in Table 6.3. Note that these patterns are the same as the non-overlapping patterns of Table 6.1, except that in Table 6.3 the first three input patterns overlap in one place. Despite the overlap these input patterns are still fairly sparse, since most of the elements are 0. The sparse-overlapping patterns can be entered using the commands `InPat=[1 0 0 0;1 1 0 0;1 0 1 0;0 0 0 1]` and `DesOut=[1;1;0;0]`. The network can be trained on these sparse-overlapping patterns, and the actual output can be computed, using either the script `HebbPatAssoc` or the one-line commands given above.

The sparse-overlapping patterns specify that output unit y_1 should be active (state 1) when input unit x_1 is active alone (pattern 1), or when input units x_1 and x_2 are active together (pattern 2), but that y_1 should be inactive (state 0) when input units x_1 and x_3 are active together (pattern 3). Also y_1 should be inactive when input unit x_4 is active alone (pattern 4). For this task we can think of the response of output y_1 to input x_1 as being contingent on inputs x_2 and x_3. These sparse-overlapping patterns could correspond to a behavioral scenario in which an organism should produce an escape response (by activating y_1) if x_1 is active either by itself or with x_2, but should not produce an escape response if x_1 is active with x_3. To properly associate these patterns, and to account for the simple contingency they imply, the weighted input of unit x_3 must counteract the weighted input of unit x_1 to the output unit.

The network trained using the classic Hebb rule fails on this simple contingency task. The actual outputs and the weights following training on the sparse-overlapping (simple contingency) patterns are shown in Tables 6.3 and 6.4, respectively. The network fails specifically on the third pattern, where it should output a 0 but outputs a 1 instead. This failure results because weight v_{13}, the weight of the connection from input unit x_3 to output unit y_1, is 0 (Table 6.4), but it should be negative to counteract weight v_{11} from input unit x_1. The classic Hebb rule fails, in part, to train the network to properly associate the

TABLE 6.4   Weight matrix after Hebb rule training on the sparse-overlapping (simple contingency) patterns

To output unit	From input unit			
	1	2	3	4
1	2	1	0	0

TABLE 6.5   Learning the sparse-overlapping (simple contingency) patterns using the covariation rule

Input patterns				Desired output patterns	Actual output patterns
1	0	0	0	1	1
1	1	0	0	1	1
1	0	1	0	0	0
0	0	0	1	0	0

The input, desired output, and actual output following training are listed for a two-layered, feedforward network of binary threshold units. The network has four input units and one output unit.

sparse-overlapping (simple contingency) patterns of Table 6.3 because it cannot produce negative (inhibitory) connection weights.

6.2   Learning a Simple Contingency Using the Covariation Rule

Other Hebbian update rules (see Chapter 4), including the covariation rule, can produce negative weights using only non-negative unit activities and can learn to associate some overlapping patterns. To illustrate this we will use the covariation rule to train the network on the sparse-overlapping (simple contingency) patterns of Table 6.3, which are reproduced in Table 6.5. (Note that the covariation rule is also known as the Hopfield rule; see Chapter 4). The following equation specifies the weight values using the covariation rule to train a pattern associator:

$$v_{ij} = \sum_l \left(2y_i^l - 1\right)\left(2x_j^l - 1\right)$$ 6.4

The covariation rule is the same as the classic Hebb rule (see Equation 6.1) except that the binary states of the post-synaptic and pre-synaptic units are converted from 1 and 0 to +1 and −1 before they are multiplied. The network can be trained using the covariation rule by appropriately modifying script `HebbPatAssoc`, or it can be trained using the one-line command `V=(2*DesOut'−1)*(2*InPat−1)`. As before, computation of the sums of the weighted inputs to the output units, and their conversion to binary, can be accomplished in one step using `Out=(V*InPat')'>0`.

The covariation rule successfully trains the network on the simple contingency task. The actual output following training is shown in Table 6.5, and the connection weights following training are shown in Table 6.6. The trained network properly associates the sparse-overlapping patterns because the weighted input from unit x_3 is able to counteract the weighted input from unit x_1. Specifically, weight v_{11} is +2 while v_{13} is −2.

TABLE 6.6   Weight matrix after covariation training on the sparse-overlapping (simple contingency) patterns

To output unit	From input unit			
	1	2	3	4
1	+2	+2	−2	−2

TABLE 6.7   Failure to learn the dense-overlapping (complex contingency) patterns using the covariation rule

Input patterns	Desired output patterns	Actual output patterns
1 0 1 0	1	1
1 1 1 1	1	1
1 1 1 0	0	1
1 0 0 1	0	0

The input, desired output, and actual output following training are listed for a two-layered, feedforward network of binary threshold units. The network has four input units and one output unit.

As its name implies, the value of a weight trained using the covariation rule is equal to the covariation of the activities of its pre-synaptic and post-synaptic elements. For binary units, the covariation is +1 whenever the pre-synaptic and post-synaptic elements both have the same state (both 1 or both 0), but the covariation is −1 whenever the pre-synaptic and post-synaptic elements have different states. Consider weight v_{11}. Its pre-synaptic and post-synaptic elements (x_1 and y_1) have the same state for patterns 1, 2, and 4, but different states for pattern 3 (see Table 6.5). The net covariation is +2, and this is the value of the weight. Similarly, the covariation of input unit x_2 with the output y_1 is +2, while the covariations of units x_3 and x_4 with the output are −2, and these determine the values of their connection weights to output unit y_1.

Because the covariation rule is able to produce negative weights, it was able to train a network to properly associate the sparse-overlapping patterns in Table 6.3 (and Table 6.5), but it can fail with other sets of patterns. To illustrate this we use the covariation rule to train the network to associate the dense-overlapping patterns in Table 6.7. Whereas the sparse-overlapping patterns are consistent with a simple contingency, the dense-overlapping patterns could represent a more complex set of contingencies. In order to successfully associate the dense-overlapping patterns the network would need to learn a relatively complex set of relationships among its inputs.

The dense-overlapping (complex contingency) patterns can be entered using the commands `InPat=[1 0 1 0;1 1 1 1;1 1 1 0;1 0 0 1]` and `DesOut=[1;1;0;0]`. The input patterns are dense because most of the elements are 1 rather than 0. The network can be trained using the covariation rule on these dense-overlapping patterns, and the actual output can be computed, using the same methods that were used for the sparse-overlapping patterns. The actual output and the connection weights following training are shown in Tables 6.7 and 6.8, respectively.

The network trained using the covariation rule fails to properly associate the dense-overlapping patterns (see Table 6.7). Specifically, it would need to activate the output unit when input units x_1 and x_3 are active together (pattern

TABLE 6.8   Weight matrix after covariation training on the dense-overlapping (complex contingency) patterns

To output unit	From input unit			
	1	2	3	4
1	0	0	2	0

1) and when all four input units are active together (pattern 2), but not activate the output unit when input units x_1, x_2, and x_3 are active together (pattern 3), or when input units x_1 and x_4 are active together (pattern 4). To properly associate these patterns it seems that the learning algorithm would have to carefully combine the inputs by establishing a precise pattern of positive and negative weights. Despite the ability of the covariation rule to produce negative weights, it is not able to do that. In fact, only one of the weights, v_{13}, is nonzero (see Table 6.8). The reason is that only input unit x_3 has a nonzero covariation with the desired output (see Table 6.7).

In order to train the network to properly associate either the sparse-overlapping (simple contingency) or the dense-overlapping (complex contingency) patterns, the learning algorithm would essentially need to learn relationships among the inputs. Neither the classic Hebb rule nor the covariation rule does this. The covariation rule trained the network to properly associate the sparse-overlapping patterns not only because it could produce negative weights, but also because the sparse-overlapping patterns were set up so that the covariations between input and output produced positive and negative weights in the correct arrangement. In contrast, the input–output covariations implied by the dense-overlapping patterns did not produce positive and negative weights in an arrangement that permitted proper pattern association. The limitations of Hebbian algorithms in training pattern associators are overcome by learning algorithms that are based not on input–output covariation but on network performance. Performance-based algorithms change connection weights according to the errors made by the network in a pattern association task.

6.3   Using the Delta Rule to Learn a Complex Contingency

Learning algorithms that are driven by network error can learn relationships among the inputs in pattern association tasks. One of the simplest and most robust of the error-driven learning algorithms is the delta rule. This rule is used to train two-layered, feedforward networks to produce pattern associations. Unlike Hebbian rules, which proceeded from ideas and observations on neural plasticity (see Chapter 4), the delta rule was derived for a specific purpose, which was to produce weight updates in two-layered neural networks that minimize the error between the desired and the actual outputs for a set of input patterns (Rumelhart et al. 1986). We will briefly consider the derivation of the delta rule before using it computationally to train neural networks.

The delta rule is perhaps the simplest of the gradient-descent learning algorithms. (Back-propagation is a more complex gradient-descent learning algorithm that we will explore in the next section.) The gradient of a multivariate function is a vector field that indicates the direction and magnitude of the maximal slope of the function at any point. For example, the vectors of the gradient for a bowl-shaped function (such as an elliptic paraboloid) would all point away from the center of the bowl, and would indicate shallow slopes near the center and progressively steeper slopes moving outward toward the rim. A more formal definition of the gradient is given in Math Box 6.1.

While a bowl exists in three dimensions, the gradient is defined for functions of arbitrary dimension. If the function relates the error measure for a neural network with the connection weights of the network, then the gradient indicates the direction and magnitude of the maximal rate of increase of the error for any set of weight values. A gradient-descent learning algorithm, such as the delta rule, first finds the gradient of network error with respect to the connection weights, and then makes changes in the weights that are propor-

ⓂATH BOX 6.1   THE GRADIENT OF VECTOR CALCULUS

The multivariate function $f(x_1, x_2, ..., x_n)$ defines a scalar field in n dimensions, which is the value of the function for every point in n-dimensional space. The gradient, denoted by $\nabla f(x_1, x_2, ..., x_n)$, is a vector field in n dimensions that indicates the slope and direction of greatest increase of the function (Schey 2005).

An analogy with a univariate function makes the multivariate case clearer. The gradient $\nabla f(x)$ is just the derivative df/dx, which is the rate of change, or slope, of $f(x)$ at any specific value of x. The derivative df/dx can be represented in one dimension as a point on a line, or as a vector drawn from the origin to this point. The length of this vector equals the magnitude of the slope, and it points in the direction in which $f(x)$ increases.

For multivariate functions the gradient $\nabla f(x_1, x_2, ..., x_n)$ is the ordered set of partial derivatives of the function $f(x_1, x_2, ..., x_n)$ with respect to each of the variables, as shown in Equation B6.1.1:

$$\nabla f(x_1, x_2, ..., x_n) = \left(\frac{\partial f}{\partial x_1}, \frac{\partial f}{\partial x_2}, \cdots, \frac{\partial f}{\partial x_n} \right) \quad \text{B6.1.1}$$

The gradient $\nabla f(x_1, x_2, ..., x_n)$ for any specific set of values of the x_i ($i = 1, ..., n$) can be represented as a point in n-dimensional space, or as a vector drawn from the origin to this point. By analogy with $\nabla f(x)$ (which is df/dx), the vector defined by $\nabla f(x_1, x_2, ..., x_n)$ [from zero to ($\partial f / \partial x_1$, $\partial f / \partial x_2, ..., \partial f / \partial x_n$)] points in the direction of maximal slope of $f(x_1, x_2, ..., x_n)$ and its length equals the magnitude of the maximal slope. Since the gradient $\nabla f(x_1, x_2, ..., x_n)$ fills n-dimensional space with such vectors it is called a vector field. The inner (dot) product (see Math Box 1.2) of the gradient with a unit vector gives the slope of the function in the direction of the unit vector. Note that $\partial f / \partial x_i$ is the component of the gradient along the x_i axis.

If the multivariate function $E(w_1, w_2, ..., w_n)$ describes the error of a neural network in the n-dimensional space defined by its connection weights w_i, then the gradient $\nabla E(w_1, w_2, ..., w_n)$ indicates the direction and slope by which the error increases maximally. Changing the weights in the direction opposite to the gradient will decrease the error. A change in an individual weight Δw_i made in the direction opposite to $\partial E / \partial w_i$ will also reduce the error. Making proportional weight changes in the direction opposite to the component of the gradient along each weight axis is the basis of gradient-descent neural network learning algorithms such as the delta rule (see Math Box 6.2) and back-propagation (see Math Box 6.5). An error gradient (vector field) with respect to the weights for a simple, two-weight neural network is depicted schematically in Figure 6.2.

tional to the opposite of the gradient. Thus, the algorithm makes larger weight changes where the gradient is steep, and smaller ones where the gradient is more shallow, and iteratively converges on a set of weights that minimizes network error.

A formal derivation of the delta rule is given in Math Box 6.2. Briefly, the derivation begins by defining the network error as a function of the differences between the desired and actual output unit responses for any given input pattern. The derivation proceeds by finding the gradient of network error with respect to the weights, and concludes by finding weight updates that move actual network output in the direction of minimal error. A graphic illustration of this process is given in Figure 6.2, which depicts the network error with respect to the weights in a hypothetical neural system having only two weights, w_1 and w_2. In the illustration, minimal error is achieved when both weights equal 2.5. The delta rule would move the weights, incrementally and iteratively, from their start values to their error-minimizing values by moving them down the gradient of network error with respect to the weights.

While the notions undergirding the derivation of the delta rule may seem rather sophisticated, the delta rule itself, and the training procedure in which it is used, is very simple. On each iteration the two-layered, feedforward network to be trained using the delta rule is presented with an input pattern, and the actual output it produces in response is compared with the desired output for that pattern. The difference between the desired response for each output unit and the actual response is the error for each output unit. In contrast with Hebbian rules, in which the weight update is based on the input activity and

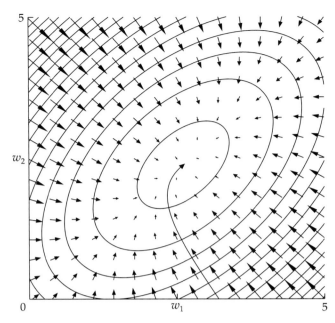

FIGURE 6.2 **Gradient descent in a neural network with only two weights:** w_1 **and** w_2 Error in this hypothetical network is minimized when $w_1 = w_2 = 2.5$. (From McClelland and Rumelhart 1989.)

output activity at a given connection, the weight update for the delta rule is proportional to input activity and output *error*. This is the essential difference between Hebbian and error-driven learning algorithms.

It is important to emphasize that the delta rule (and other supervised learning algorithms) differs from covariation (and other Hebbian algorithms) not only in being error-driven but also in being iterative. Rather than seeing each pattern only once, as do the Hebbian rules, the delta rule will see each pattern many times, generally in random order, and can make weight updates every time. The weight updates using the delta rule to train a two-layered pattern associator network are given by Equation 6.5:

$$\Delta v_{ij} = a(d_i - y_i)f'(q_i)\, x_j = ae_i\, f'(q_i)\, x_j = ag_i x_j \qquad \textbf{6.5}$$

In this equation, Δv_{ij} is the change in weight v_{ij} to unit y_i from unit x_j. The error e_i equals the desired (d_i) minus the actual (y_i) output. The term $f'(q_i)$ is the derivative of the activation function with respect to the weighted input sum q_i (see below in this section). The weight change then equals the learning rate a times the error, times the derivative of the activation function, times the state of the input unit x_j. It is convenient computationally to combine the product of the error and activation-function derivative terms into an "error signal" term g_i where $g_i = e_i f'(q_i)$. Then the weight change Δv_{ij} specified by the delta rule equals the learning rate a times the error signal g_i (for output unit y_i) times the state of input unit x_j such that $\Delta v_{ij} = ag_i x_j$. These weight changes are applied over many iterations as each pattern is presented many times and in random order, until network error has been reduced below a tolerance.

The delta rule learning procedure begins by constructing a random matrix **V** (with elements v_{ij}) connecting every input unit x_j to every output unit y_i. (Random initial weight values range uniformly from −1 to +1.) Then an input pattern is chosen from the set at random and presented to the network. The

MATH BOX 6.2   DERIVATION OF THE DELTA RULE LEARNING ALGORITHM

The delta rule (and several other learning algorithms) was derived by analytically determining how to adjust the connection weights in a network in order to achieve some objective. The delta rule is used to train two-layered, feedforward networks with input units x_j and output units y_i. (Here i and j index the output and input units, respectively.) The objective was to minimize the network error E, defined as one-half of the sum of the squared differences between the desired d_i and actual y_i outputs for any input pattern, as shown in Equation B6.2.1:

$$E = \frac{1}{2}\sum_i (d_i - y_i)^2 \qquad \text{B6.2.1}$$

The goal is to make individual weight changes Δv_{ij} so that the network error is reduced. This will occur if the weight changes are proportional to the opposite of the component of the network error gradient with respect to each weight: $\Delta v_{ij} \propto -\partial E / \partial v_{ij}$. (Gradients are described in Math Box 6.1.) The derivation begins by using the chain rule to expand the partial derivative $-\partial E / \partial v_{ij}$, as shown in Equation B6.2.2:

$$\frac{-\partial E}{\partial v_{ij}} = \frac{-\partial E}{\partial y_i}\frac{\partial y_i}{\partial q_i}\frac{\partial q_i}{\partial v_{ij}} \qquad \text{B6.2.2}$$

where q_i is the weighted input sum. The derivation continues by evaluating each term. The first term in the expansion is (the opposite of) the partial derivative of the network error with respect to the output y_i. This partial derivative, shown in Equation B6.2.3, can be found by differentiating the definition of the network error (see Equation B6.2.1) with respect to y_i:

$$\frac{-\partial E}{\partial y_i} = (d_i - y_i) \qquad \text{B6.2.3}$$

The second term in the expansion is simply the derivative of the output of the activation function y_i with respect to the input to the activation function q_i, which is shown in Equation B6.2.4:

$$\frac{\partial y_i}{\partial q_i} = f'(q_i) \qquad \text{B6.2.4}$$

(See Math Box 6.3 for the derivative of the squashing activation function.) The third term is the partial derivative of the weighted input sum q_i with respect to the weights

v_{ij}. This partial derivative is shown in Equation B6.2.5.

$$\frac{\partial q_i}{\partial v_{ij}} = \frac{\partial}{\partial v_{ij}}\sum_l v_{il}x_l = x_j \qquad \text{B6.2.5}$$

By substituting Equations B6.2.3, B6.2.4, and B6.2.5 into B6.2.2, and by including the learning rate a as a constant of proportionality, we find the delta rule weight changes shown in Equation B6.2.6:

$$\Delta v_{ij} = a(d_i - y_i)f'(q_i)x_j \qquad \text{B6.2.6}$$

In words, the weight adjustment specified by the delta rule for weight v_{ij} is computed as the learning rate a, times the difference between the desired d_i and actual y_i output, times the derivative of the activation function for weighted input sum q_i, times the input x_j. Equation B6.2.6 can be shortened by defining the error signal g_i as shown in Equation B6.2.7:

$$g_i = (d_i - y_i)f'(q_i) \qquad \text{B6.2.7}$$

in which case the delta rule can be written as in Equation B6.2.8:

$$\Delta v_{ij} = a g_i x_j \qquad \text{B6.2.8}$$

Equation B6.2.8 corresponds to Equation 6.5 in the main text. By substituting Equations B6.2.3 and B6.2.4 into Equation B6.2.7, the error signal at an output unit y_i can be written in terms of partial derivatives as in Equation B6.2.9:

$$g_i = \frac{-\partial E}{\partial y_i}\frac{\partial y_i}{\partial q_i} = \frac{-\partial E}{\partial q_i} \qquad \text{B6.2.9}$$

The error signal is useful in the derivation of back-propagation (see Math Box 6.5) and for programming purposes (see MATLAB Boxes 6.2 and 6.3). Rumelhart and coworkers (1986) provide further details on the derivation of the delta rule and back-propagation.

output response calculation begins in the usual way, by finding the weighted sum of the inputs, but the weighted input sum is then processed by the squashing activation function as shown in Equations 6.6 and 6.7:

$$q_i = \sum_j v_{ij}x_j \qquad \textbf{6.6}$$

$$y_i = \frac{1}{1+\exp(-q_i)} \qquad \textbf{6.7}$$

MATH BOX 6.3   DIFFERENTIATING THE SQUASHING FUNCTION

The squashing function, defined in Equation B6.3.1, gives the output y of a neural unit in terms of its weighted input sum q:

$$y = \frac{1}{\left(1 + e^{-q}\right)} \qquad \text{B6.3.1}$$

To differentiate the squashing function we use the following two generic derivative formulas (Equations B6.3.2 and B6.3.3):

$$\frac{d}{dx}\left(\frac{u}{v}\right) = \frac{v\frac{d}{dx}u - u\frac{d}{dx}v}{v^2} \qquad \text{B6.3.2}$$

$$\frac{d}{dx}e^u = e^u \frac{d}{dx}u \qquad \text{B6.3.3}$$

Applying the quotient formula (see Equation B6.3.2) to the squashing function (see Equation B6.3.1) we get Equation B6.3.4:

$$\frac{d}{dq}y = \frac{\left(1+e^{-q}\right)\frac{d}{dq}(1) - (1)\frac{d}{dq}\left(1+e^{-q}\right)}{\left(1+e^{-q}\right)^2} \qquad \text{B6.3.4}$$

Applying the exponential formula (see Equation B6.3.3) and simplifying we get Equation B6.3.5:

$$\frac{d}{dq}y = \frac{e^{-q}}{\left(1+e^{-q}\right)^2} \qquad \text{B6.3.5}$$

Equation B6.3.5 gives us the derivative of the squashing function in terms of the weighted input sum q, but an even simpler expression can be derived by first rewriting the right hand side of Equation B6.3.5 as in Equation B6.3.6.

$$\frac{e^{-q}}{\left(1+e^{-q}\right)^2} = \frac{1}{\left(1+e^{-q}\right)}\frac{e^{-q}}{\left(1+e^{-q}\right)} \qquad \text{B6.3.6}$$

By the definition of the squashing function (see Equation B6.3.1), we see that first term on the right-hand side of Equation B6.3.6 is just y. The second term is just $1 - y$. Thus, the derivative of the squashing function can be written, as in Equation B6.3.7, in terms of its value y:

$$y = \frac{1}{\left(1+e^{-q}\right)} \;\Rightarrow\; \frac{d}{dq}y = y(1-y) \qquad \text{B6.3.7}$$

The squashing function and its derivative are shown in Figure 6.3.

In Equations 6.6 and 6.7, q_i is the weighted input sum collected by each output unit y_i. The squashing function then ensures that the output unit responses to their weighted input sums will be bounded from 0 to 1. The squashing function smoothly simulates the cut-off and saturation properties of real neurons (see Chapter 1).

The squashing activation function is used with the delta rule, rather than the simple threshold function used with Hebbian rules, because it is smooth and therefore differentiable. (The instantaneous jump from 0 to 1 implied by the threshold function is not differentiable.) The delta rule provides a method for decreasing the error between the desired and actual outputs of a two-layered network, but its derivation (see Math Box 6.2) requires that the unit activation function be differentiable. The derivative of the squashing function is simply $f'(q_i) = y_i(1 - y_i)$ (see Math Box 6.3). The values of the squashing function and its derivative over a range of net inputs (e.g., weighted input sums) are illustrated in Figure 6.3A and B. The s-shaped squashing function is also known as the sigmoid function, and units that employ it are called sigmoidal units.

On each cycle of delta rule learning, an input pattern is chosen at random and the squashed actual response of each (sigmoidal) output unit y_i is computed according to Equations 6.6 and 6.7. The actual response of each output unit y_i is compared with the desired output d_i for that pattern to form the error e_i, and the error value is used to modify the connection weights to the corresponding output units according to Equation 6.5. At intervals, the error for all output units and all patterns is determined, and the absolute maximum

(A)   (B)

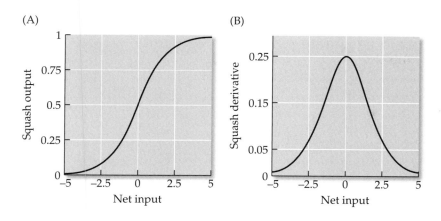

FIGURE 6.3   The squashing function (A) and its derivative (B) over the range −5 to +5. The net input could represent, for example, the sum of the weighted inputs to a unit. The s-shaped squashing function is also known as the sigmoid function.

error is compared to a tolerance. Learning ceases when the absolute maximum error is less than the preset tolerance.

The following example illustrates one weight update using the delta rule (implementing Equations 6.5–6.7). Consider a simple neural system composed only of one input unit x_1 and one output unit y_1, with connection weight v_{11}. Assume that, at the start of an iteration of delta rule learning, the value of v_{11} happens to be 0.20 (we will round values to the nearest hundredth in this numerical example). The next pattern chosen at random specifies that input x_1 should be 1 and that desired output d_1 should also be 1. The net input to the output unit is $q_1 = v_{11}x_1 = (0.20)(1) = 0.20$, and the resulting activation of the output unit, after passing q_1 through the squashing function, is $y_1 = 1 / [1 + \exp(-q_1)] = 1 / [1 + \exp(-0.20)] = 0.55$. The derivative at this output activation is $f'(q_1) = y_1(1 - y_1) = 0.55(1 - 0.55) = 0.25$. The error is $e_1 = d_1 - y_1 = 1 - 0.55 = 0.45$, and the error signal is $g_1 = e_1 f'(q_1) = (0.45)(0.25) = 0.11$. With learning rate $a = 1$, the delta rule update for this weight would be $\Delta v_{11} = a\, g_1\, x_1 = (1)(0.11)(1) = 0.11$. The new value of the weight is $v_{11} + \Delta v_{11} = 0.20 + 0.11 = 0.31$. This update makes intuitive sense. Because the actual output was too small, the delta rule specifies a positive weight adjustment. Conversely, it would specify a negative weight adjustment if the actual output had been too large. Computing error by subtracting the actual from the desired output (rather than the other way around) ensures that the weight updates will be of the appropriate sign.

The delta rule method for training a two-layered neural network pattern associator is implemented by script `deltaRuleTrain`, which is listed in MATLAB Box 6.2. To use the script to associate the dense-overlapping patterns in Table 6.7, the patterns can be entered using `InPat=[1 0 1 0;1 1 1 1;1 1 1 0;1 0 0 1]` and `DesOut=[1;1;0;0]`. The script will determine the numbers of input (`nIn`) and output (`nOut`) units directly from the input (`InPat`) and desired output (`DesOut`) patterns. The learning rate is set to 1 (`a=1`) and the tolerance is set to 0.1 (`tol=0.1`).

While there is considerable flexibility in setting the learning rate and tolerance parameters, some facts are worth noting. If we think of the delta rule as a feedback, error-driven mechanism that regulates the values of connection weights, then we can think of the learning rate a as the strength of that regulation. Real feedback mechanisms, which encounter some time delay in the feedback they receive about their performance, can become unstable if their effect on the variable they regulate is too strong. Consider, for example, what would happen to your car if the steering corrections you made on the basis of direction errors were too large. Because of the delay inherent in iterative algorithms, training using the delta rule can become unstable if the learning rate is too high. A learning rate of 1 is relatively high, but it will work for this example. For harder

MATLAB® BOX 6.2   This script trains two-layered networks of sigmoidal units to associate patterns using the delta rule.

```
% deltaRuleTrain.m
% input InPat and desired output DesOut patterns
% must be supplied in workspace

a=1; % set the learning rate
tol=0.1; % set the tolerance
nIts=10000; % set the maximum number of allowed iterations
[nPat,nIn]=size(InPat); % find numbers of patterns and inputs
[nPat,nOut]=size(DesOut); % find numbers of patterns and outputs
V=rand(nOut,nIn)*2-1; % set initially random connectivity matrix
maxErr=10; % set the maximum error to an initially high value

for c=1:nIts, % for each learning iteration (cycle)
    pIndx=ceil(rand*nPat); % choose pattern pair at random
    d=DesOut(pIndx,:)'; % set desired output d to chosen output
    x=InPat(pIndx,:)'; % set input x to chosen input pattern
    q=V*x; % find the weighted sum q of the inputs
    y=1./(1+exp(-q)); % squash that to compute the output y
    dy=y.*(1-y); % compute the derivative of the squashing function
    e=d-y; % find the error e for the chosen input
    g=e.*dy; % find output error signal g
    deltaV=a*g*x'; % compute delta rule weight update
    V=V+deltaV; % apply the weight update
    if rem(c,(5*nPat))==0, % after several updates check maximum error
        Q=(V*InPat')'; % compute the weighted input sum for all patterns
        Out=1./(1+exp(-Q)); % squash to compute output for all patterns
        maxErr=max(abs(DesOut-Out)); % find max error over all patterns
    end % end max error computation
    if maxErr<tol, break, end % break if max error is below tolerance
end % end learning loop
```

problems we will generally use a smaller learning rate (but we will use a very high learning rate for a specific purpose in Chapter 10).

In setting the tolerance, the characteristics of the squashing function are relevant (see Figure 6.3A). The squashing function asymptotically approaches 0 or 1 as the weighted input sum approaches negative or positive infinity, respectively. If desired outputs are binary, then tighter tolerances will require weights onto output units with larger absolute values. Because learning rates need to be kept relatively small in order to prevent instability, it can take many iterations to achieve weights with large absolute values. Because of the asymptotic characteristics of the squashing function, a small tightening (reduction) in the tolerance can result in a disproportionate increase in the number of training cycles required to reach it. A tolerance of 0.1 is typical for binary desired outputs. We will tighten the tolerance for problems that require a closer fit to real-valued desired outputs in the midrange of the squashing function.

The script `deltaRuleTrain` first randomizes the weights in matrix V by setting its elements to uniformly distributed random numbers between –1 and +1 using `V=rand(nOut,nIn)*2-1`. On each learning cycle the script chooses an input pattern at random by drawing a random integer `pIndx` from 1 to the number of patterns (`nPat`). It then uses `pIndx` as an index into the input and desired output arrays, and sets the input vector using `x=InPat(pIndx,:)'`, and the desired output vector using `d=DesOut(pIndx,:)'`. It finds the output `y` according to Equations 6.6 and 6.7 in vector-matrix form using `q=V*x`

TABLE 6.9   **Weight matrix after delta rule training on the dense-overlapping (complex contingency) patterns**

To output unit	From input unit			
	1	**2**	**3**	**4**
1	−6.71	−4.48	+8.94	+4.49

and $y=1./(1+exp(-q))$. (The command $1./vec$ finds the reciprocal of every element of a vector vec.) It then updates the weights according to Equation 6.5.

Note that deltaRuleTrain uses vector and matrix computations. For example, the script finds the output unit error signal vector using $g=e.*dy$, where the symbol string $.*$ produces element-by-element multiplication of the error vector e and the vector dy, which holds the derivatives of the squashing function for the outputs. Because e and dy are both columns their element-wise product is also a column. The script then computes the matrix of weight updates using $deltaV=a*g*x'$. In this command, input vector x is transposed from a column to a row, and the outer product between the error signal vector g, expressed as a column, and row vector x' produces the matrix of all products of output error signals and input states. (See Math Box 4.2 for a brief summary of the outer product between two vectors.) This outer product matrix, which is scaled by learning rate a, has the same dimensions as weight matrix V, so all of the weights can be updated in one step using $V=V+deltaV$.

Script deltaRuleTrain will train the network for nIts iterations, unless network performance falls within tolerance, at which point the script will break out of the learning loop. The script checks network performance every $5*nPat$ learning cycles. After training, the script uses the learned weights in V to find the array of weighted input sums to all output units using $Q=(V*InPat')'$, and squashes this whole array Q to find the output array using $Out=1./(1+exp(-Q))$. Note that these matrix commands can accommodate input and output layers of any size. In this example we have four input units but only one output unit.

Recall that we began this section with the goal of using the delta rule to train the network on the complex contingency (dense-overlapping) input–output patterns (see Table 6.7). The final connection weights following training using the delta rule on the dense-overlapping patterns are shown in Table 6.9, and the actual outputs of the trained network are shown in Table 6.10.

TABLE 6.10   **Learning the dense-overlapping (complex contingency) patterns using the delta rule**

Input patterns				Desired output patterns	Actual output patterns
1	0	1	0	1	0.90
1	1	1	1	1	0.90
1	1	1	0	0	0.09
1	0	0	1	0	0.09

The input, desired output, and actual output following training are listed for a two-layered, feedforward network of squashing function (sigmoidal) units. The network has four input units and one output unit.

TABLE 6.11   Failure to learn the exclusive-OR (XOR) patterns using the delta rule

Input patterns			Desired output patterns	Actual output patterns
0	0	1	0	0.50
1	0	1	1	0.58
0	1	1	1	0.49
1	1	1	0	0.57

The input, desired output, and actual output following training are listed for a two-layered, feedforward network of sigmoidal units. The network has three input units and one output unit.

(For ease of presentation, actual output values are rounded down to the nearest hundredth.) The trained network produces the correct output pattern for every input pattern within the tolerance of 0.1. Thus, it has learned to associate the dense-overlapping patterns, and it has thereby learned to accomplish the complex contingency task.

The delta rule has trained input units x_3 and x_4 to drive the output, by giving them positive weights, and it has trained input units x_1 and x_2 to counteract this drive by giving them negative weights to y_1 (see Table 6.9). This appropriately weighted combination of the inputs produces the required transformation. For example, strong excitatory drive from input unit x_3 overpowers the inhibition from input unit x_1 on input pattern 1, and produces the required output unit activation near 1, but inhibition from input unit x_1 counteracts the weaker excitatory drive from input unit x_4 on input pattern 4, and produces the required output unit activation near 0. Three-way and four-way interactions are required to produce the desired outputs for input patterns 3 and 2, respectively (see Table 6.10). The delta rule pattern associator is successful in associating the dense-overlapping (complex contingency) patterns. This success can be attributed to the ability of the algorithm to use network error to learn relationships among the inputs.

Although the delta rule is a more powerful pattern associator than the Hebbian rules, its ability to learn relationships between inputs is limited. This is illustrated using the input and desired output patterns shown in Table 6.11. The third input unit has state 1 in all of the patterns. It can be considered as a bias unit, which allows the outputs to learn to bias their activities either positively or negatively, depending on the value of the bias input weight. Such ability can be of great benefit in learning certain transformations in networks of sigmoidal units. The first and second input units and the output unit specify a logical relationship known as "exclusive-OR" (XOR). This logical operator is true (i.e., 1) if and only if one *or* the other of its inputs is true. The XOR operator is false (i.e., 0) if both of its inputs are at the same state, either true or false. This is an important operator for pattern associators, since many larger problems have XOR as a sub-problem. The XOR is a tough problem for a pattern associator because the output has to be 1 when *either* input unit x_1 or x_2 is 1, but 0 when *both* of the inputs are 1. In principle, an algorithm that can learn the relationships among inputs should be able to train a network on the XOR. As we shall see, the delta rule is not quite up to the task.

The script `deltaRuleTrain` can be used to train a two-layered network on the XOR patterns shown in Table 6.11. The patterns can be entered using the commands `InPat=[0 0 1;1 0 1;0 1 1;1 1 1]` and `DesOut=[0;1;1;0]`. Again, the learning rate is `a=1` and the tolerance is `tol=0.1`. The number of allowed training iterations is `nIts=100000`. The network trained with the delta rule fails to learn the XOR in this number of iterations. The actual outputs and the connection weights, following 100,000 cycles of training using the delta rule on the XOR, are shown in Tables 6.11 and 6.12, respectively. The network clearly fails to produce the desired output for each of the input patterns. The error still exceeds the tolerance of 0.1 after 100,000 iterations. Even with a bias unit available (input unit x_3), the network is incapable of producing an output near 1 when either x_1 or x_2 has state 1, but of producing an output near 0 when both x_1 and x_2 have state 1.

TABLE 6.12 **Weight matrix after delta rule training on the XOR patterns**

To output unit	From input unit		
	1	2	3
1	+0.03	−0.04	+0.01

The reason the two-layered network trained using the delta rule fails to learn the XOR patterns is that it has only an input and an output layer. To properly represent the relationships among the inputs required for the XOR transformation, the network would need an additional layer of units between the input and the output layers. The delta rule can be used only to train the weights to units for which an error value can be assigned (see Equation 6.5). The delta rule by itself cannot assign error signals to units in intervening layers. The back-propagation learning algorithm was specifically derived to overcome this limitation.

6.4 Learning Interneuronal Representations using Back-Propagation

The delta rule is limited by having only two layers of processing units (and one layer of weights). The computational abilities of neural networks composed of nonlinear processing units can be extended by including layers that intervene between input and output. (This is not true for multilayered networks of *linear* processing units; see Math Box 6.4.) As indicated at the beginning of this chapter, units in intervening layers, which are neither input nor output units, are called hidden units. Hidden units can correspond to interneurons in real neural systems. We will add a layer of processing units to the two-layered networks. A generic, three-layered pattern associator neural network is shown in Figure 6.4. Three-layered networks have layers x_j, y_i, and z_k. Layer x_j projects

Input units   Hidden units   Output units

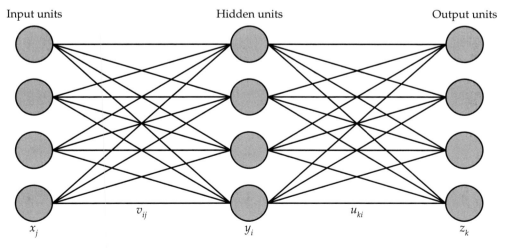

x_j v_{ij} y_i u_{ki} z_k

FIGURE 6.4 **A generic, three-layered feedforward neural network** Input units x_j project to hidden units y_i over connections with weights v_{ij}. Hidden units y_i then project to output units z_k over connections with weights u_{ki} ($j = 1, ..., n_x$, $i = 1, ..., n_y$, and $k = 1, ..., n_z$, where n_x, n_y, and n_z are the numbers of input, hidden, and output units, respectively).

MATH BOX 6.4 MULTILAYERED NETWORKS OF LINEAR PROCESSING UNITS

Feedforward networks with more than two layers are useful only if the units have nonlinear activation functions. Consider the three-layered, feedforward network shown in Figure 6.4, in which input units x_j project to hidden units y_i over connections with weights v_{ij}, and hidden units y_i then project to output units z_k over connections with weights u_{ki}. (Note that i, j, and k index the hidden, input, and output units, respectively.) We compute the activation of each unit in the usual way, by finding the value of its activation function $f(q)$ with its weighted input sum (q_i for y_i, or q_k for z_k) as the argument. Hidden and output unit activations are shown in Equations B6.4.1 and B6.4.2:

$$q_i = \sum_j v_{ij} x_j, \quad y_i = f(q_i) \qquad \text{B6.4.1}$$

$$q_k = \sum_i u_{ki} y_i, \quad z_k = f(q_k) \qquad \text{B6.4.2}$$

A linear activation function $f(q)$ involves nothing more than multiplication of its argument by a constant C, as in Equations B6.4.3 and B6.4.4:

$$q_i = \sum_j v_{ij} x_j, \quad y_i = C q_i \qquad \text{B6.4.3}$$

$$q_k = \sum_i u_{ki} y_i, \quad z_k = C q_k \qquad \text{B6.4.4}$$

In Equations B6.4.3 and B6.4.4 we scale the weighted input sums (q_i or q_k) by C to compute the unit activations (y_i or z_k). Equivalently, we could have scaled the weights (v_{ij} and u_{ki}) by C first, and then computed the unit activations (y_i or z_k) directly as weighted input sums (without computing intermediate variables q_i or q_k) using the scaled weights. Without loss of generality concerning the point we are making in this Math Box, we can assume that the constant equals 1 ($C = 1$). Then the activation of

each unit is computed directly as its weighted input sum using unscaled weights.

Weighted input sums can be computed via matrix and vector multiplication (see Math Box 1.2). For the three-layered network (see Figure 6.4) the unit states can be represented as vectors $\mathbf{x}$, $\mathbf{y}$, and $\mathbf{z}$, and the weights as matrices $\mathbf{V}$ and $\mathbf{U}$. Given linear activation functions with $C = 1$, the weighted input sums can be represented in matrix notation as $\mathbf{y} = \mathbf{Vx}$ and $\mathbf{z} = \mathbf{Uy}$. Substituting for $\mathbf{y}$ we find that $\mathbf{z} = \mathbf{UVx}$. The same applies for $C \neq 1$ because in that case the $\mathbf{U}$ and $\mathbf{V}$ matrices are simply scaled first by C. Thus, if the unit activation functions are linear, then processing in a three-layered network is equivalent to processing in a two-layered network in which the input–output weight matrix of the two-layered network is the matrix product (see Math Box 4.3) of the hidden–output and the input–hidden weight matrices of the three-layered network.

Note that the weight matrix of connections out of a layer of n units has n columns, while the weight matrix of connections into a layer of n units has n rows. What this means for feedforward networks is that the weight matrix out of a layer always conforms to the weight matrix into a layer, in that order (see also Math Box 4.3). For example, in the expression $\mathbf{z} = \mathbf{UVx}$ that we derived above, the hidden-output weight matrix $\mathbf{U}$ precedes the input-hidden matrix $\mathbf{V}$ in the product. Because of this conformability, the weight matrices between any number of additional hidden layers can be included in the product if the units are linear. Thus, multiple layers in feedforward neural networks are useful only if the unit activation functions are nonlinear.

to layer y_i over weights v_{ij}, as before, while layer y_i projects to layer z_k over weights u_{ki}. Units y_i, formerly the output units in two-layered networks, have become the hidden units (interneurons) in three-layered networks. Note that i, j, and k respectively index the hidden, input, and output units in three-layered networks (and $k = 1, \ldots, n_z$ where n_z is the number of output units in three-layered networks). We will compose the three-layered networks of sigmoidal (squashing function) units.

The challenge in training multilayer networks is in knowing how to assign error to units in intermediate (hidden) layers, for which desired values do not exist and indeed cannot be known *a priori*. The back-propagation algorithm meets this challenge by determining the error signal at the output layer and propagating it back to intermediate layers, in such a way that the error signals assigned to hidden units reflects their contribution to output error. Back-propagation, like the delta rule, is a gradient-descent learning algorithm. The derivation of back-propagation is a generalization of the derivation of the delta rule to feedforward networks of nonlinear units having arbitrarily many layers (Rumelhart et al. 1986). The derivation of the back-propagation learning algorithm is summarized in Math Box 6.5.

MATH BOX 6.5   DERIVATION OF THE BACK-PROPAGATION LEARNING ALGORITHM

Back-propagation can be thought of as an extension of the delta rule to feedforward networks with one or more layers of nonlinear hidden units that intervene between the input and output layers (see Figure 6.4). We consider a feedforward network with three layers: input units x_j, hidden units y_i, and output units z_k. (Here i, j, and k index the hidden, input, and output units, respectively.) As for the delta rule, the objective for back-propagation is to minimize the network error E, defined as one-half of the sum of the squared differences between the desired d_k and actual z_k outputs for any input pattern, as described in Equation B6.5.1:

$$E = \frac{1}{2}\sum_k \left(d_k - z_k\right)^2 \qquad \text{B6.5.1}$$

In the three-layered network, weights v_{ij} connect the input to the hidden units, and weights u_{ki} connect the hidden to the output units. The goal of back-propagation is to make changes to these weights that are proportional to the opposite of the network error gradient with respect to each weight, as shown in Equations B6.5.2 and B6.5.3:

$$\Delta v_{ij} \propto \frac{-\partial E}{\partial v_{ij}} \qquad \text{B6.5.2}$$

$$\Delta u_{ki} \propto \frac{-\partial E}{\partial u_{ki}} \qquad \text{B6.5.3}$$

Updates for both weights take the same form, as shown in Equations B6.5.4 and B6.5.5. They are composed as the product of learning rate a, the pre-synaptic activity (x_j or y_i), and the post-synaptic error signal (g_i or g_k):

$$\Delta v_{ij} = a\, g_i\, x_j \qquad \text{B6.5.4}$$

$$\Delta u_{ki} = a\, g_k\, y_i \qquad \text{B6.5.5}$$

Note that in three-layered networks the z_k are output units, while the y_i are hidden units. The error signal g_k and the weighed input sum q_k for the outputs z_k are distinguished from those for the hidden units y_i by their subscript k. Then the output error signal for the three-layered network, shown in Equation B6.5.6, is analogous to that for the two-layered network (see Math Box 6.2):

$$g_k = \frac{-\partial E}{\partial q_k} = \frac{-\partial E}{\partial z_k}\frac{\partial z_k}{\partial q_k} = \left(d_k - z_k\right)f'\left(q_k\right) \qquad \text{B6.5.6}$$

Determination of the error signal at the hidden layer is much trickier. Using the chain rule, the hidden unit error signal can be written as in Equation B6.5.7:

$$g_i = \frac{-\partial E}{\partial q_i} = \frac{-\partial E}{\partial y_i}\frac{\partial y_i}{\partial q_i} \qquad \text{B6.5.7}$$

As for the delta rule (see Math Box 6.2), the second term on the right of Equation B6.5.7 is the derivative of the unit activation function with respect to the weighted input sum, as shown in Equation B6.5.8:

$$\frac{\partial y_i}{\partial q_i} = f'\left(q_i\right) \qquad \text{B6.5.8}$$

Evaluation of the first term on the right of Equation B6.5.7 involves a summation over all of the output units z_k (see Rumelhart et al. 1986 for details). This summation is shown in Equation B6.5.9:

$$\frac{-\partial E}{\partial y_i} = -\sum_k \frac{\partial E}{\partial q_k}\frac{\partial q_k}{\partial y_i} \qquad \text{B6.5.9}$$

The first term in the summation is the opposite of the output error signal (see Equation B6.5.6), so that in Equation B6.5.10 we have:

$$-\sum_k \frac{\partial E}{\partial q_k}\frac{\partial q_k}{\partial y_i} = \sum_k g_k \frac{\partial}{\partial y_i}\sum_l u_{kl}y_l = \sum_k g_k u_{ki} \qquad \text{B6.5.10}$$

Equation B6.5.10 specifies that a component of the error signal at hidden unit y_i is the sum of all the output unit error signals g_k that are weighted by the weights u_{ki} that connect hidden unit y_i to each of the output units z_k. In other words, the output unit error signals are *back-propagated* down the connections by which the hidden units project up to the output units. By substituting Equation B6.5.10 into B6.5.9, and Equations B6.5.9 and B6.5.8 into B6.5.7, the hidden unit error signal, described in Equation B6.5.11, is found to be:

$$g_i = f'\left(q_i\right)\sum_k g_k u_{ki} \qquad \text{B6.5.11}$$

Substituting B6.5.11 and B6.5.6 into Equations B6.5.4 and B6.5.5 gives the back-propagation updates with the error signal terms g_i and g_k written out. Equations B6.5.6 and B6.5.11 correspond to Equations 6.8 and 6.9 of the main text, and Equations B6.5.5 and B6.5.4 are the same as Equations 6.10 and 6.11 of the main text, respectively.

The error signal at the output layer is the same for three-layered networks as for two-layered networks, except that the output units are the z_k rather than the y_i, so the relevant index is k as shown in Equation 6.8:

$$g_k = \left(d_k - z_k\right) f'\left(q_k\right) = e_k f'\left(q_k\right)$$ **6.8**

The error signal g_k equals the output error $(d_k - z_k)$, multiplied by the derivative of the squashing function for output state z_k, which is $f'(q_k) = (z_k)(1 - z_k)$ (see Math Box 6.3). The error signal at the hidden layer index (i) takes a rather different form, as shown in Equation 6.9:

$$g_i = f'\left(q_i\right) \sum_k g_k u_{ki}$$ **6.9**

The error signal g_i equals the derivative of the squashing function for hidden unit state y_i, which is $f'(q_i) = (y_i)(1 - y_i)$, times a summation term. The summation term is the sum of the products of the output unit error signals g_k (in the output layer indexed by k), weighted by the weights u_{ki} connecting unit y_i in the hidden layer (with index i) to all the units in the output layer. This weighting goes in the direction opposite the one that determines the usual weighted input sum to a unit. Note that the output error signals in Equation 6.9 are propagated backward over the connections from the hidden units, scaled by the same weights that scale the hidden unit activity that is propagated forward over these same connections. This crucial step, which determines the contribution of the hidden units to output error, is what has given the back-propagation algorithm its name. In principle, back-propagation of error can take place over arbitrarily many layers of hidden units. We will use only one layer of hidden units in this book.

After the error signals at the output and hidden layers are calculated, the updates for the hidden–output weights u_{ki} are computed as in Equation 6.10:

$$\Delta u_{ki} = a g_k y_i$$ **6.10**

Likewise the updates for the input–hidden weights v_{ij} are computed as in Equation 6.11:

$$\Delta v_{ij} = a g_i x_j$$ **6.11**

In these equations g_k and g_i are the output and hidden unit error signals, y_i and x_j are the hidden and input unit states, and a is the learning rate. The training sequence for back-propagation is the same as that for the delta rule, except that now an intervening layer is involved. In determining network activation, the hidden layer must be activated before the output layer can be activated. (We will use the squashing function as the activation function for hidden and output units in three-layered networks; see Equations 6.6 and 6.7.) Similarly, concerning assignment of hidden unit contribution to the error, the output layer error signal (see Equation 6.8) must be computed before the error signal at the hidden layer can be computed (see Equation 6.9).

The computations involved in back-propagation will be illustrated using a very simple example, in which we will implement Equations 6.6–6.11 (for ease of presentation we will round values to the nearest hundredth). Consider a network composed only of one input unit x_1, one hidden unit y_1, and two output units z_1 and z_2. The weight v_{11} connects x_1 to y_1, and weights u_{11} and u_{21} connect y_1 to z_1 and z_2, respectively. Assume that, at the start of an iteration of back-propagation learning, the value of v_{11} happens to be 0.50, and the values of both u_{11} and u_{21} are 0.70. The next pattern chosen at random specifies that input x_1 should be 1 and that both desired outputs d_1 and d_2 should also be 1. The net input to the hidden unit is $q_{y1} = v_{11}x_1 = (0.50)(1) = 0.50$, and the resulting activation of the hidden unit, after passing q_{y1} through the squash-ing function, is $y_1 = 1 / [1 + \exp(-q_{y1})] = 1 / [1 + \exp(-0.50)] = 0.62$. The derivative at this hidden unit activation is $f'(q_{y1}) = y_1(1 - y_1) = 0.62(1 - 0.62) = 0.24$. The net input to output unit z_1 is $q_{z1} = u_{11}y_1 = (0.70)(0.62) = 0.43$, and the resulting activation of output unit z_1, after passing q_{z1} through the squashing function, is $z_1 = 1 / [1 + \exp(-q_{z1})] = 1 / [1 + \exp(-0.43)] = 0.61$. The derivative at this output unit activation is $f'(q_{z1}) = z_1(1 - z_1) = 0.61(1 - 0.61) = 0.24$. The net input to output unit z_2, its resulting activation, and its derivative are the same as for z_1. The error for output unit z_1 is $e_1 = d_1 - y_1 = 1 - 0.61 = 0.39$. The error e_2 for output unit z_2 is the same. The error signal at output unit z_1 is $g_{z1} = e_1 f'(q_{z1}) = (0.39)(0.24) = 0.09$, and the same for the error signal g_{z2} at z_2.

The computation of the error signal at the hidden unit involves the output unit error signals, each weighted by the weight of the connection from the hidden unit to each output unit, that are essentially propagated back from the output layer to the hidden layer where they are summed. This weighted sum is multiplied by the derivative of the hidden unit activation to compute the hidden unit error signal. Thus, the error signal at the hidden unit is $g_{y1} = f'(q_{y1}) (u_{11}g_{z1} + u_{21}g_{z2}) = (0.24)[(0.70)(0.09) + (0.70)(0.09)] = 0.03$. Note that this is the back-propagation step in this simple numerical example.

With learning rate $a = 1$ the back-propagation update for weight u_{11}, which connects hidden unit y_1 to output z_1, would be $\Delta u_{11} = a \, g_{z1} \, y_1 = (1)(0.09)(0.62) = 0.06$. The new value of the weight is $u_{11} + \Delta u_{11} = 0.70 + 0.06 = 0.76$. The weight u_{21} is updated by the same value. The back-propagation update for weight v_{11}, connecting input x_1 to hidden unit y_1, would be $\Delta v_{11} = a \, g_{y1} \, x_1 = (1)(0.03) (1) = 0.03$. The new value of the weight is $v_{11} + \Delta v_{11} = 0.50 + 0.03 = 0.53$. These updates make sense. Because both actual outputs were too small, and because there is only one hidden unit to drive both output units, back-propagation specifies that all the connection weights, including the input–hidden weight v_{11} and both hidden–output weights u_{11} and u_{21}, should be increased.

The method for computing weight updates in a three-layered pattern asso-ciator using back-propagation is implemented by script `backPropTrain`, which is listed in MATLAB Box 6.3. The script is similar in basic outline to `deltaRuleTrain` (see MATLAB Box 6.2), but is necessarily more compli-cated. Script `backPropTrain` relies more than `deltaRuleTrain` on vec-tor and matrix operations and it takes several short cuts. For example, the states of the hidden units in vector y are updated using the command `y=1./ (1+exp(-V*x))`, where the weighted input sum for all hidden units is expressed directly as `V*x`, rather than by first assigning the weighted input sums to the intermediate vector variable q and using that as the argument of the squashing function. For convenience, the script `backPropTrain` handles bias units internally, and appends the bias to input and hidden unit state vec-tors. For example, the command `y=[y' b]'` appends the bias to the hidden unit state vector after it is updated.

In script `backPropTrain` the weight update computations begin by converting the state vectors from columns to rows (`x=x'`, `y=y'`, and `z=z'`). The error signal at the output zg is computed using the command `zg=e.*(z.*(1-z))`, where the error vector e, which is the difference between the desired and actual output state vectors, is multiplied by the deriv-ative of the squashing function at the output states `(z.*(1-z))`. Note again that the `.*` command specifies element-by-element multiplication of vectors, not their inner or outer products. The error signal yg at the hidden layer is computed using `yg=(y.*(1-y)).*(zg*U)`. The command `(y.*(1-y))` computes the derivative of the squashing function at the hidden unit states. The command `zg*U` implements the back-propagation step in script `backPropTrain`. Note that this command specifies multiplication of a (row)

MATLAB® BOX 6.3   This script trains three-layered networks of sigmoidal units to associate patterns using back-propagation.

```
% backPropTrain.m
% input InPat and desired output DesOut patterns
% must be supplied in workspace

a=0.25; % set the learning rate
tol=0.1; % set the tolerance
b=1; % set the bias
nIts=100000; % set the maximum number of allowed iterations
nHid=2; % set the number of hidden units
[nPat,nIn]=size(InPat); % find numbers of patterns and inputs
[nPat,nOut]=size(DesOut); % find numbers of patterns and outputs
V=rand(nHid,nIn+1)*2-1; % set initial input-hidden weight matrix
U=rand(nOut,nHid+1)*2-1; % set initial hidden-output weight matrix
deltaV=zeros(nHid,nIn+1); % define input-hidden change matrix
deltaU=zeros(nOut,nHid+1); % define hidden-output change matrix
maxErr=10; % set the maximum error to an initially high value

for c=1:nIts, % for each learning iteration
    pIndx=ceil(rand*nPat); % choose pattern pair at random
    d=DesOut(pIndx,:); % set desired output to chosen output
    x=[InPat(pIndx,:) b]'; % append the bias to chosen input
    y=1./(1+exp(-V*x)); % compute the hidden unit response
    y=[y' b]'; % append the bias to the hidden unit vector
    z=1./(1+exp(-U*y)); % compute the output unit response
    e=d-z'; % find the error vector
    if max(abs(e))>tol, % train if any error exceeds tolerance
        x=x';y=y';z=z'; % convert column to row vectors
        zg=e.*(z.*(1-z)); % compute the output error signal
        yg=(y.*(1-y)).*(zg*U); % compute hidden unit error signal
        deltaU=a*zg'*y; % compute the change in hidden-output weights
        deltaV=a*yg(1:nHid)'*x; % change in input-hidden weights
        U=U+deltaU; % update the hidden-output weights
        V=V+deltaV; % update the input-hidden weights
    end % end the training conditional
    if rem(c,(5*nPat))==0, % every so often check network performance
        Inb=[InPat b*ones(nPat,1)]; % append bias to input patterns
        Hid=(1./(1+exp(-V*Inb')))'; % find hid response to all patterns
        Hidb=[Hid b*ones(nPat,1)]; % append bias to all hidden vectors
        Out=(1./(1+exp(-U*Hidb')))'; % output response to all patterns
        maxErr=max(abs(abs(DesOut-Out))); % find max overall error
    end % end max error computation
    if maxErr<tol, break, end, % break if all errors within tolerance
end % end training loop
```

vector and a matrix, in that order (see Math Box 4.3). Because the columns of U are the weights from each hidden unit to every output unit, the command zg*U computes the sum of the output error signals (in row vector zg) weighted by the weights from each hidden unit to every output unit (each column of U). Thus, zg*U computes the summation in Equation 6.9 for each hidden unit. The matrices of weight updates are computed as for the delta rule using the outer product commands: deltaU=a*zg'*y and deltaV=a*yg(1:nHid)'*x. Note that in the command for deltaV the sub-

TABLE 6.13   **Learning the XOR patterns using back-propagation**

Input patterns	Desired output patterns	Actual output patterns
0 0	0	0.09
1 0	1	0.90
0 1	1	0.90
1 1	0	0.09

The input, desired output, and actual output following training are listed for a three-layered, feedforward network of sigmoidal, squashing function units. The network has two input units, two hidden units, and one output unit.

command `yg(1:nHid)`, where `nHid` is the number of hidden units, removes some bias-related terms from the outer product matrix. Since the bias units do not receive connections (by definition) there are no connection weights onto them that need to be updated. The hidden–output and input–hidden weights are updated using `U=U+deltaU` and `V=V+deltaV`.

To use the script `backPropTrain` to associate the XOR patterns, the patterns can be entered using commands `InPat=[0 0;1 0;0 1;1 1]` and `DesOut=[0;1;1;0]`. The script will determine the required numbers of input and output units from the patterns, but the required number of hidden units must be specified. Set `nHid=2` for the XOR problem. Set other parameters as follows: bias `b=1`, tolerance `tol=0.1`, learning rate `a=0.25`, and maximum number of iterations `nIts=100000`. The script trains the weights in matrices `V` and `U` and stores the actual outputs for each input pattern in array `Out`.

The XOR is a hard problem for this network configuration. It took over 20,000 cycles (iterations) for this run of the algorithm to reach tolerance. However, the number of iterations required to reach tolerance depends heavily on the values in the initially random weight matrices and can vary widely. Following training, the actual outputs, along with the input and desired XOR patterns, are shown in Table 6.13, and the final connection weights are shown in Table 6.14.

The network trained with back-propagation learns to associate the XOR patterns, and produces the correct output pattern for every input pattern within the tolerance of 0.1 (see Table 6.13). The solution that back-propagation finds to the XOR problem can be appreciated by examining the connection weights

TABLE 6.14   **Weight matrices after back-propagation training on the XOR patterns**

	From input unit		From bias unit
To hidden unit	**1**	**2**	**1**
1	−4.62	+4.50	−2.60
2	+4.47	−4.57	−2.56

	From hidden unit		From bias unit
To output unit	**1**	**2**	**1**
1	+6.03	+6.02	−3.05

(see Table 6.14). The hidden and output units all receive an inhibitory bias, so their states would be close to 0 with 0 input. Each hidden unit can be activated by one of the inputs, and either hidden unit is capable of overcoming the inhibitory bias on the output and driving the output unit by itself. The important feature of the solution is that each input unit excites one hidden unit and inhibits the other, so that when both inputs are 1, each cancels the effect of the other on the hidden units. Thus, neither hidden unit is activated when both inputs are 1, nothing counteracts the inhibitory bias on the output, and the output unit state is again 0. Back-propagation has developed an elegant solution to the XOR problem.

This solution is not unique. The back-propagation algorithm can develop other solutions to the XOR problem. The exact solution depends on the nature of the initial, random connectivity matrix, and on the random order of presentation of the patterns. This in itself is an interesting feature of error-driven learning algorithms such as back-propagation. The algorithm seeks a goal, there are numerous ways to achieve it, and the algorithm will find one of those ways in solving the problem.

6.5 Simulating Catastrophic Retroactive Interference in Learning

The ability of back-propagation to train a three-layered neural network to solve the XOR problem demonstrates its power as a learning algorithm. The example in this section also demonstrates the power of three-layered networks as pattern associators. It can be proven mathematically that a pattern associator with one layer of hidden units can learn to approximate any continuous function, provided there are sufficiently many hidden units and each has a monotonically increasing, nonlinear transfer function (such as the sigmoidal squashing function). This is the universal approximation theorem (Cybenko 1989). The theorem proves that a three-layered network of nonlinear units trained using back-propagation is a powerful computational device.

The universal approximation property can be demonstrated by using back-propagation to train a three-layer pattern associator to approximate the sine [$\sin(x)$] and the exponential [$\exp(-x)$] functions. We begin by generating input–output patterns for $\sin(x)$ and $\exp(-x)$ over the same range of x but at different, alternating values. The range from 0 to π is sampled at discrete intervals and divided into alternating sets. Values of the sine function are computed for one set (odd indices), while the values of the exponential function are computed for the other set (even indices). The following MATLAB commands can be used to set these inputs and desired outputs: `x=linspace(0,pi,43)',indx=1:43,odd=find(rem(indx,2)~=0),` `even=find(rem(indx,2)==0),si=x(odd),so=sin(si),ei=x(even),` and `eo=exp(-ei)`.

To get an idea of the power of back-propagation in training networks to approximate functions, the actual output of an untrained network to the sine input (`InPat=si`) is compared with the desired sine output (`DesOut=so`) in Figure 6.5A. The untrained network has random input–hidden and hidden–output weights distributed uniformly between −1 and +1. Commands for randomizing the weight matrices and computing hidden and output unit responses (along with those for back-propagation training) are available in script `backPropTrain` (see MATLAB Box 6.3). The script first finds the number of patterns nPat using `[nPat,nIn]=size(InPat)`, which also finds the number of inputs nIn, and `[nPat,nOut]=size(DesOut)`, which also finds the number of outputs nOut. The number of hidden units is set to nHid=10. Then

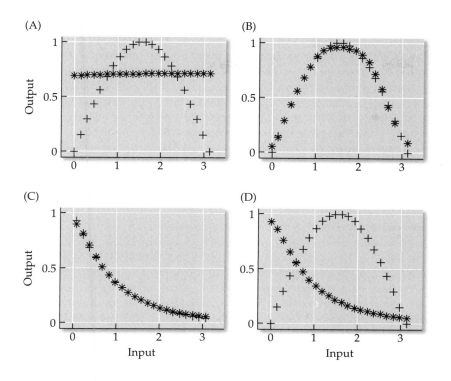

FIGURE 6.5   Demonstrating catastrophic interference Each panel compares the desired (+) and actual (∗) output of a three-layered, feedforward network with one input, one output, and ten hidden units. (A) Testing on sine before any training has taken place (initial weights are random). (B) Testing on sine after training on sine. (C) Testing on exponential after training on exponential (start weights were not random; training on exponential began using weights that had already been trained on sine). (D) Retesting on sine after training on exponential. Learning on sine has been destroyed.

the input-hidden and hidden-output weight matrices are randomized using `V=rand(nHid,nIn+1)*2-1` and `U=rand(nOut,nHid+1)*2-1`. The output of the untrained three-layered network is found by first setting up an input pattern array with an appended bias using `Inb=[InPat b*ones(nPat,1)]` where bias `b=1`. The hidden unit responses are computed using `Hid=(1./(1+exp(-V*Inb')))'`. Then a bias is also appended to the hidden unit activation array using `Hidb=[Hid b*ones(nPat,1)]`, and the output unit activation array is found using `Out=(1./(1+exp(-U*Hidb')))'`. These commands can be run outside the script from the MATLAB command line. The actual output can be compared graphically with the desired output using `plot(InPat,DesOut,InPat,Out)`.

The actual output of the untrained network is a line with a shallow slope; hardly a sine or an exponential. To use `backPropTrain` to train the network on the input and desired sine output patterns (`InPat=si` and `DesOut=so`), set the learning rate `a=0.1`, the tolerance `tol=0.05`, and the number of iterations `nIts=100000` (the number of hidden units should be `nHid=10` and the bias should be `b=1`). Note that we have tightened our tolerance to achieve more accurate learning on these real-valued patterns, with values closer to the midrange of the squashing function. Training on these patterns can easily take all 100,000 iterations and still not reach this tight tolerance (but it should get close). Following training with back-propagation, you should notice that the actual output matches the desired sine function output quite well. An example is shown in Figure 6.5B.

Now that the network has been trained on the sine function, we will train it on the exponential function. We will *not* first randomize the connection weights, but will leave the weights at the values they developed in learning to approximate the sine function. In this way we can see not only if the network can learn to approximate the exponential function, but also if it can retain its ability to approximate the sine function after being trained on the exponential function. To train the network on the input and desired exponential output patterns, set `InPat=ei` and `DesOut=eo`. Following training with back-propagation, you should notice that the actual output now matches the desired exponential function output quite well. An example is shown in Figure 6.5C. These results demonstrate that three-layered pattern associators with nonlinear units can be trained by back-propagation to approximate various nonlinear functions.

After being trained on the exponential function, we can retest the network on the sine input set. (See above and also script `backPropTrain` in MATLAB Box 6.3 for commands that will test the network following training.) Remember that the sine input set alternates with the exponential input set so that, in principle, the network could have learned to associate the sine outputs with one input set and the exponential outputs with the other input set. However, for the sine input set, the network now produces the exponential, not the sine, as shown in Figure 6.5D. Thus, the representation of the sine function has been destroyed in the process of learning the exponential.

This phenomenon, in which new learning destroys old learning in networks trained using back-propagation, has been called "catastrophic interference." It can be thought of as an extreme form of retroactive interference in learning (see Chapter 14 for background on catastrophic interference). Real brains do not seem to suffer from catastrophic interference (but they show the effects of retroactive interference), and the fact that networks trained with back-propagation do suffer catastrophic interference has called their neurobiological relevance into question. Modelers have responded with various solutions. One possibility is a scheme that involves the relearning of previously learned patterns along with the new patterns (see Chapter 14 for a detailed discussion of this scheme). Another possibility involves expanding the input layer to include units that indicate the context in which a particular pattern association is being learned. This possibility is explored in Exercise 6.3.

6.6 Simulating the Development of Non-Uniform Distributed Representations

By accomplishing pattern associations of increasing difficulty, the foregoing sections of this chapter have illustrated the processing power of three-layered networks of nonlinear units trained using back-propagation. As mentioned at the beginning of the chapter, back-propagation is an unlikely model of the learning process that occurs in the brain, because the backward propagation of error signals is unlikely to occur in the real nervous system. However, neurobiologically plausible mechanisms for accomplishing error-driven learning have been proposed (e.g., Zipser and Rumelhart 1990; O'Reilly 1996), and it is certainly possible that the brain utilizes error-driven learning in some form. We can use the back-propagation algorithm as a tool to set the connection weights in multilayered neural networks and thereby construct brain-like models of real neural systems. We will use back-propagation in the construction of a brain-like representation in the example in this section.

In neural networks having many hidden units, back-propagation will develop a structure in which network processing becomes distributed over the available units, in a manner not unlike what actually appears to occur in many parts of the brain. This is demonstrated best by using a very simple computational problem. We will train networks on the simple input and desired output patterns in Table 6.15. You might recognize these patterns as being similar to those of the labeled-line scenario of the first example (see Table 6.1).

The simple labeled-line patterns of Table 6.15 can be entered using the commands `InPat=[0 0;1 0;0 1]` and `DesOut=[0;1;1]`. We will first associate these patterns using a network having two input units, one hidden

TABLE 6.15   Learning the simple labeled-line patterns using
                back-propagation

Input patterns	Desired output patterns	Actual output patterns	Hidden unit responses
0 0	0	0.09	0.16
1 0	1	0.90	0.86
0 1	1	0.90	0.86

The input, desired output, actual output, and hidden unit responses following training are listed for a three-layered, feedforward network of sigmoidal units. The network has two input units, one hidden unit, and one output unit.

unit, and one output unit. Again, the script `backPropTrain` will determine the required numbers of input (`nIn`) and output (`nOut`) units from the patterns, but the required number of hidden units must be set in the script as `nHid=1`. Set the other parameters as follows: bias `b=1`, tolerance `tol=0.1`, learning rate `a=0.1`, and number of iterations `nIts=100000`. You should find that back-propagation will learn this simple transformation quite a bit faster than it learned the XOR (parameter `c` in `backPropTrain` keeps track of the number of learning cycles, or iterations). For this run the back-propagation algorithm reached tolerance after about 10,000 iterations. The actual output and hidden unit responses, along with the inputs and desired outputs for the simple labeled-line patterns, are shown in Table 6.15, and the final weights are shown in Table 6.16.

The hidden and output units have an inhibitory bias, which ensures that their states are near 0 when the input unit states are 0. Each input unit has a strong, excitatory connection to the hidden unit, which in turn has a strong, excitatory connection to the output unit. This allows either input unit to drive the output state near 1 when the input state is 1. Different weight configurations will emerge with randomization of the weight matrices and retraining on the simple labeled-line patterns, but all of the trained networks that can produce this transformation will share an important feature in common. Because the single hidden unit must drive the output unit to have equal responses to both inputs, the single hidden unit must also respond equally to both inputs (see Table 6.15). This situation becomes more interesting when the number of hidden units is increased.

The network is retrained on the simple labeled-line patterns using the same parameters, except that the number of hidden units is expanded to 50 (`nHid=50`). The network reaches tolerance after about 2500 iterations. Thus, the network learns the transformation much faster with 50 than with one hid-

TABLE 6.16   Weight matrices after back-propagation training
                on simple labeled-line patterns

	From input unit		From bias unit
To hidden unit	1	2	1
1	+3.90	+3.94	−2.07
	From hidden unit		From bias unit
To output unit	1		1
1	+5.87		−2.86

FIGURE 6.6   Simulating a non-uniform distributed representation A feedforward neural network with two input units, one output unit, and 50 hidden units is trained on the simple labeled-line patterns. The output (+) and the 50 hidden unit (•) responses to the two inputs are plotted against each other. Responses falling near the dashed line have roughly equal sensitivities to inputs from input units 1 and 2. Most hidden units respond to the inputs unequally, yet the network produces an output with nearly equal sensitivities.

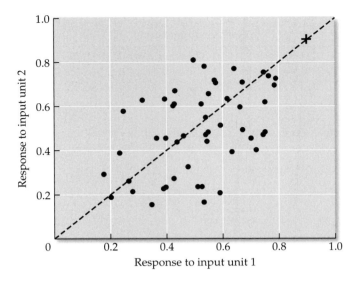

den unit. The hidden and output responses to each of the inputs are shown in Figure 6.6. The response to input unit 1 (input pattern 2) is plotted against the response to input unit 2 (input pattern 3) for the output unit (+) and each hidden unit (•). The plot can be generated using the MATLAB command `plot(Hid(2,:),Hid(3,:),'*',Out(2,:),Out(3,:),'*')`.

This plot shows that, although the output unit responds with strength near 1 for both inputs, as demanded by training, the hidden units vary in their responses to the two inputs. Some prefer one input over the other. No two hidden units respond in exactly the same way. This plot provides a simple example of a non-uniform distributed representation. It is distributed because it is mediated by many hidden units operating in parallel. It is non-uniform because of the variability in the response properties of the hidden units.

This particular representation is not unique; there are infinitely many representations that would accomplish the same pattern association. This representation resulted from a series of weight adjustments, brought about by back-propagation, which started from a random initial weight configuration and ended when training reached tolerance. A different random initial configuration would result in a different non-uniform distributed representation. As with the XOR, so with the simple labeled-line: back-propagation begins with some initial configuration and seeks a goal. There are numerous ways to achieve that goal, and the algorithm will find one of those ways. The reason the network learns faster with 50 than with one hidden unit is that the random initial weight configuration offers more possible solutions in the larger network.

Non-uniform distributed representations can result when the number of hidden units is larger than the minimal number required to produce the input–output transformation. We see this in the simple labeled-line example in this section. When the transformation is produced by one hidden unit, that hidden unit responds uniformly to the two inputs. In contrast, when the transformation is distributed over 50 hidden units, those hidden units respond non-uniformly and vary widely in the proportions with which they combine the two inputs. Similar non-uniform distributed representations are found neurophysiologically in many parts of the brain (see next section), and it is possible that real neural systems also distribute their processing over an abundance of interneurons. As we saw in this section with artificial networks and hidden units, real neural systems might need an abundance of interneurons to increase their speed of error-driven learning. (We will consider the learning speed issue again in Chapter 14.) Also, having surplus interneurons would make real networks robust to damage, and would make it more likely that a network can successfully retrain itself in the event that it loses some interneurons. In Chapter 8 we will consider another benefit to a neural system of having an abundance of interneurons.

6.7   Modeling Non-Uniform Distributed Representations in the Vestibular Nuclei

As pointed out in the first section of this chapter, the desired output patterns are generally different from the input patterns in a pattern associator, so a trained pattern associator network can be said to transform inputs into outputs. Whether at the level of the reflex or at higher cognitive levels, the nervous system can also be said to transform inputs into outputs. Neural networks that associate patterns serve as models for many neural systems. In this section we briefly review models of real neural systems that are based on three-layered pattern associators.

The vestibulo-oculomotor system is a frequent subject of modeling studies because it has been well characterized neurophysiologically (Wilson and Melvill Jones 1979; Robinson 1989). The vestibulo-oculomotor system is diagrammed in Figure 6.7. The function of the vestibulo-oculomotor system is to rotate the eyes in three dimensions in order to keep the eyes on target (or more precisely, to keep the target on the foveae). The complexity of this system, evident in the diagram, will necessarily be reduced in modeling it using three-layered pattern associator neural networks.

The vestibulo-ocular reflex (VOR) forms the backbone of the vestibulo-oculomotor system. The function of the VOR is to stabilize the retinal image by producing eye rotations that counterbalance for head rotations. Head rotation is transduced by the semicircular canal receptors of the inner ear. The left and right horizontal canals (LHC and RHC) are oriented horizontally and transduce head rotations in the horizontal plane. The left and right anterior (LAC and RAC) and posterior (LPC and RPC) canals are oriented vertically and transduce head rotations outside the horizontal plane. Neural signals from the semicircular canals are transmitted into the brainstem by semicircular canal primary afferent sensory neurons.

Eye rotations are ultimately produced by the eye muscles. The left eye and its extra-ocular muscles are depicted in Figure 6.7. Eye rotations in the horizontal plane are produced by the lateral and medial rectus (LR and MR) muscles, while eye rotations outside the horizontal plane are produced by the superior and inferior rectus (SR and IR) and oblique (SO and IO) muscles. The eye muscles are innervated by motoneurons that originate in brainstem nuclei and project to the eye muscles over the sixth (to LR), the fourth (to SO), and the third (to MR, SR, IR, and IO) cranial nerves. The VOR (and the vestibulo-oculomotor system generally) is organized bilaterally and operates in push–pull. For example, a head rotation in the horizontal plane to the left will activate afferents from the left horizontal canal and suppress afferents from the right horizontal canal. The VOR would produce a compensatory (counterbalancing) movement of the left eye by activating medial rectus motoneurons and suppressing lateral rectus motoneurons. (A mirror-symmetric arrangement pertains for the right eye, which is omitted for clarity.)

Neurons in the vestibular nuclei in the brainstem are the interneurons of the VOR pathway, and they play a central role in VOR function (see Figure 6.7). Vestibular nucleus neurons receive head rotation signals from the semicircular canal afferents and transmit them to the motoneurons. While semicircu-

FIGURE 6.7 Schematic diagram of the vestibulo-oculomotor system Inputs to the vestibular nuclei include afferents from the six semicircular canals and projections from the left and right pursuit system. Inhibitory interneurons of the commissural system and some inhibitory vestibular nucleus neurons are shown with filled circles. Outputs from the vestibular nuclei go to the motorneurons of the eye muscles. Abbreviations are: LAC, LPC, LHC, RAC, RPC, RHC, left or right anterior, posterior, and horizontal semicircular canal or primary afferent; III, IV, VI, oculomotor, trochlear, and abducens nuclei (these nuclei contain the eye-muscle motoneurons). The model represents the left eye only. The arrangement for the right eye is mirror-symmetric and is omitted because the essential features of the model can be illustrated by reference to only one eye. Note that the inferior oblique eye muscle is beneath the eye and is not visible in this diagram. (After Anastasio and Robinson 1989a.)

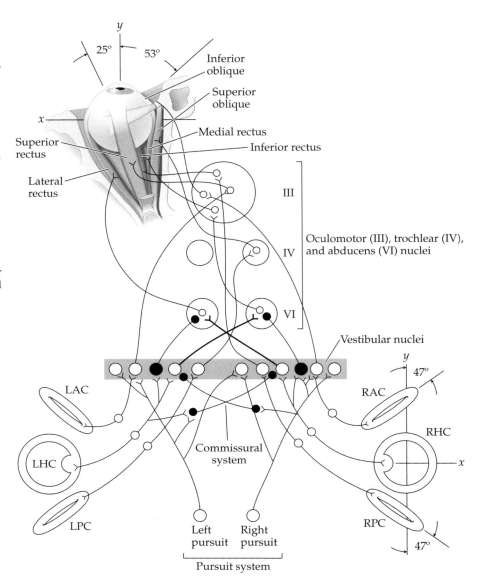

lar canal afferents project directly to vestibular nucleus neurons on the same (ipsilateral) side, they project indirectly, over the neurons of the vestibular commissural system, to the opposite (contralateral) side.

The manner in which vestibular nucleus neurons represent the signals they receive is intriguing. Insight into the representation has been gained through neural systems modeling. One example involves the way in which vestibular nucleus neurons represent signals from more than one oculomotor subsystem. Vestibular nucleus neurons transmit signals not only from the vestibular receptors, which drive the VOR, but they also transmit command signals from other oculomotor subsystems such as the pursuit system, which moves the eyes in order to track moving targets (Robinson 1989). The pursuit system also works in push–pull, as depicted in Figure 6.7. The question arises as to how vestibular nucleus neurons represent these two different command signals. Does each vestibular nucleus neuron carry both signals with equal strength? Alternatively, are certain vestibular nucleus neurons specialized for individual commands? Some pertinent experimental results are shown in Figure 6.8.

Each panel of Figure 6.8 shows head position, eye position, and the action potential (spike) discharge of a vestibular nucleus neuron in a behaving mon-

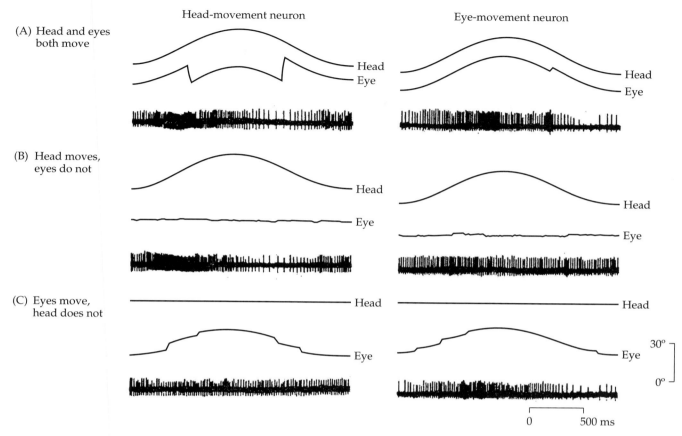

FIGURE 6.8   Vestibulo-oculomotor related behavior of vestibular nucleus neurons The data show the activity of two vestibular nucleus neurons, one encoding primarily head movement (on the left) and the other encoding primarily eye movement (on the right). Recordings were made from a behaving monkey. Neural activity is shown as representative spike trains. Horizontal head angular position and eye angular position are shown as curves marked Head and Eye, respectively. (After Keller and Kamath 1975.)

key (Keller and Kamath 1975). Data are shown for two different vestibular nucleus neurons. According to a classification scheme to be explained, the data on the left side of Figure 6.8 were recorded from a head-movement neuron, while the data on the right were recorded from an eye-movement neuron.

The behaving monkey is seated in a primate chair with its head fixed to the chair, and it is viewing a target, such as a banana. The reference frame is the room in which the chair and the banana are situated. The activities of the two neurons are recorded under three different conditions. In condition A, the primate chair is rotated sinusoidally but the banana is stationary relative to the room. In this condition the monkey produces compensatory eye movements, so both the head and the eyes are rotating. In condition B the banana rotates with the chair. In this condition the monkey does not need to move his eyes to follow the banana, so the head rotates but the eyes do not rotate. In condition C the chair is stationary but the banana is moved from side to side sinusoidally. In this condition the monkey rotates his eyes to follow the banana, but the head does not rotate.

Of interest are changes in the rate of action potential discharge (firing rate) that are correlated with head and/or eye rotation. The neuron on the left of Figure 6.8 modulates its activity when both the head and the eyes are rotating (A), and it modulates its activity when the head alone is rotating (B), but it does not modulate its activity when the eyes alone are rotating (C), so this neuron is classified as a head-movement neuron. The neuron on the right of Figure 6.8 also modulates its activity when both the head and the eyes are rotating (A), and it modulates its activity when the eyes alone are rotating (C), but it does not modulate its activity when the head alone is rotating (B), so this neuron is classified as an eye-movement neuron.

From these data alone one might conclude that vestibular nucleus neurons are specialized for specific eye movement commands; head-movement neurons would be specialized for vestibular commands and eye-movement neurons would be specialized for pursuit commands. Further experimentation and analysis revealed that this is not the case (e.g., Fuchs and Kimm 1975; Tomlinson and Robinson 1984). While some vestibular nucleus neurons do carry pure vestibular or pure pursuit commands, others carry vestibular and pursuit commands at roughly equal strength, but most carry vestibular and pursuit commands at unequal strengths. These findings indicate that vestibular nucleus neurons vary widely in the proportions with which they combine vestibular and pursuit commands. Furthermore, while most vestibular nucleus neurons carry vestibular and pursuit commands that would drive the eyes in the same direction, some vestibular nucleus neurons even carry vestibular and pursuit commands that would drive the eyes in opposite directions. Despite this diversity of behavior patterns, some researchers maintained the view that individual vestibular nucleus neurons were specialized for specific functions, and attempted to classify them into an expanded set of categories (e.g., Tomlinson and Robinson 1984). Neural systems modeling provided a different view.

The horizontal vestibulo-oculomotor system was modeled as a three-layered pattern associator trained using back-propagation to represent vestibular and pursuit commands (Anastasio and Robinson 1989a, b). The push–pull, vestibular and pursuit patterns are reproduced in Table 6.17. The network had four input units, two vestibular (LHC and RHC) and two pursuit (LP and RP). It had two output units, representing the horizontal recti motoneurons of the left eye (LR and MR), and 40 hidden units, representing vestibular nucleus neurons. The vestibular-pursuit patterns specified that the input and output units should have spontaneous activities of 0.50, and that the output units should produce push–pull activity patterns of size and direction appropriate to drive vestibular and pursuit eye movements. Because the neurons that control vestibular and pursuit eye movements operate over a roughly linear activity range (Robinson 1989), the push–pull modulations of the vestibular-pursuit patterns occurred over the approximately linear midrange of the sigmoidal squashing function (see Figure 6.3).

The network learned to operate properly by adjusting its connection weights so that actual output was equal to the pursuit input, and equal but opposite to the vestibular input (within tolerance). Because the function of the vestibulo-oculomotor system is to keep the target on the foveae, targets will slip off the foveae if the vestibulo-oculomotor system fails to operate properly. Such a "retinal slip" error signal is provided over several pathways to neurons in the real vestibular nuclei (Wilson

TABLE 6.17   Input and desired output patterns for the vestibular-pursuit simulation

Condition	Input patterns				Desired outputs	
	LP	LHC	RHC	RP	LR	MR
Head still	0.50	0.50	0.50	0.50	0.50	0.50
Pursue left	0.60	0.50	0.50	0.40	0.60	0.40
Pursue right	0.40	0.50	0.50	0.60	0.40	0.60
Head left	0.50	0.60	0.40	0.50	0.40	0.60
Head right	0.50	0.40	0.60	0.50	0.60	0.40

These patterns are also used in Exercise 6.4. Abbreviations: LP and RP, left and right pursuit commands; LHC and RHC, left and right horizontal canal afferents; LR and MR, lateral and medial rectus eye muscle motoneurons.

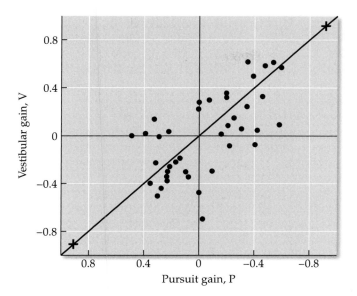

FIGURE 6.9   Simulating the non-uniform distributed representation of vestibular and pursuit commands in the vestibular nuclei The vestibular-pursuit, feedforward neural network model has two output units and 40 hidden units. The vestibular (V) and pursuit (P) gains (sensitivities) of hidden and output units are plotted against each other. (After Anastasio and Robinson 1989a.)

and Melvill Jones 1979; Berthoz and Melvill Jones 1985). Thus, output error in the model corresponds to retinal slip error in the real vestibulo-oculomotor system. Following error-driven learning on the vestibulo-oculomotor task the vestibular and pursuit activities of the hidden and output units in the model were determined and used to compute unit response gains. (Gain is a measure of the sensitivity of the units to the different types of inputs.)

Vestibular or pursuit gain is defined as $(y_r - y_s) / (x_r - x_s)$ for the hidden units and as $(z_r - z_s) / (x_r - x_s)$ for output units, where x_s, y_s, and z_s are the spontaneous activities of input, hidden, or output units (x_s always equals 0.50 as specified in Table 6.17), y_r and z_r are the responses of hidden or output units to vestibular or pursuit inputs, and x_r is the response of the left input unit of the pair that carries either the vestibular or the pursuit signals. (The left input unit of each pair is chosen arbitrarily to provide a common reference for computing and comparing gains.) The output (+) and hidden (•) units are located according to their vestibular and pursuit gains in Figure 6.9. Because a head rotation signal should produce an oppositely directed eye rotation, but a pursuit command should produce an eye rotation in the same direction, a unit that produces vestibular and pursuit eye rotations in the same direction should have opposite vestibular and pursuit gains. Because most units do produce vestibular and pursuit eye rotations in the same direction, the pursuit axis in Figure 6.9 is reversed for illustrative purposes.

The output units (+) lie along the diagonal line, because they have equal and opposite vestibular and pursuit gains, as demanded by training (see Table 6.17). Most hidden units (•) lie on or around the diagonal line, indicating that they have both vestibular and pursuit activity, although usually in unequal proportions. Hidden units falling along the horizontal or vertical axis can be considered as pure pursuit or pure vestibular units, respectively. Most hidden units fall in quadrants one and three and encode vestibular and pursuit eye rotations in the same direction, but the few hidden units falling in quadrants two and four actually encode vestibular and pursuit eye rotations in opposite directions. All of these response patterns had long been known through experimental observation (e.g., Fuchs and Kimm 1975; Tomlinson and Robinson 1984). Rather than falling into separate functional categories, the hidden units seem to mediate both functions as a population, over which the vestibular and pursuit commands are distributed non-uniformly. Thus, a non-uniform distributed representation occurring at the level of the vestibular nuclei may explain the diverse activity patterns observed among real vestibular nucleus neurons.

The view of vestibular organization offered by the neural network simulation was at odds with the one that attempted to fit the various responses into a rigid set of discrete categories (e.g., Tomlinson and Robinson 1984). The modeling results led to the alternative idea that the diversity of response patterns among the population of vestibular neurons was a natural consequence of a non-uniform distributed representation in the vestibular nuclei. To some this idea seemed counterintuitive, perhaps because of the way in which we normally conceive of organization in groups.

To illustrate this, let us take a rather wide digression. Consider the fable of Stone Soup, which promotes the idea that small contributions made by many individuals can add up to something wonderful. The fable begins with hungry travelers who stop in a small village and build a cooking fire, upon which they place a large pot filled with water and into which they add a stone. Curious villagers come by and quickly realize that soup made from a stone will not be very satisfying. Inspired by generosity, the villagers begin to contribute ingredients to the soup. A woman brings a cabbage, a boy brings half a dozen carrots, a man brings five potatoes, and so on. Together, by each contributing a little, they end up with a huge pot of rich, flavorful soup to share.

Notice in telling the tale that each villager brings only one type of item, as though each one falls neatly into a discrete category: cabbage woman, carrot boy, potato man, and so on. We could just as easily imagine that the woman brings half a cabbage, a carrot, and two potatoes, the boy brings half a cabbage, two carrots, and a potato, and the man brings no cabbage, but brings three carrots and two potatoes. In other words, we could imagine that the ingredients were divided up and distributed non-uniformly among the villagers, who then combined them in proportions appropriate to make a delicious soup. In fact, there are infinitely many ways to divvy up the various ingredients among the villagers and get exactly the same delicious soup at the end. Although it may make for a cleaner story, the single-item for each-villager distribution is just one of the many possible distributions of ingredients.

Likewise in the vestibular nuclei, there are an infinite number of ways in which the vestibular neurons could represent eye-movement commands and get the same correct eye movement behavior through their collective action. The hypothetical representation in which all neurons fall into discrete, single-command categories is just one of those ways, and apparently it is an unlikely way, since it has never been observed in an experimental animal. We may be inclined to think in terms of discrete categories, but a non-uniform distributed representation, in which neurons mix and match signals in seemingly random ways that defy categorization, is consistent with the way in which eye movement commands are distributed in the vestibular nuclei.

Another example of a distributed representation involves the manner in which vestibular nucleus neurons represent spatial sensorimotor transformations (Anastasio and Robinson 1989a, 1990). As shown in Figure 6.7, the sensorimotor transformation required for the horizontal VOR is relatively simple, since the horizontal canals and the horizontal recti motoneurons all lie in the horizontal plane. The situation is different for the vertical VOR, because the vertical canals and the vertical eye muscles lie in different planes, and because the vertical eye muscles do not lie in orthogonal planes.

The semicircular canal afferents can be characterized according to the vector of rotation about which their response is the most sensitive (with polarity determined according to the right-hand rule). An afferent sensitivity vector is perpendicular to the plane of the semicircular canal by which the afferent

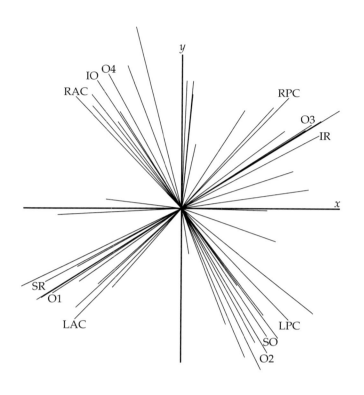

FIGURE 6.10   Simulating the non-uniform distributed representation of sensorimotor activation vectors in the vestibular nuclei The feedforward neural network model of the vertical VOR has four input units (representing the vertical semicircular canal afferents), four output units (representing the vertical eye-muscle motoneurons of the left eye), and 40 hidden units (representing vestibular nucleus neurons). The activation vectors of the hidden units have a diversity of magnitudes and directions. The canal activation vectors are LAC, LPC, RAC, and RPC (left or right anterior or posterior canal). The activation vectors of the motoneurons are O1, O2, O3, and O4. The rotation vectors of the muscles are SR, SO, IR, and IO (superior or inferior rectus or oblique). The rotation vectors of the muscles do not coincide with the motoneuron activation vectors because the muscles form a skewed coordinate system. (After Anastasio and Robinson 1990.)

is activated. The rotation vector of an eye muscle is the vector about which the eye rotates when that muscle acts alone (again with polarity determined by the right-hand rule). However, the muscles must act together. Because the muscles do not lie in orthogonal planes, the activation vectors of the eye muscles (or motoneurons), which they express when working together to rotate the eye, are not the same as their rotation vectors (see Anastasio and Robinson 1990 for details). In any case, the question arises as to how vestibular nucleus neurons represent this sensorimotor transformation. Do the activation vectors of vestibular nucleus neurons line up along the afferent sensitivity vectors? Do they lie along the muscle activation vectors? Alternatively, do they lie along some unique vectors that are intermediate between the afferent sensitivity vectors and the motoneuron activation vectors?

To explore this sensorimotor transformation, the vertical VOR was modeled as a three-layered network having four input units representing afferents from the vertical semicircular canals (LAC, LPC, RAC, and RPC), four output units representing the motoneurons of the vertical muscles of the left eye (SR, SO, IR, and IO), and 40 hidden units representing vestibular nucleus neurons. The model was trained to produce input and desired output patterns that were consistent with compensatory eye rotations for head rotations about eight axes spaced 45 degrees apart in the horizontal plane (see Anastasio and Robinson 1990 for further details). Following training, the activation vectors of the hidden and output units were determined, and are shown in Figure 6.10. The activation vectors of the output units (O1, O2, O3, and O4) fall near the motoneuron activation vectors, as demanded by training. Rather than fall along any particular vectors, the hidden unit vectors are dispersed in many directions. The spray of hidden unit activation vectors resembles that of the activation vectors of real vestibular nucleus neurons, as shown in Figure 6.11.

The diversity of response types observed for vestibular nucleus neurons is consistent with the hypothesis that they represent signals in a non-uniform, distributed manner. Similarly diverse representations, whether of response

FIGURE 6.11 The non-uniform distributed representation of sensorimotor activation vectors in the real vestibular nuclei (A) The activation vectors of real vestibular nucleus neurons in the cat. (B) The sensitivity vectors for the left horizontal, anterior, and posterior semicircular canals. (After Baker et al. 1984.)

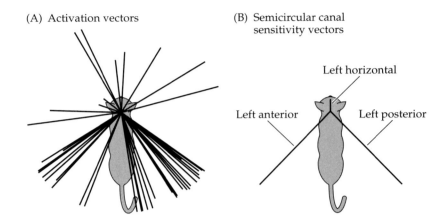

(A) Activation vectors

(B) Semicircular canal sensitivity vectors

Left horizontal

Left anterior   Left posterior

combinations as in the vestibular-pursuit example, or of spatial response vectors as in the vertical VOR example, are observed in various regions throughout the oculomotor system (Anastasio 1991). These non-uniform distributed representations are characteristic of the representations that develop in three-layered pattern associator neural networks trained using back-propagation. Similar models have been used to simulate the coordinate transformations that occur in the posterior parietal cortex (Zipser and Anderson 1988; Xing and Anderson 2000), and the local bending reflex of the leech, in which the ability to identify individual neurons has facilitated the derivation of experimentally testable predictions from the models (Lockery et al. 1989; Lockery and Sejnowski 1993). The three-layered pattern associator trained using back-propagation is a model that captures many of the essential features of the input–output transformations produced by real neural systems.

Supervised learning is not the only way to train a neural network to produce a non-uniform distributed representation. Distributed representations that can be described as non-uniform also arise in networks trained using unsupervised learning, in cases where more than one stimulus feature is being represented. The multisensory map model we considered in Chapter 5 offers a case in point. Units in that model represent every possible combination of the three sensory modalities: visual, auditory, and somatosensory. It is as though those three input types are divided up and distributed non-uniformly among the units in the network (see also Anastasio 1991). The orientation map in striate cortex can also be seen as a non-uniform distributed representation, in which retinal position, and components of orientation in the horizontal and vertical directions, are divided up and distributed non-uniformly among the units.

The multisensory and orientation representations we studied in Chapter 5 arose in networks trained using the self-organizing map algorithm, so output units with similar preferred inputs were located near each other in arrangements that simulated brain maps. The non-uniform distributed representations we considered in this chapter arose in networks trained using back-propagation, so they learned to produce desired input–output transformations that simulated sensorimotor transformations. Although the two types of learning (supervised and unsupervised) have different goals, they share in common the need to represent their inputs over a population of units. Real neural systems have the same requirement, and could develop map-like or non-uniform distributed representations through diffferent mechanisms that nevertheless meet their common need to adequately represent their inputs. We will consider this issue in more depth in Chapter 8.

Exercises

6.1 At the beginning of the chapter we saw that Hebbian training was able to associate non-overlapping (labeled-line) patterns but not overlapping patterns, and that covariation training was able to associate sparse-overlapping (simple contingency) but not dense-overlapping (complex contingency) patterns. Try using the pre-synaptic and post-synaptic rules to associate these patterns. Given inputs and desired outputs in arrays `InPat` and `DesOut`, connectivity weight matrices can be made using the pre-synaptic and post-synaptic rules using the commands `VPr=(2*DesOut'-1)*InPat` and `VPo=DesOut'*(2*InPat-1)`. Their thresholded outputs following training can be found using `OutPr=(VPr*InPat')'>0` and `OutPo=(VPo*InPat')'>0`. Do the pre-synaptic and post-synaptic rules outperform Hebb? Do they perform as well as covariation? Do they produce the same weight matrices?

6.2 Train three-layered networks of sigmoidal units having different numbers of hidden units on the XOR problem. This can be done using `backPropTrain` and the input and desired output patterns in Table 6.13, with `nHid` set for different numbers of hidden units. What is the relationship between number of hidden units and number of training cycles needed to learn the XOR transformation?

6.3 In the catastrophic interference example, training the network to approximate the exponential function [exp(−*x*)] destroyed its previously trained ability to approximate the sine function [sin(*x*)] over the same input range (0 to π), even though the two functions were trained using alternating values of the input. To design a network that can approximate either the sine or the exponential function, add two input units, of which one takes value 1 for sine and 0 for exponential, while the other takes value 1 for exponential and 0 for sine. The third input unit will take the arguments of the functions, while the desired output will be either the sine or the exponential of the argument, accordingly as either function is specified by the first two input units. One way to do this is to make array `InPat` to have three columns, in which the first column is 1 for all odd and 0 for all even indices, the second column is 1 for all even and 0 for all odd indices, and the third column holds a series of real numbers from 0 to π. (The command `rad=linspace(0,pi,nPts)'` will make such a series in column vector `rad` that is `nPts` elements long.) Then make array `DesOut` a column vector in which the elements with odd indices are the sine of the corresponding elements of `rad`, while the elements with even indices are the exponential of the corresponding (but negative) elements of `rad`. Train a three-layered pattern associator on `InPat` and `DesOut` using `backPropTrain` with `nHid=10` and other parameters as set in the catastrophic interference example in Section 6.5. Following training, the performance of the network on this dual-function approximation task can be visualized using `plot(indx,DesOut,'+',indx,Out,'*')`, where `indx=1:nPts`. How would you evaluate this strategy for overcoming catastrophic interference?

6.4 Reproduce the modeling results of Figure 6.9 by training a three-layered feedforward network of sigmoidal units on the vestibular-pursuit patterns in Table 6.17. The network will need to have four input units and two output units. The input units will represent the left and right pursuit commands (LP and RP) and the head rotation signal from the left and right horizontal semicircular canals (LHC and RHC). The outputs will represent the lateral and medial rectus (LR and MR) motoneurons of the left eye. All inputs and desired outputs have a spontaneous rate of 0.50. Like the actual vestibulo-oculomotor system, the network model is organized bilaterally and operates in push–pull. For example, a leftward head rotation is signaled by an increase in LHC to 0.60 and a decrease in RHC to 0.40. The compensatory vestibular command that produces a rightward eye movement is encoded by a decrease in LR to 0.40 and an increase in MR to 0.60. Vestibular or pursuit gain is defined as $(y_r - y_s) / (x_r - x_s)$ for the hidden units and as $(z_r - z_s) / (x_r - x_s)$ for output units, where x_s, y_s, and z_s are the spontaneous activities of input, hidden, or output units (x_s always equals 0.50), y_r and z_r are the responses of hidden or output units to vestibular or pursuit inputs, and x_r is the response of the left input unit of the pair that carries either the vestibular or the pursuit signals. Assume, for example, that hidden unit y_1 has a spontaneous rate of 0.55, and its response to a head-left input is 0.65. Then the vestibular gain of y_1 is $(0.65 - 0.55) / (0.60 - 0.50) = 1$. Note that the spontaneous rates of the hidden and output units (their activity when the head is still and the input units are all at 0.50) must be determined before their gains can be determined. To use `backPropTrain` on this problem, set `InPat` and `DesOut` according to the values in Table 6.17. Because the units are operating away from the extremes of the squashing function, you can set a tight tolerance of `tol=0.001` and you can use a large learning rate of `a=1`. The network should reach tolerance well within `nIts=100000` iterations. To compute their gains, use the hidden and output responses to leftward head rotations or pursuit signals. Noting that the gain of the reference input (left member of each input pair) is always 0.1 in these cases simplifies hidden and output unit gain computations. For example, following training, the hidden unit vestibular gain can be computed using `HidVG=(Hid(4,:)-Hid(1,:))/0.1`, and output unit vestibular gain can be computed using `OutVG=(Out(4,:)-Out(1,:))/0.1`. Pursuit gains are computed similarly. Plotting the pursuit versus vestibular gains of all the hidden and output units should reproduce Figure 6.9, after the polarity of the pursuit gains is reversed.

References

Anastasio TJ (1991) Distributed processing in vestibulo-ocular and other oculomotor subsystems in monkeys and cats. In: Arbib MA, Ewert J-P (eds) *Visual Structures and Integrated Functions*. Springer-Verlag, New York, pp 95–110.

Anastasio TJ, Robinson DA (1989a) Distributed parallel processing in the vestibulo-oculomotor system. *Neural Computation* 1: 230–241.

Anastasio TJ, Robinson DA (1989b) The distributed representation of vestibulo-oculomotor signals by brainstem neurons. *Biological Cybernetics* 61: 79–88.

Anastasio TJ, Robinson DA (1990) Distributed parallel processing in the vertical vestibulo-ocular reflex: Learning networks compared to tensor theory. *Biological Cybernetics* 63: 161–167.

Baker J, Goldberg J, Hermann G, Peterson B (1984) Optimal response planes and canal convergence in secondary neurons in vestibular nuclei of alert cats. *Brain Research* 294: 133–137.

Berthoz A, Melvill Jones G (eds) (1985) *Adaptive Mechanisms in Gaze Control: Facts and Theories*. Elsevier, Amsterdam.

Cybenko G (1989) Approximation by superpositions of a sigmoidal function. *Mathematics of Control, Signals, and Systems* 2: 303–314.

Fuchs AF, Kimm J (1975) Unit activity in the vestibular nucleus of the alert monkey during horizontal angular acceleration and eye movement. *Journal of Neurophysiology* 38: 1140–1161.

Gallistel CR (1980) *The Organization of Action: A New Synthesis*. Lawrence Erlbaum, Hillsdale, NJ.

Hull R, Vaid J (2007) Bilingual language lateralization: A meta-analytic tale of two hemispheres. *Neuropsychologia* 45: 1987–2008.

Keller EL, Kamath BY (1975) Characteristics of head rotation and eye movement related neurons in alert monkey vestibular nucleus. *Brain Research* 100: 182–187.

Lockery SR, Sejnowski TJ (1993) The computational leech. *Trends in Neuroscience* 16: 283–290.

Lockery SR, Wittenberg G, Kristan WB, Cottrell GW (1989) Function of identified interneurons in the leech elucidated using neural networks trained by back-propagation. *Nature* 340: 468–471.

McClelland JL, Rogers TT (2003) The parallel distributed processing approach to semantic cognition. *Nature Reviews Neuroscience* 4: 310–322.

McClelland JL, Rumelhart DE (1989) *Explorations in Parallel Distributed Processing: A Handbook of Models, Programs, and Exercises*. MIT Press, Cambridge, MA, pp 83–159.

Orchard GA, Phillips WA (1991) *Neural Computation: A Beginner's Guide*. Lawrence Erlbaum, London, pp 63–91.

O'Reilly RC (1996) Biologically plausible error-driven learning using local activation differences: The generalized recirculation algorithm. *Neural Computation* 8: 895–938.

Robinson DA (1989) Control of eye movements. In: Brooks VB (ed) *Handbook of Physiology, Section 1: The Nervous System, Vol II, Part 2*. American Physiological Society, Bethesda, pp 1275–1320.

Rumelhart DE, Hinton GE, Williams RJ (1986) Learning internal representations by error propagation. In: Rumelhart DE, McClelland JL, PDP Research Group (eds) *Parallel Distributed Processing: Explorations in the Microstructure of Cognition, Vol 1: Foundations*. MIT Press, Cambridge, MA, pp 318–362.

Schey HM (2005) *Div, Grad, Curl, and All That: An Informal Text on Vector Calculus. Fourth Edition*. WW Norton, New York.

Sejnowski TJ, Rosenberg CR (1987) Parallel networks that learn to pronounce English text. *Computational Systems* 1: 145–168.

Tomlinson RD, Robinson RA (1984) Signals in vestibular nucleus mediating vertical eye movements in the monkey. *Journal of Neurophysiology* 51: 1121–1136.

Wilson VJ, Melvill Jones G (1979) *Mammalian Vestibular Physiology*. Plenum Press, New York.

Xing J, Andersen RA (2000) Models of the posterior parietal cortex which perform multimodal integration and represent space in several coordinate frames. *Journal of Cognitive Neuroscience* 12: 601–614.

Zipser D, Anderson RA (1988) A back propagation programmed network that simulates response properties of a subset of posterior parietal neurons. *Nature* 33: 679–684.

Zipser D, Rumelhart DE (1990) The neurobiological significance of the new learning models. In: Schwartz EL (ed) *Computational Neuroscience*, MIT Press, Cambridge, MA, pp 192–200.

Reinforcement Learning and Associative Conditioning

Reinforcement learning algorithms can simulate certain types of associative conditioning and train neural networks to form non-uniform distributed representations

t is a matter of common knowledge that individuals learn to increase the reward they receive from the world and to minimize the punishment, but this seemingly obvious statement has never been proven directly. Even in experimental animals, the pleasure of reward and the pain of punishment are impossible to measure (Robbins and Everitt 1996). Yet an extensive body of experimental work has established that the behavioral responses of an animal can be conditioned through reinforcements in the form of stimuli that the animal would normally approach or avoid. Indirect evidence strongly suggests that certain neural systems act as internal reward or punishment systems that can guide a wide array of types of learning in various contexts (Robbins and Everitt 2003).

The first evidence of such an internal reward system in the brain was provided by the experiments of Olds and Milner (1954). They implanted an electrode in the septal area of a rat's brain and (after it recovered from surgery) placed the rat in a Skinner box, which is a box with ample room for a rat that has a bar on one side that a rat can press. They arranged this Skinner box so that a bar-press would cause electric current to flow through the electrode. They then observed that the rat not only pressed the bar, but did so "with remarkable vigor and persistence" (Milner 1970).

The normal exploratory behavior of a rat is such that it will eventually press the bar in a Skinner box. In the operant conditioning experiments of Skinner (see also Section 7.5), a rat learns to press the bar to receive a food morsel, and the learning is apparently driven by the motivational value of the food. The fact that a rat will bar-press to receive electric stimulation of the septal region implies that the stimulation itself is motivating. One possible interpretation of this finding is that animals are motivated to consummate actions that promote survival or reproduction because their brains provide them with experiences of reward when they do so, and that electric stimulation of brain regions such as the septal area produces an experience of reward similar to that normally produced by the consummation of those actions.

Further research demonstrated that rats would bar-press to cause current flow through many brain regions, implicating them as reward centers (Milner 1970). Alternatively, they would bar-press to prevent current flow through other brain regions, implicating them as punishment centers (Robbins and Everitt 2003). Most of these sites correspond either to the origins or the destinations of bundles of axons that carry neuromodulatory neurotransmitters from midbrain structures to other regions of the brain. For example, projections originating from the locus coeruleus carrying norepinephrine constitute a reward system, while projections originating from the raphe nucleus carrying serotonin constitute a punishment system (Robbins and Everitt 2003). The septal area, which was the target of the first self-stimulation studies, receives projections from the locus coeruleus (Milner 1970).

The most intensely studied of the intrinsic reinforcement systems originates from the ventral tegmental area. Its projections carry the neurotransmitter dopamine to a wide range of destinations throughout the brain (Schultz 2007). Dopamine is a classic neuromodulatory neurotransmitter in that it can be released along axonal varicosities and can influence the activity of many synapses by diffusing locally through a volume of brain tissue. The dopamine neurons operate over a wide range of time scales, and the secreted dopamine binds with a variety of receptor types, giving the dopamine system a considerable repertoire. It appears to play a role in reward, punishment, salience, learning, cognition, and many other processes (Schultz 2007). We will consider the special role of dopamine as a signal of reward prediction in Chapter 11. This chapter will concern reward and punishment signals in a more general way, as the providers of positive or negative reinforcement signals that guide learning.

In the strict sense, reinforcement learning involves learning to choose actions so as to maximize rewards or minimize punishments (Sutton and Barto 1998; Dayan and Balleine 2002). We will consider reinforcement learning in the strict sense in the second half of this chapter, where we will use it to simulate the acquisition of a conditioned avoidance response. In the more general sense, reinforcement learning can include forms of learning in neural systems that are guided by one or a few signals that are broadcast to every synapse (connection weight) in the network, rather than by error signals that are specific to each synapse. In this way we can distinguish reinforcement learning from supervised learning (see Chapter 6). Reinforcement learning can be considered as a weak form of supervised learning, but one that is also more neurobiologically plausible.

Reinforcement learning overcomes the major neurobiological implausibility of back-propagation, which is that error signals are propagated backwards down axons. With reinforcement learning, a reward (or punishment) signal is broadcast to all synaptic connections in the network. Several reinforcement signals may be available at the same time. Individual connections may or may not use a given reinforcement signal, but the same reinforcement signals are available to all units and all synapses. The reinforcement signals are used to guide connection weight changes that improve network performance. In the strict sense of reinforcement learning, the weight changes alter network behavior so as to increase positive reinforcement (reward) and/or decrease negative reinforcement (punishment). The broadcast reinforcement signals in neural models correspond to the reward and punishment neuromodulatory systems in the real brain.

Neural systems that learn through reinforcement face two major challenges. The first concerns the management of delays between network events, such as responses to stimuli or elicitations of actions, and the reinforcements associated with those events. In Chapter 11 we will consider a general mechanism for learning in the context of temporal disparities between events and reinforcements. In this chapter we will confine our study to neural systems that receive reinforcement after every event (response or action).

The second challenge concerns balancing the exploitation of the currently learned set of weight values and exploration of alternative values that might increase reward or decrease punishment. In the second half of this chapter we will study a model of avoidance conditioning wherein the activity of one of the elements is associated with the need for exploration. We will see how the behavior of this element matches that observed for certain neurons in the limbic system of the brain. In the first half of this chapter we will consider neural networks that continuously explore weight space by making random perturbations of their connection weights. Such a scheme is plausible neurobiologically.

From Brownian motion to the quantal release of transmitter, real synapses are awash in randomness. Perhaps the most important source of synaptic randomness from the viewpoint of reinforcement learning involves spike-time-dependent plasticity. The strength of a synaptic connection is modified according to differences in the order and timing of pre-synaptic and post-synaptic spikes over a window of tens of milliseconds (Caporale and Dan 2008). Because spike trains have a significant random component on this time scale (Kostal et al. 2007), synaptic strength fluctuates randomly on a continuous basis. Of critical importance for reinforcement learning, plasticity due to spike-time dependence can be regulated by neuromodulators (Caporale and Dan 2008). It is reasonable to suppose that real synapses can vary randomly in strength, and that fluctuations that improve the performance of the overall neural system can be retained over a longer term through reinforcement.

Naturally occurring synaptic weight fluctuations can be simulated as random connection weight perturbations in neural network models. We will consider various forms of learning by weight perturbation in this chapter. We will use weight perturbation to estimate the gradient of network error that we computed explicitly in Chapter 6 as part of supervised learning, but instead of back-propagating the network error signal we will broadcast it to all the connection weights. We will consider gradient estimation mainly by way of leading up to perturbative reinforcement learning. In perturbative reinforcement learning, connection weights undergo random perturbations, and if a perturbation increases positive reinforcement or decreases negative reinforcement it is retained, otherwise it is discarded. We will see that perturbative reinforcement learning actually works best when all weights are perturbed simultaneously but in different directions and by different amounts. We will use this simple and plausible method to train a three-layered neural network to form a non-uniform distributed representation.

While reinforcement learning may be more neurobiologically plausible than back-propagation, it is also less efficient. Certain pattern associations that are learned quickly (i.e., in few training cycles) and reliably (i.e., from almost any initial weight configuration) using supervised methods are learned more slowly and unreliably using perturbative reinforcement. In some cases this shortcoming can be overcome by pre-structuring the neural system prior to learning, and we will also explore the importance of structure in reinforcement learning problems.

The model of avoidance conditioning we will study in the second half of this chapter will be based on schemata, which are elements of neural systems models that represent groups of neurons. Structure in the form of organization of the schemata will enable them to simulate avoidance conditioning, and the exploration that is necessary in order to acquire the avoidance response. In the first half of this chapter, which concerns perturbative learning, structure will take the form of pre-set neural network connection weights. We turn our attention first to perturbative learning in neural networks.

7.1 Learning the Labeled-Line Task via Perturbation of One Weight at a Time

For our first example we will explore a form of learning that could be considered reinforcement learning in its less strict sense. Here the reinforcement signal is related to the error of a neural network on a pattern association task. More specifically, the signal in this case will be the change in network error due to weight perturbation. This signal can be positive or negative, and would correspond to an opposed reward/punishment form of reinforcement learning (Milner 1970; Robbins and Everitt 2003). The same change in network error signal will be available to all the connections in the network, and each one could potentially use it to estimate the component of the network error gradient with respect to its own weight. As we saw in Chapter 6, the true error gradient can be used to derive changes to the weights of a neural network that move the error down the gradient and so reduce it. In Chapter 6 we used the delta rule (two-layered feedforward networks) or back-propagation (three-layered feedforward networks) to compute exactly the gradient of network error with respect to each individual weight. Here we will use weight perturbation to estimate (rather than compute exactly) the component of the gradient with respect to a weight. We will use gradient estimates to derive weight updates that should, on average, reduce the error.

The gradient of the error with respect to the weights is schematized, for a very simple neural network having only two weights, in Figure 7.1. The diagram in Figure 7.1 is the same as in Figure 6.2 to emphasize that perturbative learning (this chapter) and exact computation (previous chapter) are two different methods for descending the same error gradient. The first task for any gradient descent learning procedure is to find the gradient $\partial E / \partial w_{ij}$ of network error E with respect to weight w_{ij} (where w_{ij} stands for any weight to a unit i from a unit j). The gradient $\partial E / \partial w_{ij}$ basically indicates the direction in which a change in the weight will produce an increase in the error, so to decrease the error the weight should be moved in the opposite direction. Thus, the gradient can be used to derive the weight update Δw_{ij}, which is the opposite of the gradient scaled by the learning rate a: $\Delta w_{ij} = -a(\partial E / \partial w_{ij})$. Whereas the delta rule and back-propagation exactly compute the gradient $\partial E / \partial w_{ij}$, where the symbol ∂ denotes the partial derivative, the gradient could also be estimated as $\delta E / \delta w_{ij}$, where the symbol δ denotes a small, discrete change.

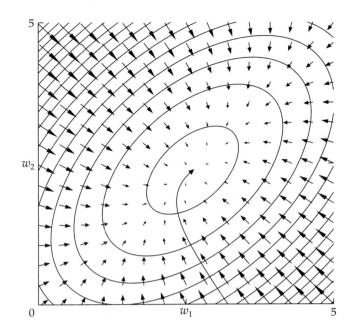

FIGURE 7.1   Gradient descent in a neural network with only two weights: w_1 **and** w_2 Error in this hypothetical network is minimized when $w_1 = w_2 = 2.5$. (From McClelland and Rumelhart 1989.)

Gradient estimation can be carried out by making a small change in a weight δw_{ij}, while holding fixed the values of all the other weights, and observing the resulting change δE in network error as shown in Equation 7.1:

$$\frac{\delta E}{\delta w_{ij}} = \frac{E\left(\mathbf{W} + \delta\,\mathbf{W}_{ij}\right) - E\left(\mathbf{W}\right)}{\delta w_{ij}} \qquad\qquad \textbf{7.1}$$

This estimate involves perturbation by δw_{ij} of the single weight w_{ij} in weight matrix $\mathbf{W}$. In Equation 7.1 this perturbation is made by adding to $\mathbf{W}$ the matrix $\delta\mathbf{W}_{ij}$, which is of the same dimensions as $\mathbf{W}$ and has all 0 elements except for element (i, j), which equals δw_{ij}. The weight update based on the gradient estimate in Equation 7.1 is shown in Equation 7.2:

$$\Delta w_{ij} = -a\frac{\delta E}{\delta w_{ij}} \qquad\qquad \textbf{7.2}$$

This method assumes a non-negative measure of network error E. Recall from Chapter 6 that for the delta rule and back-propagation E was taken as the summed squared differences between the desired and actual outputs (see Math Boxes 6.2 and 6.5). Here we can simply take E as equal to the summed absolute values of these differences. Note that for gradient estimation the weight change is explicitly proportional to the opposite of the gradient (shown by the minus sign in Equation 7.2), whereas for delta rule and back-propagation the sign change is implicit in the formula for the error signal (see Math Boxes 6.2 and 6.5). This method of gradient estimation via perturbation of a single weight (see Equations 7.1 and 7.2) seems crude but it is guaranteed to work provided that two conditions are satisfied. First, the perturbation size δw_{ij} and the learning rate a must be small enough that the estimate is meaningful and the weight update does not overshoot the minimum of the error function. Second, all of the other weights in the network must be held fixed while only the single weight to be updated is perturbed.

A simple numerical example illustrates how this method can be used to update the weights in a neural network. Consider a neural network having only one linear output unit y and two input units x_1 and x_2 with connection weights onto y of w_1 and w_2. The gradient depicted in Figure 7.1 could apply to this simple network. (For notational simplicity in this example, we drop the first subscript $i = 1$ from the weights.) Assume that, at a certain point in training, both w_1 and w_2 have value 1. Assume also that the task this network must learn is to transform the input pattern [1 1] to the desired output $d = 5$. The actual output is $y = w_1x_1 + w_2x_2 = (1)(1) + (1)(1) = 2$, and the network error for this weight configuration is $E(w_1,w_2) = |d - y| = |5 - 2| = 3$. Now we hold the value of w_2 fixed at 1 but we perturb weight w_1 by $\delta w_1 = 1$, so the actual output becomes $y = (w_1 + \delta w_1)x_1 + w_2x_2 = (1 + 1)(1) + (1)(1) = 3$, and the network error with w_1 perturbed is $E(w_1 + \delta w_1, w_2) = |d - y| = |5 - 3| = 2$. We can use these values to estimate the error gradient with respect to weight w_1 as $\delta E / \delta w_1 = [E(w_1 + \delta w_1, w_2) - E(w_1, w_2)] / \delta w_1 = (2 - 3) / 1 = -1$. If the learning rate a equals 1, then the update is $\Delta w_1 = -a(\delta E / \delta w_1) = -(1)(-1) = 1$, and the new, updated value of weight w_1 is $w_1 + \Delta w_1 = 1 + 1 = 2$. Updating w_1 from 1 to 2 has decreased the error from 3 to 2. The value of w_2 is updated similarly. In this very simple example we were able to use a large weight perturbation and learning rate but, in practice, values that are small relative to the size of the average weight should be used.

The reinforcement learning methods we will consider in this chapter are iterative in that they progress by making small weight changes over many learning cycles. The example we consider in this section involves error-gradient estimation through perturbation of one weight at a time. For this method, a single weight is chosen at random and perturbed using a small increment that is of random sign, but of fixed size, on each learning cycle. (We will relax these methodological restrictions in later examples.) The network error measure is found before and after the perturbation and used to compute the change in network error δE due to the perturbation. When computed using the one-at-a-time method, the signal δE is relevant only to the single connection that underwent the weight perturbation. That connection can use the δE signal, along with the learning rate a, and the amount δw_{ij} by which its weight was perturbed, to estimate the gradient and compute an update according to Equation 7.2. The perturbed weight is then updated, a new weight is chosen at random, and the process is repeated until the error is reduced below a tolerance.

The restriction of this method to one weight at a time seems implausible neurobiologically. We will address this issue in the next section. Otherwise the method is plausible. We can assume that each weight "knows" the amount δw_{ij} by which it was perturbed, and also "knows" the learning rate a. If each weight receives the change in error δE, then the perturbed weight (but not the other weights) could use that to estimate the gradient and compute an update according to Equation 7.2. Given the change in error signal δE that is broadcast to all connections as a neuromodulatory signal, the process of computing and applying the weight update Δw_{ij} is local. This method assumes that individual synapses are capable of simple computations, but these are not out of the question for real synapses. We will consider the issue of "smart synapses" in detail in Chapter 14.

In this section we will use error-gradient estimation, through perturbation of one weight at a time, to train a two-layered, feedforward network of sigmoidal units. Recall from Chapter 6 that sigmoidal units y_i compute the weighted sum q_i of their inputs and bound that sigmoidally between 0 and 1 using the squashing function (Equations 7.3 and 7.4):

$$q_i = \sum_j v_{ij} x_j \qquad\qquad 7.3$$

$$y_i = \frac{1}{1 + \exp(-q_i)} \qquad\qquad 7.4$$

Input units   Output units

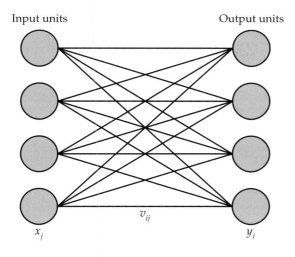

x_j v_{ij} y_i

FIGURE 7.2   A generic, two-layered feedforward neural network Input units x_j project to output units y_i over connections with weights v_{ij}. (Indices are $j = 1, …, n_x$ and $i = 1, …, n_y$, where n_x and n_y are the numbers of input and output units, respectively.)

(Recall also from Chapter 6 that Equation 7.3 is equivalent to $\mathbf{q} = \mathbf{Vx}$.) A generic two-layered network, with input units x_j, output units y_i, and input–output weights v_{ij} is depicted in Figure 7.2. Note that i ($i = 1, …, n_y$) and j ($j = 1, …, n_x$) index the n_y output and the n_x input units, respectively. We considered the same two-layered network architecture in Chapter 6 (see Figure 6.1). To facilitate explanation of the one-at-a-time weight perturbation method and its implementation in MATLAB®, the network we consider in this example will have only one output unit. Script `pertGradientOneByOne`, listed in MATLAB Box 7.1, will train two-layered, feedforward networks having multiple input units, but only one output unit, to associate patterns using gradient estimation through perturbation of one weight at a time.

The weights in script `pertGradientOneByOne` are held in matrix `V`. Because this two-layered, feedforward network has only one output unit, matrix `V` is just a row vector with as many elements as input units. This script randomly chooses the index of the single weight to be updated using `vChoose=ceil(nIn*rand)` where `nIn` is the number of input units. On each iteration it generates a weight perturbation of absolute value `pSize=0.005` but of random sign (positive or negative) using `pert=pSize*sign(randn)` and perturbs the single, randomly chosen weight using `V(vChoose)=V(vChoose)+pert`. Note that `pert` corresponds to δw_{ij} in Equations 7.1 and 7.2. After each single weight perturbation the script finds the actual output for all of the patterns in the training set using `Q=V*InPat'` and `Out=1./(1+exp(-Q))`, and finds the new error over all of the patterns in the set using `newErr=sum(abs(DesOut-Out'))`. Note that network error is the sum of the absolute differences between the desired and actual outputs. In these commands `InPat` is the array of input patterns, `Q` is the array of weighted input sums, and `Out` and `DesOut` are the arrays of actual and desired outputs, respectively. The script then uses the previous, unperturbed network error in variable `error` to find the change in error using `delErr=newErr-error`, and estimates the gradient using `estGrad=delErr/pert` (see Equation 7.1). The script computes the weight update using `vDelta=-a*estGrad` (see Equation 7.2) and finally updates the randomly chosen weight using `V(vChoose)=V(vChoose)+vDelta`.

We will use gradient estimation through perturbation of one weight at time to train a network having four input units and one output unit on the input and desired output patterns shown in Table 7.1. The output unit is sigmoidal. (Since the input states are specified their activation function is irrelevant.) The patterns correspond to the non-overlapping, labeled-line patterns we used in

MATLAB® BOX 7.1   **This script trains two-layered networks of sigmoidal units (with only one output unit) to associate patterns using perturbation to estimate the error gradient at one weight at a time.**

```
% pertGradientOneByOne.m
% initial weight matrix V, and input InPat and desired
% output DesOut patterns, must be supplied in workspace

[nPat,nIn]=size(InPat); % determine numbers of patterns and inputs
[nPat,nOut]=size(DesOut); % determine number of output units
Out=zeros(nPat,nOut); % set up output hold array
a=0.01; % set learning rate
pSize=0.005; % set perturbation size
tol=0.1; % set error tolerance within which training is adequate
count=0; % set the iteration counter to zero
countLimit=100000; % set count limit over which training stops

Q=V*InPat'; % find the weighted input sums for all patterns
Out=1./(1+exp(-Q)); % squash to find the output for all patterns
error=sum(abs(DesOut-Out')); % find initial error over all patterns

while error>tol, % while actual error is over tolerance
    pert=pSize*sign(randn); % generate a single weight perturbation
    vChoose=ceil(nIn*rand); % choose one weight from V at random
    V(vChoose)=V(vChoose)+pert; % perturb this weight
    Q=V*InPat'; % find the weighted input sum for all the patterns
    Out=1./(1+exp(-Q)); % squash to find the output for all patterns
    newErr=sum(abs(DesOut-Out')); % find new error over all patterns
    delErr=newErr-error; % find change in error due to perturbation
    estGrad=delErr/pert; % compute estimated gradient
    vDelta=-a*estGrad; % compute weight change
    V(vChoose)=V(vChoose)+vDelta; % apply weight change to weight
    error=newErr; % save new error as the error
    count=count+1; % increment the counter
    if count>countLimit, break, end % break if counter over limit
end % end training loop
```

our study of supervised learning in Chapter 6. Like the other scripts in this book, most of the parameters are set, for convenience, within the script, but some are set outside the script and must be entered into the MATLAB workspace separately from the script. For script pertGradientOneByOne the input and desired output training patterns must be set outside the script. The non-overlapping, labeled-line patterns can be entered into the MATLAB workspace using InPat=[1 0 0 0;0 1 0 0;0 0 1 0;0 0 0 1] and DesOut=[1;1;0;0]. For reasons that will become clear later, it is more convenient to set the initial connectivity matrix V outside the script also. We will start by setting the elements of V to normally distributed random deviates by issuing the command V=randn(1,4) at the MATLAB command line.

Other parameters are set in the script. Set the learning rate a=0.01. The script pertGradientOneByOne uses a while loop and will continue to update the weights either until the error falls below the tolerance tol=0.1, or until the number of iterations exceeds countLimit=100000. For this particular run the network learned the non-overlapping patterns after about 16,000 iterations. (Variable count counts the learning cycles.) Thus, the network succeeded in learning the

TABLE 7.1 **Learning the labeled-line patterns using gradient estimation at one weight at a time**

Input patterns				Desired output patterns	Actual output patterns
1	0	0	0	1	0.98
0	1	0	0	1	0.97
0	0	1	0	0	0.03
0	0	0	1	0	0.02

The input, desired output, and actual output following training are listed for a two-layered, feedforward network of sigmoidal units. The network has four input units and one output unit (a 4-by-1 network). Note that the labeled-line input patterns are non-overlapping.

labeled-line task using gradient estimation through perturbation of one weight at time. The actual output after training is also shown in Table 7.1, and the final weights are shown in Table 7.2. Note that, because of the randomness inherent in perturbative learning, the results will differ from simulation to simulation. All of the results presented in this chapter are, therefore, representative of the results that are typical for each example.

Gradient estimation via weight perturbation as we have implemented it so far is simple, but its plausibility is diminished by its restriction to one weight perturbation per training cycle. It is unrealistic to suppose, in a real neural system, that all of the synapses remain fixed while a single synapse is perturbed. This would require a level of communication and coordination between synapses far beyond anything that has been described. Fortunately, gradient estimation works well, and in some cases even better, when all connection weights undergo simultaneous perturbation. We consider that in the next section.

7.2 Perturbing All Weights Simultaneously and the Importance of Structure

Fortunately, the restriction to perturbation of single weights in the gradient estimation procedure can be dropped. If all of the weights in a neural network were contained as the elements w_{ij} of a matrix **W**, then they could all be perturbed simultaneously and in parallel by adding to **W** a matrix of perturbations δ**W** of the same dimensions as **W**. Then the network error gradient with respect to the single weight w_{ij} could be estimated as in Equation 7.5:

$$\frac{\delta E}{\delta w_{ij}} = \frac{E(\mathbf{W} + \delta\mathbf{W}) - E(\mathbf{W})}{\delta w_{ij}}$$

7.5

Weight updates could be derived from this gradient as before using Equation 7.2. Equation 7.5 would seem to give inaccurate estimates of the error gradi-

TABLE 7.2 **Weight matrix after training on the labeled-line (non-overlapping) patterns using gradient estimation at one weight at a time**

To output unit	From input unit			
	1	2	3	4
1	+3.71	+3.62	−3.42	−3.97

MATH BOX 7.1   THE BROWNIAN MOTION ALGORITHM

A neural network can be trained to minimize its error in producing a desired output by adjusting its weights so that network error moves down the error gradient with respect to the weights. This gradient can be calculated exactly (using delta rule or back-propagation, for example; see Chapter 6) or it can be estimated, essentially by "jiggling" a weight and noting the effect of the jiggle on network error. More formally, if $E(\mathbf{W})$ is the error measure for a network with generic weight matrix $\mathbf{W}$, then the true gradient of the network error with respect to any weight w_{ij} is $\partial E / \partial w_{ij}$ (∂ designates the partial derivative). The true error gradient can be estimated by perturbing w_{ij} by δw_{ij} (δ denotes "a small change in") and measuring the change in network error δE as the entire weight matrix $\mathbf{W}$ except for the element w_{ij} is held constant. This relationship is shown in Equation B7.1.1:

$$\frac{\partial E}{\partial w_{ij}} \approx \frac{\delta E}{\delta w_{ij}} = \frac{E(\mathbf{W}+\delta\mathbf{W}_{ij})-E(\mathbf{W})}{\delta w_{ij}} \quad \text{B7.1.1}$$

In Equation B7.1.1, $E(\mathbf{W})$ is the error of the unperturbed network, and $\delta\mathbf{W}_{ij}$ is a matrix of the same dimensions as $\mathbf{W}$ that contains all 0s but has δw_{ij} at element (i, j), so that $E(\mathbf{W} + \delta\mathbf{W}_{ij})$ is the error of the network with the single weight w_{ij} perturbed by adding perturbation δw_{ij} to it. The change in error in Equation B7.1.1 could be used to compute an update for weight w_{ij} according to Equation B7.1.2:

$$\Delta w_{ij} = -a\frac{\delta E}{\delta w_{ij}} \quad \text{B7.1.2}$$

where a is the learning rate. While this method is straightforward and is guaranteed to work, the idea that all of the other synapses in a real neural system would be held fixed while only one is perturbed seems unrealistic. To make the same estimate by perturbing all of the weights simultaneously, we would first generate a matrix $\delta\mathbf{W}$ of the same dimensions as $\mathbf{W}$ and in which every element is a perturbation of fixed absolute value but random sign, and add this matrix of perturbations to the weight matrix

$\mathbf{W}$. We then estimate the error gradient $\partial E / \partial w_{ij}$ with respect to any weight w_{ij} using Equation B7.1.3:

$$\frac{\partial E}{\partial w_{ij}} \approx \frac{\delta E}{\delta w_{ij}} = \frac{E(\mathbf{W}+\delta\mathbf{W})-E(\mathbf{W})}{\delta w_{ij}} \quad \text{B7.1.3}$$

It would seem that Equation B7.1.3 would give us an inaccurate estimate of the gradient, because we perturb all of the weights to estimate the gradient with respect to a single weight. Alspector and coworkers (1993) showed how Equation B7.1.3 actually provides an accurate gradient estimate on average. They performed a Taylor series expansion of Equation B7.1.3 and, ignoring higher order terms, found:

$$\frac{\delta E}{\delta w_{ij}} = \frac{\partial E}{\partial w_{ij}} + \sum_{kl \neq ij}\left(\frac{\partial E}{\partial w_{kl}}\right)\left(\frac{\delta w_{kl}}{\delta w_{ij}}\right) \quad \text{B7.1.4}$$

Thus, the gradient estimate $\delta E / \delta w_{ij}$, generated by simultaneously perturbing all the weights, is equal to the true gradient $\partial E / \partial w_{ij}$ plus a summation term that is a function of all the weight perturbations. The important point is that the summation term has mean value 0 because, with perturbations of fixed size but random sign, the last term in parentheses is as likely to be +1 as −1. The implication is that if each synapse has access to a signal proportional to the resulting change in error due to simultaneous weight perturbation, then it can adjust its weight by assuming it was the only weight perturbed. The analysis shows that the weight change rule in Equation B7.1.2, incorporating the gradient estimate $\delta E / \delta w_{ij}$ found using simultaneous, parallel weight perturbation as in Equation B7.1.3, will follow the true gradient on average, but with the noise implied by the summation term in Equation B7.1.4 (and to a smaller extent by the higher-order terms that we have ignored). Equations B7.1.1, B7.1.2, and B7.1.3 correspond with Equations 7.1, 7.2, and 7.5 of the main text, respectively.

ent, because all of the weights are perturbed to find the gradient at a single weight. As shown by Alspector and coworkers (1993), Equation 7.5 actually tracks the true error gradient on average, provided that the perturbations have random sign but uniform absolute value. Their analysis is summarized in Math Box 7.1. The learning algorithm based on this analysis is called the Brownian motion algorithm. Thus, gradient estimation via weight perturbation works even when all the weights in a neural network are perturbed simultaneously, which is more plausible than perturbation of one weight at a time. Another benefit of parallel weight perturbation is that all weights can be updated simultaneously, and this makes learning more efficient. Our next example will concern gradient estimation via parallel weight perturbation, and simultaneous weight update, using the Brownian motion algorithm.

MATLAB® BOX 7.2 **This script trains two-layered networks of sigmoidal units to associate patterns using perturbation to estimate the error gradient at all weights simultaneously.**

```
% pertGradientParallel.m
% initial weight matrix V, and input InPat and desired
% output DesOut patterns, must be supplied in workspace

[nPat,nIn]=size(InPat); % determine numbers of patterns and inputs
[nPat,nOut]=size(DesOut); % determine number of output units
Out=zeros(nPat,nOut); % set up output hold array
a=0.01; % set learning rate
pSize=0.005; % set perturbation size
tol=0.1; % set error tolerance within which training is adequate
count=0; % set the iteration counter to zero
countLimit=100000; % set count limit over which training stops

Q=V*InPat'; % find the weighted input sums for all patterns
Out=1./(1+exp(-Q)); % squash to find the output for all patterns
error=sum(sum(abs(DesOut-Out'))); % initial error over all patterns

while error>tol, % while actual error is over tolerance
    Pert=pSize*sign(randn(nOut,nIn)); % parallel weight perturbation
    V=V+Pert; % apply perturbation to all weights in parallel
    Q=V*InPat'; % find the weighted input sum for all the patterns
    Out=1./(1+exp(-Q)); % squash to find the output for all patterns
    newErr=sum(sum(abs(DesOut-Out'))); % new error over all patterns
    delErr=newErr-error; % find change in error due to perturbation
    estGrad=delErr./Pert; % compute matrix of estimated gradients
    deltaV=-a*estGrad; % compute matrix of weight changes
    V=V+deltaV; % apply weight change matrix to weight matrix
    error=newErr; % save new error as the error
    count=count+1; % increment the counter
    if count>countLimit, break, end % break if counter over limit
end % end training loop
```

Script `pertGradientParallel`, listed in MATLAB Box 7.2, will train two-layered, feedforward networks of sigmoidal units on pattern association tasks by estimating the network error gradient using parallel weight perturbation, and by updating all network weights simultaneously. This script is similar to the one-weight-at-a-time script `pertGradientOneByOne`, except that all weights are perturbed and updated simultaneously. Also the network is not limited to one output unit only. On each learning cycle a matrix of perturbations, of the same dimensions as weight matrix V, in which each element has absolute value `pSize=0.005` but random sign, is generated using `Pert=pSize*sign(randn(nOut,nIn))`. Note that variable `Pert` in script `pertGradientParallel` is an entire matrix of weight perturbations, not a single perturbation value as for variable `pert` in `pertGradientOneByOne`. The script perturbs the entire weight matrix V using `V=V+Pert`.

After each entire weight matrix perturbation the script finds the actual output for all of the patterns in the training set, as before, using `Q=V*InPat'` and `Out=1./(1+exp(-Q))`, and finds the new network error over all of the patterns in the set using `newErr=sum(sum(abs(DesOut-Out')))`. Note that this command can compute error in networks having more than one output unit. The script then uses the previous, unperturbed network error in vari-

TABLE 7.3   Learning the labeled-line patterns using gradient estimation at all weights in parallel

Input patterns				Desired output patterns	Actual output patterns
1	0	0	0	1	0.98
0	1	0	0	1	0.98
0	0	1	0	0	0.02
0	0	0	1	0	0.04

The input, desired output, and actual output following training are listed for a two-layered, 4-by-1 feedforward network of sigmoidal units. Note that the labeled-line input patterns are non-overlapping.

able `error` to find the change in error using `delErr=newErr-error`, and computes the matrix of gradient estimates using `estGrad=delErr./Pert` (see Equation 7.5). Note that in the second command a scalar (`delErr`) is divided element-wise by the matrix of weight perturbations (`Pert`) yielding a matrix of estimates of the same dimensions as weight matrix `V`. The script then computes the matrix of weight changes as `deltaV=-a*estGrad`, and finally updates the entire weight matrix using `V=V+deltaV`.

We will first use parallel gradient estimation to train a network having four input units and one output unit on the non-overlapping, labeled-line patterns, which are reproduced in Table 7.3. As for `pertGradientOneByOne`, the input and desired output patterns `InPat` and `DesOut`, and the initial weight matrix `V`, must be set outside of script `pertGradientParallel`. The training patterns can be entered using `InPat=[1 0 0 0;0 1 0 0;0 0 1 0;0 0 0 1]` and `DesOut=[1;1;0;0]`. As before, set the elements of `V` to normally distributed random deviates using `V=randn(1,4)`. The other parameters are set in the script.

With learning rate `a=0.01` as before, the network learns the non-overlapping patterns to within tolerance `tol=0.1` in about 5000 iterations using the Brownian motion algorithm. As with gradient estimation through perturbation and update of one weight at time, the network succeeded in learning the labeled-line task using gradient estimation through perturbation and update of all weights simultaneously. Note that the number of required iterations for parallel gradient estimation is far fewer than the approximately 16,000 iterations required for one-weight-at-a-time gradient estimation. The actual outputs following training are also shown in Table 7.3, and the final weight values are shown in Table 7.4. The final weights produced by parallel gradient estimation are roughly the same as those produced by one-weight-at-a-time gradient estimation (see Table 7.2).

For both forms of gradient estimation, parallel and one-weight-at-a-time, the perturbations have random sign but uniform absolute value. Uniformity of perturbation size appears to be necessary for gradient estimation (see Alspec-

TABLE 7.4   Weight matrix after training on the labeled-line (non-overlapping) patterns using gradient estimation at all weights in parallel

To output unit	From input unit			
	1	2	3	4
1	+4.04	+3.81	−3.82	−3.18

TABLE 7.5   **Failure to learn the complex contingency patterns using gradient estimation at all weights in parallel**

Input patterns	Desired output patterns	Actual output patterns
1 0 1 0	1	1.00
1 1 1 1	1	1.00
1 1 1 0	0	1.00
1 0 0 1	0	0.00

The input, desired output, and actual output following training are listed for a two-layered, 4-by-1 feedforward network of sigmoidal units. Note that the complex contingency input patterns overlap substantially.

tor et al. 1993 for further details). The scripts that implement these methods (see MATLAB Boxes 7.1 and 7.2) compute the error over the entire set of training patterns. It is not necessary in general for perturbative learning to compute the error over the entire training set, and perurbative learning also works if updates occur after each pattern is presented (Alspector et al. 1993). Computation of the error over the entire training set is convenient here because we use relatively few training patterns.

Both forms of gradient estimation, parallel and one-weight-at-a-time, succeeded in training neural networks on the non-overlapping, labeled-line patterns. Recall from Chapter 6 that covariance learning was also capable of training two-layered, feedforward neural networks on the non-overlapping pattern set, but it failed on a dense overlapping pattern set that we characterized as a complex tangle of input–output contingencies. In contrast, the delta rule was capable of training the network on the dense, overlapping pattern set. Since gradient estimation, like the delta rule, is an error-driven learning procedure it should, in principle, also succeed in training a two-layered network on the dense overlapping (complex contingency) pattern set. The dense-overlapping pattern set (Orchard and Phillips 1991) is reproduced in Table 7.5. We test the ability of the Brownian motion algorithm on this pattern set in the next example.

The overlapping patterns can be entered into the MATLAB workspace using the commands `InPat=[1 0 1 0;1 1 1 1;1 1 1 0;1 0 0 1]` and `DesOut=[1;1;0;0]`. The elements of `V` are reinitialized to normally distributed random deviates using `V=randn(1,4)` from the command line. Within the script the learning rate is again set to `a=0.01`. For this particular simulation, which is representative of the majority of simulations using the overlapping patterns, the network did not reach tolerance `tol=0.1` before the number of iterations exceeded `countLimit=100000`. The actual output after 100,001 unsuccessful iterations is also shown in Table 7.5, and the weights are shown in Table 7.6. The network fails to learn the third pattern.

TABLE 7.6   **Weight matrix after unsuccessful training on the complex contingency (overlapping) patterns using gradient estimation at all weights in parallel**

To output unit	From input unit			
	1	2	3	4
1	–2.36	+3.99	+9.64	–4.59

TABLE 7.7 Successfully learning the complex contingency patterns using gradient estimation at all weights in parallel

Input patterns				Desired output patterns	Actual output patterns
1	0	1	0	1	0.98
1	1	1	1	1	0.97
1	1	1	0	0	0.04
1	0	0	1	0	0.02

The input, desired output, and actual output following training are listed for a two-layered, 4-by-1 feedforward network of sigmoidal units. Training began from an initial random state different from that which generated the unsuccessful learning results in Table 7.5.

Due to the randomness inherent in perturbative learning, the results can differ greatly from one simulation to the next. To see this, we again reinitialize the weight matrix from the command line using V=randn(1,4) and retrain the network using parallel gradient estimation at the same learning rate a=0.01. This time the Brownian motion algorithm succeeds in reducing the error below tolerance tol=0.1. Training requires about 33,000 iterations. Thus, the network succeeded in learning the complex contingency task using gradient estimation through perturbation and update of all weights simultaneously. The actual output after training is shown in Table 7.7, and the final weights are shown in Table 7.8.

The reason that the network failed in its first attempt to learn the overlapping patterns but succeeded in its second attempt is due to the configuration of the initial weight matrix. Note that the final weight matrix, which for a network of four input units and one output unit is a four-element row vector, has negative numbers as its first two elements and positive numbers as its second two elements (see Table 7.8). This is significant, because the initially random weight matrix, which was **V** = [−2.39 +0.26 +0.58 +0.90], had its first two numerical elements less than its second two. Similarly successful results are obtained starting from **V** = [−1 −1 +1 +1], and from other starting configurations in which the first two numerical elements are less than the second two. This suggests that the structure of the initial weight matrix plays an important role in perturbative learning. This level of sensitivity to the initial weight matrix is not also observed for supervised learning mechanisms such as the delta rule and back-propagation. Thus, perturbative learning appears to be less robust than supervised learning, but its main advantage, that of greater neurobiological plausibility, is not diminished by its greater reliance on the

TABLE 7.8 Weight matrix after successful training on the complex contingency (overlapping) patterns using gradient estimation at all weights in parallel

To output unit	From input unit			
	1	2	3	4
1	−10.69	−7.45	+14.84	+6.86

Training began from an initial, random state different from that which generated the unsuccessful learning results in Table 7.5. The weights in this table are different from those in Table 7.6.

starting configuration of the weight matrix. Rather than starting from a completely random state, it is reasonable to assume that real neural systems, even those capable of adaptive synaptic plasticity, start learning with some structure already available to them due to genetic and developmental processes. The theme of initial structure will reemerge in some of the other examples of reinforcement learning that we will consider in this chapter.

7.3 Plausible Weight Modification using Perturbative Reinforcement Learning

Contemplation of the simple two-weight error gradient shown in Figure 7.1 suggests another method for implementing perturbative learning. It seems possible that learning could be achieved, and network error minimized, simply by perturbing the weights, either one at a time or all simultaneously, and retaining the perturbation if the error is reduced but discarding the perturbation otherwise. That such is indeed possible in a related context was demonstrated by Venkatesh (1993), who showed that any matrix of binary weights could be learned through perturbation by flipping them (0 to 1 or vice-versa), either singly or in subsets chosen at random. In the directed drift algorithm (Venkatesh 1993), input patterns are presented to the network, and one or several randomly chosen weights have their binary values flipped if the output is in error, but the weights are left unperturbed otherwise. Directed drift is proven to work in this restricted context (Venkatesh 1993). We explore its use for real-valued weights in the next example.

Script `pertDirectedDrift`, listed in MATLAB Box 7.3, will train two-layered, feedforward networks of sigmoidal units to associate patterns using a real-valued adaptation of the directed drift algorithm. It is similar to the previously considered gradient estimation script `pertGradientParallel` in that all of the weights are perturbed in parallel, but it differs from the gradient estimation method in that network error is not used to estimate the gradient. Instead, it is used as a (negative) reinforcement signal. Thus, the version of directed drift we use here is an example of reinforcement learning in the strict sense, and we can also call it perturbative reinforcement learning.

Script `pertDirectedDrift` generates a matrix of perturbations of fixed absolute value but random sign using `Pert=a*sign(randn(nOut,nIn))` where `a=0.01` is the learning rate. Note that the learning rate value is the same for directed drift as for gradient estimation, but it is used as the size (absolute value) of the perturbation in directed drift, rather than the scale factor for weight updates as in gradient estimation. On each iteration the directed drift routine first saves the current weight matrix using `holdV=V`. It then applies the weight matrix perturbation using `V=V+Pert` and determines the error over the whole pattern set as in gradient estimation. The script then implements two, sequential if-then conditionals. If the perturbation does not reduce the error, then it is removed by restoring the weights to their unperturbed values using `V=holdV`. If the perturbation does reduce the error, then it is retained and the error is reset to the new, lower value using `error=newErr`, as before.

We will train the network using perturbative reinforcement learning on the overlapping patterns, which can be entered into the workspace as before using the commands `InPat=[1 0 1 0;1 1 1 1;1 1 1 0;1 0 0 1]` and `DesOut=[1;1;0;0]`. The elements of `V` are reinitialized to normally distributed random deviates using `V=randn(1,4)` at the command line. For this particular simulation, which is representative of the majority of simulations using directed drift to train on the overlapping patterns, the network did not reach tolerance `tol=0.1` before the number of iterations exceeded

MATLAB® BOX 7.3   This script trains two-layered networks of sigmoidal units to associate patterns by perturbing all weights simultaneously.

```
% pertDirectedDrift.m
% initial weight matrix V, and input InPat and desired
% output DesOut patterns, must be supplied in workspace

[nPat,nIn]=size(InPat); % determine numbers of patterns and inputs
[nPat,nOut]=size(DesOut); % determine number of output units
Out=zeros(nPat,nOut); % set up output hold array
a=0.01; % set learning rate
tol=0.1; % set error tolerance within which training is adequate
count=0; % set the iteration counter to zero
countLimit=100000; % set count limit over which training stops

Q=V*InPat'; % find the weighted input sums for all patterns
Out=1./(1+exp(-Q)); % squash to find the output for all patterns
error=sum(sum(abs(DesOut-Out'))); % initial error over all patterns

while error>tol, % while actual error is over tolerance
    Pert=a*sign(randn(nOut,nIn)); % weight perturbation matrix
    holdV=V; % hold the current weight matrix
    V=V+Pert; % apply perturbation to all weights in parallel
    Q=V*InPat'; % find the weighted input sum for all the patterns
    Out=1./(1+exp(-Q)); % squash to find the output for all patterns
    newErr=sum(sum(abs(DesOut-Out'))); % new error over all patterns
    if newErr>=error, % if the perturbation increases the error
        V=holdV; % then restore the unperturbed weights
    elseif newErr<error, % leave perturbation if it decreased error
        error=newErr; % and save new error as the error
    end % end conditional
    count=count+1; % increment the counter
    if count>countLimit, break, end % break if counter over limit
end % end training loop
```

countLimit=100000. Like gradient estimation, it seems that directed drift has similar difficulties with the dense-overlapping (complex contingency) pattern set.

Considering the benefits we experienced with weight pre-structuring using gradient estimation, we reinitialize the weight matrix using V=[-1 -1 +1 +1] and retrain using directed drift. As for gradient estimation, directed drift succeeds in training the network on the overlapping patterns starting from this more commodious initial weight configuration. The actual outputs following training are shown in Table 7.9, and the final weights are shown in Table 7.10. The weights learned using directed drift (perturbative reinforcement learning) are very close to those learned using gradient estimation (see Table 7.8).

While the final results of parallel gradient estimation and parallel directed drift are comparable, directed drift learns in fewer iterations. Starting from $\mathbf{V} = [-1\ -1\ +1\ +1]$ the directed drift algorithm required only about 5000 cycles (stored in count) to reduce error below the tolerance of tol=0.1. This can be compared with the approximately 33,000 iterations required by gradient estimation on this problem with a similar starting weight configuration. Thus directed drift, which is even simpler than gradient estimation, learns faster.

TABLE 7.9   Successfully learning the complex contingency patterns using parallel, pertubative reinforcement learning

Input patterns				Desired output patterns	Actual output patterns
1	0	1	0	1	0.98
1	1	1	1	1	0.97
1	1	1	0	0	0.03
1	0	0	1	0	0.02

The input, desired output, and actual output following training are listed for a two-layered, 4-by-1 feedforward network of sigmoidal units. On each training cycle, the parallel weight perturbation was followed by retention of the perturbation or restoration of the unperturbed weights if reinforcement was positive or negative, respectively. The initial weight matrix was $\mathbf{V} = [-1\ -1\ +1\ +1]$.

Directed drift is also more robust than parallel gradient estimation (Brownian motion) in the sense that it can also work with parallel weight perturbations that differ not only in sign but also in absolute value (see Exercise 7.1). Considering that it is simpler, faster, and more robust than Brownian motion, directed drift (perturbative reinforcement learning) appears to be preferable as a neural network learning algorithm.

It seems counterintuitive that the Brownian motion algorithm, and much less that directed drift, should work at all. These algorithms seem to do the opposite of what one should do in trying to adjust multiple parameters in order to achieve a goal. Consider an experimental situation. A careful scientist would adjust one parameter at a time, holding all others constant. This methodical, systematic approach is completely at odds with the parallel weight update strategies we have used in the previous two examples, in which all of the parameters are tweaked at the same time but in random directions. Still, the viability both of the Brownian motion and the directed drift algorithms are supported by theory (Alspector et al. 1993; Venkatesh 1993), and we have used them successfully to train neural networks on pattern association tasks. Although these algorithms seem to operate differently than we would want them to operate in a controlled laboratory setting, they are a lot like real life, in which we often have to take on whole situations that are characterized by multiple factors beyond our control. When we move in with a new roommate or take a new job, we experience an unavoidable tweaking of many of our parameters all at once. Most of the time we have no option other than to try a situation, and if it works then we stay with it, but if it fails we move on. We could extrapolate from these algorithms to suggest, not entirely whimsically, that some forms of learning in our brains, like our changing circumstances in life, are like a directed drift.

TABLE 7.10   Weight matrix after successful training on the complex contingency (overlapping) patterns using parallel, perturbative reinforcement learning

To output unit	From input unit			
	1	2	3	4
1	−10.80	−7.32	+14.76	+6.96

The initial weight matrix was $\mathbf{V} = [-1\ -1\ +1\ +1]$.

The version of directed drift we use here, which we can also refer to as perturbative reinforcement learning, is neurobiologically plausible. As argued at the beginning of the chapter, it is reasonable to suppose that the strengths of the synaptic weights in real neural systems undergo random perturbations, and that a reinforcement signal related to performance is available to all synapses. The individual synapses would require some mechanism for restoring the previous values of their weights in case of negative reinforcement, but such ability is not out of the question for real synapses. A perturbative reinforcement strategy similar to that described in this section, in which the overall amount of input activity arriving at the cerebellum is used as a negative reinforcement signal, has been used to train a model of the cerebellar control of the vestibulo-ocular reflex (Anastasio 2001). That learning strategy, called the input minimization algorithm, is discussed in detail in Chapter 14. Our next example in this chapter also concerns the vestibulo-oculomotor system.

7.4 Reinforcement Learning and Non-Uniform Distributed Representations

Simultaneous perturbative reinforcement learning is effective not only in two-layered but also in three-layered neural networks. Input–hidden, hidden–output, and bias weights can all be perturbed simultaneously. We will use perturbative reinforcement learning (the directed drift algorithm) in this section to show how two different input signals are distributed over the hidden units in a three-layered, feedforward neural network. Specifically, we will use perturbative reinforcement learning to reproduce the results on the formation of a non-uniform distributed representation that we obtained in Chapter 6 using back-propagation. This simulation was a simplified version of a neural network model of distributed parallel processing in the vestibulo-oculomotor system (see Chapter 6).

A generic three-layered network, with input units x_j, hidden units y_i, and output units z_k, is depicted in Figure 7.3. Input units connect to hidden units

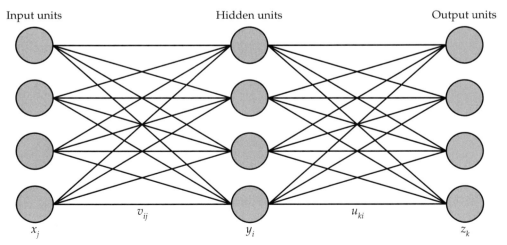

Input units   Hidden units   Output units

x_j v_{ij} y_i u_{ki} z_k

FIGURE 7.3 **A generic, three-layered feedforward neural network** Input units x_j project to hidden units y_i over connections with weights v_{ij}. Hidden units y_i then project to output units z_k over connections with weights u_{ki}. (Indices are $j = 1, \dots, n_x$, $i = 1, \dots, n_y$, and $k = 1, \dots, n_z$, where n_x, n_y, and n_z are the numbers of input, hidden, and output units, respectively.)

over input–hidden weights v_{ij}, and hidden units connect to output units over hidden–output weights u_{ki}. Note that i ($i = 1, ..., n_y$), j ($j = 1, ..., n_x$), and k ($k = 1, ..., n_z$) now index the n_y hidden, the n_x input, and the n_z output units, respectively. The y_i, which were the output units of two-layered networks, have become the hidden units in three-layered networks. We considered the same three-layered network configuration in Chapter 6 (see Figure 6.4). Script `pertDistributedRep`, listed in MATLAB Box 7.4, will use perturbative reinforcement learning to train three-layered networks of sigmoidal units to associate patterns. This script is similar to script `pertDirectedDrift`, except that it perturbs both input–hidden (matrix `V`) and hidden–output (matrix `U`) weights simultaneously.

Script `pertDistributedRep` generates two perturbation matrices with elements that vary randomly not only in sign but also in absolute value: `PertV=a*randn(nHid,nIn+1)` and `PertU=a*randn(nOut,nHid+1)`. Note that the extra column in each matrix represents built-in bias weights. The script holds both unperturbed matrices (`holdV=V` and `holdU=U`). Then it perturbs both matrices (`V=V+PertV` and `U=U+PertU`), and it restores the unperturbed matrices (`V=holdV` and `U=holdU`) if the error increases, but retains the perturbations otherwise. For convenience, the script generates random initial start matrices automatically. (This script is unlike the other scripts we have used so far in this chapter, which required that the initial weight matrices be set outside the script and available in the workspace before running the script.) The number of hidden units `nHid` is set in the script, but the numbers `nIn` and `nOut` of input and output units are determined by the script from the input and desired output pattern arrays, `InPat` and `DesOut`, which must be provided outside of the script, as usual.

The three-layered, feedforward network will have two input units and one output unit. It will be trained on the labeled-line patterns reproduced in Table 7.11. These patterns can be entered using `InPat=[0 0;1 0;0 1]` and `DesOut=[0;1;1]`. To observe the *non*-distributed (single hidden unit) representation of the two input signals, set the number of hidden units to `nHid=1`. The network reduces the error below the tolerance `tol=0.1`, and so learns the labeled-line transformation, in about 4000 iterations. The actual outputs after training, as well as the responses of the single hidden unit, are also shown in Table 7.11. The final weights are shown in Table 7.12. Like the output unit, the hidden unit responds strongly to both input units. Because the output unit responses can only be weighed versions of the responses of the single hidden unit, the hidden unit must represent both input signals equally in order to accomplish the transformation. This situation changes when the number of hidden units is increased.

We increase the number of hidden units to `nHid=50` and retrain the network on the labeled-line patterns. Perturbative reinforcement trains the net-

TABLE 7.11 Learning the simple labeled-line patterns using parallel, perturbative reinforcement

Input patterns	Desired output patterns	Actual output patterns	Hidden unit responses
0 0	0	0.06	0.08
1 0	1	0.98	0.91
0 1	1	0.98	0.90

The input, desired output, actual output, and the responses of the hidden unit following training are listed for a three-layered, feedforward network of sigmoidal units. The network has two input, one hidden, and one output unit.

MATLAB® BOX 7.4 **This script trains three-layered networks of sigmoidal units to develop a distributed representation using parallel, perturbative reinforcement learning.**

```matlab
% pertDistributedRep.m
% input InPat and desired output DesOut patterns must be supplied

nHid=50; % set number of hidden units
[nPat,nIn]=size(InPat); % determine number of input units
[nPat,nOut]=size(DesOut); % determine number of output units
Hid=zeros(nHid,nPat); % define hidden unit hold array
Out=zeros(nOut,nPat); % define output unit hold array
V=randn(nHid,nIn+1); % randomize input-hidden weights V
U=randn(nOut,nHid+1); % randomize hidden-output weights U
b=1; % set the bias
B=b*ones(nPat,1); % set up a bias vector
INb=[InPat B]'; % concatenate bias to the inputs
a=0.01; % set learning rate
tol=0.1; % set error tolerance within which training is adequate
count=0; % zero the counter
countLimit=10000; % set count limit over which training stops

Qhid=V*INb; % find weighted input sum to hidden units
Hid=1 ./(1+exp(-Qhid)); % squash to find hidden unit responses
HidB=[Hid' B]'; % concatenate bias to hidden unit responses
Qout=U*HidB; % find weighted input sum to output units
Out=1 ./(1+exp(-Qout)); % squash to find output unit responses
error=sum(sum(abs(DesOut-Out'))); % initial error over all patterns

while error > tol, % while actual error is over tolerance
    PertV=a*randn(nHid,nIn+1); % make perturbation matrix for V
    PertU=a*randn(nOut,nHid+1); % make perturbation matrix for U
    holdV=V; % hold the current input-hidden weight matrix V
    holdU=U; % hold the current hidden-output weight matrix U
    V=V+PertV; % apply perturbation to weights in V
    U=U+PertU; % apply perturbation to weights in U
    Qhid=V*INb; % find weighted input sum to hidden units
    Hid=1./(1+exp(-Qhid)); % squash to find hidden responses
    HidB=[Hid' B]'; % concatenate bias to hidden unit responses
    Qout=U*HidB; % find weighted input sum to output units
    Out=1./(1+exp(-Qout)); % squash to find output unit responses
    newErr=sum(sum(abs(DesOut-Out'))); % new error over all patterns
    if newErr>=error, % if the perturbation increases the error
        V=holdV; % then restore unperturbed weights for V
        U=holdU; % and restore unperturbed weights for U
    elseif newErr<error, % leave perturbation if it decreased error
        error=newErr; % and save new error as the error
    end % end conditional
    count=count+1; % increment the counter
    if count>countLimit, break, end % break if counter over limit
end % end training loop
```

work to reduce the error below tolerance tol=0.1 in about 1000 iterations. The network learns the transformation considerably faster with 50 than with only one hidden unit. It is generally the case that networks with greater numbers of hidden units learn faster. Because larger networks have more ways available to accomplish a given transformation, a learning algorithm requires

TABLE 7.12   Weight matrices after perturbative reinforcement training on the simple labeled-line patterns

	From input unit		From bias unit
To hidden unit	**1**	**2**	**1**
1	+4.72	+4.62	−2.50

	From hidden unit	From bias unit
To output unit	**1**	**1**
1	+8.11	−3.33

less iteration to find a workable weight configuration (but see Exercise 7.3). We will again consider the relationship between hidden unit number and speed of neural network learning in a genetic algorithm example in Chapter 13.

The main point of this example is to use perturbative reinforcement learning to produce a non-uniform distributed representation of input signals 1 and 2. That we have achieved this is illustrated in Figure 7.4, in which the responses of the single output unit, and each of the 50 hidden units, to inputs 1 and 2 are plotted against each other. The output unit (plus sign) has large and equal responses to inputs 1 and 2, as demanded by training. In contrast, the hidden units (dots) vary greatly in their responses to the two input signals. Some hidden units have roughly equal responses to the two inputs, and fall near the same diagonal (dashed) line as the output unit. Other hidden units have very strong responses to input 1 but very weak responses to input 2, or vice-versa. Most hidden units respond to both inputs in some unequal proportion. In that they combine the two inputs in a great variety of ways, the responses of the hidden units resemble the responses to vestibular (V) and pursuit (P) inputs of neurons in the vestibular nuclei (see Chapter 6 for background on these responses).

This response diversity was also reproduced in three-layered neural network models of the vestibulo-oculomotor system trained using back-propagation (see Figure 6.9). We explored a simpler version of this model in Chapter 6 (see Figure 6.6; see also Exercise 6.4). A comparison between Figures 6.6 and 7.4 suggests that perturbative reinforcement learning produces an even wider

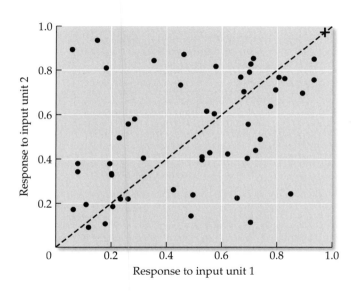

FIGURE 7.4   Simulating a non-uniform distributed representation A three-layered, feedforward neural network with two input units, one output unit, and 50 hidden units is trained on the simple labeled-line patterns using perturbative reinforcement learning (directed drift). The output (+) and the 50 hidden unit (•) responses to the two inputs are plotted against each other. Responses falling near the dashed line have roughly equal sensitivities to input units 1 and 2. Most hidden units respond to the inputs unequally, yet the network produces an output with nearly equal sensitivities.

diversity of hidden unit responses than back-propagation. Thus, not only is perturbative reinforcement learning more neurobiologically plausible than back-propagation, but it produces non-uniform distributed representations that are even more diverse and so provide a stronger match to actual data. The comparison suggests perturbative reinforcement learning as a viable alternative to back-propagation as a model of certain forms of learning in real neural systems. Although reinforcement learning is not typically applied in modeling the vestibulo-oculomotor system, it has often been employed in the context of models of associative conditioning. We will consider a reinforcement learning model of a specific type of associative conditioning in the last two sections of this chapter.

7.5 Reinforcement in a Schema Model of Avoidance Conditioning

Reinforcement approaches have been used to model data generated under a variety of experimental learning paradigms (Dayan and Balleine 2002). The most thoroughly studied form of animal learning is associative conditioning (Mackintosh 1983). In classical associative conditioning, an animal learns to form an association between two types of stimuli: the unconditioned stimulus (US) and the conditioned stimulus (CS). The unconditioned response (UR) is evoked normally by the unconditioned stimulus, but it is not normally evoked by the conditioned stimulus. Repeated pairing of the unconditioned and the conditioned stimulus will produce associative conditioning, such that the behavioral response is eventually evoked by presentation of the conditioned stimulus alone. A response evoked by a conditioned stimulus is called a conditioned response (CR). Associative conditioning was first demonstrated by Ivan Pavlov and his famous dog. Pavlov paired the presentation of meat (US) with a ringing bell (CS) to his dog. The dog normally salivated (UR) when it saw the meat. After repeated pairings of meat and bell, the dog salivated when Pavlov rang the bell (CR), even if he proffered no meat. Pavlov had conditioned the dog to associate the bell (CS) with the meat (US).

Operant conditioning is a form of learning in which a response is conditioned by reinforcement. The response is operant in the sense that it is a behavior that the animal elicits spontaneously. Repeatedly following the operant response with reinforcement will alter the frequency with which the response is elicited. The operant response will occur more or less frequently as the reinforcement that follows it provides reward or punishment, respectively. Operant conditioning was made popular by B. F. Skinner. He found that rats placed in a box with a bar will spontaneously press the bar as part of their natural, exploratory (operant) behavior. If Skinner proffered a food-pellet reward each time the rat pressed the bar, the frequency of bar-presses increased. This apparatus became known as the Skinner box.

There are many subtle differences between associative and operant conditioning, and these differences can have important implications for models of learning processes (Dayan and Balleine 2002). Yet classical and operant conditioning are similar in that both seem to involve the association between an event (such as a stimulus or a response) and anticipated rewards (or punishments). Thus, Pavlov's dog learned to associate the bell with meat. Even though Pavlov did not necessarily give the dog the meat to eat, we can assume that the presentation of meat caused the dog to anticipate reward. Skinner's rat learned to associate bar pressing with food-pellets, which we can assume are rewarding for the rat. Associations between events and punishments (negative rewards) can also be formed. As we discussed at the beginning of the chapter, we must infer that the stimuli presented by the experimenter are rewarding or punishing, since what is actually experienced as reward or punishment cannot be measured. With this caveat we can use the terms "reward" and "punishment" to describe the likely experiences of an animal.

Eye-blink conditioning has been studied extensively by Richard Thompson (Thompson and Kim 1996). In this type of conditioning, a rabbit learns to associate a tone with an air puff delivered to the eye. The air puff normally elicits an eye blink. With repeated pairing of tone and air puff, the rabbit learns to blink whenever it hears the tone. Eye-blink conditioning seems to involve a combination of classical and operant conditioning. The rabbit learns to associate the tone with the air puff (classical), and to associate the blink with avoidance of contact between the air puff and its eye (operant). The common factor in both of these aspects of eye-blink conditioning is that they are both driven by reinforcement.

The brain circuitry responsible for this behavior is schematized in Figure 7.5. The air puff (US) normally evokes an eye blink (UR) via a reflex pathway through the trigeminal nucleus of the brainstem. Auditory signals related to the tone (CS) are not sent to the trigeminal nucleus, which is primarily a somatosensory and motor structure. Thompson discovered that signals related to

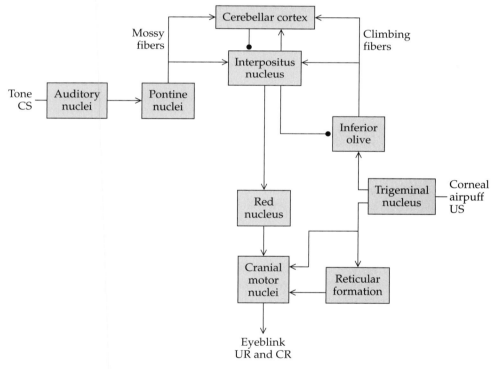

FIGURE 7.5   Schematic of the brain circuitry involved in conditioning the eye-blink response An airpuff delivered to the cornea (US) elicits an eye blink (UR) through a reflex pathway involving the trigeminal nucleus, the reticular formation, and cranial motoneurons. The corneal signal arrives at the cerebellum (cerebellar cortex and interpositus nucleus of the cerebellum) via a pathway through the inferior olive. A tone (CS) activates neurons in the auditory nuclei (also called the cochlear nuclei in mammals). The auditory signal also arrives at the cerebellum (cortex and interpositus nucleus) but along a different pathway through the pontine nuclei. Because the corneal and auditory signals meet in the cerebellum they can be associated there and, through associative conditioning, the tone can be made to elicit an eye blink (CR) via the cerebellum and red nucleus. Arrowheads and filled circles represent excitatory and inhibitory connections, respectively. (After Thompson and Kim 1996.)

FIGURE 7.6 Multiunit responses of neurons in the medial geniculate nucleus and the anterior and posterior cingulate cortex during avoidance conditioning in rabbits The neurons respond to a tone (CS) that predicts shock, and the rabbit can avoid the shock by taking a step in its walking wheel. The learning stages shown are: pre-training; training begins; first response (the rabbit begins to respond to the CS by taking a step); and trained (about 80% correct avoidance responding). The multiunit response to the tone changes very little with training in the medial geniculate nucleus of the thalamus. The multiunit activity in the posterior cingulate cortex progressively increases with training, while that in the anterior cingulate cortex increases at the beginning and then decreases. Note also that the time course of the response in the medial geniculate, which drives auditory responses in the cortex, is short in temporal duration as compared with the responses in the cingulate cortex. (After Talk et al. 2004.)

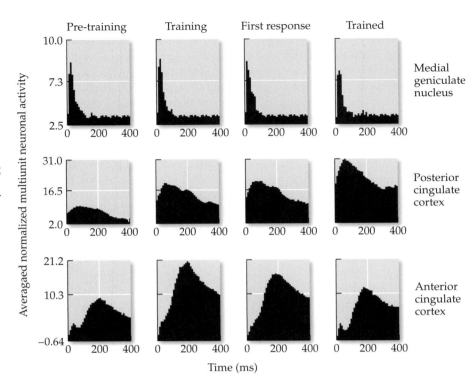

the air puff and to the tone come together in the cerebellum, specifically in the cerebellar cortex and the interpositus nucleus (one of the deep cerebellar nuclei). With conditioning, neurons in the interpositus nucleus develop increased responses to the tone and, through efferent motor pathways from the cerebellum, these responses can produce eye blink (CR). Thus, the cerebellum is the neuroanatomical substrate for associative conditioning of the eye-blink response. The example of eye blink conditioning illustrates the importance of structure for reinforcement learning in the real nervous system.

Neurophysiological studies have provided neural correlates of many types of associative conditioning, and these data can be modeled computationally using reinforcement approaches. The type of associative conditioning we will consider in this chapter is avoidance of foot shock in rabbits. This experimental paradigm also seems to involve both classical and operant conditioning. A rabbit is placed in a metal walking wheel, the floor of which can be electrified to deliver a mild electric shock to its feet. During training, the shock is preceded by a tone, and the shock is withheld if the rabbit takes a step and rotates (spins) the wheel. The rabbit soon learns to associate the tone and the shock (classical conditioning), and to spin the wheel when it hears the tone to avoid the shock (operant conditioning). We can assume that this learning is driven by reinforcement, and that avoiding the shock is rewarding to the rabbit.

Multiunit recordings reveal that neurons in regions of the limbic system, including the limbic parts of the thalamus, the amygdala, and the cingulate cortex, change their responses to the tone during the course of acquisition of the avoidance response (Gabriel 1993; Kubota et al. 1996; Talk et al. 2004). A representative sample of this multiunit data is reproduced in Figure 7.6, which compares training-induced response changes in the medial geniculate nucleus of the thalamus, and in the anterior and posterior cingulate cortex (Talk et al. 2004). Response changes in the medial geniculate are very small. In contrast, the response to the tone in the posterior cingulate increases as learning proceeds. Response increases with training are also observed in other limbic regions (Gabriel 1993), and could be related to the production of motor commands that drive or initiate the specific avoidance behavior being trained. Using single-unit rather than multiunit recording (not shown), some limbic neurons are observed to decrease their response to the tone as training proceeds (Kubota et al. 1996). Response decreases with training might be related to suppression of those motor commands that would otherwise drive behaviors that are inconsistent with the specific avoidance behavior being trained. Interestingly, the response to the tone in the anterior cingulate increases but then decreases again as training proceeds (see Figure 7.6). In this and the next section we will explore a reinforcement learning model that offers a possible explanation for this puzzling finding.

The model we will use to simulate avoidance learning is different from most of the models we employ in this book in that its elements are schemata rather than neural units. Schemata are interactive and functional elements that represent neuronal organization at a level above that of the individual neuron, and can stand for groups of neurons or whole networks (Arbib 2003). Schema theory is most readily applied in cases where the neural system under study is composed of many interacting regions whose neuron-level behavior is not known in detail. Schema theory is a modeling paradigm well suited to data sets such as that on decision-making, which involve various experimental techniques including lesioning, pharmacological manipulation, microdialysis, and functional imaging (e.g., Doya 2008). These techniques probe neural function at a level above that of individual neurons. Schema theory is also an appropriate tool with which to simulate the multiunit data on avoidance learning. These data record the changes in the responses to tones of whole groups of neurons in the limbic system during acquisition of the avoidance response.

Like a neural network, the structure of a schema-theoretic model is critical to its function, but schema-based models typically have a more complex and heterogeneous structure than neural network models. The connectivity among the schemata, their modes of interaction, and even some of the connection weights will be pre-specified in the model we will use to simulate avoidance learning. A simple version is depicted in Figure 7.7. It is based on two sche-

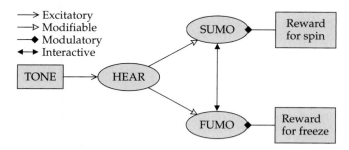

FIGURE 7.7   Simple schema theoretic model of avoidance conditioning Neural schemata are represented as ovals. Other elements are represented as rectangles. Connections can be excitatory, modifiable (and excitatory), modulatory, or signifying a competitive interaction. The connection types are indicated using different arrow styles (inset). The TONE element provides an auditory input that activates the HEAR schema. The SUMO and FUMO schemata represent upper motoneurons that can elicit wheel spinning or freezing (no spin) actions, respectively. These schemata both receive input from HEAR, and they compete with each other. The action taken (spin or freeze) is determined by whichever of SUMO or FUMO has the larger response to the tone, except that the opposite action is sometimes taken according to a fixed probability of exploration. The connections from HEAR to SUMO or FUMO are modified by reinforcement signals that depend on the rewards for spinning or freezing, respectively.

mata that represent high-level motor control neurons (or neural subsystems). Such neurons are sometimes referred to as upper motoneurons because they are situated far upstream of actual motoneurons in the nervous system. We will assume that activation of these upper motoneurons elicits, or at least facilitates, operant behavioral responses. There must be many types of operant behavioral responses in rabbits, but we will consider only two of the responses that we might expect would be made by a rabbit in a wheel. One behavioral response we will consider is stepping, or spinning of the wheel, while the other is the freezing response common to rabbits and other rodents. We will refer to the upper motoneurons that elicit the "spin" and "freeze" responses as the spin upper-motoneuron (SUMO) and the freeze upper-motoneuron (FUMO), respectively.

We will assume that both SUMO and FUMO receive auditory input and respond to the tone. We will further assume that the behavioral response of the rabbit will be determined by whichever upper-motoneuron schema has the larger response to the tone. For example, if the response of SUMO is greater than that of FUMO, then SUMO will win the competition for control of the behavioral response, and the rabbit will spin the wheel rather than freeze. However, since there is an element of randomness in behavior, we will assume that the rabbit will sometimes innovate (i.e., explore). This means that the rabbit will sometimes produce the behavior represented by the upper-motoneuron schema that loses the competition for behavioral control. Finally, we assume that the rabbit can learn to change its behavioral response to the tone by adjusting the sizes of the responses of SUMO and FUMO to the tone. We assume that this learning is driven by reinforcement signals, and that the overall rabbit model expresses reinforcement learning by acquiring a simulated version of the avoidance response. The ability of the model to simulate this form of reinforcement learning depends entirely on its structure.

The model will incorporate a HEAR schema that represents the auditory system. We will design the model so that the weights of the excitatory connections from the HEAR schema to either upper-motoneuron schema are modifiable. On each trial, the weight that is modified will be the one associated with the connection from HEAR to whichever upper motoneuron represented the behavioral response produced by the simulated rabbit. For example, if the rabbit spins the wheel, then the weight of the connection to SUMO from HEAR will be modified. The amount of this modification will be proportional to the difference between a reinforcement signal and the current weight value. Thus the weights from HEAR, and so the responses of SUMO and FUMO to the tone, will track the reinforcement associated with a spin or a freeze response, respectively.

Specifically, if the simulated rabbit spins the wheel, then the update for the weight to SUMO from HEAR, which is w_{sh}, is given by Equation 7.6:

$$w_{sh}(c+1) = w_{sh}(c) + a\left[r_s - w_{sh}(c)\right] \qquad \textbf{7.6}$$

where r_s is the reward for spinning, a is the learning rate, and c indexes the learning cycles (which correspond to learning trials). (Note that terms of the form $w(c)$ are read as "the value of weight w on update cycle c.") If the rabbit spins the wheel, then the weight to FUMO from HEAR, which is w_{fh}, would remain unchanged. However, if the rabbit freezes instead, then w_{sh} remains unchanged but w_{fh} is updated according to Equation 7.7:

$$w_{fh}(c+1) = w_{fh}(c) + a\left[r_f - w_{fh}(c)\right] \qquad \textbf{7.7}$$

where r_f is the reward for freezing. Note that in both cases (see Equations 7.6 and 7.7), weight adjustments stop (or become 0) when the value of the modifiable weight equals the value of reinforcement for either behavior. The model is designed to simulate learning of conditioned avoidance. Hopefully, the responses of the schemata during the learning process will reflect those of real neurons. To the extent that they do, the model should provide us with additional insight into the neural basis of avoidance conditioning.

Script `avoidanceLearn`, listed in MATLAB Box 7.5, simulates the avoidance learning situation and implements Equations 7.6 and 7.7. All of its variables are set within the script. The model has two phases of learning: pretraining and training. The number of learning trials in the whole training period is set in variable `nTrials`, while the number of those trials that are pre-training trials is set in variable `preTrInt`. The rewards for a spin or a freeze are held in variables `rews` and `rewf`, respectively. Shock follows the tone during the training period, but can be avoided by spinning the wheel, so the rewards for spin and freeze are 1 and 0 during training (`rews=1` and `rewf=0`). Shock does not follow the tone during pre-training. Since the rabbit would needlessly expend energy by spinning during pre-training, the rewards for spin and freeze are 0 and 1 during pre-training (`rews=0` and `rewf=1`).

MATLAB® BOX 7.5 This script simulates avoidance conditioning as reinforcement learning.

```
% avoidanceLearn.m

nTrials=2000; % set number of learning trials
preTrInt=800; % set pretraining interval
a=0.01; % set learning rate
bprob=0.005; % set baseline probability of exploration
wsh=0; % set initial modifiable weight to sumo from hear
wfh=0; % set initial modifiable weight to fumo from hear
hear=1; % set response of hear

for c=1:nTrials, % for each trial of avoidance learning
    if c<=preTrInt,      % if during pretraining interval
        rews=0; rewf=1; % set rewards for pretraining
    else                 % if during training interval
        rews=1; rewf=0; % set rewards for training
    end % end reward set conditional
    sumo=wsh*hear; % compute response of sumo
    fumo=wfh*hear; % compute response of fumo
    spin=sumo>fumo; % spin if sumo is larger than fumo
    prob=bprob; % set exploration probability to its baseline
    if prob>rand, spin=1-spin; end % explore sometimes
    sumorec(c)=sumo; % save responses of sumo
    fumorec(c)=fumo; % save responses of fumo
    spinrec(c)=spin; % save the spin actions
    if spin==1,                % if a spin was produced
        wsh=wsh+a*(rews-wsh); % update the hear-sumo weight
    else                       % if the rabbit froze instead
        wfh=wfh+a*(rewf-wfh); % update the hear-fumo weight
    end % end update conditional
end % end main training loop
```

In script `avoidanceLearn` (as in the model; see Figure 7.7) the responses of `sumo` and `fumo` are determined by their weighted inputs from `hear`. (Note that we print schema names in `monotype` when they refer to variable names in scripts, but in CAPS when they refer to model elements.) In the script, the modifiable weights to `sumo` and `fumo` from `hear` are designated as `wsh` and `wfh`, respectively. These weights are updated as `wsh=wsh+a*(rews-wsh)` and `wfh=wfh+a*(rewf-wfh)`, which implement Equations 7.6 and 7.7, respectively, with learning rate `a`. Because rewards `rews` and `rewf` take values of 0 or 1 only (`rews=0` and `rewf=1` pre-training; `rews=1` and `rewf=0` training), the values of `wsh` and `wfh` range between 0 and 1. The responses of `sumo` and `fumo` to the tone are `sumo=wsh*hear` and `fumo=wfh*hear`. The response of `hear` to the tone is simply set to 1, so the responses of `sumo` and `fumo`, reflecting the values of `wsh` and `wfh`, also range between 0 and 1. The rabbit will spin if `sumo` is greater than `fumo` (in which case `spin` equals 1), but will freeze otherwise (in which case `spin` equals 0). However, the rabbit will innovate according to the probability of exploration (`prob`), which is set to a baseline probability (`bprob`). The script uses if-then structures to evaluate the conditions under which events such as spins and weight updates should occur. The logical `spin==1`, used in the weight update conditional, returns 1 if `spin` equals 1 but returns 0 otherwise.

To get a feeling for the behavior of the model we run script `avoidanceLearn` with the parameters set as: `nTrials=2000`, `preTrInt=800`, `wsh=0`, `wfh=0`, `a=0.01`, and `bprob=0.005`. The responses of `sumo` and `fumo` on each trial, and the occurrences of spins, are stored in arrays `sumorec`, `fumorec`, and `spinrec` and are plotted in Figure 7.8. (Note that the response of `sumo` or `fumo` on each training cycle is a single scalar value, not an entire response time-course as for the data in Figure 7.6.) The avoidance behavior is acquired at the point at which the response of `sumo` exceeds that of `fumo` because, at that point, the simulated rabbit is most likely to spin the wheel in response to the tone. Specifically, if the response of `sumo` exceeds that of `fumo`, then the rabbit spins the wheel except at the low baseline probability of exploration `bprob=0.005`, at which it freezes instead. Different levels of shading in Figure 7.8 separate the pre-training from the training intervals. For the run depicted in Figure 7.8, it seems that the simulated rabbit has acquired the avoidance response after about 400 training trials.

The response of `fumo` increases during pre-training, but during training the response of `fumo` decreases while that of `sumo` increases. The changes in the responses of `sumo` and `fumo` are direct consequences of the changes in modifiable weights `wsh` and `wfh`, which in turn depend both on the reinforcements `rews` and `rewf` and on the behavior of the simulated rabbit. When the response is greater for `fumo` than for `sumo`, as during pre-training, spins are few and occur only at the low probability of exploration. The response of `fumo` increases rapidly during pre-training as weight `wfh` moves toward the pre-training freeze reward `rewf=1` with each freeze action. During training, the rewards for spins and freezes reverse. In the early training period, the response of `fumo` decreases rapidly because the reward for a freeze is now `rewf=0`, and freezes are still frequent because `fumo` is greater than `sumo`. The response of `sumo` increases during training as weight `wsh` moves toward the training spin reward `rews=1`. The `sumo` response increases very slowly during the early training period because `sumo` is still less than `fumo` and spins are infrequent. However, the `sumo` response increases rapidly in the later training period because, after avoidance behavior has been acquired, `sumo` is greater than `fumo` and spins are frequent.

Exploration is critical in the avoidance learning model. Were it not for exploration (or innovation), the simulated rabbit would never try a spin dur-

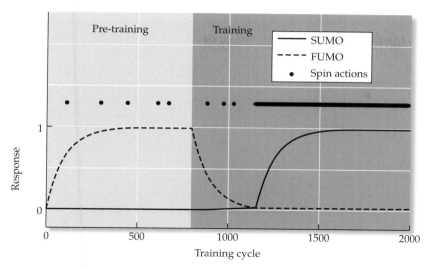

FIGURE 7.8   Simulation of avoidance conditioning The simulation is based on the schema model in Figure 7.7. The weights of the connections from HEAR to SUMO or FUMO are modifiable. The action of spin or freeze (no spin) is determined by whichever of SUMO or FUMO, respectively, has the larger response to HEAR, except that the opposite action is taken with probability of exploration of 0.005. The total number of 2000 learning cycles is divided (as indicated by shading) into 800 pre-training cycles (no shock follows the tone) and 1200 training cycles (shock follows the tone). Reinforcement (reward) for spin or freeze is, respectively, 0 or 1 during pre-training, and 1 or 0 during training. The modifiable weights onto SUMO or FUMO track the reward for spin or freeze, respectively, and their responses change accordingly. The system learns to freeze during pre-training and to spin during training, except for occasional innovations due to exploration. Solid and dashed lines illustrate the responses of SUMO and FUMO, respectively, and the dots denote spins.

ing training, and it would never discover the reward for a spin during the training period. Even worse, it would never experience an increase in weight `wsh`, so the response of `sumo` would never exceed that of `fumo` and the simulated rabbit would never acquire the avoidance response. To demonstrate the importance of exploration in the model, we increase the baseline probability of exploration to `bprob=0.05`. The responses over the course of pre-training and training of `sumo` and `fumo`, and the occurrences of spins, are plotted in Figure 7.9 (in which shading differences again separate the pre-training and training intervals). With the increased baseline exploration probability, the onset of the avoidance response has advanced up to around trial 200 of training, a doubling of the speed of acquisition.

The simulation in this section illustrates an important aspect of adaptive behavior, that which involves a trade-off between exploitation of a learned, successful behavior and exploration of other, possibly more successful behaviors. The baseline probability sets the proportion of exploration relative to exploitation in the avoidance learning simulation. While in the simulated rabbit this proportion is fixed, it is possible that the propensity of a real animal to explore is not fixed but changes with the circumstances. If the behavioral responses of an animal are successful in a particular situation, it would tend to persist in those responses. Under those circumstances, the proportion of exploration relative to exploitation is likely to be low. However, if the situation changes and the previously established behaviors are no longer appropriate, then the animal may be inclined to try different responses, even choosing among alternative responses at random. In these new circumstances the pro-

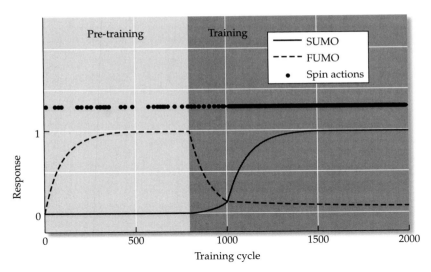

**FIGURE 7.9   Simulation of avoidance conditioning at a higher level of explora-
tion** The simulation is based on the schema model in Figure 7.7. The parameters
of the simulation are the same as those for the simulation illustrated in Figure 7.8,
except that the probability of exploration has been increased ten times, to 0.05. The
model acquires the avoidance behavior during training (darker shading) at the point
at which the response of SUMO exceeds that of FUMO. At this point the model is
most likely to produce a spin in response to the tone. Note that the number of training cycles (trials) required to reach acquisition is lower here (about 200) with the
exploration probability at 0.05, than in the previous simulation (about 400) with the
exploration probability at 0.005 (see Figure 7.8). Solid and dashed lines illustrate the
responses of SUMO and FUMO, respectively, and the dots denote spins.

portion of exploration relative to exploitation might be high. To simulate this,
we will add an additional schema type to the simulation. This schema, which
we will designate as CALL, will track the pain experienced by the rabbit and
will serve as a call to exploration in the network.

7.6 Exploration and Exploitation in a Model of Avoidance Conditioning

In this section we will extend the avoidance learning simulation by adding
a schema CALL that can increase the proportion of exploration relative to
exploitation. The extended model is depicted in Figure 7.10. Since we are interested here in simulating avoidance conditioning, we will leave out the details
concerning how a schema such as CALL could actually implement increased
exploration in a neural system. Instead, we will simply use the response of
CALL to augment the probability of exploration.

As for SUMO and FUMO, we will assume that CALL receives input from
HEAR, and the modifiable weight of this connection will be designated as w_{ch}.
To make the response of CALL track the pain experienced by the simulated
rabbit, we can update the value of w_{ch} according to Equation 7.8:

$$w_{ch}(c+1) = w_{ch}(c) + a\left[r_p - w_{ch}(c)\right] \qquad \textbf{7.8}$$

where r_p designates the state of the PAIN schema and serves as a (negative)
reinforcement signal. Equation 7.8 would update w_{ch} until it equaled r_p, but

FIGURE 7.10   Schema theoretic model of avoidance conditioning in which the probability of exploration can be augmented The model in Figure 7.7 is extended with the addition of a schema designated as CALL, the function of which is to increase the probability of exploration. This is depicted by the modulatory connection from CALL to the interactive connection between SUMO and FUMO. Like SUMO and FUMO, CALL receives a modifiable connection from the HEAR schema. The modifiable connection onto CALL is adjusted according to a reinforcement signal that depends on the pain variable, which is represented by the PAIN schema. Pain results from shock, which occurs following the tone unless the spin action is taken. The SPIN element inhibits the SHOCK element.

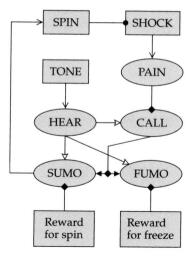

→ Excitatory
—• Inhibitory
—▷ Modifiable
—◆ Modulatory
◀—▶ Interactive

the state of PAIN will depend on the behavior of the simulated rabbit. Since the simulated rabbit should learn to avoid pain, the state of the PAIN schema should not stay constant. Therefore, the value of w_{ch}, and likewise the response of CALL, will track a moving target (changing reinforcement signal). This will have important consequences for the time course of training-induced changes in the responses of the CALL schema, as we shall see.

It is important to point out that the avoidance model weight update equations (see Equations 7.6–7.8) do track quantities that represent reinforcement signals, but they do not implement reinforcement learning by themselves. Instead, the weight update equations, as part of the overall structure of the simulated rabbit, enable that structure to accomplish reinforcement learning and to simulate acquisition of the avoidance response. As we discussed at the beginning of this chapter, reinforcement learning in the strict sense involves learning to choose actions that maximize rewards or minimize punishments (Sutton and Barto 1998; Dayan and Balleine 2002). The simulated rabbit *as a whole* accomplishes reinforcement learning in the strict sense, because it learns to minimize punishment by acquiring the avoidance response. The mechanism by which the simulated rabbit acquires the avoidance response involves the tracking of reinforcement signals (see Equations 7.6–7.8) by some of the schemata that control its behavior.

Script `avoidanceLearnCall`, listed in MATLAB Box 7.6, will implement the extended avoidance learning model that includes the `call` schema. As for `sumo` and `fumo`, the response of `call` is determined by its weighted input from `hear`. The modifiable weight is designated as `wch`. The script updates the weight to `call` from `hear` using `wch=wch+a*(pain-wch)`, which implements Equation 7.8. Note that `pain` will always be 0 during pre-training, and it will be 0 during training if the rabbit spins the wheel but will be 1 if it freezes instead. The value of `wch` therefore ranges between 0 and 1. The response of `call` is computed as `call=wch*hear`. Since `hear` is 1, the response of `call` also ranges between 0 and 1 (as do the responses of `sumo` and `fumo`). We can use `call` to augment the probability of exploration using `prob=bprob+bprob*call`. (Since `call` ranges between 0 and 1, this command will yield a valid probability value for `prob` provided `bprob` is 0.5 or less.)

Script `avoidanceLearnCall` assumes that pre-training has already occurred, so the parameter `preTrInt` is irrelevant, and the modifiable weight to `fumo` from `hear` is set at `wfh=1`. The other modifiable weights are initially set to 0: `wsh=0` and `wch=0`. The parameters are set as in the simulation without `call` (`avoidanceLearn`) except that the learning rate is `a=0.005`. The baseline probability of exploration is reset to `bprob=0.005`. Script `avoidanceLearnCall` saves the responses of `call` on each trial in array `callrec` (and also saves the responses of `sumo`, `fumo`, and the spins as in `avoidanceLearn`).

MATLAB® BOX 7.6   This script simulates avoidance conditioning as reinforcement learning with automatic adjustment of exploration.

```
% avoidanceLearnCall.m

nTrials=2000; % set number of learning trials
a=0.005; % set learning rate
bprob=0.005; % set baseline probability of exploration
wsh=0; % set initial modifiable weight to sumo from hear
wfh=1; % set initial modifiable weight to fumo from hear
wch=0; % set initial modifiable weight to call from hear
hear=1; % set response of hear

for c=1:nTrials, % for each trial of avoidance learning
    if c<=nTrials/10,   % if during pretraining interval
        rews=0; rewf=1; % set rewards for pretraining
    else                % if during training interval
        rews=1; rewf=0; % set rewards for training
    end % end reward set conditional
    call=wch*hear; % compute response of call
    sumo=wsh*hear; % compute response of sumo
    fumo=wfh*hear; % compute response of fumo
    spin=sumo>fumo; % spin if sumo is larger than fumo
    prob=bprob+bprob*call; % compute probability of exploration
    if prob>rand, spin=1-spin; end % explore sometimes
    callrec(c)=call; % save responses of call
    sumorec(c)=sumo; % save responses of sumo
    fumorec(c)=fumo; % save responses of fumo
    spinrec(c)=spin; % save the spin actions
    if c<=nTrials/10,                 % if pretraining
        pain=0;                       % no pain is delivered
    elseif c>nTrials/10 & spin==1,    % if spin during training
        pain=0;                       % pain is avoided
    elseif c>nTrials/10 & spin==0,    % if no spin during training
        pain=1;                       % pain is not avoided
    end % end pain conditional
    wch=wch+a*(pain-wch); % update the hear-call weight
    if spin==1,                       % if a spin was produced
        wsh=wsh+a*(rews-wsh);         % update the hear-sumo weight
    else                              % if the rabbit froze instead
        wfh=wfh+a*(rewf-wfh);         % update the hear-fumo weight
    end % end update conditional
end % end main training loop
```

Following the simulation the responses of SUMO, FUMO, and CALL, and the spin occurrences are plotted in Figure 7.11. It seems that the simulated rabbit has acquired the avoidance response (the point at which the response of SUMO exceeds that of FUMO) after about 700 training trials (the first 200 trails are pre-training). The responses of SUMO and FUMO respectively increase and decrease during training, as before. The responses of CALL increase and then decrease again during training. These changes in response are due to changes in the modifiable weights, which are due, in turn, to the reinforcement signals and the behavior of the simulated rabbit.

During simulated avoidance conditioning, the responses of SUMO, FUMO, and CALL, reflecting their input weights from HEAR, track their associated reinforcement signals. The rewards for spin and freeze, which are tracked by SUMO and FUMO, are 1 and 0 during training. The CALL schema tracks pain, which is 1 during training, unless the rabbit spins. In the early training period FUMO exceeds SUMO and, since the CALL response is small early on, the rabbit explores (and spins) rarely, freezes mostly, and experiences pain. Thus, FUMO rapidly decreases and CALL rapidly increases. The increase in CALL causes an increase in exploration. With a larger CALL response the rabbit will explore more often, and the frequency of spins will increase even though FUMO still exceeds SUMO. Thus the response of SUMO will slowly increase. After SUMO exceeds FUMO the rabbit will mostly spin. The response of SUMO then increases rapidly, but the avoidance of pain will cause the response of CALL to decrease again. After avoidance behavior is acquired, the call to exploration provided by CALL is no longer needed. The changes in the responses of SUMO, FUMO, and CALL over the course of simulated avoidance learning can be compared with those of real neurons.

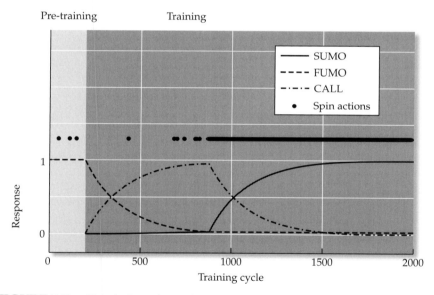

FIGURE 7.11   Simulation of avoidance conditioning with an adjustable probability of exploration The simulation is based on the model in Figure 7.10. The HEAR schema excites SUMO and FUMO, as before, and also excites the CALL schema, which increases the probability of exploration (innovation) in the model. The modifiable weight from HEAR to CALL tracks PAIN which, during training, is 0 if the tone is followed by a spin and 1 if it is not. The action of spin or freeze (no spin) is determined predominantly by whichever of SUMO or FUMO, respectively, has the larger response. Schema SUMO has the larger response after the point of acquisition of the avoidance behavior, at about 700 training cycles (trials). Note that the first 200 cycles shown here represent the end of a pre-training interval, as indicated by lighter shading. The response of CALL increases before avoidance acquisition, because pain is usually experienced, and decreases again after acquisition, because pain is usually avoided. Solid, dashed, and dot-dashed lines illustrate the responses of SUMO, FUMO, and CALL, respectively, and the dots denote spins.

Real neurons in the limbic system show changes in the sizes of their responses to the tone during the acquisition of avoidance behavior in rabbits, but these changes vary among neurons in different regions (Gabriel 1993; Kubota et al. 1996; Talk et al. 2004). Some neurons progressively increase their responses during training. This training-induced progression is exemplified by the posterior cingulate cortex multiunit recording in Figure 7.6 and simulated by SUMO in the model. Other neurons progressively decrease their responses during training (not shown), and this progression is simulated by FUMO. Arguably the most interesting limbic neurons increase but then decrease their responses. This training-induced progression is exemplified by the anterior cingulate cortex multiunit recording in Figure 7.6 and simulated by CALL in the model.

The correspondence between the simulated and experimental results suggests that the role of the anterior cingulate is to increase exploratory behavior by increasing the probability that the real rabbit will explore behavioral alternatives rather than exploit the previously most well adapted behavior. This suggestion is supported by studies in monkeys showing that the activity of neurons in the anterior cingulate cortex is associated with shifts between exploration and exploitation in tasks in which the need to search for new strategies alternates with periods of success of previously adapted strategies (Procyk et al. 2000; Quilodran et al. 2008).

The simple schema-theoretic simulation captures salient aspects of the neural basis of avoidance conditioning. It suggests that avoidance conditioning could be driven by reinforcement associated with the outcomes of actions taken by an animal in the learning situation. It also suggests that neurons that increase and then decrease their responses as the avoidance behavior is acquired may be promoting exploration of alternative and potentially more appropriate actions. By further analogy with the model, we would not view the neurons by themselves as implementing reinforcement learning. Instead, we would see them as components of a larger system of multiple neural structures that mediates the acquisition of avoidance conditioning by the rabbit. This conditioning conforms to reinforcement learning in the strict sense, because the rabbit learns to reduce the amount of pain (foot shock) it experiences. Predictions can be derived from the model by removing individual schemata, thereby simulating the effects of lesions of specific brain regions. A post-diction from the model, in which a simulated lesion can explain a known finding, is the subject of Exercise 7.4.

Another very intriguing aspect of the data in Figure 7.6 is the long duration of the auditory responses of the neurons in the anterior and posterior cingulate cortex. Neurons in cortex receive their auditory input from the medial geniculate nucleus of the thalamus, but the response duration of medial geniculate neurons is much shorter than that of the cingulate cortex neurons (Talk et al. 2004). The responses in cingulate cortex endure from the time of the tone right up until the time at which the animal initiates an action in response to the tone (about one second). It is as though the cingulate cortex maintains its sensory responses long enough for them to be related with reinforcement from the environment concerning the outcomes of the behavioral responses of the rabbit. The long duration responses may overcome the delay inherent in this type of reinforcement learning. In Chapter 2 we saw how positive feedback mechanisms can prolong sensory responses. We have suppressed this and other details of neural mechanism in our schema-based model. Specifically, the responses on each trial of the schemata in the model are scalars (single numbers), not whole response time-courses (as in Figure 7.6). Yet the response properties of real neurons often have functional significance. Response prolongation occurs in many parts of the real brain and could occur in the cingulate cortex and other parts of the limbic system for the purposes of reinforcement learning.

As we discussed at the beginning of the chapter, one of the challenges of reinforcement learning is managing delayed reinforcement. In Chapter 11 we will study a general mechanism for learning despite temporal disparities between events (including sensory cues) and reinforcement. The particular case of avoidance learning that we studied in this chapter may reveal a specific mechanism for managing delay. In avoidance conditioning to an auditory cue, the delay between the sensory input (tone) and the reinforcement is bridged by the prolonged auditory responses of neurons in the limbic system (see Figure 7.6). Combined with the possibility suggested by the model, that the anterior cingulate may adjust the level of exploration in a learning situation, it seems that the limbic system may be designed to meet two of the major challenges of reinforcement learning: the trade-off between exploitation and exploration, and the delay of reinforcement. This possibility, like all of the possibilities suggested by the models in this book, is a hypothesis that requires experimental validation.

Exercises

7.1 In `pertGradientParallel` and `pertDirectedDrift` (see MATLAB Boxes 7.2 and 7.3, respectively), all of the weights are perturbed simultaneously, and the individual perturbations can have different signs but they all have the same absolute value. Try each algorithm using completely random perturbations in which individual perturbations can vary both in sign and in absolute value. To do this in `pertGradientParallel`, replace the first command of the while loop `Pert=pSize*sign(randn(nOut,nIn))` with the command `Pert=pSize*randn(nOut,nIn)`. To make it easier, use the non-overlapping (labeled-line) patterns. Does it work? To try it in `pertDirectedDrift`, replace the first command of the while loop `Pert=a*sign(randn(nOut,nIn))` with `Pert=a*randn(nOut,nIn)`. Do you get better performance with purely random, parallel perturbations using the gradient estimation or the directed drift algorithm? Which algorithm seems more robust?

7.2 In script `pertDirectedDrift` (see MATLAB Box 7.3) all of the weights in `V` are perturbed simultaneously. Try this algorithm using one-weight-at-a-time perturbation. To make it easier, use the non-overlapping (labeled-line) patterns. To do perturbative reinforcement one-weight-at-a-time, replace the matrix perturbation commands with single weight perturbation commands. To generate a single weight perturbation use `pert=a*sign(randn)`. Choose the index of one weight at random (for a network with one output unit) using `vChoose=ceil(nIn*rand)`. Hold this value in `vHold=V(vChoose)` and perturb it using `V(vChoose)=vHold+pert`. Evaluate the effect of this single perturbation as for the parallel perturbations. If performance does not improve, as when `newer>=error` is true, then restore the unperturbed weight using `V(vChoose)=vHold`. Which method, one at a time or all weights simultaneously, learns faster? Which seems the more neurobiologically plausible?

7.3 We used perturbative reinforcement learning to train a three-layered, feedforward neural network on a simple labeled-line task. We found that the network could accomplish this task with only one hidden unit. When it had 50 hidden units, the network also accomplished the task and created a non-uniform distributed representation of the inputs resembling that observed in many real neural systems (as discussed in Chapter 6). We also saw that the network with 50 hidden units seemed to learn the task in fewer iterations than the network with only one hidden unit. Do a test specifically to examine the effects of hidden unit number. Run `pertDistributedRep` (see MATLAB Box 7.4) ten times each for networks with 10, 100, and 1000 hidden units. It might be convenient to comment out the statement that sets `nHid` in the script so you can set it in another script that calls `pertDistributedRep`. Does the network, on average, learn in fewer iterations when it has more hidden units? Is learning with many hidden units reliable? Does there appear to be a trade-off between speed and trainability associated with number of hidden units?

7.4 Using script `avoidanceLearnCall` (see MATLAB Box 7.6) we simulated the effects of a hypothetical neural type (`call`) that increased the probability of exploration in the presence of negative reinforcement (`pain`). Lesioning of certain regions of the limbic system, such as the anterior cingulate, can delay but not prevent avoidance learning (Gabriel 1993). To explore this in the model, "lesion" the `call` unit by replacing the command `call=wch*hear)*hear` with `call=0` in script `avoidanceLearnCall`. What happens? Does the model still simulate avoidance learning? Is the time altered for the onset of the avoidance response?

References

Alspector J, Meir R, Yuhas B, Jayakumar A, Lippe D (1993) A parallel gradient descent method for learning in analog VLSI neural networks. In: Hanson SJ, Cowan JD, Giles CL (eds) *Advances in Neural and Information Processing Systems 5*. Morgan Kaufmann, San Francisco, pp 836–844.

Anastasio TJ (2001) Input minimization: A model of cerebellar learning without climbing fiber error signals. *NeuroReport* 12: 3825–3831.

Arbib MA (2003) Schema theory. In: Abrib MA (ed) *The Handbook of Brain Theory and Neural Networks. Second Edition*. MIT Press, Cambridge, MA, pp 993–998.

Caporale N, Dan Y (2008) Spike timing-dependent plasticity: A Hebbian learning rule. *Annual Review of Neuroscience* 31: 25–46.

Dayan P, Balleine BW (2002) Reward, motivation, and reinforcement learning. *Neuron* 36: 285–298.

Doya K (2008) Modulators of decision making. *Nature Neuroscience* 11: 410–416.

Gabriel M (1993) Discriminative avoidance learning: A model system. In: Vogt BA, Gabriel M (eds) *Neurobiology of the Cingulate Cortex and Limbic Thalamus: A Comprehensive Handbook*. Birkhäuser, Boston, pp 478–523.

Kostal L, Lansky P, Rospars JP (2007) Neuronal coding and spiking randomness. *European Journal of Neuroscience* 26: 2693–2701.

Kubota Y, Wolske M, Poremba A, Gabriel M (1996) Stimulus-related and movement-related single-unit activity in rabbit cingulate cortex and limbic thalamus during performance of discriminative avoidance behavior. *Brain Research* 72: 22–38.

Mackintosh NJ (1983) *Conditioning and Associative Learning*. Clarendon Press, Oxford.

McClelland JL, Rumelhart DE (1989) *Explorations in Parallel Distributed Processing: A Handbook of Models, Programs, and Exercises*. MIT Press, Cambridge, MA, pp 83–159.

Milner PM (1970) *Physiological Psychology*. Holt, Rinehart and Winston, New York, pp 378–412.

Olds J, Milner P (1954) Positive reinforcement produced by electrical stimulation of septal area and other regions of rat brain. *Journal of Comparative and Physiological Psychology* 47: 419–427.

Orchard GA, Phillips WA (1991) *Neural Computation: A Beginner's Guide*. Lawrence Erlbaum, London, pp 63–91.

Procyk E, Tanaka YL, Joseph JP (2000) Anterior cingulate activity during routine and non-routine sequential behaviors in macaques. *Nature Neuroscience* 3: 502–508.

Quilodran R, Rothé M, Procyk E (2008) Behavioral shifts and action valuation in the anterior cingulate cortex. *Neuron* 7: 314–325.

Robbins TW, Everitt BJ (1996) Neurobehavioral mechanisms of reward and motivation. *Current Opinion in Neurobiology* 6: 228–236.

Robbins TW, Everitt BJ (2003) Motivaiton and reward. In: Squire LR, Bloom FE, McConnell SK, Roberts JL, Spitzer NC, Zigmond MJ (eds) *Fundamental Neuroscience. Second Edition*. Academic Press, Orlando, FL, pp 1109–1126.

Rumelhart DE, Hinton GE, Williams RJ (1986) Learning internal representations by error propagation. In: Rumelhart DE, McClelland JL, PDP Research Group (eds) *Parallel Distributed Processing: Explorations in the Microstructure of Cognition, Vol 1: Foundations*. MIT Press, Cambridge, MA, pp 318–362.

Schultz W (2007) Multiple dopamine functions at different time courses. *Annual Review of Neuroscience* 30: 259–288.

Sutton RS, Barto AG (1998) *Reinforcement Learning: An Introduction*. MIT Press, Cambridge, MA.

Talk A, Kashef A, Gabriel M (2004) Effects of conditioning during amygdalar inactivation on training-induced neuronal plasticity in the medial geniculate nucleus and cingulate cortex in rabbits (*Oryctolagus cuniculus*). *Behavioral Neuroscience* 118: 944–955.

Thompson RF, Kim JJ (1996) Memory systems in the brain and localization of memory. *Proceedings of the National Academy of Sciences* 93: 13438–13444.

Venkatesh SS (1993) Directed drift: A new linear threshold algorithm for learning binary weights on-line. *Journal of Computer and Systems Science* 46: 198–217.

8

Information Transmission and Unsupervised Learning

Unsupervised learning algorithms can train neural networks to increase the amount of information they contain about their inputs and simulate the properties of sensory neurons

In order for the brain to process information it must first "contain" information. We will define information content precisely in the next section, but even without a precise definition it would seem that neural systems in general, and sensory systems in particular, would need to acquire and, in some sense, contain information about the world in order to make that information available for further processing. Work at the interface between theoretical and experimental neuroscience suggests that sensory systems do indeed acquire and contain information about the world. Neural network learning algorithms have been developed that train output units to increase the amount of information they contain about their inputs. In so doing, these algorithms cause the output units to adopt response properties that closely resemble those of real sensory neurons. In this chapter we will explore simple neural networks that learn to increase the amount of information that is transmitted from their input units and contained by their output units.

As we discussed at length in Chapter 5, neurons in real sensory systems are often organized as maps in which neurons that respond to similar input features are located near each other in the map. Neural network learning algorithms that explicitly train output units to maximize the information they contain about their inputs, and cause their output units to adopt realistic response properties, do not generally also form maps. In contrast, the self-organizing map algorithm (and similar map-forming Hebbian schemes), which were not designed explicitly to maximize information, can actually increase the amount of information transmitted from input to output in a network. Simulations show that information transmission can be increased independently of map formation in neural networks trained using the self-organizing map algorithm on orthogonal (non-overlapping) input patterns, which preclude map formation. Together these modeling results suggest that map formation in the brain may be incidental, and may emerge out of the need for information acquisition by neural networks. In this chapter we will demonstrate that unsupervised learning algorithms can increase the amount of information that a neural network acquires from its inputs and contains in its outputs, regardless of whether or not a map is formed.

Although the brain must contain information in order to process information, more information content is not necessarily better. Clearly, a small amount of useful information is of greater behavioral relevance to an organism than a large amount of useless information. The distinction between useful and useless information depends on the "meaning" of the information to the organism. An example from everyday life illustrates the difference between the amount and the meaning of information.

Suppose that your brother wakes up every morning and eats a bowl of cornflakes. Then on any given morning, the event that your brother eats a bowl of cornflakes is not very informative, because you knew beforehand that he would most likely get up and eat a bowl of cornflakes. Consider instead the event that your brother finds $1000 in his morning bowl of cornflakes. This event contains a lot of information, because the occurrence of this event was very unlikely. This event is also meaningful because the receipt of $1000 is quite relevant for your brother, especially considering his questionable financial circumstances.

Now consider the event that, on a particular morning, your brother has in his breakfast bowl a cornflake in the shape of the state of Illinois. The occurrence of a cornflake of exactly that shape is highly unlikely, so this event also contains a lot of information. However, the event is meaningless, because your brother will just drown this special cornflake in milk and gobble it up, along with all the other cornflakes in his bowl. This example shows that the amount of information conveyed by an event can be large but the information itself can be meaningless.

There is an important technical difference between information and meaning. Information, as we will see in the next section, can be precisely defined and objectively quantified in terms of the probabilities associated with events. While meaning can also be precisely defined and quantified, it is entirely a matter of the goals and objectives of the user of the information. For your brother, with his particular set of goals and objectives, the event that he acquired a cornflake in the shape of the state of Illinois was meaningless because he just gobbled it up anyway. That this event would be meaningful given a different set of goals and objectives is proven by the fact that someone actually sold a cornflake in the shape of the state of Illinois for more than $1000 over the Internet. Apparently, another enterprising individual sold over the Internet a potato chip in the shape of the state of Florida.

In this chapter we will not only quantify the amount of information that a neural network can transmit from its input to its output, but will also quantify the meaning of that information in terms of the operational objectives of the neural system that the network is meant to simulate. We will explore the consequences of background activity, which is ubiquitous in the brain, on self-organization and show how map-forming algorithms can increase information transmission despite high background levels. Before we begin our simulations we will review some basic concepts in information theory (for in-depth treatments see Cover and Thomas 1991; Applebaum 1996).

8.1   Some Basic Concepts in Information Theory

The concept of information is closely related to the concept of probability (Applebaum 1996). Stated informally, the occurrence of an event contains information, but the occurrence of an improbable event contains more information than the occurrence of a probable event. Consider an input X that has only two possible states, $X = 0$ and $X = 1$. Imagine that we can observe the input, and over repeated observations we note that X takes state 0 or state 1 seemingly at random. Thus, we can describe X as a (binary) random variable, and we can quantify its behavior by assigning probabilities to the states of X, denoted $P(X = x)$, where P is probability and x is some particular value of the state of X. In words, the expression $P(X = x)$ is the probability that random variable X takes specific value x. The probability $P(X = x)$ can take any value in the range $0 \leq P(X = x) \leq 1$, and the sum of the probabilities of all possible states of a random variable must sum to 1. For example, if binary random variable X is in state 0 for 50% of the time and in state 1 for the other 50% of the time, then $P(X = 0) = 0.5$ and $P(X = 1) = 0.5$, and $P(X = 0) + P(X = 1) = 1$. Furthermore, we can say that $[P(X = 0) = 0.5, P(X = 1) = 0.5]$ is the (discrete) probability distribution for binary random variable X.

Given the probabilities associated with the states of X, the information content of the event that X takes one of its specific states can be quantified. The information content of the generic event that $X = x$ can be quantified in units of bits using Equation 8.1 (Cover and Thomas 1991; Applebaum 1996):

8.1
$$I(X = x) = -\log_2 P(X = x)$$

where $\log_2$ is log to the base 2 (if $x = 2^y$ then $y = \log_2 x$). For the simple probability distribution we defined above, in which $P(X = 1) = 0.5$, the event that $X = 1$ contains $-\log_2(0.5) = 1$ bit of information. Thus, 1 bit is the amount of information contained in a 50-50 occurrence, like the flip of a fair coin. Now imagine that the input is in state 1 only 25% of the time. Then $P(X = 1) = 0.25$, and the event that $X = 1$ now contains 2 bits of information. The less probable event contains more information. Taking it to an extreme, imagine the input is in state 1 for 0% of the time, so that $P(X = 1) = 0$. Then the impossible event that $X = 1$ would carry infinite information. At the other extreme, imagine that the input is in state 1 for 100% of the time, so that $P(X = 1) = 1$. The now inevitable event that $X = 1$ contains 0 information, because it was already certain that X would be in state 1. Thus, the more certainty that is associated with an event, the less information it contains.

The uncertainty of a random variable X (also called its entropy) is the average of its information content. It is defined in Equation 8.2:

$$H(X) = -\sum_{X} P(X = x)\log_2 P(X = x)$$
8.2

where, by definition, $P(X = x) \log_2 P(X = x) = 0$ when $P(X = x) = 0$. The summation is over all possible states of X. In general, X can be a single variable or a vector, and it can have any number of discrete states. In our simple case, X

is a single binary random variable, so it has only two states, and Equation 8.2 can be written out in full as in Equation 8.3:

$$H(X) = -P(X = 1)\log_2 P(X = 1) - P(X = 0)\log_2 P(X = 0) \qquad \textbf{8.3}$$

Equation 8.3 can be evaluated for different probability distributions for binary variable X. When $P(X = 1) = 1$ and $P(X = 0) = 0$, then $H(X) = 0$ bits. Likewise, $H(X) = 0$ bits when $P(X = 1) = 0$ and $P(X = 0) = 1$. When $P(X = 1) = 0.25$ and $P(X = 0) = 0.75$, then $H(X) = 0.81$ bits. When $P(X = 1) = 0.5$ and $P(X = 0) = 0.5$, then $H(X) = 1$ bit. The binary random variable X reaches its maximal uncertainty (1 bit) when both of its states are equally probable. It may seem strange that the average information content of a random variable is the same as its uncertainty. This relationship can be understood by realizing that "uncertainty represents 'potential information' in the sense that when a random variable takes on a value we gain information and lose uncertainty" (Applebaum 1996).

When measured in bits, another way of thinking about the uncertainty (entropy) of a random variable is in terms of the number of yes/no questions required to know its state. If you want to know the state of a single binary random variable X when both states are equally probable [$P(X = 1) = 0.5$, $P(X = 0) = 0.5$], then all you need is one question: Is the state 1? (Or equivalently: Is the state 0?) So the binary random variable with probability distribution [$P(X = 1) = 0.5$, $P(X = 0) = 0.5$] has uncertainty of 1 bit, and this is maximal. If the variable is always in state 1, so that [$P(X = 1) = 1$, $P(X = 0) = 0$], then you know the state of the variable without asking. Thus, the binary random variable with distribution [$P(X = 1) = 1$, $P(X = 0) = 0$] (and similarly [$P(X = 1) = 0$, $P(X = 0) = 1$]) has the minimal uncertainty of 0 bits. For binary random variables with uncertainty between maximal (1 bit) and minimal (0 bits), you would need, on average, between zero questions and one question to know its state.

To take another example from everyday life, we can ask how many questions, on average, it takes to guess the value of an integer chosen uniformly at random from the range between 1 and 100. Now X is a uniformly distributed random variable with $n = 100$ states x, and all are equally probably so that $P(X = x) = 1/n$. By applying Equation 8.2 to the uniformly distributed random variable we have the relationships shown in Equation 8.4:

$$H(X) = -\sum_X P(X = x)\log_2 P(X = x) = -n(1/n)\log_2(1/n) = \log_2(n) \qquad \textbf{8.4}$$

Since $\log_2(100)$ is between $\log_2(64)$ and $\log_2(128)$, we know even without a calculator that it should take between six and seven questions, on average, to guess an integer chosen uniformly at random in the range from 1 to 100. With a little more precision, for a uniformly distributed random variable with 100 states, $H(X) \cong 6.64$ bits.

In applying ideas from information theory to neural systems, it is useful to consider the states of the input units as random variables and, in the simplest case, as binary random variables. Consider a neural network, such as the two-layered feedforward network in Figure 8.1, which has two input units, x_1 and x_2. If they are both binary, then the input layer of the network has four states: $(x_1 = 0, x_2 = 0)$, $(x_1 = 1, x_2 = 0)$, $(x_1 = 0, x_2 = 1)$, and $(x_1 = 1, x_2 = 1)$. The random variables representing the two input units are X_1 and X_2. If we assume that both random input variables are distributed with maximal entropy, then $P(X_1 = 1) = P(X_1 = 0) = P(X_2 = 1) = P(X_2 = 0) = 0.5$. If the two random variables are statistically independent of one another, then their joint probability (considered again later in this section) is just the product of their individual probabilities. In the maximum entropy case, the joint probability of any state of the two-unit input layer is $P(X_1 = x_1, X_2 = x_2) = P(X_1 = x_1)P(X_2 = x_2) = (0.5)(0.5) = 0.25$. Thus, all four states of the input layer in this case have probability

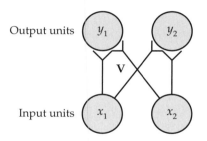

Output units y_1 y_2

V

Input units x_1 x_2

FIGURE 8.1   Two-input/two-output, feedforward network   Units are binary, threshold elements. Input units x_1 and x_2 project to output units y_1 and y_2 over weights in matrix **V**, which has elements v_{ij} that connect x_j to y_i ($i = 1, 2$ and $j = 1, 2$).

0.25. Applying Equation 8.2, we find that $H(X_1, X_2) = -4[P(X_1 = x_1, X_2 = x_2)$ $\log_2 P(X_1 = x_1, X_2 = x_2)] = -4[0.25 \log_2(0.25)] = 2$ bits. The result that (X_1, X_2) is a 2-bit input makes intuitive sense. Since both inputs are maximally uncertain, we would need one question to know the state of X_1, and another question to know the state of X_2.

In this chapter it will be more convenient to refer to the states of the input layer as a whole, rather than refer to the states of individual units. Henceforth, we will use random variable X to represent the states of the input layer as a whole. If the input layer is composed of two input units whose states are random variables X_1 and X_2, then $X = (X_1, X_2)$ and a particular value of X would be $x = (x_1, x_2)$. For the network with two binary units, the four states of X are just as we listed them in the previous paragraph [$(x_1 = 0, x_2 = 0)$, $(x_1 = 1, x_2 = 0)$, $(x_1 = 0, x_2 = 1)$, and $(x_1 = 1, x_2 = 1)$], and $H(X) = H(X_1, X_2)$. As for the input layer, we can use random variable Y (with particular values y) to represent the states of the output layer as a whole, no matter how many units compose the output layer or how may discrete states each unit may have. The issue then becomes how much of the input information $H(X)$ is contained by the outputs with information $H(Y)$. That issue is the main concern of this chapter.

Of central importance in the study of neural systems is the extent to which the responses of the output neurons in a network represent the information contained in its input. Representation of input information is a necessary prerequisite for information processing, and it is an essential task in itself. A critically important job for the sensory systems is to increase the amount of information available to the brain concerning the external environment. Stated differently, the responses of the sensory systems should decrease the uncertainty (entropy) of the brain regarding the stimuli that evoke those responses. The amount by which one random variable, such as output Y, can reduce the uncertainty associated with another random variable, such as input X, is measured by the conditional entropy as shown in Equation 8.5:

$$H(X \mid Y) = -\sum_Y P(Y) \sum_X P(X \mid Y) \log_2 P(X \mid Y)$$

8.5

In this equation we employ a shorthand in which X can stand for $X = x$ and Y can stand for $Y = y$ in probability expressions. By this shorthand $P(X)$ and $P(X = x)$ both denote the probability that $X = x$. This shorthand does not apply to the informational measures we use, such as $H(X)$, which is the average information content over all states of a random variable X. Because writing $X = x$ and $Y = y$ can be cumbersome for long expressions we will switch back and forth between the long and short forms for probability expressions.

The conditional entropy $H(X \mid Y)$, defined in Equation 8.5, measures the average uncertainty remaining about the state of X after the state of Y is known. It is possible that Y contains complete information about X, in which case $H(X \mid Y) = 0$. It is also possible that Y contains no information about X, in which case $H(X \mid Y) = H(X)$. The ability of Y to contain information about X depends, in part, on the number of states that Y has available to encode the states of X. Obviously, Y cannot contain complete information about X if Y has fewer states than X. In a real neural system, the number of available states of the output depends on the number of neurons in the network, and on the number of distinguishable (by the brain) states of each neuron. While the former is measurable using neuroanatomical techniques, the latter is more elusive and is still a matter of debate in neuroscience.

The ability of Y to contain information about X also depends on how the states of Y depend statistically on the states of X. This dependency is described by the conditional probability of Y given X. The conditional probability $P(Y = y \mid X = x)$ is the probability of observing some $Y = y$ given that $X = x$. If Y is independent of X, then $P(Y \mid X) = P(Y)$. The dependence (or independence) of two random variables works both ways. If Y is independent of X, then X is independent of Y, and $P(X \mid Y) = P(X)$, so that knowing Y tells us nothing about X. If Y is independent of X, then Y contains no information about X, and Y cannot decrease our uncertainty about X, so that $H(X \mid Y) = H(X)$. Conversely, if Y depends on X, then Y does contain information about X so that Y does tell us something about X. If Y depends on X then we gain information about X by knowing Y. This implies that Y can decrease our uncertainty about X so that $H(X \mid Y) < H(X)$. Thus, information gain is equivalent to a reduction in uncertainty.

The amount of information gained about X due to Y can be quantified as a reduction in uncertainty as in Equation 8.6:

$$I(X;Y) = H(X) - H(X \mid Y) \qquad \textbf{8.6}$$

The information gain $I(X;Y)$ is also called the mutual information between X and Y. The mutual information $I(X;Y)$ is the information that X and Y share, so $I(X;Y) = I(Y;X)$. Consider, for example, the output responses Y of a simple, two-layered, feedforward neural network that receives input X (such as in Figure 8.1). By the mutual information $I(X;Y)$, the output response Y provides information concerning input X. But mutual information implies a two-way relationship. By the same mutual information $I(X;Y)$, which equals $I(Y;X)$, the input X contains as much information about Y as Y contains about X. Thus, mutual information is symmetric, even though the operation of a feedforward neural network is not.

The mutual information $I(X;Y)$ can be computed using Equation 8.6 from the entropy $H(X)$ and the conditional entropy $H(X \mid Y)$. Another way to compute $I(X;Y)$, which is often more convenient when studying neural systems, makes use of the relationship between the statistical dependence of two random variables and the information they provide about each other. To use this measure we employ the joint probability $P(X = x, Y = y)$, which is the probability that $X = x$ *and* $Y = y$. The joint probability and the conditional probability are related through the definition of conditional probability (Equation 8.7):

$$P(X,Y) = P(X \mid Y)P(Y) = P(Y \mid X)P(X) = P(Y,X) \qquad \textbf{8.7}$$

If X and Y are independent, then $P(X \mid Y) = P(X)$, and $P(X,Y) = P(X)\,P(Y)$. It follows that if X and Y are independent, then for any specific values x and y the logarithm of the ratio $P(X = x, Y = y) / P(X = x)\,P(Y = y)$ is 0. However, if X and Y are dependent, then the log of this ratio takes nonzero values. Taking the average of this quantity is another way to compute mutual information:

$$I(X;Y) = \sum_X \sum_Y P(X,Y) \log_2 \left(\frac{P(X,Y)}{P(X)P(Y)} \right) \qquad \textbf{8.8}$$

Equations 8.6 and 8.8 compute the same measure, but Equation 8.8 requires knowledge only of the joint probability distribution for variables X and Y. Equation 8.8 is convenient for our purposes, because it is often straightforward to determine the joint distribution for models of neural systems. We will use the concepts of entropy and mutual information to study information transmission in simple, two-layered feedforward neural network models, by first determining the joint probability distribution of the inputs to the network and the responses of the output units.

8.2 Measuring Information Transmission through a Neural Network

In our first example we will evaluate the ability of the two-input/two-output (2-by-2) feedforward network shown in Figure 8.1 to extract information from its inputs by computing the mutual information between inputs and outputs. The inputs x_1 and x_2 are binary, for simplicity. The outputs y_1 and y_2 are simple summing units with a threshold, so they also have binary states. The output unit states depend deterministically on the inputs, and this affords a simplification in computing the mutual information between inputs and outputs (see below in this section and also Section 8.3). In that they are deterministic, the output units are like the units we have used in previous chapters. Unlike the networks in previous chapters, the input units will be stochastic (i.e., their states will be random variables).

If we want the output units to contain as much information as possible concerning the inputs, we might suppose that we should connect both input units to both output units with strong connection weights. We can set up the network, find its responses to all possible inputs, and compute the mutual information between the inputs and outputs to evaluate our supposition. The first step is to set up the two-layered feedforward network. To model complete connectivity between inputs and outputs, we will have each input unit project to both output units with weights of 1. The weighted input sums to both output units are computed as $\mathbf{q} = \mathbf{V}\mathbf{x}$, where $\mathbf{q} = [q_1\ q_2]^T$, $\mathbf{x} = [x_1\ x_2]^T$, and $\mathbf{V}$ is a 2-by-2 matrix as in Equation 8.9:

$$\begin{bmatrix} q_1 \\ q_2 \end{bmatrix} = \begin{bmatrix} v_{11} & v_{12} \\ v_{21} & v_{22} \end{bmatrix} \begin{bmatrix} x_1 \\ x_2 \end{bmatrix} \qquad \textbf{8.9}$$

The weights v_{ij} connect input unit x_j to output unit y_i ($i = 1, 2$ and $j = 1, 2$). For the case of complete connectivity, which we study in this example, $v_{ij} = 1$ for all i and j. The matrix multiplication in Equation 8.9 will produce the net input q_i to each output unit. This output must be thresholded to yield the actual output y_i as shown in Equation 8.10:

$$y_i = \begin{cases} 1, & q_i > \theta \\ 0, & q_i \leq \theta \end{cases} \qquad \textbf{8.10}$$

The threshold θ will be set to 0.7. In this simple case, with binary input states and all connection weight values equal to 1, any θ such that $0 \leq \theta < 1$ would ensure that an input of 1 will bring the output unit above threshold. Our choice of $\theta = 0.7$ will facilitate comparisons we will make with other networks later in the chapter. Since the two inputs are binary, the combined input X has four possible states: (0, 0), (1, 0), (0, 1), and (1, 1). Because the outputs are thresholded, the combined output Y will also have the same four possible states. The input–output behavior of the network can be determined simply by finding the (thresholded) output of the network to each of the four input states. Script `info2by2`, which is listed in MATLAB® Box 8.1, will do this computation.

Arrays `InPat` and `Out` in script `info2by2` hold the input and output states, respectively. The script implements Equations 8.9 and 8.10 by first set-

M̲ATLAB® BOX 8.1   **This script computes input–output mutual information in a feedforward network with two stochastic, binary input units and two deterministic, binary output units.**

```
% info2by2.m

px1=0.8; px2=0.7; % set input probabilities
% set network connectivity
V=[1,1;1,1]; % complete connectivity
% V=[1,1;0,1]; % almost-complete connectivity
% V=[1,0;0,1]; % identity connectivity
% V=[0,1;1,0]; % flipped-identity connectivity
% V=[1,0;0,0]; % minimal connectivity

% find network responses and set conditional probability table
thr=0.7; % set threshold
InPat=[0,0;1,0;0,1;1,1];% set input patterns
Out=zeros(4,2); % zero output array
y=zeros(2,1); % zero output vector
condi=zeros(4); % zero conditional probability table
for l=1:4, % for each input pattern (letter l indexes patterns)
    x=InPat(l,:)'; % set input x to next pattern
    q=V*x; % find the weighted input sum q
    y=q>thr; % find thresholded output y
    if y==[0;0], condi(1,1)=1; % output 0,0 is state one
    elseif y==[1;0], condi(2,1)=1; % output 1,0 is state two
    elseif y==[0;1], condi(3,1)=1; % output 0,1 is state three
    elseif y==[1;1], condi(4,1)=1; end % output 1,1 is state four
    Out(l,:)=y'; % save output in output array
end % end of network response and conditional probability loop

% compute the input probability distribution
pX=zeros(4,1); % zero the input probability vector
pX(1)=(1-px1)*(1-px2); % find the probability of input state one
pX(2)=px1*(1-px2); % find the probability of input state two
pX(3)=(1-px1)*px2; % find the probability of input state three
pX(4)=px1*px2; % find the probability of input state four

% compute informational measures using function infoCOMP
[hX hY mi]=infoCOMP(pX,condi);
```

ting input x to pattern l using `x=InPat(l,:)'` (note that the letter l indexes the patterns). It then computes q using `q=V*x` and thresholds q to get y using `y=q>thr` where the threshold is set to `thr=0.7`. Connectivity matrix V can be configured for complete connectivity using `V=[1,1;1,1]`. The input and resulting output states when the matrix V is configured for complete connectivity are shown in Table 8.1A. For this network input state (0, 0) produces output state (0, 0). All the other input states produce the output state (1, 1). Thus, both outputs are activated when either one or both of the inputs are active. These responses, along with the probabilities we will assign to the input units, will be used to measure information transmission in the network.

The central task in quantifying the information that a network extracts from its inputs is to determine the joint probability distribution of the inputs and outputs (e.g., Equation 8.8). The joint distribution can be determined from the input probabilities, which we set directly, and from the conditional prob-

TABLE 8.1 Probabilistic characterization of the 2-by-2, deterministic feedforward network of binary, threshold units with complete input–output connectivity

(A) Input-output table for the 2-by-2 network with complete connectivity

Input state X	(0, 0)	(1, 0)	(0, 1)	(1, 1)
Output state Y	(0, 0)	(1, 1)	(1, 1)	(1, 1)

(B) Input probabilities for the network with complete connectivity

Input state X	(0, 0)	(1, 0)	(0, 1)	(1, 1)
Probability $P(X)$	0.06	0.24	0.14	0.56

(C) Conditional probability table for the network with complete connectivity

	Input state X			
	(0, 0)	(1, 0)	(0, 1)	(1, 1)
Output state Y				
(0, 0)	1	0	0	0
(1, 0)	0	0	0	0
(0, 1)	0	0	0	0
(1, 1)	0	1	1	1

(D) Joint probability $P(X,Y)$ for the network with complete connectivity

	Input state X			
	(0, 0)	(1, 0)	(0, 1)	(1, 1)
Output state Y				
(0, 0)	0.06	0	0	0
(1, 0)	0	0	0	0
(0, 1)	0	0	0	0
(1, 1)	0	0.24	0.14	0.56

(E) Output probabilities for the network with complete connectivity

Output state Y	(0, 0)	(1, 0)	(0, 1)	(1, 1)
Probability $P(Y)$	0.06	0	0	0.94

abilities of the outputs given the inputs, which we can find from the network responses. In order for the probability distribution of the input states to be valid, the probabilities of the four possible states of input X [(0, 0), (1, 0), (0, 1), (1, 1)] must sum to 1. The simplest way to ensure that they do is to set the probabilities of each input (x_1 and x_2) separately, and to assume they are independent of one another. If binary input x_1 takes value 1 with probability p_{x1}, then it takes value 0 with probability $(1 - p_{x1})$. Similarly, we can have binary input x_2 take values 1 and 0 with probabilities p_{x2} and $(1 - p_{x2})$, respectively. If the two inputs are independent, then the probability of each combined, two-element state $X = (X_1, X_2)$ is just the product of the probabilities of each separate element (see Section 8.1). Thus, the probability of input state (0, 0), which we can write as $P(X = (0, 0))$, is equal to the product $(1 - p_{x1}) (1 - p_{x2})$. Similarly for the three other input states: $P(X = (1, 0)) = p_{x1} (1 - p_{x2})$, $P(X = (0, 1)) = (1 - p_{x1}) p_{x2}$, and $P(X = (1, 1)) = p_{x1} p_{x2}$. Note that the probabilities of the four input states are the product of the following two sums: $[p_{x1} + (1 - p_{x1})] [p_{x2} + (1 - p_{x2})]$. Since each sum [terms in brackets] obviously equals 1, we know their product must equal 1, so we are guaranteed that the probabilities of the four inputs states will also sum to 1. Knowing the probability distribution of the inputs allows us to compute the entropy (uncertainty) of the inputs, which is also the amount of information contained by the inputs (see Equation 8.2).

For example, if the probabilities are $p_{x1} = 0.8$ and $p_{x2} = 0.7$ that the individual inputs take value 1, then the four input state probabilities are: $P(X = (0, 0)) = 0.06$, $P(X = (1, 0)) = 0.24$, $P(X = (0, 1)) = 0.14$, and $P(X = (1, 1)) = 0.56$. Note that these four values constitute the probability distribution $P(X)$ for input state variable X. The probabilities that the individual binary inputs take value 1 can be set in `info2by2` as `px1=0.8` and `px2=0.7`. The script `info2by2` computes and stores the input probability distribution of the four combined input states in vector variable `pX`. For example, the first element of `pX` is the probability of the first input state $P(X = (0, 0))$. It is computed using `pX(1)=(1-px1)*(1-px2)`. The other elements of `pX` are computed similarly. The input probability distribution $P(X)$ is shown in Table 8.1B.

The entropy of X is computed using Equation 8.2, where the summation occurs over all four states of X: $H(X) = -[0.06 \log_2(0.06) + 0.24 \log_2(0.24) + 0.14 \log_2(0.14) + 0.56 \log_2(0.56)] = 1.60$ bits. This is the amount of information contained by the inputs. For convenience in this chapter, the informational measures of input and output entropy, and input–output mutual information, are computed using the function `infoCOMP`, which is listed in MATLAB Box 8.2. All of the scripts in this chapter will call `infoCOMP`. The input entropy $H(X)$ is computed by `infoCOMP` and stored in scalar variable `hX`. The function computes input entropy by first defining (and zeroing) the vector `log2pX=zeros(nX,1)`, where `nX` is the number of input states, and then by finding the logs for all nonzero values of the input probability distribution `pX` using `log2pX(find(pX~=0))=log2(pX(find(pX~=0)))`. (The `find` command is used in this way to find nonzero values throughout `infoCOMP`.) With `pX` and `log2pX` both available, the function computes input entropy using `hX=-sum(pX.*log2pX)`, which implements Equation 8.2.

In order to determine the mutual information between the input and the output of the network, we need to determine the joint probability distribution $P(X,Y)$ of the input and output (see Equation 8.8). The joint input–output distribution can be determined from the input state probabilities $P(X)$, which we set above, and from the conditional probabilities of the outputs given the inputs $P(Y|X)$ (see Equation 8.7). Because the outputs are deterministic, the conditional probabilities can be determined directly from the responses of the network to each of the inputs, and can be represented as entries in a conditional probability table, as shown in Table 8.1C.

The conditional probability table will have as many rows as output states Y and as many columns as input states X. In the case of a 2-by-2 network of binary elements, there will be four input states and four output states, so the conditional probability table will have four rows and four columns. Every column of the conditional probability table will indicate the conditional probability of each output state Y given a specific input state X. For example, the first column of the conditional probability table shown in Table 8.1C indicates the probability of each possible output state $[(0, 0), (1, 0), (0, 1), (1, 1)]$ given the input state $(0, 0)$. The other columns indicate the probability of each possible output state given the input states $(1, 0)$, $(0, 1)$, and $(1, 1)$ (see Table 8.1C). The conditional probabilities of the deterministic output states given each input state will contain a single 1 in each column, with the other entries all 0.

Script `info2by2` (see MATLAB Box 8.1) uses the network responses to construct the conditional probability table and stores it in array `condi`. Of the four possible output states, two of them, $(1, 0)$ and $(0, 1)$, occur with 0 probability. Note that the rows of the conditional probability table (see Table 8.1C) that correspond to output states $(1, 0)$ and $(0, 1)$ contain all 0s. Thus, the output

MATLAB® BOX 8.2   **This function computes the input and output entropy and the input–output mutual information for a neural network.**

```
% infoCOMP.m
% this funciton takes the input probability distribution pX and
% the conditional probability table condi as arguments, and computes
% input entropy hX, output entropy hY, and mutual information mi

function [hX hY mi] = infoCOMP(pX,condi) % declare function

[nY nX]=size(condi); % find numbers of input and output states

% compute input entropy (input information content)
log2pX=zeros(nX,1); % zero vector for log2 of input probability
log2pX(find(pX~=0))=log2(pX(find(pX~=0))); % log2 of probability
hX=-sum(pX.*log2pX); % compute the input entropy

% find joint and marginal probability distributions
joint=zeros(nY,nX); % zero the joint probability table
for j=1:nX, joint(:,j)=condi(:,j)*pX(j); end % compute the joint
pY=sum(joint')'; % compute marginal of the output

% compute output entropy (output information content)
log2pY=zeros(nY,1); % zero vector for log2 of output probability
log2pY(find(pY~=0))=log2(pY(find(pY~=0))); % log2 of probability
hY=-sum(pY.*log2pY); % compute the output entropy

% compute mutual information
pprod=pY*pX'; % compute matrix of probability products
jprat=zeros(nY,nX); % zero the ratio of joint to prob product matrix
jprat(find(pprod~=0))=joint(find(pprod~=0))./pprod(find(pprod~=0));
ljprat=zeros(nY,nX); % zero matrix for log2 of ratio
ljprat(find(jprat~=0))=log2(jprat(find(jprat~=0))); % log2 of ratio
mi=sum(sum(joint.*ljprat)); % compute mutual information
```

does not utilize all of its available states to represent the input. This is a clue that the output in this case does not contain complete input information. We can quantify this precisely by computing the mutual information.

From the definition of conditional probability shown in Equation 8.7, we know that $P(X,Y) = P(Y \mid X) P(X)$. Therefore, to compute the joint probability distribution from the conditional probability table, we need only multiply each entry in the conditional probability table by the appropriate input probability. Note that each column of the conditional probability table specifies the conditional probability of each of the states of the output Y given one of the states of the input X. Multiplication of each of the columns of the conditional probability table by the corresponding value of $P(X)$ will accomplish the conversion to the joint distribution. The function infoCOMP (see MATLAB Box 8.2) will use the conditional probability table condi to determine the numbers of input states nX and output states nY using [nY nX]=size(condi). The function will then compute the joint distribution and store it in array variable joint. It does this by first defining and zeroing the array joint=zeros(nY,nX), and then it computes each column of joint in a loop: for j=1:nX, `joint(:,j)=condi(:,j)*pX(j); end`. The joint distribution $P(X,Y)$ for the 2-by-2 network with complete connectivity is shown in Table 8.1D.

Summing the elements in each row of the joint probability table will yield the unconditional probability distribution of the output $P(Y)$. Output probability distribution $P(Y)$ is also called the marginal distribution of Y because it is found along the margin of the joint probability table, after summing its row elements. Function `infoCOMP` computes $P(Y)$ from $P(X,Y)$ using `pY=sum(joint')'`. The output probability distribution $P(Y)$ is shown for the case of complete connectivity in Table 8.1E.

Now the joint probability distribution $P(X,Y)$, and the marginal distribution $P(Y)$ computed from it, along with the input probability distribution $P(X)$ already specified, can be combined using Equation 8.8 to compute the mutual information $I(X;Y)$ between the input X and the output Y. Specifically, to complete our numerical example, we note that $P(X) = [0.06, 0.24, 0.14, 0.56]$ (see Table 8.1B) and $P(Y) = [0.06, 0, 0, 0.94]$ (see Table 8.1E). We note further that the joint distribution $P(X,Y)$ has only four nonzero values (see Table 8.1D). By definition in computing informational measures, $(0) \log_2(0) = 0$. Thus we need only four terms to compute the mutual information. These are the terms associated with the four nonzero joint probabilities, which are $P(X = (0, 0), Y = (0, 0))$, $P(X = (1, 0), Y = (1, 1))$, $P(X = (0, 1), Y = (1, 1))$, and $P(X = (1, 1), Y = (1, 1))$. The mutual information is then computed as $I(X;Y) = 0.06 \log_2(0.06 / (0.06)(0.06)) + 0.24 \log_2(0.24 / (0.24)(0.94)) + 0.14 \log_2(0.14 / (0.14)(0.94)) + 0.56 \log_2(0.56 / (0.56)(0.94)) = 0.33$ bits.

The numerical example illustrates how the input–output mutual information for a neural network can be computed from the input probability distribution and the conditional probabilities of the outputs given the inputs. Function `infoCOMP` (see MATLAB Box 8.2) will take as arguments the input probability distribution `pX` and the conditional probability table `condi`, and will compute the mutual information $I(X;Y)$ and store it in variable `mi`. As we have warned previously, $\log_2(0)$ is $-\infty$, so `infoCOMP` finds (using `find`) 0 probability values before taking logs and sets $\log_2(0) = 0$. The function computes mutual information `mi` by breaking Equation 8.8 down into components. Function `infoCOMP` also computes the input entropy $H(X)$ and output entropy $H(Y)$ and stores them in variables `hX` and `hY`, respectively. Calls to the function are made using `[hX hY mi]=infoCOMP(pX,condi)`. The function `infoCOMP` will be called in this way from all of the scripts in this chapter.

We calculated the value of $I(X;Y)$ for the 2-by-2 network with complete connectivity between input and output to be 0.33 bits (the value of `mi` calculated by `info2by2` using `infoCOMP` for the case of complete connectivity is the same). The information gained at the output is much less than the information content of the input, since the mutual information $I(X;Y) = 0.33$ bits is almost five times smaller than the entropy of the input $H(X) = 1.60$ bits. The output Y clearly does not contain complete information about the input X in this network with complete input–output connectivity. Our supposition was that, in order to convey as much information as possible to the outputs from the inputs, both input units should connect to both output units with connection weights strong enough that either input unit could produce an above-threshold activation of both output units. This supposition is not valid.

In light of our previous result, it would be interesting to see if a network with incomplete input-output connectivity actually extracts more information from its inputs than a network with complete input–output connectivity. To explore this, we will keep the input probabilities the same ($p_{x1} = 0.8$ and $p_{x2} = 0.7$), but change element v_{21} in the connectivity matrix from 1 to 0. Now matrix **V** has all elements equal to 1 except for element v_{21}, which equals 0. It can be set in script `info2by2` using `V=[1,1;0,1]`. We can call this the almost-complete connectivity matrix. Because the input probabilities are unchanged, the information content of the input will be the same as before. However, changing the connectivity matrix will change the input–output behavior of the network, and may also change its ability to convey information about its inputs to its outputs.

The input to, and output from, the network with almost-complete connectivity is shown in Table 8.2B. Input states (0, 0) and (1, 0) produce the corresponding states of the output, but input states (0, 1) and (1, 1) both produce the output state (1, 1). The network with almost-complete connectivity uses three of its possible four states to represent the input. We would therefore expect an improvement in its ability to transfer information from input to output over that measured for the network with complete connectivity, which used only two of its possible output states. (The input–output table for the network with complete connectivity is reproduced for convenience in Table 8.2A.) We can make a more precise assessment by comparing the mutual information (variable `mi` in script `info2by2`) between input and output in the networks with complete and almost-complete connectivity.

The value of $I(X;Y)$ for the 2-by-2 network with almost-complete connectivity between input and output is 1.10 bits. The information gained at the output in this network is much greater than that of the previous network with complete connectivity, but it is still less than the information content (entropy) of the input, which is 1.60 bits. The output Y does not contain complete information about the input X in this network that has almost-complete input–output connectivity.

We will keep the input probabilities the same ($p_{x1} = 0.8$ and $p_{x2} = 0.7$), but further reduce the input–output connectivity in the network by changing ele-

---

TABLE 8.2   Input–output tables for the 2-by-2, deterministic feedforward network of binary units with various patterns of input–output connectivity

(A) With complete connectivity matrix

Input state X	(0, 0)	(1, 0)	(0, 1)	(1, 1)
Output state Y	(0, 0)	(1, 1)	(1, 1)	(1, 1)

(B) With almost-complete connectivity matrix

Input state X	(0, 0)	(1, 0)	(0, 1)	(1, 1)
Output state Y	(0, 0)	(1, 0)	(1, 1)	(1, 1)

(C) With identity connectivity matrix

Input state X	(0, 0)	(1, 0)	(0, 1)	(1, 1)
Output state Y	(0, 0)	(1, 0)	(0, 1)	(1, 1)

(D) With minimal connectivity matrix

Input state X	(0, 0)	(1, 0)	(0, 1)	(1, 1)
Output state Y	(0, 0)	(1, 0)	(0, 0)	(1, 0)

(E) With flipped-identity connectivity matrix

Input state X	(0, 0)	(1, 0)	(0, 1)	(1, 1)
Output state Y	(0, 0)	(0, 1)	(1, 0)	(1, 1)

ment v_{12} from 1 to 0. Now the connectivity matrix **V** is the 2-by-2 identity matrix (V=[1,0;0,1] in script info2by2). The input to and output from the network with identity connectivity is shown in Table 8.2C. Each state of the input produces the corresponding state of the output. Thus, the network with identity connectivity uses all of its available output states to represent the input, and we would therefore expect a further improvement in its ability to transfer information from input to output. The value of $I(X;Y)$ for the 2-by-2 network when connectivity matrix **V** is the identity matrix is 1.60 bits, which is equal to the information content of the inputs. (Entropy $H(X) = 1.60$ bits.) In this case, where the connectivity matrix is the identity matrix, the output Y does contain complete information about the input X.

Because entropy is a non-negative quantity, it follows directly from Equation 8.6 that $I(X;Y) = H(X) - H(X \mid Y) \leq H(X)$. Since $I(X;Y) = I(Y;X)$, it is also the case that $I(X;Y) = H(Y) - H(Y \mid X) \leq H(Y)$. This proves that the mutual information $I(X;Y)$ between random variables X and Y can never be greater than the information content $H(X)$ or $H(Y)$ of either variable (Cover and Thomas 1991). The consequence of this in our context is that a neural network cannot transfer more information from input to output than is contained in the input. The previous result therefore shows us that we cannot possibly configure connectivity matrix **V** to give us more information transmission than is provided by the identity connectivity matrix. However, the previous result might lead us legitimately to wonder whether we could further reduce the connectivity of matrix **V** and still obtain complete information transmission from input to output.

To explore this possibility we will keep the input probabilities the same ($p_{x1} = 0.8$ and $p_{x2} = 0.7$), but change element v_{22} from 1 to 0 (V=[1,0;0,0] in script info2by2). Now the connectivity matrix **V** is a 2-by-2 matrix of 0s with a 1 at element v_{11}. We can call this the minimal-connectivity matrix. The input to and output from this network is shown in Table 8.2D. The input states (0, 0) and (0, 1) both produce the state (0, 0) at the output, and the input states (1, 0) and (1, 1) both produce the state (1, 0) at the output. Thus, the network with minimal connectivity only uses two of its possible four output states to represent the input. This provides us with a strong indication that the network with minimal connectivity transfers less information than the network with identity connectivity.

The value of $I(X;Y)$ for the 2-by-2 network with the minimal connectivity matrix is 0.72 bits. In this case the output Y does not contain complete information about the input X. The minimal connectivity matrix transmits more input information than the complete connectivity matrix, but less than the almost-complete matrix. Of course, the minimal matrix conveys less information than the identity matrix, which conveys complete information from input to output.

The reason that the network with the identity connectivity matrix can transmit complete input information is *not* that it produces a perfect match between input and output states, but that it assigns a unique output state to each input state. To see this we can keep the same input probabilities ($p_{x1} = 0.8$ and $p_{x2} = 0.7$), but set matrix **V** to be the flipped 2-by-2 identity matrix (V=[0,1;1,0] in script info2by2). The input to and output from the network with flipped-identity connectivity is shown in Table 8.2E. Input states (0, 0) and (1, 1) produce the corresponding states of the output, but input state (1, 0) produces output state (0, 1) and vice-versa. The correspondences between the input and output states are different here than they were for the identity matrix network. However, the output still produces a unique state for every input state. The value of $I(X;Y)$ for the 2-by-2 network with connectivity matrix **V** equal to the flipped-identity matrix is also 1.60 bits, the same as the value of the input

we considered in the previous section, the script constrains V to have all positive elements by applying the command V(find(V<0))=0 after each weight update. It does not constrain b. To compare the behavior of sigmoidal networks trained using the Bell–Sejnowski algorithm with the binary, threshold networks from the previous section, a threshold is applied after squashing the output activations in the sigmoidal network. This makes the output responses binary. The threshold is *not* applied during training.

We will use the Bell–Sejnowski algorithm implemented in infoMax2by2 to maximize information transfer in this simple, two-layered feedforward neural network. The script will first initialize the connectivity matrix V and the bias vector b to uniformly distributed random values between 0 and 1 using V=rand(2) and b=rand(2,1). We will set the threshold (to be applied after squashing) to 0.51. This is an appropriate value to use with sigmoidal units, since their output is 0.5 for an input of 0.

For purposes of comparison, we will first examine the behavior of the network before training. The input–output behavior of the network with randomized connectivity weights and biases is determined by finding the squashed and thresholded output state for each input state. (This can be done using Equations 8.12 and 8.13, followed by a threshold step as in Equation 8.10, as though the output of the squashing function was still denoted by q_i and must be thresholded to finally give y_i.) Note that the code for evaluating network behavior before training is not shown in the listing for script infoMax2by2, but it is the same as the code that evaluates network behavior after training (see MATLAB Box 8.3). The input–output behavior of the network before training is shown in Table 8.3A. Different initially randomized weight matrices and bias vectors will produce different initial input–output relationships. This particular randomized network produces output state (1, 1) in response to all four input states. The inability of the output to distinguish among the different states of the input implies that the information transfer ability of the initially random network is extremely poor.

To challenge the Bell–Sejnowski algorithm we will set the individual input probabilities to $p_{x1} = 0.5$ and $p_{x2} = 0.5$ using px1=0.5 and px2=0.5. The information content of this input, equal to its entropy $H(X)$, is maximal at 2 bits. Now we will set the learning rate to a=0.01 and train the network for 3000 iterations using the Bell–Sejnowski algorithm. Rather than set them afresh on each training cycle, script infoMax2by2 sets the inputs for all iterations before training and stores them in sample array sam, with two rows and nSam=3000 columns, using commands sam=zeros(2,nSam), sam(1,:)=rand(1,nSam)<px1, and sam(2,:)=rand(1,nSam)<px2.

TABLE 8.3 Input–output tables for a 2-by-2, deterministic feedforward network of sigmoidal units following training with the Bell–Sejnowski infomax algorithm

(A) With initially randomized connectivity matrix

Input state X	(0, 0)	(1, 0)	(0, 1)	(1, 1)
Output state Y	(1, 1)	(1, 1)	(1, 1)	(1, 1)

(B) With connections trained using the Bell–Sejnowski algorithm

Input state X	(0, 0)	(1, 0)	(0, 1)	(1, 1)
Output state Y	(0, 0)	(0, 1)	(1, 0)	(1, 1)

(Setting the input as samples ahead of time is a technique useful for completing Exercise 8.2.) Note that script `infoMax2by2` does *not* apply the threshold to the output responses during training. Only the squashing function is applied during training. The threshold is something we have added on after the sigmoidal nonlinearity to facilitate comparisons with networks of threshold units.

When training a network with initially random connection weights, whether we use the Bell–Sejnowski algorithm or any other algorithm, the specific results will depend on the values of the initially random weights. When training a network from an initially random connectivity, we will present results that are representative of, but not necessarily the same as, those that you will observe in your simulations. In this particular case, the bias inputs are both about −1.5 following 3000 training iterations with the Bell–Sejnowski algorithm. The connectivity matrix after training is shown in Equation 8.16:

$$\mathbf{V} = \begin{bmatrix} 0.03 & 3.03 \\ 3.09 & 0.03 \end{bmatrix} \qquad\qquad \textbf{8.16}$$

This matrix has the form of the flipped-identity connectivity matrix. Each output unit gets a strong connection from one input unit and a very weak, almost-zero connection from the other input unit. Thus, each output unit is set to respond briskly to one input unit, and this increases the individual entropy of each output unit. Also, each output unit is specialized for only one input unit, and that decreases the mutual information between the outputs. This connectivity matrix seems to have maximized the joint entropy of the output units, so it should also have maximized the information transfer from input to output.

After training, script `infoMax2by2` evaluates the input–output behavior of the network by finding the squashed and thresholded output state for each input state. (The script implements Equations 8.12 and 8.13, followed by Equation 8.10 as though the output of the squashing function was still denoted by q_i.) The input to and output from the trained network is shown in Table 8.3B. Input states $(0, 0)$ and $(1, 1)$ produce the corresponding states of the output, but input state $(1, 0)$ produces output state $(0, 1)$ and vice-versa. The correspondences between input and output states are the same here as they were for the network with the flipped-identity connectivity matrix that we studied in the previous section (see Table 8.2E). As in that network, the output of the network trained using the Bell–Sejnowski infomax algorithm produces a unique output state for every input state. Note that the Bell–Sejnowski algorithm does not always produce a connectivity matrix in the flipped-identity form. It just as often produces a connectivity matrix in the identity form. The important point is that the algorithm always produces a matrix that separates the input connections to the output units, and this enables the outputs to produce a unique state for each input state.

Script `infoMax2by2` (see MATLAB Box 8.3) will use the output responses, where the weighted input sum at the output is first passed through the sigmoidal squashing function and then thresholded, to construct the conditional probability table `condi`. As in script `info2by2` (listed in MATLAB Box 8.1), script `infoMax2by2` will also assemble the input probability distribution `pX`. (Recall that we set `px1=0.5` and `px2=0.5` to achieve maximum input entropy in order to challenge the algorithm.) The script will then use `pX` and `condi` to find the input entropy `hX`, the output entropy `hY`, and the input-output mutual information `mi` using the function call `[hX hY mi]=infoCOMP(pX,condi)`. To recap, the function `infoCOMP` (see MATLAB Box 8.2) will multiply each column of the conditional probability table $P(Y \mid X)$ by the corresponding input probability $P(X)$ to find the joint distribution $P(X,Y)$. It will use the joint to compute the (marginal) output probability distribution $P(Y)$, and finally compute the mutual information $I(X;Y)$ according to Equation 8.8. The function will also use $P(X)$ and $P(Y)$, respectively, to find the input $H(X)$ and output $H(Y)$ entropies. We can gauge information transmission in the network by comparing the information content of the input $H(X)$ with the input–output mutual information $I(X;Y)$, where we may also note that for deterministic networks $I(X;Y) = H(Y)$.

For purposes of comparison we can compute the input–output mutual information for the 2-by-2 network with its connection weights and biases initially randomized, as they were before training using the Bell–Sejnowski algorithm. Given the network responses shown in Table 8.3A for the initially randomized network, the mutual information $I(X;Y)$ is 0. Thus, the untrained, randomized network is incapable of transferring information from input to output. In contrast, the value of $I(X;Y)$ is 2 bits for the network trained using the Bell–Sejnowski algorithm (Table 8.3B). (Note that the output entropy $H(Y)$ is equal to the mutual information $I(X;Y)$, as expected for this deterministic network.) Since the information content of the input $H(X)$ is also 2 bits, the output of the trained network contains complete information concerning the input. Thus, the Bell–Sejnowski infomax algorithm has successfully maximized mutual information $I(X;Y)$ in this network.

As is the case for many neural network learning algorithms, infomax algorithms including the Bell–Sejnowski algorithm have been widely used both as tools to construct models of neural systems and in technological applications. One of the most compelling technological applications of the Bell–Sejnowski infomax algorithm is called blind source separation, in which a mixture of signals from statistically independent sources is separated by a neural network into its original components. An example adapted from Haykin (1999), in which a sine wave is separated from random noise, is illustrated in Figure 8.2. Using the Bell–Sejnowski algorithm to implement this separation of signals is the subject of Exercise 8.2. In that the algorithm separates the mixture into its

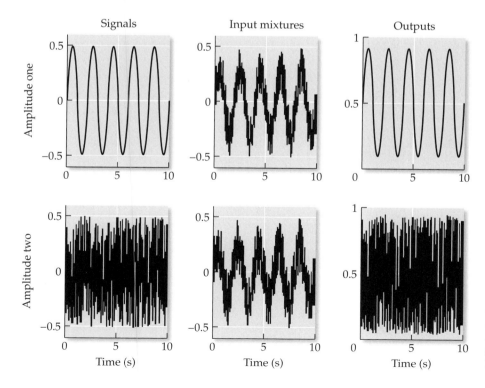

FIGURE 8.2   Blind source separation using the Bell–Sejnowski information maximization algorithm Each column of panels shows the amplitudes of two simulated, temporal signals. The two original signals are a sine wave, nominally at 0.5 cycles per second, and uniformly distributed random noise. The inputs to the network are mixtures of these original signals. After training, the outputs are unmixed (separated) versions of the original signals. (After Haykin 1999.)

statistically independent components, it constitutes an example of a technique that is known more generally as independent components analysis.

One of the most compelling applications of infomax algorithms to the modeling of neural systems is the simulation of the formation of the response properties of neurons in primary visual cortex. Olshausen and Field (1996) trained a set of basis functions to represent natural images by simultaneously satisfying two goals: to minimize the error of reconstruction of the images, and to maximize the efficiency of the representation. These goals can be cast in information-theoretic terms. If the basis functions are thought of as the weights from a two-dimensional array of input units to each output unit in a two-layered network, then the Olshausen–Field algorithm corresponds to simultaneous maximization of the input–output mutual information and minimization of the output entropy (see Bell and Sejnowski 1997 for discussion). The resulting basis functions constituted a minimum-entropy, or sparse, code. The basis functions (weight arrays) that result from the application of the Olshausen–Field algorithm to real images take the form of oriented, two-dimensional Gabor functions. (See Chapter 3 for a summary of the Gabor function.) As such, the basis functions, shown in Figure 8.3, resemble the orientationally selective receptive fields of neurons in primary visual cortex, shown in Figure 8.4. The correspondence between the simulated and experimental results suggests that visual cortical neurons have orientationally selective (Gabor-like) receptive fields in order to represent maximally the information contained in the visual environment. The results of Olshausen and Field further suggest that real sensory systems not only maximize the information that they contain about the sensory environment, but they do so in an efficient manner.

Information maximization algorithms do not depend on the sparseness constraint in order to produce input–output weight arrays that resemble the orientationally selective receptive fields of neurons in primary visual cortex. Networks trained on natural images using the Bell–Sejnowski algorithm also produce input–output weight arrays that resemble orientated Gabor functions, leading to the interpretation that orientationally selective receptive fields are the independent components of the visual environment. Training neural networks on natural images using the Bell–Sejnowski algorithm requires

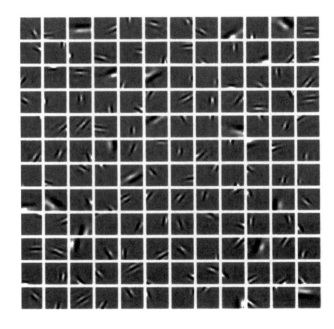

FIGURE 8.3 Learning a sparse code for natural images Each panel illustrates one member of a set of 144 basis functions that were trained on 16-by-16 pixel patches extracted from images of natural scenes. The basis functions can be thought of as the weights of the connections from a two-dimensional, 16-by-16 array of input units onto each one of 144 output units. The responses of the output units to patches of the images can be saved, and the output unit responses can be played back through the weights to reconstruct the images. The basis functions were trained using an algorithm that optimally achieved two objectives: to minimize the error of reconstruction, and to do so with minimal output unit activity. The algorithm simultaneously maximized information transmission from input to output, and maximized output activity sparseness, thus achieving a minimal-entropy code. The figure shows the 144 basis functions (square weight arrays) following 400,000 image-patch training presentations. The resulting basis functions resemble the orientationally selective receptive fields of neurons in primary visual cortex. (From Olshausen and Field 1996.)

FIGURE 8.4 **The receptive fields of neurons in primary visual cortex are well described using two-dimensional Gabor functions** The data (left column) are examples of the visual receptive fields of neurons in the primary visual (striate) cortex. The fit (right column) are real-valued (i.e., approximate) two-dimensional Gabor functions (see Chapter 3 for details) whose parameters are adjusted so that the summed squared differences between the data and the functions are minimized. (From Ringach 2002.)

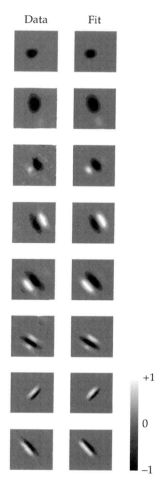

additional procedures, such as pre-filtering, which we will not consider here (see Bell and Sejnowski 1997 for details), but it demonstrates that the Bell–Sejnowski algorithm, designed explicitly to maximize information transmission through a neural network without a sparseness constraint, is also capable of simulating the development of orientationally selective receptive fields. As we have seen in previous chapters (especially Chapters 4 and 6), sparse activity patterns do offer advantages in terms of accuracy of storage and recall in adaptive networks. Thus, sparseness is a desirable quality, but sparseness is not essential to the ability of infomax algorithms to create output representations that resemble those observed in real sensory systems.

Whether or not they include a sparseness constraint, the output representations developed by infomax algorithms generally fail to reproduce an important feature of many real sensory representations. Unlike the neurons in primary visual cortex, the output units in these information maximizing networks are not organized spatially according to preferred input features. These infomax procedures may produce orientationally selective receptive fields (e.g., Olshausen and Field 1996; Bell and Sejnowski 1997; Harpur and Prager 2000), but they do not reproduce map-like structures such as the orientation-pinwheels that are actually observed in primary visual cortex.

In Chapter 5, we studied neural network models of the visual cortical map of orientation selectivity that were trained using Hebbian map-forming algorithms, including the self-organizing map (SOM) algorithm (Kohonen 1997). The purpose of the SOM (and related algorithms) is to create feature maps, not to increase input–output mutual information. However, it has been demonstrated that Hebbian map-forming algorithms similar to the SOM can produce output units with orientationally selective receptive fields that resemble Gabor functions (provided that Hebbian training is appropriately constrained and augmented with additional mechanisms; see Linsker 1986, 1990 for details). It has also been demonstrated that map-forming SOM-like algorithms can increase information transfer from input to output (Linkser 1989, 1990). The information transfer ability of the SOM itself can be illustrated more simply in the context of a model not of a single (e.g., visual) sensory representation, but of a multisensory representation.

The deep layers of the superior colliculus are multisensory in that they receive input from the visual, auditory, and somatosensory systems (Wallace and Stein 1996). One might suppose that all neurons in the deep colliculus should receive heavily weighted input from all three sensory systems, in order to maximize the amount of sensory information that can be represented by the responses of collicular neurons. As we saw in Section 8.2, that supposition would be misguided. The mutual information between the input and output of a network depends on the number of distinct states that the output uses to represent the input. Complete and heavily weighted input–output connectivity might cause any input unit to activate all the output units, but it is unlikely to produce the diversity of output response states that would be necessary to encode the diversity of input states.

In fact, the vast majority of neurons in the deep colliculus do *not* receive input from all three sensory systems. Instead, an individual neuron in the deep colliculus can be selective for any of the possible combinations of the three modalities. Unisensory neurons respond to visual, auditory, or somatosensory stimulation. Bisensory neurons respond to visual or auditory, visual or somatosensory, or auditory or somatosensory stimulation. Only trisensory neurons respond to stimulation in all three modalities. As shown in Figure 8.5, fewer than 10% of deep collicular neurons in cats or monkeys are trisensory. In cats, about 50% of deep collicular neurons are multisensory (bisensory or trisensory), while in monkeys only about 25% are multisensory (Wallace and Stein 1996). It is possible that the diversity of modality selectivities observed among neurons in the deep colliculus is necessary for it to represent the information present in its inputs.

The colliculus is also organized topographically. A topographic, multisensory map model of the colliculus, trained using the SOM, was presented in Chapter 5. This map exhibited a modality-pinwheel structure that was analogous to the topographically organized orientation-pinwheel structure of primary visual cortex. An information-theoretic analysis of a similar multisensory map is shown

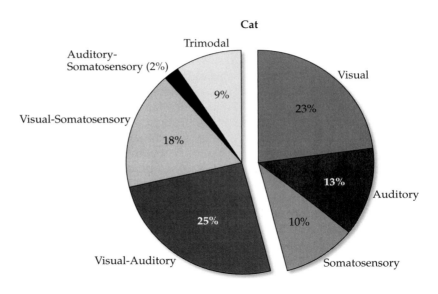

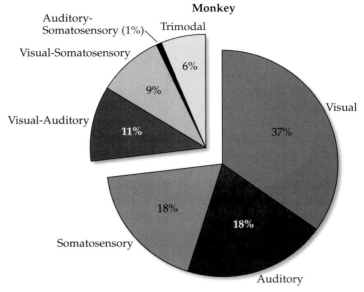

FIGURE 8.5 Percentages of neurons in the deep layers of the superior colliculus having each of seven different selectivities for stimulus modality The unisensory selectivities are visual, auditory, and somatosensory. The multisensory selectivities are visual-auditory, visual-somatosensory, auditory-somatosensory, and visual-auditory-somatosensory. Many neurons are unisensory despite the availability of multisensory input. In cat, about 50% of neurons in the deep colliculus are multisensory, while in monkey only about 25% are multisensory. (After Wallace and Stein 1996.)

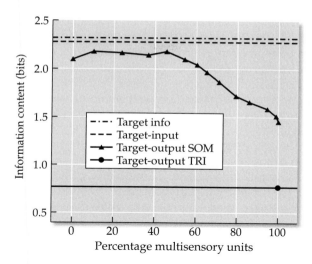

FIGURE 8.6   Information extraction and percentages of multisensory units in a superior colliculus model Self-organizing map (SOM) training causes a model of the superior colliculus to extract most of the information contained in its inputs, but only when the percentage of multisensory units is between about 10% and 50%. The colliculus is modeled as the output layer of a two-layered, feedforward network trained using the SOM to represent inputs of three sensory modalities: vision, audition, and somatosensation (see Anastasio and Patton 2003 for details). Weights below a threshold are pruned (set to zero) following SOM training, and the modality selectivity of each output unit is determined according to the modality (or modalities) of the inputs from which it receives nonzero input weights. Each data point is the average of the estimated output information content of ten networks, each trained from a random initial condition. For each network, the percentage of multisensory units is varied by changing the pruning threshold. The stochastic inputs (dashed line) contain most of the target information (dot-dashed line). The information content of the network is highest for percentages of multisensory units from about 10% to 50%. Information content steadily decreases for multisensory percentages above 50%, and approaches the low information content of a uniformly trisensory network, in which each output unit has connections of exactly the same weight from inputs of each of the three modalities. (After Anastasio and Patton 2003.)

in Figure 8.6. The units in the map receive inputs that represent the visual, auditory, and somatosensory inputs to the deep colliculus (Anastasio and Patton 2003). All inputs are stochastic, like the inputs to the networks in this chapter. The connection weights are trained using the SOM. Connections with weights that fall below a threshold are pruned following SOM training. The modality selectivity of an output unit is determined from the modalities of its input connections that remain after pruning. The percentage of multisensory output units can be controlled by adjusting this pruning threshold.

The network contains 100 model colliculus neurons (output units). Even after thresholding their responses to make them binary, there are 2^{100} output states potentially available to contain input information. Explicitly measuring the input–output mutual information, as we did above for 2-by-2 networks, is impossible with 100 output units. Instead, the output state is taken simply as the number of model collicular neurons that are active above some threshold (Anastasio and Patton 2003). The resulting informational measures are therefore approximate but still instructive.

The stochastic inputs encode the sensory characteristics of a target that can present any one of the seven modality combinations at random. As shown in Figure 8.6, the stochastic inputs contain almost as much information as the target. Following training, the responses of the model colliculus neurons contain almost as much information as the inputs, but only when the percentage of multisensory (bisensory and trisensory) neurons is between about 10% and 50%. As the percentage of multisensory units increases above 50%, information content decreases and approaches the low information content of the uniformly trisensory network. Interestingly, the range of high information content, from 10% to 50% multisensory, encompasses the multisensory percentages actually observed in cats and monkeys (Wallace and Stein 1996; see also Figure 8.5).

As explained in Chapter 5, the specific prediction that a modality map exists in the deep superior colliculus, which is based on simulations using the SOM algorithm, remains to be tested. If a modality map is discovered there, then the finding would lend support to the more general hypothesis that the purpose of cooperative, activity-dependent processes in the brain, which we simulate using the SOM, is not to form maps per se, but to increase the information content of sensory representations. We will explore this hypothesis in the next two sections.

The SOM algorithm simulates the activity-dependent processes that shape map-like neural representations, and it has two components: competitive and cooperative. The competitive component causes different output units to become specialized for different inputs. The resulting segregation or separation of the inputs is similar to that produced by the Bell–Sejnowski infomax algorithm, and we would expect that the competitive component of the SOM should likewise produce some increase in information transmission. The cooperative component, implemented over a neighborhood of output units during SOM training, is what leads to map formation, but we will show that the cooperative component may also play a role in information transmission. In the next section we will consider the ability of the purely competitive component of the SOM to increase information transmission in neural networks. In Section 8.5 we will evaluate the added benefit to information transmission of the cooperative component.

8.4   Information Transmission and Competitive Learning in Neural Networks

As we recall from Chapter 5 (see Equations 5.1–5.3), Kohonen (1997) expressed the three steps in the SOM algorithm as shown in Equations 8.17–8.19:

$$\mathbf{y} = \mathbf{V}\mathbf{x} \qquad \textbf{8.17}$$

$$y_m = \max_i \{y_i\} \qquad \textbf{8.18}$$

$$\mathbf{V}_{\text{row } h}(c+1) = \frac{\mathbf{V}_{\text{row } h}(c) + a\mathbf{x}^{\text{T}}(c)}{\left\| \mathbf{V}_{\text{row } h}(c) + a\mathbf{x}^{\text{T}}(c) \right\|_2} \qquad \textbf{8.19}$$

Equations 8.17– 8.19 specify that the output unit response vector **y** is the product of connectivity matrix **V** and input (column) vector **x**, and that the connection weights to unit y_m having the maximal response (the winner), and to any other output units in the training neighborhood indexed by h, are updated by adding to them the (transposed) input vector **x** that has been scaled by the learning rate a. To prevent growth of connection weights without bound, and to enhance specialization, this row vector is normalized by dividing it by its Euclidean norm (two-norm; see Math Box 5.1). Variable c indexes the update cycles. In this section we explore purely competitive learning, where the weights are trained only to the winning output unit, not to its neighbors. For purely competitive learning, the only output unit indexed by h is m. We will use competitive learning to train 2-by-2 networks as in Figure 8.1. Script `competitive2by2`, listed in MATLAB Box 8.4, will implement this training.

The 2-by-2 networks we will study in this section are the same as those we studied in Section 8.2. The units compute the weighted sum of their inputs $\mathbf{q} = \mathbf{V}\mathbf{x}$, where $\mathbf{q} = [q_1 \ q_2]^T$, $\mathbf{x} = [x_1 \ x_2]^T$, and $\mathbf{V}$ is the connectivity matrix, and the activities of the outputs $\mathbf{y} = [y_1 \ y_2]^T$ are made binary by thresholding, as in Equations 8.9 and 8.10. Note that the competitive learning algorithm (and the SOM, Equations 8.17–8.19) does *not* threshold the output unit activations during training. Thresholding of output unit activations is used in this chap-

---

MATLAB® BOX 8.4 **This script trains a 2-by-2, feedforward network using competitive, unsupervised learning, and finds the input–output mutual information.**

```
% competitive2by2.m

px1=0.5; px2=0.5; % set input probabilities
thr=0.7; % set threshold
nIts=1000; % set number of training iterations
a=1; % set learning rate
InPat=[0,0;1,0;0,1;1,1]; % set input patterns
V=rand(2); % initialize connection weight matrix

% train weights
for c=1:nIts, % for each training iteration
    x=[rand<px1; rand<px2]; % set the input
    y=V*x; % find the output
    [winVal,winIndx]=max(y); % find the winning output
    hld=V(winIndx,:)+a*x'; % update winner's weights
    V(winIndx,:)=hld/norm(hld); % normalize
end % end competitive training loop

% find responses and set conditional prob after training
y=zeros(2,1); % zero output vector
out=zeros(4,2); % zero output array
condi=zeros(4); % zero conditional probability table
for l=1:4, % for each input state (pattern, indexed by letter l)
    x=InPat(l,:)'; % set the input from patterns
    q=V*x; % compute the weighed input sum
    y=q>thr; % threshold the weighted input sum
    if y==[0;0], condi(1,l)=1; % output 0,0 is state one
    elseif y==[1;0], condi(2,l)=1; % output 1,0 is state two
    elseif y==[0;1], condi(3,l)=1; % output 0,1 is state three
    elseif y==[1;1], condi(4,l)=1; end % output 1,1 is state four
    out(l,:)=y'; % save output in output array
end % end of network response and conditional probability loop

% compute input probability distribution and info measures
pX=zeros(4,1); % zero the input probability vector
pX(1)=(1-px1)*(1-px2); pX(2)=px1*(1-px2); % find probs
pX(3)=(1-px1)*px2; pX(4)=px1*px2;          % of input states
[hX hY mi]=infoCOMP(pX,condi); % compute info measures
```

ter to simplify the computation of informational measures and to facilitate comparisons between the performances of different network types. Note also that bias inputs and the squashing activation function, which were used in the context of the Bell–Sejnowski infomax algorithm in Section 8.3, are generally not used in the context of competitive learning or SOM training and will not be used again in this chapter.

The goal of the example in this section is to determine whether competitive learning will increase information transfer in a simple, two-layered feedforward neural network. The procedure is to measure the information transfer in a network with initially random input–output connectivity, and then see whether information transfer is increased after competitive training. (Note that the code for evaluating the network before training is not included in the listing for `competitive2by2` in MATLAB Box 8.4, but it is the same as the code that evaluates the network after training, which is listed, and is explained later in this section.) Before training, script `competitive2by2` initializes weight matrix V by setting its elements to uniformly distributed random numbers between 0 and 1 (`V=rand(2)`). The threshold θ is set at `thr=0.7`, as in Section 8.2, but in this section such a high threshold is needed to eliminate responses due to equivocal weights that can sometimes develop using competitive learning (and SOM training). The input and output states of the randomized network before training, computed using Equations 8.9 and 8.10, are shown in Table 8.4A. This network produces output state (0, 0) in response to the first three input states, and produces output state (1, 0) in response to the fourth input state (1, 1). The inability of the output to distinguish among most of the input states implies that the information transfer ability of the random network is poor.

The input–output relationships of the initially random network are used to construct its conditional probability table. With that, the mutual information between input and output for any input probability distribution can be computed (see below in this section). With individual input probabilities set at $p_{x1} = 0.5$ and $p_{x2} = 0.5$, the input entropy $H(X)$ is maximal at 2 bits. Given the responses of the initially random network, the mutual information $I(X;Y)$ is 0.81. Thus, the untrained, randomized network is able to transfer very little of the input information to the output.

With the learning rate set at 1 (`a=1`), and the input probabilities set at `px1=0.5` and `px2=0.5`, the network is trained for `nIts=1000` iterations of competitive training using script `competitive2by2`. On each iteration the script sets the input according to the input probabilities using `x=[rand<px1; rand<px2]`, finds output vector `y=V*x`, and finds the index `winIndx` of the winning output unit using `[winVal,winIndx]=max(y)`. (Note that `winVal` is the winning value.) The script then updates the weight vector of the winner using two commands and intermediate variable `hld` as follows: `hld=V(winIndx,:)+a*x'` and `V(winIndx,:)=hld/norm(hld)`. The weight matrix after training from the initially random configuration for this representative case is shown in Equation 8.20:

$$\mathbf{V} = \begin{bmatrix} 0.98 & 0.18 \\ 0.00 & 1.00 \end{bmatrix} \qquad \textbf{8.20}$$

This connectivity matrix has the form of the identity matrix. Competitive learning in this case has segregated the input connections because it causes the output units to specialize for different inputs. Competitive learning is not explicitly an infomax algorithm, so it is not surprising that weight matrices trained using competitive learning are not as cleanly segregated as those

TABLE 8.4   Input-output tables for a 2-by-2, deterministic feedforward network of binary threshold units following training using the competitive learning algorithm

(A) With initially randomized connectivity matrix				
Input state X	(0, 0)	(1, 0)	(0, 1)	(1, 1)
Output state Y	(0, 0)	(0, 0)	(0, 0)	(1, 0)

(B) With connections trained using competitive learning algorithm				
Input state X	(0, 0)	(1, 0)	(0, 1)	(1, 1)
Output state Y	(0, 0)	(1, 0)	(0, 1)	(1, 1)

trained using the Bell–Sejnowski algorithm. Still, competitive training tends to increase information transmission by causing output units to specialize.

The input to and output from the trained network is shown in Table 8.4B. As for the network with the identity connectivity matrix that we studied in Section 8.2, each state of the input produces the corresponding state of the output. Competitive learning does not always produce a connectivity matrix with the form of the identity matrix. Sometimes it has the form of the flipped-identity matrix, and sometimes it looks more like an almost-complete connectivity matrix. However, weight matrices adapted through competitive learning generally produce a unique output state for every input state. This allows the network to increase its information transfer from input to output.

Script `competitive2by2` uses the input probabilities `px1=0.5` and `px2=0.5` to compute the input probability distribution `pX` as described in Section 8.2. The script also uses the input–output behavior of the network to construct the conditional probability table `condi`, and then computes informational measures using `[hX hY mi]=infoCOMP(pX,condi)` (see MATLAB Boxes 8.2 and 8.4). The value of $I(X;Y)$ for the network trained using competitive learning is 2 bits. Since the information content of the input $H(X)$ is also 2 bits, the output of the trained network contains complete information concerning the input.

Although competitive learning performs well for the input probabilities chosen ($p_{x1} = 0.5$ and $p_{x2} = 0.5$), it does not perform as well for other input probability distributions. While it is usually able to increase the amount of information transfer, it is often unable to convey complete input information. This sub-maximal performance is not surprising, since competitive learning was not designed to maximize information transfer in neural networks. The point of the simulations in this section is to demonstrate that, by causing output units to specialize for specific inputs, competitive learning can substantially increase information transmission from input to output in a neural network.

8.5   Information Transmission in Self-Organized Map Networks

Like the infomax algorithms we considered in Section 8.3, the competitive learning algorithm we studied in Section 8.4 was able to increase information transmission in a neural network. This increase occurred even though competitive learning was not designed to be an infomax algorithm. Also like the infomax algorithms, the competitive learning algorithm does not form a map. In this section we explore a possible connection between information transfer and feature maps in networks trained using the SOM, which combines both competitive and cooperative mechanisms. Theoretical studies have shown that the size of the neighborhood of cooperation in networks trained using the SOM determines the amount of information transmitted from input to output following training (Ritter and Schulten 1986; Villmann and Claussen 2006). Here we will explore how the cooperative component of the SOM can substantially increase input–output information transmission in the presence of input background activity. This ability is neurobiologically significant, because most of the sensory inputs to real brain maps have substantial spontaneous background activity. While maps are formed by the cooperative component of the SOM, our examples will suggest that information acquisition, and not map formation, is the real purpose of cooperation in the activity-dependent processes that produce map-like neural representations.

The two-layered network we will study in this section will serve as a model of a real neural structure. The feedforward network has 20 (or more) input units and 30 output units, as shown in Figure 8.7. The linear array of input units constitutes a one-dimensional representation of the visual environment. The environment is stochastic in that targets appear at random locations within it. The linear array of output units represents a one-dimensional version of the superior colliculus. The function of the superior colliculus is to detect and localize the targets of orienting movements such as saccadic eye movements (Wurtz and Goldberg 1989). We will use the SOM algorithm to train the network on input patterns that encode targets at various locations, and then measure the amount of target information contained in the resulting output representation. Casting the network as a model of a real neural structure with a well-described function will also allow us to assess the information content of the network in terms of the operational objectives of that structure. Specifically, we will quantify the results of SOM training both descriptively, in terms of input–output mutual information, and functionally, in terms of the probability of error in localizing targets. Thus, we will ascribe meaning to the information contained in the output layer.

The target can appear anywhere within the simulated environment with uniform probability. Target location is encoded by the input units using a spatial code, and there is one input unit at each potential target location. When the target appears at a given location, it drives the input at the corresponding location, and a number of input units on either side of that location according to the input spatial tuning field. (The spatial tuning field accounts for the receptive fields of real visual sensory neurons, as described in Chapter 3.) The input units that are driven by the target take value 1. The input units that are not driven by the target have nonzero, spontaneous background activity.

The script `infoSOMbackground`, listed in MATLAB Box 8.5, will train a SOM network on this input. The background is specified by variable `bg`,

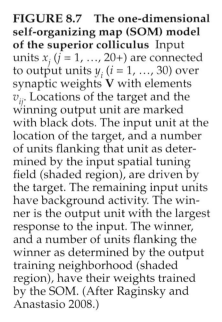

FIGURE 8.7 The one-dimensional self-organizing map (SOM) model of the superior colliculus Input units x_j (j = 1, ..., 20+) are connected to output units y_i (i = 1, ..., 30) over synaptic weights **V** with elements v_{ij}. Locations of the target and the winning output unit are marked with black dots. The input unit at the location of the target, and a number of units flanking that unit as determined by the input spatial tuning field (shaded region), are driven by the target. The remaining input units have background activity. The winner is the output unit with the largest response to the input. The winner, and a number of units flanking the winner as determined by the output training neighborhood (shaded region), have their weights trained by the SOM. (After Raginsky and Anastasio 2008.)

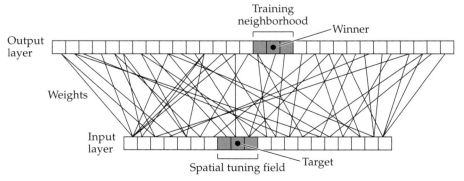

and the input background is set using `x=ones(nIn,1)*bg` were `nIn` is the number of input units. The input spatial tuning field is specified by variable `stf`. When `stf=0`, only the input unit at the location corresponding to the target is driven. When `stf=1`, the input unit at the corresponding location and the flanking input unit on either side are driven. Actually, to simplify programming of script `infoSOMbackground`, there is an offset of one unit in the input representation of the target. Specifically, on each training cycle, the target location (target position `rTpos`) is chosen uniformly at random using

MATLAB® BOX 8.5 This script trains a self-organizing map network and finds informational measures, including estimated distortion, following training.

```
% infoSOMbackground.m

nX=20; % set the number of input states
stf=1; % set the input spatial tuning field
nIn=nX+stf*2; % find the number of input units
nOut=30; % set the number of output units
bg=0.1; % set the input background rate
nHood=0; % set neighborhood size for SOM
a=1; nIts=1000; % set learning rate and iterations for SOM
V=rand(nOut,nIn); % randomize connectivity matrix
for i=1:nOut, V(i,:)=V(i,:)/norm(V(i,:)); end % normalize V

for c=1:nIts, % for each SOM training iteration
    x=ones(nIn,1)*bg; % set the input background activity
    rTpos=ceil(rand*nX); % choose a target location at random
    x(rTpos:rTpos+stf*2)=ones(stf*2+1,1); % set input driven activity
    y=V*x; % compute the output vector
    [winVal winIndx]=max(y); % find the winning output response
    fn=winIndx-nHood; % set the first neighbor for SOM training
    ln=winIndx+nHood; % set the last neighbor for SOM training
    if fn < 1, fn=1; end, % keep the first neighbor in bounds
    if ln > nOut, ln=nOut; end, % keep last neighbor in bounds
    for h=fn:ln, % for each output unit in neighborhood
        hld=V(h,:)+a*x'; % update its weight vector
        V(h,:)=hld/norm(hld); % normalize weight vector
    end % end neighborhood loop
end % end training loop

condi=zeros(nOut,nX); % zero the conditional probability table
for s=1:nX, % for each input state
    x=ones(nIn,1)*bg; % set the input background activity
    x(s:s+stf*2)=ones(stf*2+1,1); % set input driven activity
    y=V*x; % compute the output vector
    y=double(y==max(y)); % find the winning outputs
    condi(:,s)=y/sum(y); % share conditional prob among winners
end % end loop for finding conditional probability table
[maxprob,pref]=max(condi); % find preferred inputs for each output
pX=ones(nX,1)/nX; % find the (uniform) input probability
[hX hY mi]=infoCOMP(pX,condi) % find informational measures
% estimate distortion
d=fsolve(@(d)log2(nX)+d*log2(d)+(1-d)*log2(1-d)-d*log2(nX-1)-mi,...
    [0.5],optimset('Display','off')); d=real(d);
```

`rTpos=ceil(rand*nX)`, where `nX` is the number of input states, which is equal to the number of target locations. Then the input is generated using `x(rTpos:rTpos+stf*2)=ones(stf*2+1,1)`. The one-unit offset has no effect on the network behavior we are simulating in this example. The variously generated input vectors x will constitute the input patterns that the SOM will train the network to represent.

To take account of spatial tuning field `stf`, the number of input units `nIn` must be larger than the number of target locations (or number of input states `nX`), and specifically `nIn=nX+stf*2`. Since the input state (target location) probability distribution is uniform it is found using `pX=ones(nX,1)/nX`. Because the input probability distribution is uniform, input entropy could be computed according to Equation 8.4 using `hX=log2(nX)`, but in `infoSOMbackground` it will be computed, along with the other informational measures, using function `infoCOMP`.

Script `infoSOMbackground` will use the SOM to train the superior colliculus model with learning rate a and neighborhood size `nHood` according to the same procedures as in Chapter 5 (see MATLAB Box 5.1). The only exception is that the initially randomized connectivity matrix `V=rand(nOut,nIn)` will be normalized before training using the following loop: `for i=1:nOut, V(i,:)=V(i,:)/norm(V(i,:)); end`, where `nOut` is the number of output units. (Normalizing the initially random connectivity matrices makes the results in this section more consistent.) The spatial tuning field, which determines whether or not the input patterns overlap, together with the training neighborhood size will determine whether or not the SOM is able to form a map of the input at the output. The training neighborhood size and the level of input background activity will both have important consequences for the ability of the SOM to increase information transfer in the model.

The output is modeled as winner-take-all, and this process is implemented directly by finding the responses of the output units to the input and simply choosing the output unit having the maximal response. (We could use recurrent connections dynamically to produce the winner as in Chapter 3, but we will omit this step for simplicity.) Because the output is modeled as winner-take-all, the only allowed output states are those in which a single output unit takes value 1, and the rest take value 0. This form of output simplifies the computation of information transfer, because the output can only have as many states as there are output units. Thus, variable `nOut` is the number both of output units and output states in `infoSOMbackground`.

The input is similarly simple. Regardless of the spatial tuning field, the number of input states equals the number of possible target locations, which is specified in variable `nX` in `infoSOMbackground`. Because the conditional probability table for a neural network has numbers of rows and columns equal to the numbers of output and input states, respectively, the conditional probability table for the colliculus model will have `nOut=30` rows and `nX=20` columns. With 20 input states and 30 possible output states, the network has more than enough potential output states to use to represent the input. The extent to which it actually uses them will depend primarily on input background level and training neighborhood size, as we shall see over the course of our simulations.

The computation of the conditional probability table is similar to that in previous examples, except that the winner-take-all output states are simpler. To form the conditional probability table the output of the superior colliculus model, held in output response vector **y**, is computed and processed as follows. (Note that we do not use thresholding in this example.) The responses of the output units to the input pattern **x** at each target location are determined as **y** = **Vx**, and the winner is found. The activation of the winner is set to 1, and the activation of all other output units is set to 0. Because it is possible for more than one output unit to have the maximal response, the output response vector is scaled so that its elements sum to 1. For example, if the maximal response to a given input was shared between two output units, then the processed response vector would have activations of 0.5 for those two output units, and 0s for all others. These processed response vectors indicate which output unit or units will be the winner(s) for each specific input state. Because the only allowed output states are winner-take-all states, each element of the response vector corresponds to an output state, so the processed response vectors are the conditional probabilities of all the output states given each input state. The processed response vectors (conditional probability distributions), one for each input state, are inserted as columns into the conditional probability table.

In script `infoSOMbackground`, construction of the conditional probability table is carried out as follows. The output vector is computed using `y=Vx` and the winner(s) are found using `y=double(y==max(y))`. The output vector is scaled (in case there is more than one winner) and inserted as a column of the conditional probability table using `condi(:,s)=y/sum(y)`, where s indexes the space units in the one-dimensional environment and so also indexes the input states (target locations). Again, each column of the conditional probability table can have more than one nonzero value.

Because two or more output units can probabilistically share the winning response, the network in this case is not always deterministic. The conditional probability table and the input probability distribution are used as before to compute the input and output entropies, and the input–output mutual information (using `infoCOMP`, which is called from `infoSOMbackground`). Because the network is not always deterministic, the mutual information will not always equal output entropy. Information transfer is maximal when the network assigns a unique output state to each target state. Whether it does or not depends on input background activity, and on the neighborhood employed for SOM training.

The inputs in this example spatially encode target location, and the outputs encode target location in terms of the identity of the winning output unit, so the quantity of interest is the mutual information $I(T;W)$ between the target T and the winning output unit W. Note that, since the target determines the input state, the input state and target location are equivalent, and $H(X)$ is the entropy both of the input and the target: $H(T) = H(X)$. Also, since the output is winner-take-all, the location of the winner and the output state are equivalent, and $H(Y)$ is the entropy both of the output and the winner: $H(W) = H(Y)$. Because of the equivalences between target location and input state, and between output state and winner, the input–output mutual information $I(X;Y)$ is the same as the target–winner mutual information $I(T;W)$, so we can use $I(T;W)$ and $I(X;Y)$ interchangeably. Thus, script `infoSOMbackground`, using the command `[hX hY mi]=infoCOMP(pX,condi)`, computes `hX` [equivalent to $H(X)$ or $H(T)$], `hY` [equivalent to $H(Y)$ or $H(W)$] and mutual information `mi` [equivalent to $I(X;Y)$ or $I(T;W)$]. Using $I(T;W)$ to denote mutual information in this model emphasizes the relationship between the winner and the target and focuses attention on the operational objectives of the network.

To assess the functional significance of this information, we will use $I(T;W)$ to compute the distortion D_0, which is the probability of error in determining the location of the target given the identity of the winning output unit. The distortion D_0 can be computed from the mutual information $I(T;W)$ by solving Equation 8.21 for D_0 (see Math Box 8.2 for details):

$$I(T;W) = \log_2(n) + D_0 \log_2(D_0) + (1 - D_0)\log_2(1 - D_0) - D_0 \log_2(n - 1) \quad \textbf{8.21}$$

MATH BOX 8.2 RATE-DISTORTION THEORY

The information rate of a channel is the amount of information transmitted with each use of the channel. We can think of a neural network as a channel that transmits information from its input to its output. Rate-distortion theory (Berger 1971) relates informational measures like entropy and mutual information to the operational characteristics of information-processing systems such as neural networks. It thereby endows the information being processed with "meaning."

The basic object of rate-distortion theory is the rate-distortion function of an information source. Let T ("target") be a random variable taking specific values t_S in Γ and distributed according to $P(T)$ [shorthand for $P(T = t_S)$]. Define the distortion measure by Equation B8.2.1:

$$d(t_S, \tilde{t}_S) = \begin{cases} 0, & t_S = \tilde{t}_S \\ 1, & t_S \neq \tilde{t}_S \end{cases}$$ B8.2.1

We can think of $\tilde{t}_S$ as a version of t_S that we want to be as similar to t_S as possible. Let $\tilde{T}$ be a random variable taking values $\tilde{t}_S$ in Γ and related to T via conditional probability $P(\tilde{T} \mid T)$. Then the expected value of $d(T, \tilde{T})$ is the probability that $T \neq \tilde{T}$, as shown in Equation B8.2.2:

$$E_{T,\tilde{T}}\left[d(T,\tilde{T})\right] = \sum_T \sum_{\tilde{T}} P(T)P(\tilde{T} \mid T)d(T,\tilde{T}) = \sum_T \sum_{\tilde{T} \neq T} P(T)P(\tilde{T} \mid T) \equiv P(T \neq \tilde{T})$$ B8.2.2

where $E[\cdot]$ is the expectation operator so $E_{T,\tilde{T}}[d(T,\tilde{T})]$ is the mean value of $d(T,\tilde{T})$. The rate-distortion function $R(D)$ of T is defined (Equation B8.2.3) as the minimum amount of mutual information between T and $\tilde{T}$ required to reproduce T by $\tilde{T}$ with probability of error at most D:

$$R(D) = \min_{P(\tilde{T} \mid T)} \left\{ I(T;\tilde{T}) : E_{T,\tilde{T}}[d(T,\tilde{T})] \leq D \right\}$$ B8.2.3

where the minimum is over all conditional probability distributions $P(\tilde{T} \mid T)$ satisfying $E_{T,\tilde{T}}[d(T,\tilde{T})] \leq D$. A typical rate-distortion function is illustrated in Figure B8.2.1.

Now suppose that we do not have direct access to $\tilde{T}$, but instead observe another random variable W ("winner") that is related to T via conditional probability $Q(W \mid T)$. We can think of Q as an information transmitting channel that accepts T as input and emits W as output with conditional probability $Q(W \mid T)$, and we must use W to estimate T. According to rate-distortion theory, the quality of our estimate is limited by the maximum amount of information that can be transmitted over channel Q regardless of the statistics of the input T. This is given in Equation B8.2.4 by the absolute channel capacity:

$$C(Q) = \max_{P(T)} I(T;W)$$ B8.2.4

Methods for estimating the absolute channel capacity $C(Q)$ over all possible distributions $P(T)$ will not be considered here. Instead, we will simply approximate $C(Q)$ as the $I(T;W)$ we measure for the uniform $P(T)$ we use in our simulations. Then the rate $R(D_0)$ at which the channel can transmit information with distortion D_0 is equal to the channel capacity $C(Q)$. Given our approximation for $C(Q)$, $R(D_0) = C(Q) = I(T;W)$.

(Continued on facing page)

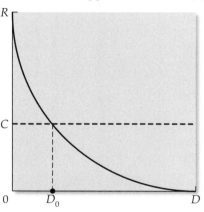

FIGURE B8.2.1 A typical rate-distortion curve The curve shows the rate R at which a channel would have to transmit information in order to recover the input from the output with distortion D, which is the probability of error in the recovering the input. The horizontal line corresponds to the capacity C of a transmission channel. In our case the channel is a neural network model of the superior colliculus that transmits target information from its input to its output. The distortion level D_0 at which $R(D_0) = C$ is the probability that the identity of the winning output unit incorrectly indicates the location of the target. The capacity C of the colliculus model is the target-winner mutual information $I(T;W)$. (After Raginsky and Anastasio 2008.)

MATH BOX 8.2   (continued)

A uniformly distributed input source, such as the target T used in the self-organizing map model of the superior colliculus (see Section 8.5), has probabilities $P(T=t_S) = 1/n$ for all $t_S = 1, \ldots, n$. The rate-distortion function for a uniform source is given in Equation B8.2.5

$$R(D) = \begin{cases} \log_2(n) - H(D) - D\log_2(n-1), & 0 \le D \le 1 - 1/n \\ 0, & D > 1 - 1/n \end{cases} \qquad \text{B8.2.5}$$

Equation B8.2.5 specifies the rate $R(D)$ by which we would need to transmit information in order to recover t_S with probability of error at most D, for error probabilities at or less than $1 - 1/n$. Because t_S appears uniformly with probability $1/n$, no information is required to estimate t_S with probability of error greater than $1 - 1/n$, so $R(D) = 0$ for $D > 1 - 1/n$. Note that D is a binary random variable, so its entropy is $H(D) = -D\log_2(D) - (1 - D)\log_2(1 - D)$. Thus, for the superior colliculus model, we measure $I(T;W)$ and solve Equation B8.2.6 to find the distortion D_0:

$$R(D_0) = I(T;W) = \log_2(n) + D_0 \log_2(D_0) + (1 - D_0)\log_2(1 - D_0) - D_0 \log_2(n - 1) \qquad \text{B8.2.6}$$

If T is target location and W is the location of the winning output unit in the self-organizing map network model of the superior colliculus, then D_0 is the probability of error in recovering T from W, given mutual information $I(T;W)$. The measure D_0 gives us an indication of the usefulness or "meaning" of the information $I(T;W)$ in terms of the operational characteristics of the self-organizing map model of the colliculus. Equation B8.2.6 corresponds to Equation 8.21 of the main text.

where n is the number of possible target states. Because Equation 8.21 would be difficult to solve using standard algebra, script `infoSOMbackground` estimates the value of D_0 using the MATLAB function solver `fsolve`. The script also determines which output unit wins the competition for each target state and stores it in vector `pref`. (In the case of a tie it chooses the output unit with the lowest index.)

We will examine representative instances of the model. The specific results depend on the initially random connectivity matrix, and on the random locations of the target during training. For each case, SOM training occurs with learning rate 1 (a=1) for 1000 iterations (nIts=1000). Following training we will use vector `pref` to construct a target–winner table. (Note that this is not the same as the conditional probability table.) The target–winner table has 2 rows and 20 columns, where each cell in the first row is marked with a target location (input state) from 1 to 20, while each cell in the second row is marked with the number of the output unit that responds best to the target location specified in the row above. We will use the target–winner table to gauge information transmission, in terms of the number of states the output uses to represent the input (target location), and to gauge map formation, in terms of the spatial arrangement of the winning output units. The target–winner tables for all cases are shown in Table 8.5. We will compare mutual target–winner information $I(T;W)$ with target entropy $H(T)$ to assess the target information content of the output, as encoded by the identity of the winning output unit. The target, which appears uniformly at random at the $n = 20$ locations, has information content (entropy) $H(T) = \log_2(20) = 4.32$ bits. We will also assess the functional significance (or meaning) of information $I(T;W)$ in terms of the distortion D_0.

Our simulations in this section will consist of a series of three comparisons. In each case we will hold the input background and spatial tuning field at set values, and will compare mutual information and distortion in networks trained either using purely competitive learning (for which the neighborhood size is 0) or using combined competitive-cooperative learning (for which the neighborhood size will be 1). (To simplify our discussion we will consider all

TABLE 8.5   Maps of the winning output unit (*W*) for each target location (*T*) in one-dimensional neural network models of the superior colliculus

(A) Input background 0.1, spatial tuning field 1, and output training neighborhood 0

T	1	2	3	4	5	6	7	8	9	10	11	12	13	14	15	16	17	18	19	20
W	4	4	5	5	10	30	30	22	22	12	12	26	26	9	9	6	6	17	2	2

(B) Input background 0.1, spatial tuning field 1, and output training neighborhood 1

T	1	2	3	4	5	6	7	8	9	10	11	12	13	14	15	16	17	18	19	20
W	22	21	30	30	28	26	24	14	16	17	18	19	13	11	9	8	1	2	4	6

(C) Input background 0.9, spatial tuning field 1, and output training neighborhood 0

T	1	2	3	4	5	6	7	8	9	10	11	12	13	14	15	16	17	18	19	20
W	16	16	16	16	16	16	16	16	16	16	16	16	16	16	16	16	16	16	16	16

(D) Input background 0.9, spatial tuning field 1, and output training neighborhood 1

T	1	2	3	4	5	6	7	8	9	10	11	12	13	14	15	16	17	18	19	20
W	12	11	9	8	6	4	2	14	16	18	18	19	20	22	24	25	27	28	29	30

(E) Input background 0.9, spatial tuning field 0, and output training neighborhood 0

T	1	2	3	4	5	6	7	8	9	10	11	12	13	14	15	16	17	18	19	20
W	20	20	20	20	20	20	20	20	20	20	20	20	20	20	20	20	20	20	20	20

(F) Input background 0.9, spatial tuning field 0, and output training neighborhood 1

T	1	2	3	4	5	6	7	8	9	10	11	12	13	14	15	16	17	18	19	20
W	8	8	8	9	30	18	20	26	14	8	8	8	16	26	22	28	7	12	8	24

The one-dimensional models of the superior colliculus, with various combinations of input background activity level, input spatial tuning field, and output training neighborhood size, were trained using the self-organizing map algorithm. These results are representative of those obtained for each of the parameter combinations. The specific results depend on the initially random state of the connectivity matrix, and on the random locations of the target during training.

learning using `infoSOMbackground` as SOM learning, regardless of training neighborhood size or spatial tuning field.) We will begin our exploration of this network by assigning a low value for input background activity of 0.1 (`bg=0.1`) and an input spatial tuning field of 1 (`stf=1`). For purely competitive training we set a neighborhood size of 0 (`nHood=0`). Following training, the target–winner table (see Table 8.5A) for this case shows that the winner-take-all output uses 11 of its possible 30 states to represent the target. Since there are 20 input (target) states, we know without computing mutual information that the output does not contain complete target information. The actual mutual information of 3.42 bits is indeed lower than the target entropy of 4.32 bits. However, in terms of the operational objectives of the network, this amount of mutual information is substantial, because the distortion D_0, which is the probability of error in using the output to localize the target, is only 0.10 in this case. Thus, with low background activity, the algorithm without its cooperative component (no neighbor training) is able to meaningfully increase input–output (target–winner) mutual information. This increase occurs by virtue of the competitive component, which promotes specialization of output unit responses. The outputs do not form a map of target location, but are ordered randomly with respect to target location. This is expected because no neighbors are trained.

Keeping the other parameters the same, we change the neighborhood size to 1 (nHood=1) and retrain the network. In this case (see Table 8.5B) it uses 19 of its possible 30 states to represent the target. Mutual information has increased to 4.22 bits, so the output contains almost complete target information. Distortion correspondingly decreases to 0.01, so the probability of error in localizing the target is practically 0. The outputs are not ordered randomly, but form a fractured map of target location. The network has developed the following five map-lets: 22–21, 30–24, 14–19, 13–8, and 1–6. The map-lets are ordered randomly, but target location changes smoothly within each. (The progression within a map-let will sometimes skip a unit.) The formation of the fractured map is the result of cooperative neighbor training (nonzero neighborhood size), and a nonzero spatial tuning field. (Fracturing could be avoided with larger spatial tuning fields; see Raginsky and Anastasio 2008.)

We now repeat the comparison between networks trained with neighborhood sizes of 0 and 1 using a high input background level of 0.9 (bg=0.9). The input spatial tuning field is again set to 1 (stf=1). Following training with a neighborhood size of 0 (nHood=0), the output uses only 1 of its 30 possible states to represent the input (see Table 8.5C). The output in this case does not distinguish between any of the different target locations. It is completely uninformative. Target–winner mutual information is 0, and distortion is essentially 1 (maximal). Thus, with neighborhood size 0, the high background activity has completely eliminated the ability of the competitive component to increase input–output information transmission in the network. As expected, with training neighborhood size 0, the network does not form a map of target location. Cooperative neighbor training dramatically changes this situation.

Following training with a neighborhood size of 1 (nHood=1), input spatial tuning field of 1 (stf=1), and a high background level of 0.9 (bg=0.9), the output uses 19 of 30 possible states to represent the target (see Table 8.5D). It forms a fractured map of target location with two map-lets, 12–2 and 14–30, in which target location changes smoothly. Target–winner mutual information jumps back up to 4.22 bits, and distortion jumps back down to 0.01. Thus, with neighbor training, mutual information is high and distortion is low, regardless of whether input background activity is high or low. The results indicate that cooperative training is more important when the input has a higher value of spontaneous background activity.

Map formation in SOM networks requires both output neighbor training and overlap among the input vectors (see Chapter 5 for a detailed exploration of map formation). In these target–localization networks, overlap between input vectors depends on a nonzero spatial tuning field. We expect map formation only when both the input spatial tuning field and the output training neighborhood are nonzero. By setting the input spatial tuning field to 0, we can explore the ability of cooperative mechanisms to increase information transmission even when no map can form.

We begin by setting the spatial tuning field to 0 (stf=0), the background to a high level (bg=0.9), and the neighborhood size to 0 (nHood=0). No map forms following this purely competitive training, as expected, and the output uses only 1 of 30 possible states to represent the input (see Table 8.5E). The target–winner mutual information is 0, and the distortion is essentially 1 (maximal). This situation is again dramatically altered by cooperative training. When trained with a neighborhood size of 1 (nHood=1), the output uses 13 of 30 possible states to represent the target (see Table 8.5F). The target–winner mutual information is 3.24 bits, and this amount of information is meaningful because the distortion is only 0.13. These considerable improvements in information transmission and target localization, brought about by training neighbors, have occurred in the absence of map formation (see Table 8.5F).

The results show that the cooperative component of SOM training is able to increase input–output mutual information even when it does not produce a feature map. (We use the term SOM to refer to training using Equations 8.17–8.19 even in cases where no map can form.) This increase in information transmission is meaningful because the distortion, which is the probability of incorrectly localizing the target given the identity of the winning output unit, decreases by nearly an order of magnitude (from essentially 1 to only 0.13) with neighbor training. The reason that neighbor training improves information transmission even with zero spatial tuning, and with the consequent absence of map formation, has to do with the nature of the input vectors when the input spontaneous background activity is close to the level of the driven activity.

When the background activity is close to the driven activity (for example, when background and driven activities are 0.9 and 1, respectively), all of the elements of the input vectors take nearly the same value, regardless of the location of the target. An output unit with the elements of its initially random input weight vector all nearly equal (a "flat" weight vector) will respond well to the input, regardless of target location. The output unit with the flattest initially random input weight vector (compared with the other output units) will win the competition for the first input, no matter the target location. Self-organizing map (SOM) training without neighbors will cause that output unit (and only that unit) to flatten its weight vector even further (i.e., make the elements of its weight vector even more nearly equal). This will make the winner even more likely to respond best to any input, regardless of target location. With high input background rate, SOM training without neighbors can result in one output unit (or a few) winning the competition for all the inputs. Information transfer is low because the output uses only one (or only a few) of its potential states to represent the target. Distortion (probability of error) is correspondingly high.

SOM training with neighbors changes this situation. Now the neighbors as well as the winner flatten their weight vectors. Since the initially random weight vectors are unlikely to be the same, training the neighbors makes them more sensitive to inputs with high background levels, and possibly also more sensitive than the winner to inputs with different target locations. The result is that the neighbors will likely be more sensitive than the previous winner to an input encoding a different target location, and the network ends up using more of its potential states to encode target location. This occurs regardless of whether or not the inputs have a nonzero spatial tuning field. If the input spatial tuning field is nonzero, then a map is formed, but information transmission is improved by cooperatively training neighbors in either case.

The deleterious effect of input background activity on information transmission in networks trained with competitive mechanisms, but without cooperative mechanisms, is also evident at intermediate background levels (i.e., between 0.1 and 0.9) as shown in Figure 8.8. When the input deterministically encodes the target, as in the examples in this section and in the simulations described in Figure 8.8, networks trained without the cooperative component (no neighbors) cannot transmit a meaningful amount of information at background levels higher than about 0.4, but can transmit meaningful information at lower background levels. However, when the input stochastically encodes target location, which is the more realistic scenario, the deleterious effect of input background on information transmission in networks trained without the cooperative component is observed at all levels of background activity (for details see Raginsky and Anastasio 2008).

In the real nervous system, input neurons have nonzero spatial tuning fields (see Chapter 3). They also have nonzero spontaneous background activities (see Chapter 2). Despite the nonzero input background activity, an SOM-type mechanism that includes a cooperative component and that operates on these

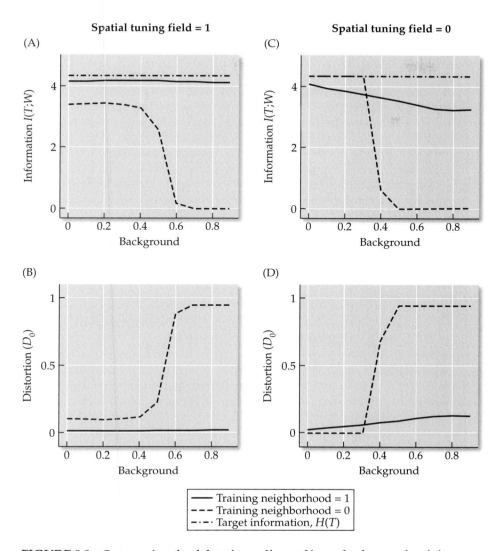

FIGURE 8.8 Overcoming the deleterious effects of input background activity on information transmission in the one-dimensional SOM model of the superior colliculus Neighbor training increases mutual information $I(T;W)$ and decreases distortion D_0 over a broad range of input background activity levels. The input spatial tuning field is either 1 (A and B) or 0 (C and D). Training neighborhood size is either 1 (solid lines) or 0 (dashed lines). With input spatial tuning 1 and neighborhood size 1, mutual information (A) is nearly maximal (i.e., nearly equal to target information $H(T)$, dot-dashed lines), and distortion (B) is nearly minimal (i.e., 0), over the entire range of input background activities. With neighborhood size 0, mutual information (A) is slightly lower, and distortion (B) slightly higher for backgrounds less than 0.4, but mutual information rapidly decreases, and distortion rapidly increases, for backgrounds greater than 0.4. With input spatial tuning 0 and neighborhood size 0, mutual information (C) is nearly maximal, and distortion (D) is nearly minimal for backgrounds less than 0.3, but mutual information rapidly decreases, and distortion rapidly increases, for backgrounds greater than 0.3. With neighborhood size 1, mutual information starts out high and decreases gradually, and distortion starts out low and increases gradually, as backgrounds increase over the range. The plots are averages over 100 simulations. (After Raginsky and Anastasio 2008.)

inputs would increase the amount of information contained in the output neuron representation. Because of the nonzero spatial tuning field, the SOM-type mechanism would also produce an output map of the feature space encoded by the inputs, but a map-like structure is not essential to the ability of the output to contain input information. As we saw in this and previous sections, the ability of the output units of a neural network to contain information about its input depends on the number of states that the output uses to represent the input, not on the particular spatial arrangement of the output units in the network. From a purely informational viewpoint, there is no requirement that the output units be organized spatially with regard to input features. The modeling results in this section suggest that map formation is incidental to the real function of the cooperative component of activity-dependent, SOM-type learning mechanisms. By promoting the full participation of all output neurons in a network, which increases the number of output states available to represent the input, the function of the cooperative component, instead of map formation, may be to increase input-output mutual information in the presence of input background activity.

8.6 Information Transmission in Stochastic Neural Networks

As we have seen so far in this chapter, a deterministic neural network is potentially capable of extracting complete information from its inputs with an output that has as many states as the input. A deterministic network is one in which a specific input always produces the same output. Real neurons, in contrast, are stochastic, in that their responses to the same input can vary randomly. Despite the "unreliability" of the responses of real neurons, they are still capable of adequately encoding their inputs. The possibility of constructing a "reliable" brain from "unreliable" neurons was suggested early on by the famous mathematician John von Neumann (1958). The key is population coding, in which one input signal is encoded by many unreliable output neurons, and the more unreliable they are the more of them are needed (Oram et al. 1998). Put in terms of information transmission, a stochastic network generally needs more output states than input states in order for the output to adequately contain input information.

In principle, a sufficiently large number of unreliable output neurons are capable of containing complete input information, provided the output and input are not statistically independent. Thus, even in a stochastic network, input–output mutual information can equal input entropy (Cover and Thomas 1991). The potential ability of a stochastic network to extract and encode complete information from its input underscores the fact that mutual information is an average quantity (see Equation 8.8). In the canonical, neurobiological example of population coding, the individual neuron provides an unreliable indication of the state of the input, but the average over the population provides a more reliable, and possibly completely reliable, indication. More generally, decoding the output of a stochastic network involves the specific relationships between the states of the output and the states of the input, as in deterministic networks. However, due to the variability inherent in the relationship between input and output in a stochastic network, stochastic and deterministic networks differ in the way in which they encode information, and in which information is decoded from them.

A deterministic network can completely encode the information contained in its input by assigning a unique output state to each input state. Such a deterministic output can be decoded directly using a "code book" that specifies

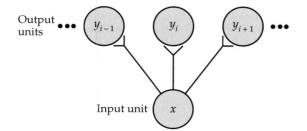

Output units $\cdots$ y_{i-1} y_i y_{i+1} $\cdots$

Input unit x

FIGURE 8.9 One-input/n-output, feedforward network Units are binary. Input unit x projects to output units y_i ($i = 1, \ldots, n$, where n is the number of output units). The connections from x to the y_i are stochastic so that output unit responses depend probabilistically on the input.

which output states correspond to which input states. In contrast, a stochastic network does not assign a unique output state to each input state. Instead, it represents the information contained in its input in terms of the statistical dependency between its output and its input. Such a stochastic output can be decoded probabilistically, by using it to infer the input state given the output state. We will consider probabilistic inference in detail in Chapter 9, where we will also demonstrate the advantages associated with inference (decoding) based on the responses of multiple unreliable neurons. What concerns us here is the ability of a stochastic network with sufficiently many output units to extract and encode input information. This can be illustrated using a network that has one stochastic input unit and an arbitrary number of stochastic output units, as shown in Figure 8.9. (This scheme can be extended to stochastic networks with arbitrarily many input units also.)

The single input unit and the multiple output units in this example are binary. Thus, the input has two states, 0 or 1, and the output has 2^n states, where n is the number of output units. We can set the probability that the input takes value 1 as p_x. Then the probability that the input takes value 0 is $1 - p_x$. The input probability distribution $P(X)$ is $[P(X = 1) = p_x, P(X = 0) = 1 - p_x]$.

The response of a stochastic output unit depends probabilistically on its input. In this example we will not try to model the real, stochastic synaptic connections between neurons. We will not even determine the output responses explicitly. For the purposes of this example we will directly specify the conditional probabilities of the outputs given the input. These conditional probabilities will determine the statistical dependencies between output states Y and input states X. We will use them to construct the conditional probability table. Note that, for a single, binary input unit ($X = X_1$), the conditional probability table will have only two columns, one for input state $X = 0$ and the other for input state $X = 1$. The conditional probability table will have 2^n rows, one for each of the 2^n output states (where n is the number of output units). For simplicity, we assume that the responses of all n output units individually ($Y_i, i = 1, \ldots, n$) have the same conditional probabilities given the input. We further assume that the responses of all n output units are statistically independent of one another.

With these simplifications, we only need to set two individual conditional probabilities. If we specify $P(Y_i = 0 \mid X = 0)$, then $P(Y_i = 1 \mid X = 0) = 1 - P(Y_i = 0 \mid X = 0)$. Similarly, if we specify $P(Y_i = 1 \mid X = 1)$, then $P(Y_i = 0 \mid X = 1) = 1 - P(Y_i = 1 \mid X = 1)$. Note that $[P(Y_i = 0 \mid X = 0), P(Y_i = 1 \mid X = 0)] = P(Y_i \mid X = 0)$ is the conditional probability distribution for Y_i given $X = 0$. Similarly, $[P(Y_i = 0 \mid X = 1), P(Y_i = 1 \mid X = 1)] = P(Y_i \mid X = 1)$ is the conditional probability distribution for Y_i given $X = 1$. If we have only one binary output unit ($Y = Y_1$), then we have only two output states, $Y = 0$ and $Y = 1$. Since we have only one binary input unit, we have only two input states, $X = 0$ and $X = 1$. In this simplest case, the conditional probability table has only two rows and two columns, and we can construct it by inserting the two conditional probability distributions we defined above as its two columns.

TABLE 8.6 Conditional and joint probability tables for stochastic, feedforward networks with one binary input unit and either one or two binary output units

(A) One binary input unit and one binary output unit

Conditional probability		Input X (0)	(1)	Joint probability		Input X (0)	(1)
Output Y	(0)	0.8	0.2	Output Y	(0)	0.4	0.1
	(1)	0.2	0.8		(1)	0.1	0.4

(B) One binary input unit and two binary output units

Conditional probability		Input X (0)	(1)	Joint probability		Input X (0)	(1)
Output Y	(0, 0)	0.64	0.04	Output Y	(0, 0)	0.32	0.02
	(1, 0)	0.16	0.16		(1, 0)	0.08	0.08
	(0, 1)	0.16	0.16		(0, 1)	0.08	0.08
	(1, 1)	0.04	0.64		(1, 1)	0.02	0.32

The conditional probability table for one binary output unit $Y = Y_1$, where $P(Y_i = 0 \mid X = 0) = 0.8$ and $P(Y_i = 1 \mid X = 1) = 0.8$, is shown in Table 8.6A. The input distribution $P(X)$ is used to convert the conditional probability table to the joint probability distribution, as before. To obtain the joint distribution, we multiply each column of the conditional probability table by the corresponding input probability. For example, the joint probability distribution $P(X,Y)$ for output Y as defined above and binary input X, where $P(X = 1) = p_x = 0.5$ (and $P(X = 0) = 1 - p_x = 0.5$), is also shown in Table 8.6A. The marginal distribution $P(Y)$ is computed from the joint distribution by summing its rows. Then the mutual information $I(X;Y)$ is computed from $P(X)$, $P(Y)$, and $P(X,Y)$ using Equation 8.8, as before.

If we have $n = 2$ output units, then we need to specify the conditional probabilities of all $2^n = 4$ output states given each of the two input states ($X = 0$ and $X = 1$). As stated above, we assume that the output units are statistically independent of one another. Then the conditional probability distribution of all of the output states can be computed by finding all possible products of the entries of the conditional probability distributions for each output unit individually, given the same input state. For example, if we have two binary output units Y_1 and Y_2, and their activities are independent of one another, then the conditional probability $P(Y_1 = 0, Y_2 = 0 \mid X = 0)$ equals the product $P(Y_1 = 0 \mid X = 0) P(Y_2 = 0 \mid X = 0)$, and so on for the other three output states given $X = 0$. The conditional probability distribution for the four possible output states given $X = 1$ is found similarly. The conditional probability table for two binary output units $Y = (Y_1, Y_2)$ where $P(Y_i = 0 \mid X = 0) = 0.8$ and $P(Y_i = 1 \mid X = 1) = 0.8$, ($i = 1, 2$) is shown in Table 8.6B. As before, the input distribution $P(X)$ is used to convert the conditional probability table to the joint distribution $P(X,Y)$. Table 8.6B also shows the joint distribution for this dual output when the single binary input X has $P(X = 1) = p_x = 0.5$ (and $P(X = 0) = 1 - p_x = 0.5$). The marginal (output) distribution $P(Y)$ is computed from the joint probability distribution, and the mutual information $I(X;Y)$ is computed from $P(X)$, $P(Y)$, and $P(X,Y)$ using Equation 8.8, as before.

This process is extended for more than two statistically independent output units $Y = (Y_1, \ldots, Y_n)$. For any number of output units n, the conditional prob-

MATLAB® BOX 8.6   This script computes informational measures for a stochastic network of binary units with one input unit and arbitrarily many output units.

```
% info1byN.m

nOut=1; % set the number of output units
px1=0.9; % set probability that input unit is 1
px0=1-px1; % find probability that input unit is 0
py0x0=0.9; % set conditional prob of output 0 given input 0
py1x1=0.9; % set conditional prob of output 1 given input 1
py1x0=1-py0x0; % find conditional prob of output 1 given input 0
py0x1=1-py1x1; % find conditional prob of output 0 given input 1

% find the conditional probability of output given input
nY=2^nOut; % compute number of output states
pyx0=1; % start off prob y given x0 vector at 1
pyx1=1; % start off prob y given x1 vector at 1
for i=1:nOut, % for as many iterations as output units
    pyx0=kron([py0x0 py1x0],pyx0); % kronecker for x0
    pyx1=kron([py0x1 py1x1],pyx1); % kronecker for x1
end  % end loop for conditional output given input probability
condi=[pyx0' pyx1']; % assemble conditional probability table

% compute input probability distribution and info measures
pX=[px0;px1]; % assemble input probability distribution
[hX hY mi]=infoCOMP(pX,condi); % find info measures
```

ability distribution of all of the 2^n output states can be computed by finding all possible products of the entries of the conditional probability distributions of each output unit individually, given either input state. The conditional probability distributions for all output states given either input state are then inserted as the columns of the conditional probability table. These conditional probability tables will all have two columns, one for $X = 0$ and another for $X = 1$, and 2^n rows where n is the number of binary output units and 2^n is the total number of binary output states. The conditional probability table is converted to the joint probability distribution using the input probability distribution, and the input, output, and joint distributions are used to compute the mutual information between the input and output, as before.

The script info1byN, listed in MATLAB Box 8.6, will compute the conditional probability table for any number of binary, stochastic, independent output units, given the same conditional probabilities of each output given the input, and will compute the input–output mutual information for the network, given a probability distribution for the single, binary, stochastic input unit. In script info1byN, the probability that the single input unit takes value 1 is held in variable px1, while the conditional probabilities that each output unit takes value 0 given input 0, or takes value 1 given input 1, are held in variables py0x0 and py1x1, respectively. It finds the complimentary conditional probabilities using py1x0=1−py0x0 and py0x1=1−py1x1. Then the conditional probability distribution for all of the binary output states given input state zero (pyx0) is computed using a loop over all nOut output units with the command pyx0=kron([py0x0 py1x0],pyx0) at each step. The conditional probability distribution for all of the output states given input state one (pyx1) is computed in the same loop using pyx1=kron([py0x1 py1x1], pyx1) at each step. The conditional probability table is then constructed using condi=[pyx0' pyx1']. The script stores the number of output states (2^n) in variable nY.

The goal of the example in this section is to use info1by N to show how a neural network can represent the information content of its input despite the stochasticity of its output units. Set the input probability to $p_x = 0.9$, and also set the conditional probabilities of the output units given the input to $P(Y_i = 0 \mid X = 0) = 0.9$ and $P(Y_i = 1 \mid X = 1) = 0.9$. These parameters are set in script info1byN using px1=0.9, py0x0=0.9, and py1x1=0.9. The script constructs condi as described above. It finds the complementary input probability using px0=1- px1, and assembles the input probability distribution using pX=[px0;px1]. Script info1byN then uses [hX hY mi]=infoCOMP(pX,condi) to compute the input and output entropy, and the input–output mutual information, as described in Section 8.2.

Begin with a network that has only one output unit by setting nOut=1. When $p_x = 0.9$ the input entropy $H(X)$ (which is the information content of the input) is 0.47 bits. For the network with one output unit and conditional probabilities $P(Y_i = 0 \mid X = 0) = 0.9$ and $P(Y_i = 1 \mid X = 1) = 0.9$, the mutual information $I(X;Y)$ between the inputs and outputs is 0.21 bits. Clearly the output does not contain complete input information in this case. It appears that one stochastic output unit is not enough.

Unlike the deterministic networks we studied in Sections 8.2–8.4, output entropy $H(Y)$ does not equal input–output mutual information $I(X;Y)$ in stochastic networks. For the network with one stochastic output unit, and with input and conditional probabilities as set above, the output entropy $H(Y)$ is 0.68 bits. The output entropy is higher than the input entropy, even though the input–output mutual information is lower. Because the output entropy is the information content of the output, we would expect it to increase as we increase the number of output units. The critical question is whether we can also increase input–output mutual information.

Keeping the input and conditional output probabilities the same, increase the output population to five units (nOut=5). The output entropy $H(Y)$ jumps up to 2.79 bits, and the mutual information $I(X;Y)$ increases to 0.44 bits. The stochastic network with five units contains almost complete input information. Now increase the number of output units to ten (nOut=10). Output entropy jumps up to 5.16 bits, and mutual information increases to 0.47 bits. With a population of ten output units, the input–output mutual information of the stochastic network equals the input information content, but only to two significant places. Further increases in mutual information accompany further increases in the number of output units, and it is possible, in principle, for enough stochastic outputs units to contain complete input information (Cover and Thomas 1991).

Considering the conditional probabilities we set above, $P(Y_i = 0 \mid X = 0) = 0.9$ and $P(Y_i = 1 \mid X = 1) = 0.9$, the output units are fairly "reliable" indicators of input activity. With conditional probabilities of $P(Y_i = 0 \mid X = 0) = 0.5$ and $P(Y_i = 1 \mid X = 1) = 0.5$, the outputs would be completely "unreliable" because their states would be statistically independent from the input states, and input–output mutual information would be zero. However, even very unreliable output units can contain some input information if there are enough of them. To see this, keep the input probability at $p_x = 0.9$, but change the output conditional probabilities to $P(Y_i = 0 \mid X = 0) = 0.6$ and $P(Y_i = 1 \mid X = 1) = 0.6$. With these more unreliable conditional probabilities the entropy of the ten output units rises to 9.81 bits, but mutual information falls to 0.10 bits. Increasing the population of these unreliable outputs to 20 units causes output entropy to increase to 19.60

bits, but mutual information increases to only 0.18 bits. Although they are greater than zero, these amounts of information transfer compare badly with the input information content of 0.47 bits. Without defining the operational objectives of the network, however, it is impossible to quantify the meaning, or usefulness, of this amount of information. Such low rates of information transfer might be adequate for some purposes.

The high levels of output entropy compared with the low levels of mutual information would seem to suggest that these are not low-entropy codes. In this simple example, the amount of output entropy can be decreased by decreasing the number of output units, or by increasing their reliability by moving the conditional probabilities of each output unit closer to $P(Y_i = 0 \mid X = 0) = 1$ and $P(Y_i = 1 \mid X = 1) = 1$ (or equivalently $P(Y_i = 0 \mid X = 0) = 0$ and $P(Y_i = 1 \mid X = 1) = 0$). (Note that the output units will be deterministic, and so completely reliable, with `py0x0=1` and `py1x1=1`, or equivalently with `py0x0=0` and `py1x1=0`, in script `info1byN`.) The responses of post-synaptic neurons to the same pre-synaptic input are known to vary, due to a variety of sources of biophysical noise (e.g., Tommershäuser et al. 2001; Franks et al. 2003). Presumably, there is some biophysical limit to the reliability of synaptic transmission between real neurons. This would limit the extent to which the entropy of individual neurons could be reduced, and would require the recruitment of additional neurons in order to ensure that the output neuron representation contains an adequate amount of input information.

The example in this section demonstrates how the output units of neural systems can contain the information present in their inputs, even when output unit activities bear a probabilistic relationship with input unit activities. When the output units are stochastic, their ability to contain the information present in their inputs depends on how many of them there are. Because the responses of real neurons depend probabilistically on their inputs (e.g., Tommershäuser et al. 2001; Franks et al. 2003), signals are encoded by entire populations of neurons in the brain (Oram et al. 1998). Thus, relatively small numbers of signals are represented by relatively large numbers of neurons, and there are many ways in which the signal components can be distributed among the neurons and still be accurately represented by the population.

The redundancy inherent in representing one or a few signals using an abundance of neurons provides many degrees of freedom for possible representational configurations. For example, if there are two signals, then one half of the population could encode one signal, and the other half could encode the other signal. Equivalently, all of the neurons in the population could encode both signals. What often appears to happen in the brain is that two or more signals are divided up and distributed non-uniformly among the neurons in a population. This leads to the kinds of non-uniform distributed representations that we studied in Chapters 6 and 7. The non-uniform distributed representations observed in many parts of the brain could reflect the need for real neural systems to adequately contain the information from relatively few sources using an abundance of unreliable (i.e., stochastic) neurons.

Distributed representations in the brain can be either topographic (arranged as a map) or non-topographic (no particular arrangement or possibly randomly arranged). As we discussed at the end of Chapter 6, both map-like and non-map distributed representations can be considered non-uniform, because input components are divided up and distributed non-uniformly over the population of neurons in either case. Both types of representation also share the need to contain information. Because of the inherent stochasticity of real neurons, that need can be satisfied only by an abundance of neurons, and the challenge for the formation of both map-like and non-map representations is to ensure the engagement of neurons in adequate numbers.

As we saw in Chapter 5, map-like representations can be formed through unsupervised learning. In Section 8.5 of this chapter, we saw that the cooperative component of the self-organizing map algorithm not only can produce maps but also tends to pull available units into the representation, thereby improving its informational adequacy. As we saw in Chapters 6 and 7, non-map representations can be formed through supervised or reinforcement learning, in which error or reinforcement drives the available units to form an adequate representation. What distinguishes these forms of learning is the presence or absence of a desired output or direct behavioral outcome. We could speculate that the difference in origin between map-like and non-map representations in the brain is that the formation of non-map representations is driven by an error or reinforcement signal, while the formation of map-like representations occurs in the absence of a direct guiding signal. This speculation is admittedly broad and would be difficult to test experimentally, but it provides a unifying framework for various learning mechanisms and the representations they form, and is based on the common need for neural representations to adequately contain information.

Exercises

8.1   In exploring the ability of deterministic, 2-by-2 feedforward networks of binary threshold units with various connectivity matrices to transmit information, we set the probabilities that the input units would take value 1 at 0.8 and 0.7 for input units X_1 and X_2, respectively. (The probabilities of value 0 were therefore 0.2 and 0.3 for X_1 and X_2, respectively.) To make the input state maximally uncertain (i.e., to make input entropy maximal), we would set the probabilities of 1 or 0 to 0.5 for both inputs. Set `px1=0.5` and `px2=0.5` in script `info2by2` (see MATLAB Box 8.1), and note the effect this has on information transmission in networks with various connectivity matrices. Is the network with segregated connectivity (i.e., the connectivity matrix that is the identity matrix) still able to transmit complete input information to the output when the input units have maximal entropy?

8.2   We used the Bell–Sejnowski infomax algorithm to maximize information transmission in deterministic, 2-by-2 feedforward networks of sigmoidal units. One of the most compelling technological applications of this algorithm is blind source separation, in which a mixture of two (or more) signals from statistically independent sources is separated by a neural network into its original components (see also Haykin 1999). Demonstrate blind source separation by modifying script `infoMax2by2` (see MATLAB Box 8.3) to separate a sine wave from random noise. Set the number of samples to 1000 (`nSam=1000`). Then set a nominal frequency of 0.5 cycles per second (`f=0.5`) and a time base of ten cycles at this frequency (`t=linspace(0, (1/f)*10,nSam)`). Then make an array of two simulated, temporal signals where `sig(1,:)=sin(2*pi*f*t)*0.5` and `sig(2,:)=rand(1,nSam)-0.5`. (Note that both signals have an amplitude range of –0.5 to +0.5.) Set a mixing matrix

`A=[0.6 0.4;0.5 0.5]`, and compute the mixture of signals as `mix=A*sig`. On any time step, input units 1 and 2 take their values from the first and second rows of `mix`, respectively. Set the initial input–output weight matrix as `V=[0.03 0.02;0.01 0.04]`, and the bias vector as `b=[0.02;0.03]`. Train the network using the Bell–Sejnowski algorithm for 2000 passes through the signal array. Performance of the algorithm is improved if it is run in batch mode, where weight changes `delV` and `delb` are accumulated over a set of time steps (50, say), and then applied as updates to `V` and `b`, respectively. After training, test the network by applying the signals in `mix` as inputs. The outputs should be squashed versions of the original signals, as in Figure 8.2.

8.3   In the example demonstrating the benefits of cooperative (neighbor) training on information transmission in self-organizing map networks, we considered neighborhood sizes of 0 (in which only the winner is trained, no neighbors) and of 1 (in which the winner and its nearest neighbor on each side are trained). Use the script `infoSOMbackground` (see MATLAB Box 8.5) to explore the effects of enlarging the neighborhood size. Set the input spatial tuning field to 1 (`stf=1`) and the input background level to 0.9 (`bg=0.9`). Run the script several times with neighborhood sizes of 1 (`nHood=1`) or 10 (`nHood=10`). Is the mutual information (`mi`) as high, and the distortion (`d`) as low, for the neighborhood of 10 as for the neighborhood of 1? Are the mutual information and output entropy (`hY`) as often the same for the neighborhood of 10 as for the neighborhood of 1? What might this indicate about the relationship between the size of the training neighborhood and information transmission in self-organizing map networks? (See Raginsky and Anastasio 2008 for further details.)

8.4   In exploring the ability of stochastic, 1-by-n networks of binary units with various numbers of output units Y_i ($i = 1, ..., n$) to transmit information, we set the probability that the single input unit X would take value 1 at 0.9. (The probability of value 0 was therefore 0.1.) With conditional probabilities of $P(Y_i = 1|X = 1) = 0.9$ and $P(Y_i = 0|X = 0) = 0.9$ for all i, 17 (or more) output units could collectively contain all the input information, at least out to four significant places. To make the input maximally uncertain (i.e., to make input entropy maximal), we would set the probability that it would take value 1 to 0.5. Set `px1=0.5` in script `info1byN` (see MATLAB Box 8.6), and note the effect this has on information transmission in networks with various conditional probabilities. Start by setting `py1x1=0.9` and `py0x0=0.9` in script `info1byN`. Can 17 output units contain all the input information now (i.e., does mutual information `mi` equal input entropy `hX`)? If not, can you increase the number of output units until they can? Now make input–output transmission more uncertain by setting `py1x1=0.8` and `py0x0=0.8`. Can you again increase the number of output units so that they collectively contain all the input information? (Be careful, increasing the number of output units too much in this exercise can be hard on your computer!)

References

Applebaum D (1996) *Probability and Information: An Integrated Approach.* Cambridge University Press, Cambridge.

Anastasio TJ, Patton PE (2003) A two-stage unsupervised learning algorithm reproduces multisensory enhancement in a neural network model of the corticotectal system. *Journal of Neuroscience* 23: 6713–6727.

Bell AJ, Sejnowski TJ (1995) An information-maximization approach to blind separation and blind deconvolution. *Neural Computation* 6: 1129–1159.

Bell AJ, Sejnowski TJ (1997) The "independent components" of natural scenes are edge filters. *Vision Research* 37: 3327–3338.

Berger T (1971) *Rate Distortion Theory: A Mathematical Basis for Data Compression.* Prentice Hall, Engelwood Cliffs, NJ.

Cover TM, Thomas JA (1991) *Elements of Information Theory.* Wiley, New York.

Franks KM, Stevens CF, Sejnowski TJ (2003) Independent sources of quantal variability at single glutamatergic synapses. *Journal of Neuroscience* 23: 3186–3195.

Haykin S (1999) *Neural Networks: A Comprehensive Foundation. Second Edition.* Prentice Hall, Upper Saddle River, NJ, pp 484–544.

Kohonen T (1997) *Self-Organizing Maps, Second Edition.* Springer-Verlag, Berlin.

Harpur G, Prager R (2000) Experiments with low-entropy neural networks. In: Baddeley R, Hancock P, Földiák P (eds) *Information Theory and the Brain.* Cambridge University Press, Cambridge, MA, pp 79–100.

Linsker R (1986) From basic network principles to neural architecture: Emergence of orientation selective cells. *Proceedings of the National Academy of Science* 83: 8390–8394.

Linsker R (1989) How to generate ordered maps by maximizing the mutual information between input and output signals. *Neural Computation* 1: 402–411.

Linsker R (1990) Perceptual neural organization: Some approaches based on network models and information theory. *Annual Review of Neuroscience* 13: 257–281.

Olshausen BA, Field DJ (1996) Emergence of simple-cell receptive field properties by learning a sparse code for natural images. *Nature* 381: 607–609.

Oram MW, Foldiak P, Perrett DI, Sengpiel F (1998) The 'Ideal Homunculus': Decoding neural population signals. *Trends in Neuroscience* 21: 259–265.

Raginsky M, Anastasio TJ (2008) Cooperation in self-organizing map networks enhances information transmission in the presence of input background activity. *Biological Cybernetics* 98: 195–211.

Ringach DL (2002) Spatial structure and symmetry of simple-cell receptive fields in Macaque primary visual cortex. *Journal of Neurophysiology* 88: 455–463

Ritter H, Schulten K (1986) On the stationary state of Kohonen's self-organizing sensory mapping. *Biological Cybernetics* 54: 99–106.

Trommershäuser J. Titz S, Keller BU, Zippelius A (2001) Variability of excitatory currents due to single-channel noise, receptor number and morphological heterogeneity. *Journal of Theoretical Biology* 208: 329–343.

Villmann T, Claussen JC (2006) Magnification control in self-organizing maps and neural gas. *Neural Computation* 18: 446–469.

von Neumann J (1958) *The Computer and the Brain.* Yale University Press, New Haven.

Wallace MT, Stein BE (1996) Sensory organization of the superior colliculus in cat and monkey. *Progress in Brain Research* 112: 301–311.

Wurtz RL, Goldberg ME (1989) *The Neurobiology of Saccadic Eye Movements.* Elsevier, Amsterdam.

9

Probability Estimation and Supervised Learning

Supervised learning algorithms can train neural units and networks to estimate probabilities and simulate the responses of neurons to multisensory stimulation

t is a commonly held belief that people are irrational. Consistent with this belief, experiments in cognitive science have revealed that people do indeed make large and systematic (i.e., non-random) errors on logical tasks (Stich 1985). This evidence might confirm our suspicions, but it might also be wrong. More recent research suggests that people are not so nutty after all. The performance of human subjects in reasoning experiments may be inconsistent with logic, but consistent with inference based on probabilities associated with exceptions to the logical premises of the experiment (Oaksford and Chater 2001). For example, a subject might be presented with the conditional premise "If A is a bird then A flies." But the human subject, with experience of the world, may have encountered evidence concerning certain birds that do not fly, and may represent the relationship between birds and flight more realistically as a probability rather than as an unqualified statement of fact. The influence of such experience, which human subjects bring with them to the experimental situation, may contribute to correct probabilistic inference but cause apparent errors in tasks involving logical reasoning.

Results such as those described above can be seen in a positive light. Rather than conclude that the brain is bad at logical reasoning, we could conclude instead that the brain is good at probabilistic inference. This positive light shines brighter as we move down the levels of processing in the brain. While the brain may be good at probabilistic inference on a higher cognitive level, it seems that the brain is *terrific* at probabilistic inference on a lower perceptual level. Brains excel at perceptual tasks, such as separating a signal from a noisy background, that confound the most powerful technological devices. It seems that the perceptual tasks brains do with the least effort are the most difficult for machines. Psychophysical experiments designed to probe this facility indicate that successful perception is based on probabilistic inference (Knill and Richards 1996). It is possible that probabilistic inference is what brains do best.

Correct probabilistic inference involves making the best of weak evidence. It also involves combining pieces of weak evidence in such a way that the integrated whole is stronger than the individual pieces of evidence considered separately. Imagine that I see you in the distance and I call out your name. Your auditory system might actually register my voice, but the difference between its response to my voice at a distance and its activity due to ambient noise might not be large enough for you to detect me. Imagine instead that I wave my arms at you. Your peripheral vision might actually register my motion, but again the difference between its response to me waving and to ambient environmental motion might not be large enough for you to notice me. Now imagine that I both call your name *and* wave my arms. In combination, the stimuli I produce might be enough for your brain to distinguish me from the background and allow you to detect me. Notice that this signal detection involved the integration of sensory inputs of different modalities (audition and vision in this case). Multisensory integration by the nervous system has become an important area of research in neuroscience. It has been studied most extensively for neurons in a region of the brain that we have encountered before in this book: the superior colliculus.

Located in the midbrain, the superior colliculus is the first place in the brain in which sensory signals of different modalities come together, and the responses of collicular neurons to multisensory stimulation is fascinatingly complex (Stein and Meredith 1993). Specifically, the response to two stimuli of different modalities (visual and auditory, for example) presented together is *not* equal to the sum of the responses to the two stimuli presented alone. Furthermore, the size of the combined-modality response relative to the single-modality responses depends on the size of the single-modality responses. Specifically, the combined-modality response is large relative to the single-modality responses when the single-modality responses are small, and vice-versa. This intriguing constellation of findings can be explained on the basis of the hypothesis that a collicular neuron uses its multisensory inputs to compute the probability that an object has appeared in its receptive field. The correspondence between the model and the data on multisensory integration by collicular neurons provides a clear indication on the neurophysiological level that some neurons may, indeed, compute probabilities. We will explore this model in detail in this chapter.

Our explorations in this chapter will also lead us into a discussion of different levels of description in neural systems modeling. As David Marr (1982) pointed out, a model of *what* a neural system does is different, in a fundamental way, from a model of *how* the neural system does it, for the reason that the same computation can be implemented in many different ways. We can study both the "what" and the "how" of neural systems function, because the neural systems models we study in this book produce a useful computation and are also implemented by neural elements (from single units to networks of many units). Our simulations in this chapter will illustrate nicely the different levels of description, first identified by Marr, on which neural systems can be modeled.

A process that often provides a bridge between levels of description is learning. For example, a neural network can learn to implement a function that is specified on the computational level. Learning will also provide a bridge between levels in this chapter. Specifically, we will show how neural systems, whether networks or single units, can be trained to implement probabilistic inferences that also can be described analytically on the computational level. The process of supervised learning will be of particular advantage in this regard, and its use in this chapter will cause us to see the objective of supervised learning in a different light.

In our exploration of supervised learning (see Chapter 6) we saw that feed-forward neural networks with three (or more) layers of sigmoidal units could be trained using back-propagation to produce almost any pattern association (input–output transformation). Often our goal was to train the output units of the networks to take the binary values of 1 or 0, given similarly binary input patterns. Of course, sigmoidal units can only take values of 1 or 0 at plus or minus infinity, but we saw that back-propagation could train network outputs to come within a very small tolerance of 1 or 0, even when the required transformation was demanding (recall the XOR problem). In binary (1, 0) pattern association tasks, it seems that we are simply training the network to give us outputs of 1 or 0 (or within tolerance of 1 or 0). What in fact occurs is more subtle. To grasp that subtlety in this chapter we will consider a specific form of pattern association known as pattern classification. This will connect our study of learning to probabilistic inference, because probabilistic inference is the best way to accomplish pattern classification (Duda et al. 2001).

The general pattern classification problem is diagrammed in Figure 9.1. Pattern classification is important technologically as well as neurologically. To clearly illustrate the idea of pattern classification we will begin this chapter with a readily understood task in the form of a simple technological application. The specific problem, depicted in Figure 9.1, is to classify fish by species automatically, according to quantities that can be measured using cameras and other artificial sensors (Duda et al. 2001).

The first and second steps involve preprocessing and feature extraction. These steps are important in technological applications and in the brain as well. We can draw a loose correspondence between preprocessing in a techno-

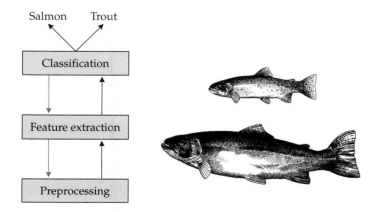

FIGURE 9.1   Flow diagram illustrating a procedure for classification of fishes In this case the fish species to be classified are salmon and trout. (Diagram after Duda et al. 2001; drawings courtesy of Bob Hines, U.S. Fish and Wildlife Service.)

logical device and sensory transduction in the nervous system, and between feature extraction in a device and sensory processes such as edge detection that we studied in Chapter 3. In this chapter we will assume that both preprocessing and feature extraction have already occurred and that the inputs to our neural systems are ready to be classified. Actual classification in the fish classifier occurs in the third step. Note in the diagram in Figure 9.1 that information flows in both directions. In this chapter we will consider only bottom-up flow. Top-down influence will be considered in detail in Chapter 12.

There are many computational systems that can act as pattern classifiers (see Duda et al. 2001), but in this chapter we will confine our attention to feedforward neural networks (or, as a special case, single neural units). Each output unit of a pattern-classifier neural network represents a different classification of its possible inputs. It is trained, using a supervised learning procedure such as back-propagation, by presenting the input patterns to be classified along with desired output patterns. In pattern classification problems the input patterns can take various forms (and generally are not binary), but any desired output pattern consists of a single 1 among 0s. Specifically, for the desired output of a pattern classification problem, the output unit corresponding to the correct class for the current input is assigned a value of 1, and all the other output units are assigned values of 0. As in the more general pattern association task, it appears again here in the pattern classification task that we are simply training the network to give 1 or 0 as outputs. Between the 1 and the 0 is where the subtlety comes in.

It has been proven analytically that any classifier (including a neural network) that minimizes a least-squares error function (as back-propagation does) produces as output an estimate of the conditional probability of each class given the input (Richard and Lippmann 1991; Bishop 1995). In other words, although we train the neural network to give us a 1 at the output unit corresponding to the correct class, and a 0 at the output unit corresponding to each incorrect class, what the trained network actually gives us is a number between 0 and 1 at each output unit that is an estimate of the probability that the given input belongs to each of the classes represented by the different output units. Thus, neural network classifiers trained via error minimization act as probability estimators that approximate probabilistic inference. Later in this chapter we will use pattern classifiers composed of single neural units as models of multisensory neurons in the superior colliculus. For our first example we will illustrate the principles involved using a simplified version of an automatic fish sorter.

9.1 Implementing a Simple Classifier as a Three-Layered Neural Network

To demonstrate the use of a neural network as a pattern classifier we will construct and train a neural network to classify fish by species according to measurements of their lengths. (This nice example is adapted from Duda et al. 2001.) This simple application is implemented by script `classifyFishBackProp`, which is listed in MATLAB® Box 9.1. The script will compose a three-layered feedforward network of sigmoidal units with 1 input, 3 output, and 12 hidden units when initialized with the following parameter settings: `nIn=1`, `nOut=3`, and `nHid=12`. A diagram of this network is provided in Figure 9.2. To make our simulated application seem a little more real, we can attach an actual fish species to each of the three classes. Specifically, we will assign output units 1, 2, and 3 (z_k, $k = 1, 2, 3$) to minnow, salmon, and marlin, respectively. The input unit x will take the value of the length of a fish to be classified. In reality, the

MATLAB® BOX 9.1   **This script trains a three-layered network of sigmoidal units using back-propagation to classify fish according to their lengths.**

```
% classifyFishBackProp.m

nIn=1; nHid=12; nOut=3; % set numbers of units
a=0.1; b=1; % set learning rate and bias
nIts=100000; % set number of training iterations
me1=2; me2=4; me3=6; % set likelihood means
sd1=1; sd2=1; sd3=1; % set likelihood standard deviations
pf1=1/3; pf2=1/3; pf3=1/3; % set priors
cumPrior=cumsum([pf1 pf2 pf3]); % find cumulative prior
maxLength=8; nLengths=30; % set max and number of fish lengths
Lvec=linspace(0,maxLength,nLengths)'; % length vector for testing

V=rand(nHid,nIn+1)*2-1; % set initial input-hidden weight matrix
U=rand(nOut,nHid+1)*2-1; % set initial hidden-output matrix
deltaV=zeros(nHid,nIn+1); % define weight change matrix for V
deltaU=zeros(nOut,nHid+1); % define weight change matrix for U

for c=1:nIts, % for each iteration
    % choose a fish type at random according to prior distribution
    indxVec=find(cumPrior>=rand); choose=indxVec(1);
    if choose==1, lFish=randn*sd1+me1; d=[1 0 0];
    elseif choose==2, lFish=randn*sd2+me2; d=[0 1 0];
    elseif choose==3, lFish=randn*sd3+me3; d=[0 0 1]; end
    % update the states of the units and compute network error
    x=[lFish b]'; % set the input with bias appended
    y=1./(1+(exp(-V*x))); y=[y' b]'; % compute hidden, append bias
    z=1./(1+(exp(-U*y))); % compute the output unit response
    e=d-z'; % find the error
    % train the network weights using back-propagation
    x=x';y=y';z=z'; % convert column to row vectors
    zg=(z.*(1-z)).*e; % compute the output error signal
    yg=(y.*(1-y)).*(zg*U); % compute the hidden error signal
    deltaU=a*zg'*y; % compute the change in hidden-output weights
    deltaV=a*yg(1:nHid)'*x; % compute change in input-hidden weights
    U=U+deltaU; V=V+deltaV; % update the hid-out and in-hid weights
end; % end training loop
% find final unit responses
Inb=[Lvec b*ones(nLengths,1)]; % append bias to all input lengths
Hid=(1./(1+exp(-V*Inb')))'; % find hid response to all lengths
Hidb=[Hid b*ones(nLengths,1)]; % append bias to all hidden vectors
Out=(1./(1+exp(-U*Hidb')))'; % find out response to all lengths
```

lengths of these fishes range from less than 1 inch to more than 100 inches, but such large input values force sigmoidal units into saturation, so fish lengths will be compressed into a narrower range. We can consider this length measurement and compression to be part of the preprocessing and feature extraction stages of our simple classifier (see Figure 9.1).

If fish of a particular species all came in one standard length, and if that length differed between species, then the classification problem would be easy. Unfortunately (from the classification standpoint), fish within a species can vary widely in length, and two individual fish of different species can have

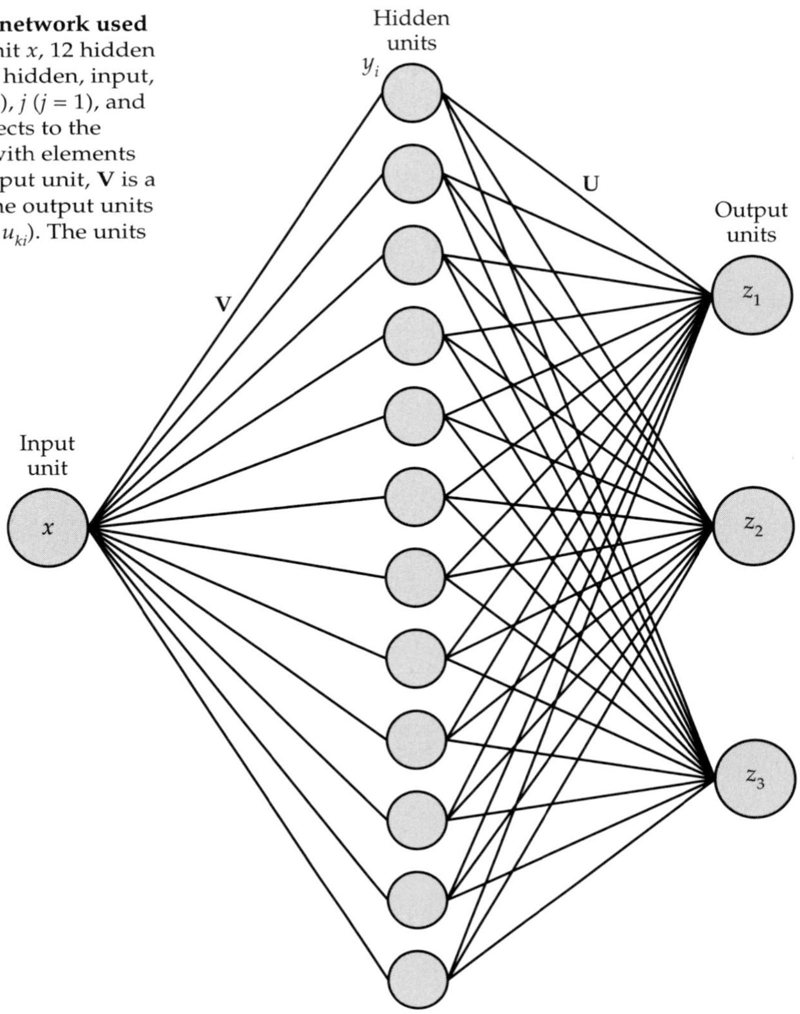

FIGURE 9.2   Three-layered, feedforward network used to classify fish by length There is 1 input unit x, 12 hidden units y_i, and 3 output units z_1, z_2, and z_3. The hidden, input, and output units are indexed by i ($i = 1,\ldots,12$), j ($j = 1$), and k ($k = 1,2,3$), respectively. The input unit projects to the hidden units over the weights in matrix $\mathbf{V}$ (with elements v_{ij}). In this case, in which there is only one input unit, $\mathbf{V}$ is a column vector. The hidden units project to the output units over the weights in matrix $\mathbf{U}$ (with elements u_{ki}). The units are sigmoidal (see Chaper 6).

the same length. What makes the pattern classification problem challenging in general is that members of different classes can have the same input patterns. Consequently, class membership cannot be determined absolutely. The best solution to the pattern classification problem is to compute the probability of each class given the input pattern, and classify the input pattern according to the class with the highest probability (Duda et al. 2001). Neural networks trained to minimize error can be used as classifiers because they estimate those class membership probabilities.

To simulate the variability in fish lengths we will use the well-known Gaussian distribution (Math Box 9.1). Specifically, we will use three separate univariate Gaussian distributions, one for each fish species. Set the mean fish lengths μ_k at 2, 4, and 6 for minnow, salmon, and marlin, respectively ($\mu_1 = 2$, $\mu_2 = 4$, $\mu_3 = 6$, where $k = 1, 2, 3$ correspond both to the output units and to the class or species of fish they represent). These means are set in `classifyFishBackProp` using `me1=2`, `me2=4`, and `me3=6`. Assume, for simplicity, that the variances σ^2 of all three Gaussians are equal to 1. Then the standard deviation, which is the square root of the variance, will be 1 for each species ($\sigma_1 = \sigma_2 = \sigma_3 = 1$). The standard deviations are set in the script using

---

MATH BOX 9.1   UNIVARIATE, MULTIVARIATE, AND BIVARIATE GAUSSIAN DISTRIBUTIONS

The univariate Gaussian probability density function for continuous random variable x is shown in Equation B9.1.1:

$$P(x) = \frac{1}{\sigma\sqrt{2\pi}}\exp\left\{-\frac{1}{2}\left(\frac{x-\mu}{\sigma}\right)^2\right\}$$
B9.1.1

where μ is the mean and σ is the standard deviation (the square root of the variance σ^2). The multivariate Gaussian probability density function for n random variables is shown in Equation B9.1.2:

$$P(\mathbf{x}) = \frac{1}{(2\pi)^{n/2}|\Sigma|^{1/2}}\exp\left\{-\frac{1}{2}(\mathbf{x}-\mu)^T\Sigma^{-1}(\mathbf{x}-\mu)\right\}$$
B9.1.2

where $\mathbf{x}$ is the vector of random variables, μ is the vector of their means, and Σ is the covariance matrix, in which the covariances between the random variables in $\mathbf{x}$ are the off-diagonal elements while the variances of each random variable in $\mathbf{x}$ are arrayed along the diagonal. The bivariate Gaussian probability density function for random variables x_1 and x_2 is described in Equation B9.1.3:

$$P(x_1,x_2) = \frac{1}{2\pi\sigma_1\sigma_2\sqrt{1-\rho^2}}\exp\left\{-\frac{1}{2(1-\rho^2)}\left[\left(\frac{x_1-\mu_1}{\sigma_1}\right)^2 - \cdots \right.\right.$$
$$\left.\left. 2\rho\left(\frac{x_1-\mu_1}{\sigma_1}\right)\left(\frac{x_2-\mu_2}{\sigma_2}\right)+\left(\frac{x_2-\mu_2}{\sigma_2}\right)^2\right]\right\}$$
B9.1.3

where μ_1 and μ_2 are the means of x_1 and x_2 and ρ is the correlation coefficient, which is defined in Equation B9.1.4:

$$\rho = \frac{\sigma_{12}}{\sigma_1\sigma_2}$$
B9.1.4

In Equations B9.1.3 and B9.1.4, σ_1 and σ_2 are the standard deviations of x_1 and x_2, and σ_{12} is their covariance (Papoulis 1991; Duda et al. 2001). Convenient formulas for generating univariate and bivariate Gaussian random deviates are given in the text in Equations 9.1 and 9.8.

`sd1=1`, `sd2=1`, and `sd3=1`. Univariate Gaussian random deviates with mean μ and standard deviation σ can be generated using Equation 9.1:

$$x = \eta(0,1)\sigma + \mu$$
9.1

where $\eta(0,1)$ is the standard (mean 0, variance 1) Gaussian deviate (Figure 9.3A). The MATLAB command `randn` will draw a random deviate (number) from a standard Gaussian (normal) distribution.

Each training iteration begins by first choosing one of the three fish species, and then by choosing the length of an individual of that species according to its length probability distribution. Both the species and the length are chosen randomly. To facilitate classification in this example we will be a bit unrealistic, on each iteration, in how we choose a species. In reality, you could catch many more minnows than salmon, and many more salmon than marlin. To keep matters simple, assume that fish of each species are encountered with equal probability. Thus, each of the three fish species has a 1/3 probability of being chosen on any given training iteration. These "encounter" probabilities are

(A)   (B)

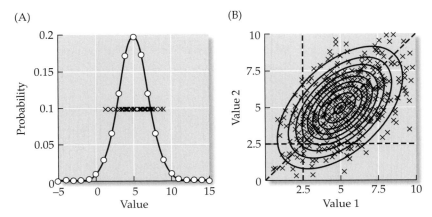

FIGURE 9.3 Univariate and bivariate Gaussian probability distributions
(A) The univariate Gaussian, computed according to Equation B9.1.1 with mean 5
and standard deviation 2, is shown as a smooth curve. The circles are the relative
frequencies of 500 random deviates generated according to Equation 9.1. The cross
symbols are 50 of those 500 deviates, plotted arbitrarily along the probability equals
0.1 line according to value. (B) The bivariate Gaussian is computed according to
Equation B9.1.3 with mean 5 and standard deviation 2 for both values and a correlation coefficient between them of 0.5. The two-dimensional Gaussian is shown as a
contour plot, in which concentric ellipsoids mark probability increasing from 0.1 on
the outside to 0.9 on the inside. The center of the innermost ellipsoid corresponds to
probability 1. The cross symbols are 500 deviates generated according to Equation
9.8 and plotted according to values 1 and 2. The dashed lines describe cuts through
the bivariate distribution. The diagonal line corresponds to the case where values 1
and 2 are equal. The horizontal line corresponds to the case where value 2 is fixed at
2.5, while the vertical line corresponds to the case where value 1 is fixed at 2.5.

known as "prior" probabilities. They are set in the script using `pf1=1/3`, and
similarly for `pf2` and `pf3`. These three values [`pf1 pf2 pf3`] constitute the
prior probability distribution for fish species. (The concept of prior probability
will be explained in more detail in the next section.) In this case the prior probability distribution is uniform. Uniform encounter (i.e., prior) probabilities
will improve classification by the network (see also Exercise 9.1).

The choice of species is accomplished in script `classifyFishBackProp`
by first finding the cumulative prior probability distribution using the command `cumPrior=cumsum([pf1 pf2 pf3])`, where `pf1`, `pf2`, and `pf3`
are the variable names for the prior probabilities of the three fish classes. The
intervals between the elements of the cumulative prior vector can be thought
of as probability "slots." To choose a fish species according to the prior probability distribution, a uniformly distributed random deviate is generated,
using `rand`, and the fish species chosen corresponds to the slot in the cumulative prior vector into which this random number falls. This is implemented
in `classifyFishBackProp` by first finding the indices of all the elements
of the cumulative prior vector that are greater than or equal to the random
deviate, using `indxVec=find(cumPrior>=rand)`. The number of the slot
into which this random number falls, which is stored in variable `choose`, is
the first of these indices: `choose=indxVec(1)`.

The value of `choose` is used to set the input and desired output on each
iteration. The desired output is set by the script to `d=[1 0 0]` for minnow, `d=[0 1 0]` for salmon, or `d=[0 0 1]` for marlin, accordingly as the
fish species chosen (i.e., the value of `choose`) is 1, 2, or 3, respectively. The
input, which corresponds to the length of a fish in our highly stylized example, is drawn from a univariate Gaussian distribution (see Equation 9.1) with

mean and standard deviation corresponding to the species of fish chosen. For example, if "minnow" is chosen, which is class 1, then the length `lFish` is drawn at random from a univariate Gaussian distribution with mean `me1` and standard deviation `sd1` using `lFish=randn*sd1+me1`, which implements Equation 9.1. As was done in script `backPropTrain` in Chapter 6 (see MAT-LAB Box 6.3), script `classifyFishBackProp` will also append a bias unit to the input and hidden unit state vectors. For example, the input is composed using `x=[lFish b]'`. Forward activation of the network is similar in script `classifyFishBackProp` as in script `backPropTrain`. Basically, each unit computes the weighted sum of its inputs and passes the result through the sigmoidal squashing funtion (see Chapter 6).

Script `classifyFishBackProp` is also similar to `backPropTrain` (see MATLAB Box 6.3) in terms of back-propagation training, except that the input patterns (single fish lengths) are drawn afresh from Gaussian distributions on each iteration, and training occurs on each iteration regardless of error. In `backPropTrain,` training occurs only when the error for a given pattern exceeds a tolerance. Training on every iteration regardless of error affords a small programming simplification and has negligable effects on the results in the classification example.

Before training, the script will randomize the input–hidden and hidden–output matrices by setting all weight values to random numbers distributed uniformly between −1 and +1. The bias, as usual, is set to `b=1`. We will train with learning rate `a=0.1` for `nIts=100000` training cycles (indexed by c). A fish species (desired output) and length (input) are chosen at random on each iteration as described above. The script `classifyFishBackProp` finds the output and hidden unit responses after training and stores them in arrays `Out` and `Hid`, respectively. The output unit responses after training are shown in Figure 9.4A. Note that, due to the several sources of randomness in this simulated application, the results will differ greatly from run to run. Figure 9.4 shows results that are typical for this simulation.

The responses of the three different output units are distinguished using different symbols (output z_1, triangle; output z_2, square; output z_3, circle). (The

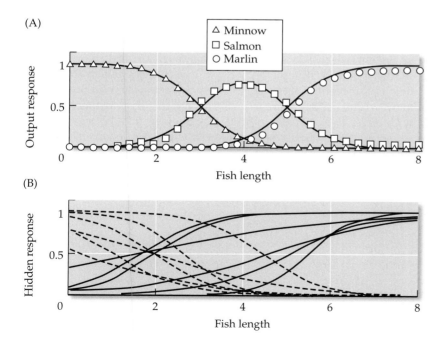

FIGURE 9.4 Classifying fish using a three-layered, feedforward network of sigmoidal units The network has 3 output units (z_1, z_2, and z_3), 12 hidden units, and 1 input unit (diagrammed in Figure 9.2). It is trained using back-propagation to classify three types of fish according to their lengths (which are artificially compressed into the range 0 to 8 to simplify training). (A) The actual output unit responses are shown as symbols (z_1, minnow, triangle; z_2, salmon, square; z_3, marlin, circle), while the smooth curves are the posterior probabilities of each class. (B) The hidden unit responses are shown as smooth curves. The responses of one group of hidden units increase with fish length (solid curves), while those of the other group decrease with fish length (dashed curves).

identities of the smooth curves drawn behind the symbols will be revealed in Section 9.3.) The response of z_1 is large for short fish lengths and decreases as length increases, while the response of z_3 is small for short fish lengths and increases as length increases. The response of z_2 is large for midrange fish lengths, and small both for short and long lengths. There are clearly ranges of the input for which the response of one output unit is larger than the responses of the other two. The response of output z_1 is larger than the responses of outputs z_2 and z_3 for short fish lengths, the response of output z_2 is larger than the responses of outputs z_1 and z_3 for medium fish lengths, and the response of output z_3 is larger than the responses of outputs z_1 and z_2 for long fish lengths. The responses of the output units can easily be read as indicating into which species of fish the network has classified the input. The class (category) determined by the network is simply the one corresponding to the output unit with the largest response. For example, inputs that produce larger responses in output unit z_1 as compared with output units z_2 and z_3 would be classified by the network as falling into class 1, which is the minnow class.

The relative sizes of the output responses reverse at certain fish length values. The relative sizes of the responses of units z_1 and z_2 reverse at a fish length value of about 3, while the relative sizes of the responses of units z_2 and z_3 reverse at a fish length value of about 5. The fish length value of 3 is midway between the means of the minnow and salmon length distributions ($\mu_1 = 2$ and $\mu_2 = 4$), while the fish length value of 5 is midway between the means of the salmon and marlin length distributions ($\mu_2 = 4$ and $\mu_3 = 6$). Examination of Figure 9.4A shows that the classifier does a bad job of classifying fish with lengths that are midway between the means we set for the length distributions of the three different species. For lengths in these regions, two of the output units will give nearly equal responses. Thus, the classifier will give an ambiguous output for fish lengths that are between the means for two different classes. The ambiguity of the output is a result of the ambiguity of the input. As we will see in the next section, the classifier network is doing about as well as it can, considering the ambiguity of the input.

The hidden unit responses are shown in Figure 9.4B. They appear to fall into two groups. In one group, the responses of the hidden units increase as their input, fish length, increases. In contrast, in the other group, the hidden unit responses decrease as their input increases. Although responses that increase with the value of an input variable seem more typical for neurons, responses that decrease as an input variable increases are not uncommon in the nervous system. With all 12 of the hidden units responding in only one of two ways, it might seem as though the network does not need them all to solve this classification problem. If the task is simply to decide class on the basis of the output unit with the maximal response, then adequate performance can be achieved with fewer than 12 hidden units (see Exercise 9.2). However, accurate estimation of class probabilities can require many hidden units (Richard and Lippmann 1991). The smooth curves drawn behind the output response symbols in Figure 9.4A are the actual probabilities of each class of fish given length as input. These conditional probabilities can be computed analytically using Bayes' rule, which is introduced in the next section.

9.2 Predicting Rain as an Everyday Example of Probabilistic Inference

Analytical methods for solving the pattern classification problem, and for making probabilistic inferences in general, are based on Bayes' rule, which is a relationship among probabilities that follows from the definition of condi-

MATH BOX 9.2   THE DERIVATION OF BAYES' RULE

Bayes' rule (more formally known as Bayes' theorem) follows from the definition of conditional probability. Consider two discrete, random variables R and C, where r and c are specific values of R and C, respectively. Then the probability that R takes value r is $P(R = r)$, the probability that C takes value c is $P(C = c)$, and the joint probability that R takes value r and C takes value c is $P(R = r, C = c)$. The conditional probability that R takes value r given that we *know* that C takes value c is given in Equation B9.2.1:

$$P(R = r \mid C = c) = \frac{P(R = r, C = c)}{P(C = c)}$$

B9.2.1

Similarly, the conditional probability that C takes value c given that R takes value r is given in Equation B9.2.2:

$$P(C = c \mid R = r) = \frac{P(C = c, R = r)}{P(R = r)}$$

B9.2.2

Since $P(R = r, C = c)$ equals $P(C = c, R = r)$, Equations B9.2.1 and B9.2.2 imply the relationship in Equation B9.2.3:

$$P(R = r \mid C = c)P(C = c) = P(C = c \mid R = r)P(R = r)$$

B9.2.3

from which Bayes' rule follows (Papoulis 1991) as shown in Equation B9.2.4:

$$P(R = r \mid C = c) = \frac{P(C = c \mid R = r)}{P(C = c)}P(R = r)$$

B9.2.4

Because R and C are discrete random variables, $P(C = c)$ can be written, according to the principle of total probability, in terms of $P(C = c \mid R = r)$ and $P(R = r)$ as in Equation B9.2.5:

$$P(C = c) = \sum_R P(C = c \mid R = r)P(R = r)$$

B9.2.5

where the summation is over all possible values of R. Thus, if we know the conditional probabilities $P(C = c \mid R = r)$, then we can use observations of C to draw inferences about R.

tional probability (Math Box 9.2). Probabilistic inference is possible because of dependencies between random variables (see Chapter 8 for background on random variables). To illustrate probabilistic inference, let us consider a problem from everyday life, that of inferring the probability of rain from an observation of cloudiness.

Assume that you are just beginning your day and it is currently not raining. Let us represent the assertion that "it will rain today" as binary random variable R where $R = 1$, and represent the assertion that "it will not rain today" as $R = 0$. Let us represent cloudiness as random variable C that takes values on an integer scale from 0 to 10, where $C = 0$ signifies a clear, cloudless sky and $C = 10$ signifies a sky overhung with dark, threatening clouds. Assume further that you live in a relatively rainy part of the country and that the chances of rain on any given day, as they would be measured and reported by your weather service, are 30%.

Chances of rain expressed as percentages are familiar to us. Probability is nothing more than assigning a number to chance that ranges between 0 and 1 rather than the more familiar percentage scale. So you begin your day with $P(R = 1) = 0.3$, which means that the probability that it will rain today is 0.3 (or chance of rain is 30%). You might also know from experience that $P(C = 3) = 0.2$, which means that the probability that cloudiness will occur at level 3 on any given day is 0.2 (or 20%). You can measure systematically, or just develop a general "feeling for," the probabilities associated with events such as $R = 1$ and $C = 3$, and so you will "know" from experience the chances of certain occurrences. Most of us are not professional meteorologists, and our knowledge of the probabilities associated with meteorological events is qualitative, but we can use our qualitative knowledge to infer meteorological outcomes to some limited degree of accuracy. For the sake of this rain prediction scenario, let us assume that we have measured and assigned numbers to the probabilities associated with certain random weather variables. Let us further assume that we have measured (to a limited degree of accuracy) not only the probabilities associated with individual random weather variables but also the dependencies between those random variables.

You remember from past rainy days that it was more likely to have been cloudy than clear. Thus, you have perceived a statistical dependency between cloudiness and rain, and you can express this dependency as a conditional probability (see Math Box 9.2 for the definition of conditional probability). For example, the conditional probability $P(C = 8 \mid R = 1) = 0.6$ means that the probability that the sky was cloudy at level 8 given that it rained that day is 0.6. Your experience might also tell you that the following is true: $P(C = 8 \mid R = 1) > P(C = 2 \mid R = 1)$. In words, given that it rained on a given day ($R = 1$), it was more likely to have been quite cloudy ($C = 8$) than mostly clear ($C = 2$). Bayes' rule allows you to put this kind of probabilistic knowledge to use for inference.

To predict rain from cloudiness, Bayes' rule would be applied as shown in Equation 9.2:

$$P(R = r \mid C = c) = \frac{P(C = c \mid R = r)}{P(C = c)} P(R = r) \qquad \textbf{9.2}$$

where r and c represent specific values of random variables R and C, respectively. Given an observation of cloudiness $C = c$, Bayes' rule can be used to infer the conditional probability $P(R = 1 \mid C = c)$ that it will rain today. In the context of Bayesian inference, the terms in Equation 9.2 have specific names as shown in Figure 9.5. The term $P(R = r)$ is called the prior probability because it is the probability assigned to the assertion $R = r$ *before* any evidence is received, such as an observation of the level of cloudiness. The conditional probability $P(R = r \mid C = c)$ is called the posterior probability, because it reflects the prior probability $P(R = r)$ *after* it has been modified by an observation. The conditional probability $P(C = c \mid R = r)$ is called the likelihood in the context of Bayesian inference, because it indicates how likely it is to observe cloudiness $C = c$ given that it will ($R = 1$) or will not ($R = 0$) rain. The evidence $P(C = c)$ is the probability of observing cloudiness $C = c$ anytime, regardless of whether it rains later or not. These naming conventions facilitate the application of Bayes' rule to inference problems.

Bayes' rule specifies how an observation can be used to modify a prior probability to yield a posterior probability. The modification term in the rain example is the ratio of the likelihood $P(C = c \mid R = r)$ and the evidence $P(C = c)$. Basically, if the level of cloudiness observed on a given morning is more likely to occur when it later will rain than it is to occur anytime, then $P(C = c \mid R = 1) > P(C = c)$ and their ratio $P(C = c \mid R = 1) \, / \, P(C = c)$ is greater than 1. According to Bayes' rule, if the modification term $[P(C = c \mid R = 1) \, / \, P(C = $

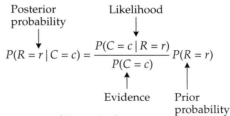

FIGURE 9.5   The anatomy of Bayes' rule

c)] is greater than 1, then the posterior probability $P(R = 1 | C = c)$ is greater than the prior probability $P(R = 1)$. Conversely, if $P(C = c | R = 1)$ / $P(C = c)$ < 1 then $P(R = 1 | C = c) < P(R = 1)$. The following numerical example (with fictitious probabilities and numbers rounded to the nearest tenth), will make these relationships clearer. It is presented in the context of a simple decision-making problem.

Suppose that you will decide to carry your umbrella on a given day if the probability that it will rain is 0.5 or greater. Because you live in a rainy region where it rains three days out of ten (30% chance of rain), the prior probability that it will rain today is 0.3. Because R is a binary variable (it will either rain or it will not rain), the prior probability that it will not rain is 0.7. The prior probability distribution for random variable R is therefore $[P(R = 1) = 0.3, P(R = 0) = 0.7]$. This is a valid probability distribution for binary random variable R because the probabilities for both possible values r of R sum to 1: $P(R = 1) + P(R = 0) = 0.3 + 0.7 = 1$. Note that the prior probability of R is the probability we assign to R *before* we have any evidence. Thus, in the absence of evidence (e.g., before you look outside at the sky to assess cloudiness) you assign prior probability $P(R = 1) = 0.3$ to the assertion that it will rain today, and since 0.3 < 0.5 you would decide not to carry your umbrella. A look at the sky could cause you to change your decision.

Suppose you look out your window and observe cloudiness of level 7. From past experience, you know that the likelihood of observing this cloudiness level given that it later will rain is 0.4, while the likelihood of observing this cloudiness level given that it later will not rain is only 0.1. In symbols, the likelihoods are $P(C = 7 | R = 1) = 0.4$ and $P(C = 7 | R = 0) = 0.1$. Knowing the likelihoods and priors you can compute the evidence $P(C = 7)$, according to the principle of total probability (see Math Box 9.2), as $P(C = 7) = P(C = 7 | R = 1)P(R = 1) + P(C = 7 | R = 0)P(R = 0) = (0.4)(0.3) + (0.1)(0.7) = 0.2$. Now you can compute the posterior probability $P(R = 1 | C = 7)$ according to Bayes' rule (see Equation 9.2) as $P(R = 1 | C = 7) = [P(C = 7 | R = 1) / P(C = 7)]P(R = 1) = (0.4 / 0.2)0.3 = 0.6$. Note that the ratio $P(C = 7 | R = 1) / P(C = 7)$, by which you modify the prior probability to get the posterior probability, is $0.4 / 0.2 = 2$. Thus, observing cloudiness of level 7 causes you to double the prior probability of 0.3 to give you a posterior probability that it will rain today of 0.6. Since 0.6 > 0.5, you decide to carry your umbrella.

9.3 Implementing a Simple Classifier Using Bayes' Rule

Bayes' rule is a simple probabilistic relationship that has profound implications. Knowing the likelihood distributions that describe the statistical relationships between an observable (or many observables) and a variable of interest, it can be shown that Bayes' rule is the optimal way to infer the probability of the variable given the value of an observable (or of many observables) (Duda et al. 2001). Its optimality explains why Bayes' rule provides the basis for the design of many data processing devices. To use Bayes' rule to classify fish F by length L we can apply it as in Equation 9.3:

$$P(F = f | L = l) = \frac{P(L = l | F = f)P(F = f)}{P(L = l)} = \frac{P(L = l | F = f)P(F = f)}{\sum_F P(L = l | F = f)P(F = f)} \quad \text{9.3}$$

where f and l are specific values of random variables F and L, respectively, and the summation in the denominator is over all values of variable F. In the example introduced above there are three fish species (minnow, salmon, and marlin). The posterior probability that the fish is, say, of class 2 (salmon) given a measurement of length 6 would be written as in Equation 9.4:

$$P(F = 2 \mid L = 6) =$$

$$\frac{P(L = 6 \mid F = 2)P(F = 2)}{P(L = 6 \mid F = 1)P(F = 1) + P(L = 6 \mid F = 2)P(F = 2) + P(L = 6 \mid F = 3)P(F = 3)} \qquad \textbf{9.4}$$

In Equation 9.4, $P(F = 1)$, $P(F = 2)$, and $P(F = 3)$ are the prior probabilities that a given fish will belong to each of the three classes. We assumed, for simplicity, that fish of each species would be encountered with equal probability [$P(F = 1) = P(F = 2) = P(F = 3) = 1/3$]. In the sea, minnows are more plentiful than salmon, and salmon more than marlin, and the prior probabilities could be changed to reflect this fact, if desired (see Exercise 9.1).

The terms $P(L = 6 \mid F = 1)$, $P(L = 6 \mid F = 2)$, and $P(L = 6 \mid F = 3)$ are the likelihoods that length $L = 6$ will be observed given that the species of fish is of class 1, 2, or 3. We modeled these likelihood distributions as univariate Gaussians with different means (but the same variance) for each fish species. (The equation describing the univariate Gaussian is given in Math Box 9.1.) It is reasonable to assume that the lengths of fish of a certain species will be Gaussian (normally) distributed, but other distribution functions could be used instead. Because the Gaussian is a continuous probability density function, it cannot be used to specify the probability of a discrete event (such as a fish having the precise length $L = 6$). However, in the context of Bayes' rule, the Gaussian can be used as a function that specifies the relative likelihoods of events, because Bayes' rule is self-normalizing. To see this, note in Equation 9.4 that the posterior probability $P(F = 2 \mid L = 6)$ is equal to the term $P(L = 6 \mid F = 2)P(F = 2)$ after it is divided by the sum of all possible such terms for which $L = 6$: $P(L = 6 \mid F = 1)P(F = 1) + P(L = 6 \mid F = 2)P(F = 2) + P(L = 6 \mid F = 3)P(F = 3)$. Thus, a likelihood function needs to describe relative likelihoods, but it does not need to describe a valid probability distribution in order to produce valid posterior probabilities using Bayes' rule. In any case, the Gaussian distributions used in the scripts in this chapter are normalized, so that they are valid probability distributions over the discrete arguments at which they are evaluated.

Bayes' rule specifies how knowledge of the prior probability and the input (observation) likelihood distributions in a classification problem can be used to compute the posterior probability of the class given some input. In Equation 9.4 we compute the posterior probability for class $F = 2$ given length $L = 6$ [$P(F = 2 \mid L = 6)$]. The other posterior probabilities are computed similarly. The point is that if we know the prior probability and likelihood distributions for a classification problem, then we can directly compute the posterior probability of the class given the input. Neural networks, when trained using adaptive algorithms that provide the network with "experience" in the world, can be useful for estimating posterior probabilities from data when the classes are known but the prior probability and likelihood distributions are not known (Bishop 1995). As we will see in later sections, simple neural models trained using adaptive algorithms to estimate posterior probabilities can also be used to simulate the responses of real neurons to sensory inputs.

The script `classifyFishBayesRule`, listed in MATLAB Box 9.2, will compute the posterior probabilities of each class of fish given the prior distribution over the species and parameters for the likelihood distributions over their lengths. In this script, as in script `classifyFishBackProp`, the prior probabilities $P(F = 1)$, $P(F = 2)$, and $P(F = 3)$ are held in variables `pf1`, `pf2`, and `pf3`. The means of the likelihood distributions are held in `me1`, `me2`, and `me3`, while the standard deviations are held in `sd1`, `sd2`, and `sd3`. The script sets vector `Lvec` of discrete fish lengths, and it computes the three

MATLAB® BOX 9.2   **This script computes the posterior probabilities of each of three hypothetical fish classes using Bayes' rule.**

```
% classifyFishBayesRule.m

% set likelihood parameters and class priors
me1=2; me2=4; me3=6; % set likelihood means
sd1=1; sd2=1; sd3=1; % set likelihood variances
pf1=1/3; pf2=1/3; pf3=1/3; % set priors (must sum to one)

% set fish lengths
maxLength=8; % set maximum fish length
nLengths=30; % set number of fish lengths
Lvec=linspace(0,maxLength,nLengths)'; % set length vector

% compute the (discretized) Gaussian likelihood distributions
plf1=(1/(sd1*sqrt(2*pi)))*exp(-1/2*((Lvec-me1)/sd1).^2);
plf2=(1/(sd2*sqrt(2*pi)))*exp(-1/2*((Lvec-me2)/sd2).^2);
plf3=(1/(sd3*sqrt(2*pi)))*exp(-1/2*((Lvec-me3)/sd3).^2);
plf1=plf1/sum(plf1); % normalize
plf2=plf2/sum(plf2); % normalize
plf3=plf3/sum(plf3); % normalize

% compute unconditional probability of length (evidence)
pl=plf1*pf1+plf2*pf2+plf3*pf3;

% compute posterior probabilities
pf1l=(plf1./pl)*pf1;
pf2l=(plf2./pl)*pf2;
pf3l=(plf3./pl)*pf3;
```

likelihoods (`plf1`, `plf2`, and `plf3`) over this vector as (discrete) univariate Gaussians (see Equation B9.1.1 in Math Box 9.1) using their respective means (`me1`, `me2`, and `me3`) and standard deviations (`sd1`, `sd2`, and `sd3`). The script normalizes these discrete likelihoods so that they are valid probability distributions. For example, script `classifyFishBayesRule` computes the Gaussian likelihood for the minnow class $P(L = l | F = 1)$ using `plf1=(1/(sd1*sqrt(2*pi)))*exp(-1/2*((Lvec-me1)/sd1).^2)`. It normalizes this distribution using `plf1=plf1/sum(plf1)`. The likelihoods over the lengths in `Lvec` for the other fish classes are computed and normalized similarly. The script computes the evidence $P(L = l)$ for the lengths in `Lvec` using the principle of total probability: `pl=plf1*pf1+plf2*pf2+plf3*pf3`.

Then the script computes the posterior probabilities (`pf1l`, `pf2l`, and `pf3l`) over the same vector of lengths `Lvec` using Bayes' rule (see Equation 9.3). For example, it computes the posterior probabilities for minnow $P(F = 1 | L = l)$ using `pf1l=(plf1./pl)*pf1`. Note that the priors are scalars, but the likelihoods and the posteriors are vectors. While Bayes' rule as expressed in Equation 9.3 suggests computation of one posterior probability for one observation of length, the script `classifyFishBayesRule` computes the posterior for all discrete lengths over a range for efficiency.

The resulting, analytically determined posterior probability curves for the fish classification problem are shown in Figure 9.6A. For comparison, the Gaussian likelihood distributions are shown in Figure 9.6B. The curves in Figure 9.6 illustrate Bayesian inference. Consider a fish of length 2. The like-

FIGURE 9.6 Classification of fish by length using Bayes' rule (A) The posterior probabilities and (B) the likelihood distributions overlap.

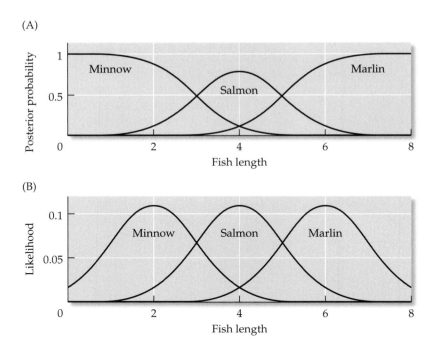

lihoods (see Figure 9.6B) indicate that this length is much more likely to be observed if the fish in question is a minnow rather than a salmon or marlin. The posteriors (see Figure 9.6A) correspondingly assign a higher probability to minnow than to salmon or marlin for a fish of length 2. Problems occur for fish of lengths that are equally likely to be of one species as another. For example, a fish of length 3 is just as likely to be a minnow as a salmon. The posteriors in this case indicate equal probability that the fish is a minnow as it is a salmon. Given equal likelihoods for fish of two species (and equal priors, see below), the Bayesian classifier does the best it can, which is to assign equal posterior probabilities in two different classes. Because Bayesian inference is optimal, the best the Bayesian classifier can do is the best that can be done given the likelihoods. One way to improve distinguishability in the fish classifier would be to provide a measure of a different attribute, such as fish color (Duda et al. 2001). In Section 9.5 we will consider Bayesian inference using observations of more than one type, in the context of a model of multisensory integration in the brain.

In this particular fish classification example, equal likelihoods lead to equal posteriors, but this is not the case in general. Unequal priors would lead to unequal posteriors in the case of equal likelihoods (this follows from Equation 9.3). For example, in the sea, minnows are much more plentiful than salmon, so the prior probability of encountering a minnow is much higher than of encountering a salmon. If the prior probability distribution reflected the relative abundance of minnows, and we observed a fish of length 3, then Bayesian inference would produce a higher posterior probability for minnow than for salmon even though a fish of length 3 is just as likely (given our highly stylized likelihood distributions) to be a salmon as a minnow. The Bayesian formulation of Equation 9.3 is completely general and is valid for any likelihood and prior distributions.

We set a uniform prior to facilitate back-propagation training of the neural network classifier in our simple application. The uniform prior probability ensures that all classes are learned equally well by the network, because it has an equal amount of experience with fishes of all three classes. Still, the posterior probabilities estimated by the network are not perfect. The same posterior probability curves in Figure 9.6A are also drawn in Figure 9.4A, behind the symbols (triangles, squares, and circles) that mark the responses of the output units in the neural network classifier. Due to the stochastic (random) nature of the problem, the output unit responses from the network will change each time it is retrained. Sometimes the network output agrees well with the analytically determined posterior probabilities, and sometimes it does not. Usually, though, the points at which the output unit responses transition will match up well with the points at which the posterior probabilities cross each other (see Figure 9.4A). Thus, classification that is near the Bayesian optimal can usually be achieved using the neural network by choosing the class corresponding to the output unit with the largest response to a given input.

The ability of a neural network to accurately estimate posterior probabilities depends on the number of hidden units it has (see Exercise 9.2). Problems with many classes may require networks with many hidden units (Richard and Lippmann 1991). Some binary classification problems are simple enough that no hidden units are required. In certain problems of neurobiological significance, single neurons are thought to act as detectors for particular target features and seem to compute the posterior probability of their feature given their inputs. In the single-neuron case, the input (and bias) weights can be trained using the delta rule. We will use the delta rule to train a single, sigmoidal unit to estimate the posterior probability that a target feature is present. The trained unit serves as a simple model of certain sensory neurons.

9.4 Modeling Neural Responses to Sensory Input as Probabilistic Inference

A neurobiological example in which real neurons may actually estimate probabilities involves neurons in the superior colliculus. The superior colliculus, especially its deeper layers, is responsible for detecting, selecting, and localizing targets (stimulus sources) in the environment and initiating orienting responses, such as saccadic eye movements, toward them (Wurtz and Goldberg 1989). In Chapter 3 we explored a simple, winners-take-all neural network as a model of the selection/localization process in the superior colliculus. Modeling work suggests that the detection process involves estimation by collicular neurons of the posterior probability that a target is present in their receptive fields, given sensory input (Anastasio et al. 2000; Anastasio and Patton 2004). We will explore that model throughout the remainder of this chapter.

The activity of real neurons has a substantial random component (see Chapters 7 and 8). Being neural, the inputs provided by the various sensory systems to brain structures such as the superior colliculus are best considered not as perfect translations of sensory events but as random variables that statistically depend on sensory events. As such, sensory inputs cannot provide a deterministic, yes/no signal to collicular neurons concerning the presence of a target, but they can provide usable evidence, and it is reasonable to suppose that collicular neurons do the best they can with the probabilistic input they receive. The model instantiates the hypothesis that collicular neurons use their sensory inputs to infer the posterior probability of a target optimally using Bayes' rule. This approach is especially useful for modeling the responses of collicular neurons to input from two sensory systems (bisensory input). We will begin the process of simulating the sensory responses of collicular neurons in this section by focusing on input from a single sensory system (unisensory input).

We will model the unisensory input as a random variable. We will simulate a collicular neuron as a single sigmoidal unit that receives this probabilistic unisensory input and a bias. (For simplicity, we will not represent the input and bias

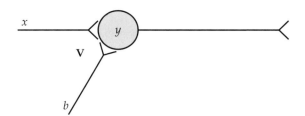

FIGURE 9.7 A single, sigmoidal unit used to simulate a unisensory neuron in the superior colliculus The unit y receives input x and bias b. The weight matrix **V** in this case is a row vector containing the weights of the two connections to y, one from x and the other from b. The unit computes the weighted sum of its inputs and passes the result through the sigmoidal squashing function (see Chapter 6). The input x could represent the visual input to the collicular neuron, and bias b could represent a constant influence on neural firing rate due to the biophysical properties of the neuron or to nonspecific inputs that are constant in combination.

explicitly as units.) The single-unit neural system is schematized in Figure 9.7. We will train it using the delta rule to estimate the posterior probability of a target. We will also evaluate the unisensory posterior probability analytically using Bayes' rule, and compare that with the responses of the single-unit model.

To set up the Bayes' rule model of the unisensory responses of collicular neurons we will need to define random variables that represent the target and the single sensory input. We will represent the target as binary variable T, where it can either be present ($T = 1$) or absent ($T = 0$). We will assume that the model neuron (unit) receives input from the visual system, and denote this as (not binary) random variable V, the value of which represents some number of neural impulses received by the unit from the visual system during a specific time period (like a second, or fraction of a second). We will denote specific values of random variable T as t_S and of random variable V as v_S. To compute the posterior probability that the target is present given visual input, Bayes' rule would be applied as in Equation 9.5:

$$P(T = 1 \mid V = v_S) = \frac{P(V = v_S \mid T = 1)P(T = 1)}{P(V = v_S \mid T = 1)P(T = 1) + P(V = v_S \mid T = 0)P(T = 0)} \qquad \textbf{9.5}$$

In Equation 9.5, $P(T = 1)$ and $P(T = 0)$ are the prior probabilities that the target is present or absent, respectively. For simplicity, we assume that a target is equally likely to be present as absent in the receptive field of the unit, so $P(T = 1) = P(T = 0) = 0.5$. The terms $P(V = v_S \mid T = 1)$ and $P(V = v_S \mid T = 0)$ are the likelihoods that a particular level of visual input $V = v_S$ will be observed given that the target is present or absent, respectively. We will model each of these likelihood distributions as a univariate Gaussian (see Math Box 9.1). We assume that a target that emits a visual stimulus will activate the visual system, so we will assign a higher mean for the target-present $P(V = v_S \mid T = 1)$ than for the target-absent $P(V = v_S \mid T = 0)$ likelihood distribution. Specifically, we will set $\mu_1 = 6$ and $\mu_0 = 3$ for the target-present and target-absent likelihood means, respectively. For simplicity, we will set the standard deviation σ equal to 1 for both cases. The discrete Gaussian we use here is a reasonable first approximation to the actual distribution of impulses received by a collicular neuron in a specific time interval, but other distribution functions could be used instead (Anastasio et al. 2000; Patton and Anastasio 2003).

The script `unisensoryBayesRule`, listed in MATLAB Box 9.3, will compute the target-present posterior probability $P(T = 1 \mid V = v_S)$ given the target prior probability distribution $[P(T = 1), P(T = 0)]$ and the visual input likelihood distributions $P(V = v_S \mid T = 1)$ and $P(V = v_S \mid T = 0)$. The procedures are similar to those described for the fish classification example in Section 9.3. In script `unisensoryBayesRule`, the priors are held in variables `pt1` and `pt0`. The target-present and target-absent likelihood means and standard deviations are held, respectively, in variables `mev1`, `mev0`, `sdv1`, and `sdv0`. The script sets up a vector `vis` representing values of visual input over a range, and it computes the target-present and target-absent likelihoods (`pvt1` and `pvt0`) over this vector as (discrete) univariate Gaussians (see Equation B9.1.1

MATLAB® BOX 9.3   **This script computes the posterior probability of a target given sensory input of one modality (i.e., visual).**

```
% unisensoryBayesRule.m

% set likelihood parameters and target priors
mev1=6; mev0=3; % set target present and absent likelihood means
sdv1=1; sdv0=1; % set target present and absent likelihood SDs
pt1=0.5; pt0=1-pt1; % set target present prior, compute absent

% set range of sensory input values
maxV=9; % set maximum sensory input value
nVals=30; % set number of sensory input values
vis=linspace(0,maxV,nVals); % set sensory (visual) input vector

% compute the Gaussian likelihoods distributions
pvt1=(1/(sdv1*sqrt(2*pi)))*exp(-1/2*((vis-mev1)/sdv1).^2);
pvt0=(1/(sdv0*sqrt(2*pi)))*exp(-1/2*((vis-mev0)/sdv0).^2);
pvt1=pvt1/sum(pvt1); % normalize
pvt0=pvt0/sum(pvt0); % normalize

% compute unconditional probability of input (evidence)
pv=pvt1*pt1+pvt0*pt0;

% compute the posterior probabilities
pt1v=(pvt1./pv)*pt1;
pt0v=(pvt0./pv)*pt0;
```

in Math Box 9.1) using their respective means (mev1 and mev0) and standard deviations (sdv1 and sdv0). As before, the script normalizes these discrete likelihoods so that they are valid probability distributions. The script uses the prior and likelihood distributions to compute the evidence pv over the vector vis. With the likelihood, evidence, and prior distributions available the script computes the posterior probability distributions (pt1v and pt0v) over the visual input vector vis using the unisensory Bayes' rule model (see Equation 9.5). The target-present posterior probability $P(T = 1 \mid V = v_S)$, and the target-present and target-absent likelihoods $P(V = v_S \mid T = 1)$ and $P(V = v_S \mid T = 0)$ over a range of visual input values are shown as smooth curves in Figure 9.8A and B, respectively.

Together the curves in Figure 9.8 illustrate the process of inferring the posterior probability of a target given sensory inputs of one modality. For example, visual input at activity level $V = 3$ is more likely given that the target is absent than present (see Figure 9.8B), and the posterior probability that the target is present is correspondingly very low (see Figure 9.8A). In contrast, visual input at activity level $V = 6$ is more likely given that the target is present than absent (see Figure 9.8B), and the posterior probability that the target is present is correspondingly very high (see Figure 9.8A). As in the fish classification example, a problem occurs when the visual input is equally likely given that the target is present or absent. At that level, the visual input indicates nothing about the target and Bayesian (i.e., optimal) inference dictates that the posterior target probability should equal the prior target probability (see Equation 9.5). To facilitate delta rule training (which we will undertake later in this section), we set the prior distribution to $[P(T = 1) = 0.5, P(T = 0) = 0.5]$ so that the target-present and target-absent priors are equal. Thus, given a

FIGURE 9.8   Unisensory probabilities computed using Bayes' rule, or estimated by a single sigmoidal unit trained using the delta rule (A) The target-present posterior probability computed using Bayes' rule is shown as a smooth curve, and estimates by the unit are shown as circles. (B) The target-present and target-absent visual input likelihood distributions are modeled using univariate Gaussians.

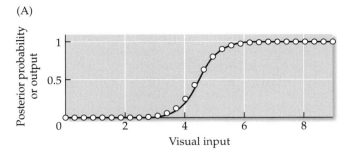

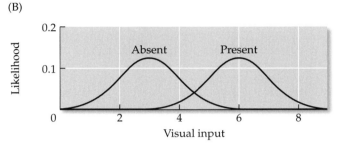

visual input that is equally likely whether the target is present or absent, the posterior target-present probability $P(T = 1 \mid V = v_S)$ is equal to 0.5. Note that the target can have any prior distribution in general.

The Bayes' rule model is essentially an hypothesis about *what* collicular neurons compute, and it posits that they compute target posterior probabilities. But the Bayes' rule model by itself indicates nothing about *how* collicular neurons might implement this computation. We will show, in principle, how a neuron could implement the computation of a posterior probability by using the delta rule to train a single sigmoidal unit, with one input weight and one bias weight, to estimate the posterior probability $P(T = 1 \mid V = v_S)$. "Target present" can be thought of as a classification of the visual input, and the single unit in this case can be thought of as a one-class classifier. Thus, we can train a single sigmoidal unit to estimate the target-present posterior probability by training it using the delta rule to classify inputs into this single class.

As discussed in detail in Chapter 6, a sigmoidal unit computes the weighted sum of its inputs and passes the result through the sigmoidal squashing function. The single sigmoidal unit depicted in Figure 9.7 computes its weighted input sum as $q = v_1 x + v_2 b$, where v_1 and v_2 are the elements of weight matrix $\mathbf{V}$ ($\mathbf{V} = [v_1\ v_2]$), and computes its activation using the squashing function as $y = 1/(1+e^{-q})$. Input x corresponds to visual input and bias $b = 1$. The delta rule will train the weights v_1 and v_2 so that y provides an estimate of the unisensory target-present posterior probability $P(T = 1 \mid V = v_S)$. (Note that the letter "v" is being used as a variable name without ambiguity, since $\mathbf{V}$ is the weight matrix containing weights v_1 and v_2, but V is a random variable representing the visual input that takes specific values v_S.) To accomplish delta rule training, parameters must be set that specify the statistical properties of the target and visual input, and the initial weights of the inputs to the sigmoidal unit.

The script `unisensoryDeltaRule`, listed in MATLAB Box 9.4, will train a single sigmoidal unit to classify its input into a single, target-present category. The required parameters, which are set in the script, include the target-present and target-absent visual input likelihood means and standard deviations (`mev1`, `mev0`, `sdv1`, and `sdv0`), and the target-present and target-absent prior probabilities (`pt1=0.5`, and `pt0` is computed in the script as `pt0=1-pt1`). The script `unisensoryDeltaRule` chooses the target state according

MATLAB® BOX 9.4 **This script trains a single sigmoidal unit using the delta rule to estimate posterior target probability given sensory input of one modality (i.e., visual).**

```
% unisensoryDeltaRule.m

nIn=1; nOut=1; % set numbers of units
a=0.1; b=1; % set learning rate and bias
nIts=100000; % set number of iterations

mev1=6; mev0=3; % set likelihood means
sdv1=1; sdv0=1; % set likelihood standard deviations
pt1=0.5; pt0=1-pt1; % set target present prior, compute absent
cumPrior=cumsum([pt1 pt0]); % find cumulative prior
maxV=9; % set maximum visual sensory input size
nVals=30; % set number of visual sensory input values
vis=linspace(0,maxV,nVals)'; % set vector of visual inputs

V=rand(nOut,nIn+1)*2-1; % set initial connectivity matrix
deltaV=zeros(nOut,nIn+1); % zero the change weight matrix

% train network using the delta-rule
for c=1:nIts,% for each iteration
    % choose target present or absent at random by prior
    indxVec=find(cumPrior>=rand); choose=indxVec(1);
    if choose==1, inV=randn*sdv1+mev1; d=1;% if target present
    elseif choose==2, inV=randn*sdv0+mev0; d=0; end % if absent
    x=[inV b]'; % set input with bias appended
    y=1./(1+exp(-V*x)); % compute the output unit response
    dy=y.*(1-y); % compute the derivative of the squashing function
    e=d-y; % find the error for the chosen input
    g=e.*dy; % find output error signal
    deltaV=a*g*x'; % compute delta rule weight update
    V=V+deltaV; % apply the weight update
end % end training loop

% find network output
Inb=[vis b*ones(nVals,1)]; % append bias to all visual inputs
Out=(1./(1+exp(-V*Inb')))'; % find output response to all inputs
```

to the cumulative prior distribution vector, as in classifyFishBackProp (see MATLAB Box 9.1), except that the cumulative prior distribution for the single-class classifier has only two "slots," one for target-present and one for target-absent. Script unisensoryDeltaRule is similar to deltaRuleTrain (see MATLAB Box 6.2), except that input patterns (single sensory input values) are drawn afresh from Gaussian distributions on each iteration, rather than being drawn from a pre-set input pattern array.

Before training, the script sets the values of the input and bias weights to random numbers between −1 and +1 using V=rand(nOut,nIn+1)*2-1 where nOut and nIn are both 1 (note that the weight matrix V containing the input and bias weights to the single unit is simply a two-element row vector). The bias unit is set to b=1, as usual. On each training iteration, the script chooses the target state (present or absent) at random with equal prior probability [$P(T=1) = P(T=0) = 0.5$], and sets the desired output accordingly: d=1 for target present, d=0 for target absent. It also draws visual input at random from a univariate Gaussian distribution with standard deviation $\sigma = 1$ (in the script set `sdv1=1` and `sdv0=1`) and mean corresponding to the chosen target state: target present mean $\mu_1 = 6$ (set `mev1=6`) and target absent mean $\mu_0 = 3$ (set `mev0=3`). The univariate Gaussian deviates are generated according to Equation 9.1, as in the fish classification example (see Section 9.1). Delta rule training occurs at a learning rate of `a=0.1` for `nIts=100000` iterations.

The actual output unit responses after training are shown in Figure 9.8A as circles. The smooth curve is the target-present posterior probability determined using Bayes' rule (see earlier in this section). This particular run of training produced a relatively good estimate of the target-present posterior. Other runs will not necessarily produce estimates that are this good, but in general the delta rule will do an adequate job of training the sigmoidal unit to estimate the target-present probability given visual input. The response of the single sigmoidal unit trained using the delta rule provides a reasonably close match to the posterior probability determined using the unisensory Bayes' rule model. The response of the unit increases as its input increases, and provides a plausible simulation of the responses of collicular neurons to inputs of one sensory modality (Stein and Meredith 1993). The correspondence between the model and the behavior of real neurons will be much more interesting in the bisensory case, as we will see in the next section. Before we get there, we will compare the single unit model trained using the delta rule with one in which the weights are determined analytically rather than learned adaptively.

As we observed previously when exploring the fish classification example, Bayes' rule can be used to compute posterior probabilities exactly when the prior and likelihood distributions are known, and networks of sigmoidal units can be trained to estimate posterior probabilities from data when the classes are known but the prior and likelihood distributions are not known. Networks of sigmoidal neural elements are not the only adaptive agents capable of such estimation. Classifiers of other forms can also estimate posterior probabilities when trained using algorithms that minimize a least-squares error function (Richard and Lippman 1991).

While it is not necessary for classification tasks in general, the sigmoidal squashing function offers important advantages for neural modeling. The sigmoidal squashing function of weighted input sum q is $f(q) = 1/(1 + e^{-q})$. It is neurobiologically plausible because it simulates the threshold and saturation properties of real neurons (see Chapter 6 for background on the sigmoidal squashing function). As we demonstrated in this section, the single sigmoidal unit, with input and bias weights trained using the delta rule, can estimate posterior probabilities. It seems that the sigmoidal function lends itself well to probability computations, and this impression can be confirmed. For simple, binary classification problems in which the priors and likelihoods are known, and in which the likelihood distributions are describable as Gaussians (or other, similarly manageable functions), it is possible analytically to determine the input and bias weight values that would allow a single, sigmoidal unit to compute the posterior probability exactly (Bishop 1995; Duda et al. 2001).

An example calculation is presented in Math Box 9.3. The example corresponds to the unisensory target detection problem, where the target-present and target-absent priors are equal [$P(T = 1) = P(T = 0) = 0.5$], and the likelihoods are Gaussian distributed, with different target-present μ_1 and target-absent μ_0 means ($\mu_1 \neq \mu_0$), but with standard deviation $\sigma = 1$ in both cases. With these simplifying assumptions, the calculation shows that the sigmoidal unit will compute the target-present posterior exactly if the weight of the sensory input equals [$(\mu_1 - \mu_0)/\sigma^2$] and if the bias weight equals [$(\mu_0^2 - \mu_1^2)/2\sigma^2$]. With the means set at $\mu_1 = 6$ and $\mu_0 = 3$, and standard deviation set at $\sigma = 1$, the analytically determined input and bias weights are +3.0 and −13.5, respec-

MATH BOX 9.3   SOLVING FOR THE INPUT AND BIAS WEIGHTS OF A SIGMOIDAL UNIT THAT COMPUTES A POSTERIOR PROBABILITY

Another benefit of using the sigmoidal squashing function (see Chapter 6) in neural systems modeling is associated with the fact that the squashing function (also called the logistic function) and the logit function are inverses. The logit of a number y between 0 and 1 is $\ln[y / (1-y)]$. If we let q be the value of the logit function, then the relationship in Equation B9.3.1 holds:

$$q = \ln\left(\frac{y}{1-y}\right) \Rightarrow y = \frac{1}{\left(1 + e^{-q}\right)}$$ (B9.3.1)

Logit function   Squashing function

This relationship can be especially useful for inference involving a binary random variable, like T (with specific values $t_S = 1, 0$), given an observation on another (not binary) random variable on which it depends, like X (with specific values x), because $1 - P(T = 1 \mid X = x) = P(T = 0 \mid X = x)$. Thus, if $q = \ln[P(T = 1 \mid X = x) / P(T = 0 \mid X = x)]$, then the squash of q would be $P(T = 1 \mid X = x)$. Making use of Bayes' rule (see Math Box 9.2), we get Equation B9.3.2:

$$q = \ln\left[\frac{P(T = 1 \mid X = x)}{P(T = 0 \mid X = x)}\right] = \ln\left[\frac{\dfrac{P(X = x \mid T = 1)P(T = 1)}{P(X = x)}}{\dfrac{P(X = x \mid T = 0)P(T = 0)}{P(X = x)}}\right]$$ (B9.3.2)

Let the likelihoods $P(X = x \mid T = t_S)$ be Gaussian distributed according to Equation B9.1.1 (see Math Box 9.1) where the mean $\mu = \mu_1$ when $T = 1$ and $\mu = \mu_0$ when $T = 0$. For simplicity, assume that the standard deviation σ is the same for both the $T = 1$ and $T = 0$ cases, and that the prior probabilities are equal, so that $P(T = 1) = P(T = 0) = 0.5$. Substituting Equation B9.1.1 into Equation B9.3.2 (with means μ_1 and μ_0 appropriately set) we arrive at Equation B9.3.3:

$$q = \left(\frac{\mu_1 - \mu_0}{\sigma^2}\right)x + \left(\frac{\mu_0^2 - \mu_1^2}{2\sigma^2}\right)b \triangleq v_1 x + v_2 b$$ (B9.3.3)

In this particular case, if a sigmoidal unit receives input x with weight $v_1 = [(\mu_1 - \mu_0)/ \sigma^2]$, and a bias input $b = 1$ with weight $V_2 = [(\mu_0^2 - \mu_1^2)/ 2\sigma^2]$, then the output y of the unit will equal the posterior probability $P(T = 1 \mid X = x)$.

tively. The script `unisensoryDeltaRule` stores the input and bias weights in matrix (row vector) V (see MATLAB Box 9.4). The input and bias weight values trained by the delta rule for the responses shown in Figure 9.8 were +2.2 and –9.1, respectively. Thus, the values found using the delta rule are reasonably close to those determined analytically.

With the mean of the target-present likelihood greater than that of the target-absent likelihood ($\mu_1 > \mu_0$), the input weight will be positive while the bias weight will be negative. Sensory inputs exert an excitatory effect on collicular neurons, while tonically (continuously) active neurons from the substantia nigra (a midbrain structure) exert an inhibitory effect on collicular neurons (Stein and Meredith 1993). It is tempting to speculate that the excitatory input and the inhibitory bias in the single-unit model correspond to sensory inputs and nigral inputs to collicular neurons, respectively. In any case, it should be emphasized that analytical computation of the weights is possible only under a restricted set of circumstances. It is likely that the connection weights mediating any probability estimation actually carried out by real neurons is learned rather than pre-set by evolution or development. Adaptability may be critical to probability estimation by real neurons. The delta rule learning scheme we implemented here is plausible neurobiologically.

As mentioned at the beginning of this section, the superior colliculus is responsible for detecting, selecting, and localizing targets in the environment and initiating orienting responses toward them (Wurtz and Goldberg 1989). Selection and localization could be mediated by a winners-take-all competition that culminates in a burst of collicular activity that initiates the orienting movement (see Chapter 3). It is not unreasonable to suppose that such a winners-take-all mechanism could also generate goal states that drive adaptive changes in the responses of collicular neurons to sensory inputs. The desired output for the single unit trained using the delta rule is simply 1 if the target is present and 0 if it is absent. A winners-take-all mechanism operating in the colliculus could generate such desired outputs for the whole population of collicular neurons by bringing some neurons to their fully active state (near 1 for sigmoidal units) and all other neurons to the inactive state (near 0 for sigmoidal units). In addition to initiating orienting movements, achievement of the winners-take-all state could also initiate adaptive processes in the superior colliculus.

Recall from Chapter 6 that weight changes Δv due to the delta rule are equal to $a(d - y)f'(q)x$, where a is the learning rate, d and y are the desired and actual outputs, x is the input, q is the weighted input sum, and $f'(q)$ is the derivative of the squashing function. (For simplicity we write this term for a single synapse so we can drop the subscripts from the variable names.) Using the formula for the derivative of the squashing function (see Math Box 6.3), the delta rule weight update equation can be written as: $\Delta v = a(d - y)y(1 - y)x$. To make use of a winners-take-all state as a desired output pattern for delta rule learning, individual synapses in the colliculus would need to store the value of the input (pre-synaptic activity x) and the initial collicular neuron response (post-synaptic activity y) prior to a winners-take-all competition, and would need to receive and utilize a signal indicating the success of the orienting movement that results from a competition. A successful orienting movement would indicate that a target was actually present and could signal to the colliculus that its pattern of activity after the winners-take-all competition corresponds to a desired output pattern. Each collicular synapse would then have the input x, actual output y, and desired output d signals it would need to compute synaptic weight adjustments according to the delta rule. (Learning rate a is just an arbitrary constant of proportionality.)

Such a multifaceted mechanism is plausible. Evidence is accumulating that neuromodulatory systems can provide reinforcement signals like those that could indicate the success of orienting movements (see Chapter 7). Evidence is also building that molecular mechanisms within synapses can play signal processing roles, compute basic functions (e.g., add and multiply), and act as simple memories (see Chapter 14). The analytical and computational approaches we explored in this section suggest not only that neurons could plausibly compute probabilities but that they could equally plausibly learn to do so.

In this section we have compared the posterior probabilities derived using Bayes' rule with the responses of a sigmoidal unit that has its input weight and bias either analytically determined or trained using the delta rule. It is important to point out that this comparison is made between modeling results on different levels of description, as distinguished by David Marr, one of the most influential of all neural systems modelers. Marr (1982) identified three levels on which neural systems can be understood. On the computational level we strive to understand the goal or objective of the processing brought about by a neural system. On the algorithmic level we strive to understand which quantities are represented by a neural system and in what way it combines them so as to achieve its goal. On the implementational level we strive to understand how the neural system accomplishes its goal in terms of neuro-biological mechanisms.

Our simple model of the unisensory responses of a collicular neuron nicely illustrates these three levels. On the computational level we hypothesize that the collicular neuron computes (or estimates) the posterior probability that a target is present in its receptive field, given its sensory input. On the algorithmic level we hypothesize that the collicular neuron can learn to represent the prior probability of the target, and the likelihood of observing sensory inputs of various amounts given that the target is present or absent. We further hypothesize, on the algorithmic level, that the collicular neuron can use those representations to infer the posterior probability of the target using Bayes' rule. On the implementational level we hypothesize that a collicular neuron can learn to adjust the weight of its sensory input and its bias (i.e., a constant influence on its activity that may be internal, external, or both), according to the parameters that describe the target prior probability and sensory likelihood distributions, and can thereby tune its responses so that they provide estimates of target posterior probability. Because the models we study in this book actually accomplish a computational goal (oscillation, memory storage, sensorimotor transformation, and so on), and because they are neural in form (from single neural units to multilayered neural networks), they can be understood on all three of Marr's levels. The models in this chapter are also similar to the other models in this book in that they are really hypotheses that need to be tested experimentally. We will address this important issue in the next section.

9.5 Modeling Multisensory Collicular Neurons as Probability Estimators

Certain datasets provide keys to modelers that open doors to new perspectives. The multisensory responses of collicular neurons constitute such a dataset. In this section we will simulate the responses of collicular neurons to sensory stimulation of two modalities, because the bisensory case easily generalizes to the multisensory case with stimuli of arbitrarily many sensory modalities (Patton and Anastasio 2003). We will describe the model on Marr's three levels: computational, algorithmic, and implementational. On the computational level, we will posit that a collicular neuron uses multisensory input to infer the probability that a target has appeared in its receptive field. On the algorithmic level, we will suggest that a collicular neuron represents target prior probabilities and sensory input likelihoods and uses them to infer target posterior probability using Bayes' rule. On the implementational level we will show how the input and bias weights to a single sigmoidal unit could be learned, or configured, to produce responses that estimate, or compute exactly, the target posterior probability. The results will give us insight into how neurons in general could function as probability computers. Clues into the multisensory function of collicular neurons can be found experimentally on the behavioral and neurophysiological levels.

Behaviorally, an animal is more likely to detect a target if it emits sensory stimuli of two or more modalities, rather than of one modality alone. Thus, the cat in Figure 9.9 detects the bird when it is both visible and audible, but not when it is only visible or only audible. These behavioral effects can be measured systematically in the laboratory (Stein and Meredith 1993) and they have neurophysiological correlates, as shown in Figure 9.10.

The superior colliculus is a layered structure (Wurtz and Goldberg 1989). While neurons in the superficial layers receive purely visual input, many neu-

FIGURE 9.9 Depiction of multisensory integration on the behavioral level The cat does not detect the bird if it provides only one sensory cue (visual or auditory), but the cat does detect the bird if it provides two cues (visual and auditory). (From Stein and Meredith 1993.)

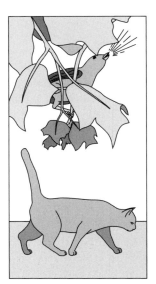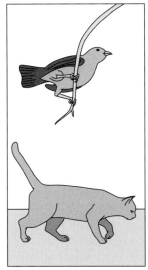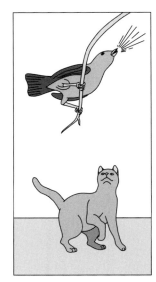

rons in the deeper layers of the superior colliculus receive input of more than one sensory modality (Meredith and Stein 1986; Stein and Meredith 1993). Multisensory collicular neurons combine their responses to multisensory input in complex and highly nonlinear ways. The responses of collicular neurons that receive inputs of two (or more) sensory modalities can be tested with stimuli of two modalities presented either separately or together. This experimental paradigm reveals that the combined-modality (cross-modal) response of collicular neurons can be larger than the dominant single-modality (modality-specific) response (see Figure 9.10). Although the cross-modal response is sometimes larger than the sum of the modality-specific responses, any increase in the cross-modal over the dominant modality-specific response is considered as multisensory enhancement. The amount of multisensory enhancement produced by the cross-modal response is quantified as a percentage of the maximal modality-specific response as in Equation 9.6:

$$\%MSE = \left(\frac{CM - MS_{\max}}{MS_{\max}} \right) \times 100 \qquad \textbf{9.6}$$

where %*MSE* is the percentage of multisensory enhancement, *CM* is the cross-modal response, and $MS_{\max}$ is the maximal (larger of the two) modality-specific responses (Stein and Meredith 1993).

Multisensory enhancement is magnitude dependent in that larger %*MSE* values are associated with smaller modality-specific responses (see Figure 9.10). In other words, %*MSE* tends to be larger when the sensory stimuli are weak and produce smaller modality-specific responses. This magnitude dependency has been termed inverse effectiveness. The elegant experimental description of these phenomena (Meredith and Stein 1986; Stein and Meredith 1993) has lead to the hypothesis on the computational level that collicular neurons use multisensory input to compute posterior probabilities (Anastasio et al. 2000). On the algorithmic level, modeling work has shown that both multisensory enhancement and inverse effectiveness can be simulated using Bayes' rule (Anastasio et al. 2000; Anastasio and Patton 2004). In the model, multisensory neurons in the superior colliculus are thought to infer the posterior probability that a target has appeared in their receptive fields, given sensory input of multiple modalities. Both multisensory enhancement and inverse effectiveness emerge from the computation of this probability. On the imple-

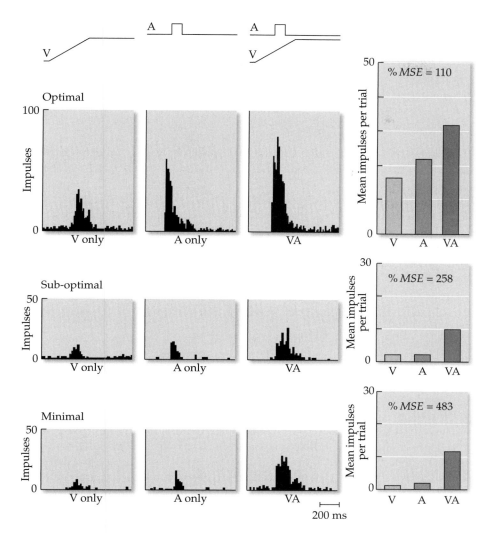

FIGURE 9.10 Neurophysiological data from cat superior colliculus illustrating the phenomena of multisensory enhancement and inverse effectiveness Stimuli V, A, and VA are visual only, auditory only, and visual and auditory combined. The V, A, and VA stimuli (shown at the top as silhouettes) are delivered at three levels of effectiveness: minimal, sub-optimal, and optimal. The neural responses (histograms) in all stimulus conditions increase as stimulus effectiveness increases. At all levels the cross-modal response (VA) is larger than either of the two modality-specific responses (V or A). The increase in the response resulting from the cross-modal combination of sensory inputs has been termed multisensory enhancement. Multisensory enhancement, expressed as a percentage (% MSE) of the larger of the two modality-specific responses, decreases with increases in stimulus effectiveness and modality-specific responses (bar charts). The inverse relationship between multisensory enhancement and stimulus effectiveness has been termed inverse effectiveness. Percentage multisensory enhancement (% MSE) is computed according to Equation 9.6. (After Meredith and Stein 1986.)

mentational level, single sigmoidal model neurons can be configured to use multiple sensory inputs to compute target posterior probabilities and thereby also simulate multisensory enhancement and inverse effectiveness (Patton and Anastasio 2003). Thus, we can describe the multisensory responses of collicular neurons on the computational, algorithmic, and implementational levels. In this section we will focus our study on versions of these models on the algorithmic and implementational levels.

We will model the bisensory responses of collicular neurons on the algorithmic level using Bayes' rule and on the implementational level by using the delta rule to train a single sigmoidal unit to estimate the posterior probability that a target is present, given bisensory input (and a bias). To construct the algorithmic model we must first determine what the model will represent. As in the unisensory case, we will again represent the target as binary random variable T, where it can either be present ($T = 1$) or absent ($T = 0$). The target-present and target-absent prior probabilities are $P(T = 1)$ and $P(T = 0)$, respectively. The two sensory input random variables will be visual V and auditory A, with specific values v_S and a_S, respectively. Unlike the unisensory case, in which the single sensory (i.e., visual) input had the univariate likelihoods $P(V = v_S \mid T = 1)$ and $P(V = v_S \mid T = 0)$, the visual and auditory inputs in the bisensory case will have the joint likelihoods $P(V = v_S, A = a_S \mid T = 1)$ and $P(V = v_S, A = a_S \mid T = 0)$ for target-present or target-absent, respectively. To compute the posterior probability that the target is present given visual and auditory input, Bayes' rule would be applied as in Equation 9.7:

$$P(T = 1 \mid V = v_S, A = a_S) =$$
$$\frac{P(V = v_S, A = a_S \mid T = 1)P(T = 1)}{P(V = v_S, A = a_S \mid T = 1)P(T = 1) + P(V = v_S, A = a_S \mid T = 0)P(T = 0)}$$

9.7

The bisensory likelihood distributions are bivariate, and involve the conjunction of V and A. We will model these likelihood distributions as bivariate Gaussians.

The bivariate Gaussian distribution can be described using five parameters: the mean of each variable, the standard deviation of each variable, and the correlation between the two variables (see Math Box 9.1). Bivariate Gaussian random deviates with means μ_1 and μ_2, standard deviations σ_1 and σ_2, and correlation coefficient ρ can be generated using Equation 9.8:

$$\begin{bmatrix} x_1 \\ x_2 \end{bmatrix} = \begin{bmatrix} \sigma_1 & 0 \\ \sigma_2 \rho & \sigma_2 \sqrt{1-\rho^2} \end{bmatrix} \begin{bmatrix} \eta(0,1) \\ \eta(0,1) \end{bmatrix} + \begin{bmatrix} \mu_1 \\ \mu_2 \end{bmatrix}$$

9.8

A contour plot showing a bivariate Gaussian distribution, and Gaussian deviates x_1 and x_2 generated using Equation 9.8 are shown in Figure 9.3B.

The main difference between the bisensory and unisensory cases of the Bayes' rule model is that the bisensory case is bivariate while the unisensory case is univariate. This obvious difference has important implications. As we shall see, the bisensory case is much more complicated than the unisensory case, although the essential form of the probabilistic model is the same in both cases. In the bisensory case, as in the unisensory case, we have two likelihood distributions: one is the target-present likelihood and the other is the target-absent likelihood. We will use subscripts 1 and 0 to denote target-present and target-absent, and subscripts V and A to denote visual and auditory. For example, the mean for the visual input when the target is present is denoted as μ_{V1}. Similarly μ_{V0} denotes the mean of the visual input when the target is absent. The target-present and target-absent means for the auditory input are denoted as μ_{A1} and μ_{A0}, respectively. Note that the sensory input random variables V and A can take nonzero values whether the target is present or absent, but we assume that their activity, on average, is higher when the target is present, so $\mu_{V1} > \mu_{V0}$ and $\mu_{A1} > \mu_{A0}$. The same subscripting conventions will be applied to the standard deviations and correlation coefficients in the bisensory case.

In simulating multisensory enhancement, we do not need to consider every possible combination of visual and auditory inputs, but can focus instead on certain combinations. The combinations correspond to the experimental conditions in which the multisensory responses of collicular neurons were tested (Meredith and Stein 1986). Note in Figure 9.10 that the visual and auditory stimuli were presented either separately or together at three levels of effectiveness: minimal, sub-optimal, and optimal. When presented together, the effectiveness levels of the two stimuli were matched. As in the unisensory case (see Section 9.4), we make the reasonable assumption that a stimulus of a certain modality drives the corresponding sensory system when it is present, but that the activity of a sensory system is spontaneous (i.e., it produces background activity) when a stimulus of its corresponding modality is absent. Thus, when a sensory input is driven we will allow its variable to take specific values over a range ($V = v_S$ or $A = a_S$), but when a sensory input is spontaneous we will set its variable to its target-absent mean ($V = \mu_{V0}$ or $A = \mu_{A0}$).

To simulate multisensory enhancement we consider the following stimulus combinations: cross-modal, in which both the visual and auditory inputs are driven equally by the target; visual-specific, in which the visual input is driven but the auditory input is spontaneous; and auditory-specific, in which the auditory input is driven but the visual input is spontaneous. Thus, rather than consider the full, two-dimensional target-present likelihood $P(V = v_S, A = a_S | T = 1)$, we need only consider the following one-dimensional cuts through it: the cross-modal $P(V = A | T = 1)$, the visual-specific $P(V = v_S, A = \mu_{A0} | T = 1)$, and the auditory-specific $P(V = \mu_{V0}, A = a_S | T = 1)$. We also consider the corresponding cuts through the target-absent likelihood $P(V = v_S, A = a_S | T = 0)$, which are the cross-modal $P(V = A | T = 0)$, the visual-specific $P(V = v_S, A = \mu_{A0} | T = 0)$, and the auditory-specific $P(V = \mu_{V0}, A = a_S | T = 0)$. It is convenient also to consider the corresponding cuts through the joint evidence distribution $P(V = v_S, A = a_S)$, which are the cross-modal $P(V = A)$, the visual-specific $P(V = v_S, A = \mu_{A0})$, and the auditory-specific $P(V = \mu_{V0}, A = a_S)$.

These cuts are illustrated using the bivariate distribution of Figure 9.3B in which both variables have mean 5. The diagonal line marks likelihoods for which both variables are equal. The horizontal and vertical lines mark likelihoods for which one variable changes over the range while the other is held fixed at a value of 2.5. The variables could be thought of as different sensory inputs that both have target-present means of 5 and target-absent means of 2.5. Then the diagonal line represents the cross-modal cut while the horizontal and vertical lines represent the two modality-specific cuts. For computational convenience, we will use the principle of total probability to compute the entire bivariate evidence distribution from the joint (visual and auditory) target-present and target-absent likelihoods, and the target prior probability distribution. Thus, we will take the cross-modal, visual-specific, and auditory-specific cuts from the bivariate target-present and target-absent likelihood and evidence distributions.

The script `bisensoryBayesRule` (MATLAB Box 9.5) will generate bivariate Gaussian likelihoods according to the parameters set in the script and will compute the target-present posterior probability $P(T = 1 | V = v_S, A = a_S)$ from the prior probability $P(T = 1)$ in the three input configurations described above (cross-modal, visual-specific, and auditory-specific). The script will also compute an analog of $\%MSE$. It does this using Equation 9.6, where the target posterior in the cross-modal case $P(T = 1 | V = A)$ stands for CM, and the larger of the visual-specific $P(T = 1 | V = v_S, A = \mu_{A0})$ or auditory-specific $P(T = 1 | V = \mu_{V0}, A = a_S)$ target posteriors stands for MS_{max}.

The script `bisensoryBayesRule` will use the same variables as script `unisensoryBayesRule` (see MATLAB Box 9.3) to hold the target prior probabilities and the means and standard deviations for the target-present and target-absent visual input. In addition, script `bisensoryBayesRule` will use `mea1`, `mea0`, `sda1`, and `sda0` to hold the means and standard deviations for the target-present and target-absent auditory input. It will also use `r1` and `r0` to hold the target-present and target-absent correlation coefficients. The script sets up vector `sVal` of (discrete) sensory input values over a range, and uses `sVal` to make the two-dimensional grids `vis` and `aud` covering the range of visual and auditory input values using `[vis,aud]=ndgrid(sVal)`. It uses `vis`, `aud`, and the likelihood means, standard deviations, and correlation parameters to compute the joint likelihoods $P(V = v_S, A = a_S | T = 1)$ and $P(V = v_S, A = a_S | T = 0)$ as (discrete) bivariate Gaussians (see Equation B9.1.3 in Math Box 9.1) and stores these in arrays `D2pvat1` and `D2pvat0`, respectively. It computes the joint evidence distribution $P(V = v_S, A = a_S)$ according to the principle of total probability (see Math Box 9.2) using `D2pva=D2pvat1*pt1+D2pvat0*pt0`. One cross-modal and two modality-specific cuts are taken from each of these two-dimensional Gaussians.

Script `bisensoryBayesRule` must necessarily use more complicated variable names than `unisensoryBayesRule` because it must take account

MATLAB® BOX 9.5 This script computes the posterior probability of a target given sensory input of two modalities (i.e., visual and auditory).

```
% bisensoryBayesRule.m

mev1=4; mev0=2; % set target present and absent visual means
mea1=3; mea0=2; % set target present and absent auditory means
sdv1=1; sdv0=1; % set target present and absent visual SDs
sda1=1; sda0=1; % set target present and absent auditory SDs
r1=0; r0=0; % set target present and absent correlation coefficients
pt1=0.5; pt0=1-pt1; % set target present prior, compute absent
maxVal=9; nVals=30; % set max and number of sensory input values
sVal=linspace(0,maxVal,nVals); % set sensory value vector
[vis,aud]=ndgrid(sVal); % make all visual/auditory value pairs

% compute the 2D Gaussian likelihood distributions
D2pvat1=(1/(2*pi*sdv1*sda1*sqrt(1-r1^2)))* ...
    exp(-(1/(2*(1-r1^2)))*(((vis-mev1)/sdv1).^2 - ...
    2*r1*(((vis-mev1)/sdv1).*((aud-mea1)/sda1))+((aud-mea1)/sda1).^2));
D2pvat0=(1/(2*pi*sdv0*sda0*sqrt(1-r0^2)))*...
    exp(-(1/(2*(1-r0^2)))*(((vis-mev0)/sdv0).^2 - ...
    2*r0*(((vis-mev0)/sdv0).*((aud-mea0)/sda0))+((aud-mea0)/sda0).^2));
D2pvat1=D2pvat1/sum(sum(D2pvat1)); % normalize
D2pvat0=D2pvat0/sum(sum(D2pvat0)); % normalize

% compute unconditional probability (evidence) of V and A
D2pva=D2pvat1*pt1+D2pvat0*pt0;

% find closest spontaneous mean indices into 2D distributions
indices=find(sVal>=mev0); spontVindx=indices(1);
indices=find(sVal>=mea0); spontAindx=indices(1);

% extract cross-modal and modality-specific likelihoods
pvat1=diag(D2pvat1); pvat0=diag(D2pvat0); pva=diag(D2pva);
pvaSPt1=D2pvat1(:,spontAindx); pvaSPt0=D2pvat0(:,spontAindx);
pvaSP=D2pva(:,spontAindx);
pvSPat1=D2pvat1(spontVindx,:); pvSPat0=D2pvat0(spontVindx,:);
pvSPa=D2pva(spontVindx,:);

% compute posterior probabilities
pt1va=(pvat1./pva)*pt1; % cross-modal
pt1vaSP=(pvaSPt1./pvaSP)*pt1; % visual specific
pt1vSPa=(pvSPat1./pvSPa)*pt1; % auditory specific

% compute BayesMSE as percentage of max mod-specific probability
if max(pt1vaSP) > max(pt1vSPa),
    BayesMSE=((pt1va-pt1vaSP)./pt1vaSP)*100;
else BayesMSE=((pt1va-pt1vSPa')./pt1vSPa')*100; end
[maxBayesMSE indxB]=max(BayesMSE);
```

of multiple stimulus configurations. For example, the cross-modal cut through the full, two-dimensional target-present likelihood $P(V = A \,|\, T = 1)$ is held in variable pvat1 and is extracted using pvat1=diag(D2pvat1). The visual-specific $P(V = v_S, A = \mu_{A0} \,|\, T = 1)$ and auditory-specific $P(V = \mu_{V0}, A = a_S \,|\, T$

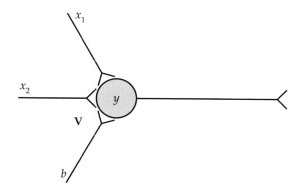

FIGURE 9.11   A single, sigmoidal unit used to simulate a bisensory neuron in the superior colliculus The unit y receives inputs x_1 and x_2 and a bias b. The weight matrix **V** is a row vector containing the weights of the three connections to y from x_1, x_2, and b. The unit computes the weighted sum of its inputs and passes the result through the sigmoidal squashing function (see Chapter 6). Inputs x_1 and x_2 could represent visual and auditory inputs, respectively, and the bias could represent constant influences on the firing rate of the collicular neuron.

=1) cuts are similarly extracted and held in variables `pvaSPt1` and `pvSPat1`, respectively. Note that `SP` in a modality-specific variable name follows the letter indicating which sensory input is spontaneous. Thus `pvaSPt1` is the target-present visual-specific likelihood because the auditory input is spontaneous. The target-absent likelihood cuts are similarly `pvat0`, `pvaSPt0`, and `pvSPat0`. The joint evidence cuts are `pva`, `pvaSP`, and `pvSPa`. With the likelihoods and evidence in place the posterior probabilities in the three different stimulus conditions can be computed. The cross-modal target-present posterior probability is computed using `pt1va=(pvat1./pva)*pt1`. The visual-specific and auditory-specific target-present posterior probabilities are computed similarly and held in variables `pt1vaSP`, and `pt1vSPa`. We will use `bisensoryBayesRule` to analytically determine posterior probability curves, which we can then compare with the responses of single sigmoidal units that are trained using the delta rule to estimate the bisensory target posterior.

A schematic of a single neural unit that receives two inputs and a bias is depicted in Figure 9.11. (As before, for simplicity, we will not represent the inputs or bias explicity as units.) The script `bisensoryDeltaRule`, which is listed in MATLAB Box 9.6, will train a single sigmoidal unit to estimate the posterior target probability by training it to "classify" its bisensory input into the single target-present class. This script is essentially the same as its unisensory counterpart (`unisensoryDeltaRule`) except that at each iteration it must draw two random deviates, one each for the visual and auditory modalities. It does this by implementing Equation 9.8. Generation of the bisensory input begins by assembling correlation matrices for the target-present and target-absent cases. The correlation matrix in the target-present case is assembled using `C1=[sdv1,0;sda1*r1,sda1*sqrt(1-r1^2)]`. Then the two-element (column) vector of visual and auditory inputs `inVA` in the target-present case can be generated using `inVA=C1*randn(2,1)+[mev1;mea1]`. Analogous procedures are used to generate the bisensory input in the target-absent case.

In the bisensory case the single sigmoidal unit, depicted in Figure 9.11, computes its weighted input sum as $q = v_1 x_1 + v_2 x_2 + v_3 b$, where v_1, v_2, and v_3 are the elements of weight matrix **V** (**V** $= [v_1\ v_2\ v_3]$), and computes its activation using the squashing function as $y = 1/(1 + e^{-q})$. Inputs x_1 and x_2 correspond to the visual and auditory inputs, respectively, and bias $b = 1$. The delta rule will train the weights v_1, v_2, and v_3 so that y provides an estimate of the bisensory target-present posterior probability $P(T = 1 \mid V = v_S, A = a_S)$. (Here **V** is the weight matrix containing weights v_1, v_2, and v_3, while V is the random variable representing the visual input that takes specific values v_S. Also without ambiguity, A is the random variable representing the auditory input that takes specific values a_S, while a is the learning rate for the delta rule.) To accomplish delta rule training, parameters must be set that specify the statistical proper-

MATLAB® BOX 9.6 **This script trains a single sigmoidal unit using the delta rule to estimate posterior target probability given sensory input of two modalities (i.e., visual and auditory).**

```
% bisensoryDeltaRule.m

nIn=2; nOut=1; % set numbers of units
a=0.1; b=1; % set learning rate and bias
nIts=100000; % set number of iterations

mev1=4; mev0=2; % set target present and absent visual means
mea1=3; mea0=2; % set target present and absent auditory means
sdv1=1; sdv0=1; % set target present and absent visual SDs
sda1=1; sda0=1; % set target present and absent auditory SDs
r1=0; r0=0; % set target present and absent correlation coefficients
pt1=0.5; pt0=1-pt1; % set target present prior, compute absent
cumPrior=cumsum([pt1 pt0]); % find cumulative prior
maxVal=9; nVals=30; % set max and number of sensory input values
sVal=linspace(0,maxVal,nVals)'; % set sensory value vector

% construct target present and absent correlation matrices
C1=[sdv1,0;sda1*r1,sda1*sqrt(1-r1^2)];
C0=[sdv0,0;sda0*r0,sda0*sqrt(1-r0^2)];

V=rand(nOut,nIn+1)*2-1; % set initial connectivity matrix
deltaV=zeros(nOut,nIn+1); % zero the change weight matrix

% train network using the delta-rule
for c=1:nIts, % for each iteration
    % choose target present or absent at random by prior
    indxVec=find(cumPrior>=rand); choose=indxVec(1);
    if choose==1, inVA=C1*randn(2,1)+[mev1;mea1]; d=1;
    elseif choose==2, inVA=C0*randn(2,1)+[mev0;mea0]; d=0; end
    x=[inVA' b]'; % set input with bias appended
    y=1./(1+exp(-V*x)); % compute the output response
    dy=y.*(1-y); % compute derivative of squashing function
    e=d-y; % find the error for the chosen input
    g=e.*dy; % find output error signal
    deltaV=a*g*x'; % compute delta rule weight update
    V=V+deltaV; % apply the weight update
end % end training loop

bVec=b*ones(nVals,1); % set bias vector
Vspont=ones(nVals,1)*mev0; Aspont=ones(nVals,1)*mea0; % set spont
Inb=[sVal sVal bVec; sVal Aspont bVec; Vspont sVal bVec]; % input
Out=(1./(1+exp(-V*Inb')))'; % compute output to all inputs
Out=reshape(Out,nVals,3)'; % reshape Out into a 2D array

% compute unitMSE for output
if max(Out(2,:)) > max(Out(3,:)),
    unitMSE=((Out(1,:)-Out(2,:))./Out(2,:))*100;
else unitMSE=((Out(1,:)-Out(3,:))./Out(3,:))*100; end
[maxunitMSE indxN]=max(unitMSE);
```

ties of the target and the visual and auditory inputs, and the initial weights of the inputs to the sigmoidal unit.

For our first simulation of multisensory enhancement we will consider a case in which the visual and auditory inputs are uncorrelated ($\rho_1 = \rho_0 = 0$), which is set using r1=0 and r0=0 in script bisensoryDeltaRule. Set the target-present and target-absent visual and auditory likelihood means as follows: μ_{V1} = 4, μ_{V0} = 2, μ_{A1} = 3, and μ_{A0} = 2 (mev1=4, mev0=2, mea1=3, and mea0=2 in the script). Note that the target-present means are larger than the target-absent means, as in the unisensory case, and the visual and auditory target-absent means are set equal to facilitate analysis of the responses. Set the standard deviations all equal at 1: $\sigma_{V1} = \sigma_{V0} = \sigma_{A1} = \sigma_{A0} = 1$ (sdv1=1, sdv0=1, sda1=1, and sda0=1). As before, set the target prior probabilities equal: $P(T = 1) = P(T = 0) = 0.5$ (set pt1=0.5, and pt0 is computed in the script as pt0=1−pt1). The bias should be set at 1 (b=1). The script will set up a single sigmoidal unit with two input weights and one bias weight (weight matrix V is a three-element row vector). Before training, the script will set the values of these weights to random numbers between −1 and +1. Set the script to run for nIts=100000 training iterations with learning rate a=0.1.

After training, script bisensoryDeltaRule determines the responses of the sigmoidal unit under the three different input configurations. In the cross-modal configuration, both the visual and auditory inputs are set equal as they are increased over the range. In the visual-specific or auditory-specific configuration, the visual or auditory input, respectively, is increased over the range while the auditory or visual input, respectively, is held fixed at its target-absent mean. The %*MSE* is computed using Equation 9.6, where the response in the cross-modal case stands for *CM* and the larger of the visual-specific or auditory-specific responses stands for MS_{max}. The script bisensoryDeltaRule stores the cross-modal, visual-specific, and auditory-specific responses in rows 1, 2, and 3, respectively, of array Out and stores the %*MSE* values in unitMSE.

The responses of the sigmoidal unit under each of the three input configurations are shown using symbols in Figure 9.12A (cross-modal, circles;

(A)

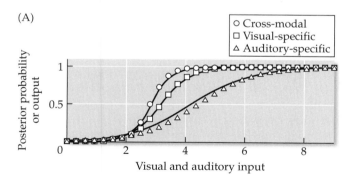

(B)

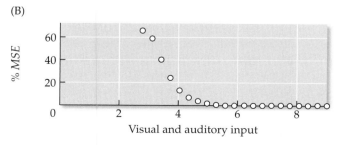

FIGURE 9.12 Bisensory probabilities computed using Bayes' rule, or estimated by a single sigmoidal unit trained using the delta rule, for uncorrelated inputs (A) The target-present posterior probabilities computed using Bayes' rule are shown as smooth curves, and estimates by the unit are shown using symbols (cross-modal, circles; visual-specific, squares; auditory-specific, triangles). (B) The percentage multisensory enhancement (%*MSE*) is computed from the unit responses according to Equation 9.6.

visual-specific, squares; auditory-specific, triangles). The smooth curves are the bisensory target-present probabilities determined analytically under each of the three input configurations using script `bisensoryBayesRule` (see MATLAB Box 9.5). This particular run of training produced a relatively good estimate of the target-present posterior. Other runs will not necessarily produce estimates that are as good. The reason that the responses of the single sigmoidal unit agree well with the actual target-present posteriors after this run is because the input and bias weights determined by the delta rule are close to the weights that can be analytically determined for the unit.

As in the unisensory case (see Math Box 9.3), the exact values of the input and bias weights to a sigmoidal unit that allow it to compute the target posterior, given Gaussian distributed likelihoods, can also be determined analytically in the bisensory case (and, indeed, in the general multisensory case; see Patton and Anastasio 2003 for details). Given the simplifying assumptions that we made for this bisensory simulation ($\sigma_{V1} = \sigma_{V0} = \sigma_{A1} = \sigma_{A0} = 1, \rho_1 = \rho_0 = 0$), the analytically derived weights take the same form for each of the two sensory inputs as they did for the single input in the unisensory case $[(\mu_1 - \mu_0)/\sigma^2]$, where μ_1 and μ_0 are the target-present and target-absent likelihood means for either modality. The values for the visual and auditory input weights due to delta rule training, which are +2.2 and +1.1, respectively, compare well with the analytically determined values of +2.0 and +1.0. The visual weight is larger than the auditory weight, reflecting its higher quality as a source of evidence concerning the target. The analytically determined bias weight formula, which is more complicated in the bisensory than in the unisensory case, specifies a bias weight of −8.5. The bias weight of −9.1 due to delta rule training in this simulation is close to that value.

Having established that a single sigmoidal unit can compute target-present posterior probabilities in the bisensory case, we examine the bisensory responses themselves (see Figure 9.12A). The responses under all three input conditions rise from 0 to 1 as the cross-modal or modality-specific inputs increase over the range, but they rise at different rates. The visual-specific response rises faster than the auditory-specific response because of the relationships between the target-present and target-absent likelihood means of the two inputs. Because the target-present and target-absent likelihood means are better separated for the visual ($\mu_{V1} = 4, \mu_{V0} = 2$) than for the auditory ($\mu_{A1} = 3, \mu_{A0} = 2$) input, the visual input provides better evidence concerning the presence of the target. As a consequence, the posterior target-present probability will change more rapidly for changes in the visual-specific than in the auditory-specific input (Anastasio et al. 2000; Anastasio and Patton 2004). These simulated responses are consistent with the actual responses of multisensory collicular neurons.

For a simulation of multisensory enhancement the focus is on the difference between the cross-modal and the modality-specific responses. In this simulation the cross-modal response rises much faster than either of the modality-specific responses (see Figure 9.12A). The %*MSE* exhibited by the unit is shown in Figure 9.12B. Note that %*MSE* values for very small output responses are not shown. Presumably, these small output values would be below the spiking threshold of a real collicular neuron and so would not show up as neural responses. Many %*MSE* values are greater than zero, indicating that the cross-modal response for the corresponding input values is larger than the visual-specific response, which is the larger of the two modality-specific responses (see Equation 9.6). The increase of the cross-modal over the maximal modality-specific response simulates multisensory enhancement. The maximal value of %*MSE* is about 66%, but %*MSE* decreases as the values of the inputs increase. Although increases in the values of the inputs cause increases in the sizes of the modality-specific responses, they cause decreases in %*MSE*. This simulates inverse effectiveness.

These results demonstrate that a single sigmoidal unit trained using the delta rule to estimate target-present posterior probabilities, given sensory input of two different modalities, can be used to simulate both multisensory enhancement and inverse effectiveness. The Bayes' rule model, which exactly computes the target posterior that is only estimated by the single sigmoidal unit, is also capable of simulating multisensory enhancement and inverse effectiveness. Thus, the Bayes' rule model provides a description of the multisensory responses of collicular neurons on the algorithmic level of Marr, while the single sigmoidal unit provides a description on the implementational level. The model on the computational level is equivalent to the hypothesis that collicular neurons use their multisensory inputs to compute target probability. The real multisensory responses of collicular neurons are consistent with this hypothesis.

The phenomena of multisensory enhancement and inverse effectiveness make sense in the context of the hypothesis of target probability computation, in which the responses of collicular neurons are seen as proportional to target posterior probability. When a stimulus of one modality is strong, the large modality-specific sensory input it generates would provide strong evidence by itself that a target is present, and the target-present probability estimated by a collicular neuron would be high. Sensory input of another modality would not increase that probability very much, so it would not be effective in producing multisensory enhancement. The response of the collicular neuron should be about the same given sensory input of two modalities (cross-modal) or of only one modality (modality-specific) when the inputs are large.

In contrast, when a stimulus of one modality is weak, the small sensory input it generates would not provide strong evidence by itself that a target is present, and the target-present probability estimated by a collicular neuron would be low. However, if the target emits a stimulus of another modality, even if it is weak and would also generate a small sensory input by itself, it could provide strong evidence that a target is present in combination with the other input. When the inputs are small, the target-present probability estimated by a collicular neuron could be much higher with two (cross-modal) than with only one (modality-specific) input. Consequently, the response of the collicular neuron should be much larger when it receives small inputs of two rather than of only one modality. The results indicate that the responses of real collicular neurons are consistent with the Bayes' rule hypothesis. The observation that small sensory inputs are much more effective in producing multisensory enhancement is consistent with the description, on the computational level, that the goal of multisensory integration is to infer target-present posterior probability given multisensory input.

The effectiveness of two sensory inputs in providing evidence concerning the presence of a target also depends on the degree to which the inputs are statistically independent. If the two sensory inputs are completely uncorrelated, as in the example we just considered, then each provides evidence that the other does not, so they would provide stronger evidence in combination. In contrast, if the two inputs are completely correlated, then the second input provides no evidence that was not already provided by the first input. Correlation between the two inputs should decrease their effectiveness and erode multisensory enhancement.

To demonstrate this relationship, we consider an example in which the visual and auditory inputs are correlated. As before, set the target-present and target-absent visual and auditory likelihood means as follows: $\mu_{V1} = 4$, $\mu_{V0} = 2$, $\mu_{A1} = 3$, and $\mu_{A0} = 2$. Set all of the standard deviations equal at 1 ($\sigma_{V1} = \sigma_{V0} = \sigma_{A1} = \sigma_{A0} =$

FIGURE 9.13   Bisensory probabilities computed using Bayes' rule, or estimated by a single sigmoidal unit trained using the delta rule, for correlated inputs (A) The target-present posterior probabilities computed using Bayes' rule are shown as smooth curves, and estimates by the unit are shown using symbols (cross-modal, circles; visual-specific, squares; auditory-specific, triangles). (B) The percentage multisensory enhancement is computed from the unit responses according to Equation 9.6. The maximum percentage multisensory enhancement (%MSE) is lower in this (correlated) example than in the previous (uncorrelated) example (see Figure 9.12). In this example, nonzero correlation between the visual and auditory inputs erodes multisensory enhancement.

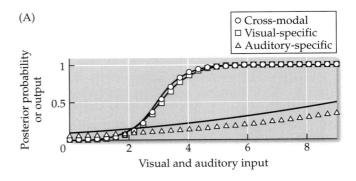

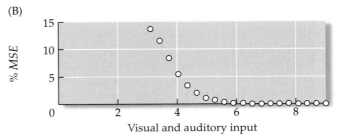

1), and set the target prior probabilities equal [$P(T = 1) = P(T = 0) = 0.5$], but now set the target-present and target-absent correlations equal at 0.4 ($\rho_1 = \rho_0 = 0.4$; in the script set r1=0.4 and r0=0.4). Script bisensoryDeltaRule will again set up a single sigmoidal unit with two input weights and one bias weight, and will set the initial values of these weights to random numbers between −1 and +1. As before, set the bias unit at 1, and train for 100,000 training iterations using the delta rule with a learning rate of 0.1.

The responses following training of the sigmoidal unit under each of the three input configurations are shown using symbols in Figure 9.13A (cross-modal, circles; visual-specific, squares; auditory-specific, triangles). The smooth curves are the bisensory target-present posterior probabilities determined by Bayes' rule under each of the three input configurations using script bisensoryBayesRule (see MATLAB Box 9.5). This particular run of training produced a relatively good estimate of the target-present posterior. Other runs will not necessarily produce estimates that are as good.

The visual-specific response is much larger than the auditory-specific response, not only because the target-present and target-absent likelihood means are better separated for the visual than for the auditory input, but also because of the nonzero correlation between the visual and auditory inputs in this example. Analytically derived formulas for the input and bias weights in the correlated bisensory case are complicated (Patton and Anastasio 2003), but a comparison of the weights between the correlated and uncorrelated cases is instructive. The visual and auditory input weights are both positive in the correlated as in the uncorrelated case. While the visual input weights are about the same in the correlated and uncorrelated cases (+2.1 and +2.2, respectively), the auditory weight is much smaller in the correlated (+0.2) than in the uncorrelated (+1.1) case. The correlation between the inputs causes the auditory weight to decrease, and so its influence on the response of the unit decreases accordingly. The bias weight is also negative but not as negative with correlated (−6.9) as with uncorrelated (−9.1) inputs, in part because the excitatory auditory input weight is smaller, so less inhibitory bias is necessary.

The most striking difference between the correlated and uncorrelated examples is that in the correlated case, the cross-modal response and the visual-specific response (the larger of the two modality-specific responses) are about the same. This is reflected by the much smaller maximum $\%MSE$ value, which is only about 14% in the correlated case compared with 66% in the uncorrelated case. The $\%MSE$ in the correlated case decreases as the values of the inputs increases (Figure 9.13B), showing that the correlated case also simulates inverse effectiveness. However, the correlation reduces the size of the cross-modal response relative to the maximal modality-specific response and seriously erodes multisensory enhancement.

The simulation using correlated bisensory inputs may help explain the responses of collicular neurons to multiple stimuli of the same sensory modality. Because the receptive fields of multisensory collicular neurons are large, it is experimentally feasible to deliver two separate sensory stimuli to the same neuron that are of the same modality, as well as of different modalities. Neurons in the superior colliculus vary with regard to the amount by which the response to one sensory input will be enhanced by another, but the amount of enhancement is much less when the two inputs are of the same rather than of different modalities (Alvarado et al. 2007). This can be explained within the context of the hypothesis that collicular neurons estimate target posterior probabilities by making the reasonable assumption that inputs of the same modality will be more highly correlated than inputs of different modalities (Patton and Anastasio 2003).

As with all of the models in this book, the one considered here is a hypothesis. The computation-level version of the hypothesis is that multisensory enhancement and inverse effectiveness result from the computation by a collicular neuron of the posterior probability that a target is present in its receptive field, given its sensory inputs. An experimentally feasible test of this hypothesis can be designed by making use of Bayes' rule, which is the algorithm-level version of the hypothesis, and of the measurable properties of collicular neurons. According to Bayes' rule, the posterior probability should depend not only on the likelihoods (which concern the sensory inputs in the case of multisensory enhancement) but also on the prior probability. The prior probability that target stimuli would fall into the receptive field of a collicular neuron should be proportional to the size of the field. The model predicts that the maximal multisensory enhancement exhibited by a multisensory neuron should be inversely proportional to the prior probability that a target stimulus would fall into its receptive field (Anastasio and Patton 2004). Testing this hypothesis is experimentally feasible because both multisensory enhancement and receptive field size are measurable for collicular neurons.

Though still hypothetical, the Bayes' rule model of multisensory enhancement provides a clear example of how the responses of neurons could be interpreted as estimates of the probability that their target feature is present. This is a relatively old hypothesis (e.g., Barlow 1969), but its application as a model of multisensory integration in the colliculus is particularly appropriate. Because inputs of different sensory modalities can be manipulated unambiguously, experimentalists studying multisensory collicular neurons were able to discover and characterize the phenomena that they called multisensory enhancement and inverse effectiveness (Meredith and Stein 1986; Stein and Meredith 1993). The correspondence between these multisensory phenomena and the behavior of the Bayes' rule model provides a strong indication that some neurons actually do compute probabilities. While it finds an especially clear expression in the multisensory context, the application of Bayesian inference in models of neural function extends well beyond multisensory integration.

As we discussed in Chapters 7 and 8, neurons and synapses are inherently noisy (with activity that is randomly varying or stochastic). The crux

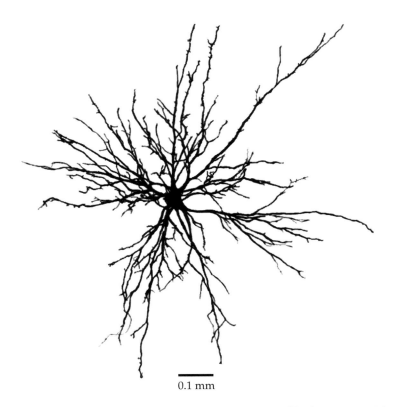

0.1 mm

FIGURE 9.14   Camera lucida drawing of a superior colliculus neuron The neuron is classified morphologically as a large multipolar radiating cell. It was found in the stratum griseum intermedium (one of the deep layers) of the superior colliculus of a cat. (From Behan et al. 1988.)

of the Bayes' rule hypothesis and similar Bayesian inference ideas is that the more stochastic inputs a neuron receives from sensory and other neurons, the more reliably it can determine the presence or absence of its target feature. In Chapter 8 we explored the ability of neural elements in a population to encode input information despite their stochastic (unreliable) relationship with the input. Bayesian inference provides a method to decode the information that is encoded by a population of stochastic neural elements. The idea that a neuron needs to integrate input from many other, noisy neurons in order to reliably detect its target feature may partly explain why neurons are so extensively interconnected. With this in mind, it is tempting to look at a neuron from the deep layers of the superior colliculus, such as the one pictured in Figure 9.14, and imagine it collecting as much input as it can over its extensive dendritic tree in order to make its best possible estimate of target posterior probability.

Ideas concerning Bayesian inference and population encoding come together in another important sense in neural systems modeling. It is possible that populations of neurons encode a probability distribution over all possible values of a random variable. This idea has been applied in modeling the responses of neurons in various brain regions (Pouget et al. 2003). For example, the population of neurons in a region of the temporal cortex specialized for processing visual motion could encode the probability of such motion in each of many possible directions simultaneously (Zemel et al. 1998). In Chapter 12 we will consider a model of a brainstem structure that computes, on every time step, the distribution of probabilities that a target is present at each (discrete) location in a simulated environment. Our examples in this chapter focused on a single neuron in the superior colliculus, but the colliculus is composed of topographically organized layers of neurons, and their receptive fields, especially in the deep, multisensory layers, are large and overlapping (Wurtz and Goldberg 1989; Stein and Meredith 1993). If each neuron computes the probability that a given target is in its receptive field, then the neurons taken together encode the probability of that target at each location in the collicular topographic representation. The population of collicular neurons could encode the target posterior probability distribution over location.

Matters get more interesting when we consider more than one target. We saw in Chapter 3 how lateral inhibitory interactions could simulate the observed reduction in the sizes of the responses of collicular neurons to targets as the number of simultaneously presented targets is increased, but this is a description on the implementational level. What is the computational goal of a representation characterized by multiple smaller peaks? It is possible that the colliculus as a whole estimates the posterior probability distribution for a single target, as though there is only ever one target in the environment. In this case each of the multiple peaks estimates the probability of the same, single target but at a different location, and the smaller amplitudes of the peaks reflect the spreading of target probability over the distribution. Alternatively, it is possible that the colliculus could somehow encode several probability distributions simultaneously, each one for a different target (Zemel et al. 1998). Whatever the case, the computation performed by the population of collicular neurons is likely to be different from that occurring in other brain structures. Most likely, different brain regions employ probabilistic population codes in different ways and for different purposes (Pouget et al. 2003). Still, the idea that populations of neurons encode probability distributions is rich with explanatory power and will continue to generate new hypotheses concerning neural systems function.

The Bayes' rule hypothesis that we explored in this chapter is most consistent with the view that each collicular neuron uses its sensory input (whether unisensory or multisensory) to estimate the posterior probability that a target is present within its receptive field. In this view the colliculus is confronted with multiple targets and its goal is to select the most probable one. It follows from the Bayes' rule hypothesis that the location of the most probable target in the environment at any time would correspond to the location on the collicular topographic map of the neuron with the largest sensory response. Reductions in the sizes of the responses due to presentation of multiple targets could be a consequence of lateral inhibitory interactions that mediate a winners-take-all competition. In Chapter 3 we used a winners-take-all network to simulate the process by which the colliculus selects and localizes a target, and generates a burst that serves as a command to make an orienting movement toward that target (Wurtz and Goldberg 1989). This process would ultimately form a multiunit burst centered on the location in the colliculus of the neuron with the largest, initial sensory response. According to the Bayes' rule hypothesis, the burst would constitute a command to make an orienting movement that would be directed toward the location having the highest target posterior probability.

Recent behavioral and neurophysiological results are compatible with this idea. Empirical findings suggest that the colliculus as a whole uses multisensory integration to generate commands for orienting movements toward those stimulus sources that indicate the most probable targets (e.g., Bell et al. 2005). The correspondences between experimental and modeling results, combined with the feasibility of directly testing the Bayes' rule hypothesis, suggest that the superior colliculus would be an auspicious brain region in which to explore ideas linking Bayesian inference and neural function.

Exercises

9.1   In the fish classification example, the prior probabilities of the three fish types were set equal. Specifically, the three fish species were minnow, salmon, and marlin, and the prior probability of catching each of the three was set at 1/3. Setting a uniform prior probability distribution would be justified if we knew nothing about fish, but we know that minnows are much more plentiful than salmon, and that salmon are much more plentiful than marlin. Try setting the prior probability distribution in a manner that better reflects the relative abundances of the three fish species. Recall that the prior distribution for the fish classification example is [$P(F = 1)$, $P(F = 2)$, $P(F = 3)$], and that the three prior probabilities must sum to 1 for the distribution to be valid. The prior probabilities of the three fish classes are held in variables `pf1`, `pf2`, and `pf3` in script `classifyFishBackProp` (see MATLAB Box 9.1). Retrain the network with your more realistic prior probabilities. What happens? How do the output and hidden unit responses compare with those that result from training with a uniform prior distribution? Would you expect this result given the nature of the training procedure? (Note that the prior probability distribution also determines how often fish of each species are presented to the network.)

9.2   We found that a three-layered network with 12 hidden units trained using back-propagation did a good job of approximating the posterior probabilities of the three fish species given their lengths (see Figure 9.4). Change the prior probability distribution back to uniform in script `classifyFishBackProp` (`pf1=1/3`, `pf2=1/3`, and `pf3=1/3`), and test the ability of the network to learn to classify fish with different numbers of hidden units (variable `nHid`). Does the network need all 12 hidden units? Do the responses of the hidden units change as you decrease their number? How does the performance of the network change as you decrease the number of hidden units?

9.3   We trained a single sigmoidal unit using the delta rule to estimate target posterior probabilities given evidence in the form of visual and auditory inputs. In our original simulation we set all standard deviations at 1, target-present and target-absent correlations at 0, and both the target-present and target-absent prior probabilities at 0.5 (uniform prior distribution). We set the target-absent visual and auditory means at 2. We also set the target-present visual mean at 4 and the target-present auditory mean at 3, and we found that maximum %*MSE* was about 66%. Keeping all other parameters the same, increase the target-present visual mean to 5 and the target-present auditory mean to 4. These increases in the visual and auditory target-present means can be made in script `bisensoryDeltaRule` (see MATLAB Box 9.6) using `mev1=5` and `mea1=4`. Ensure that the visual and auditory target-absent means are kept the same as before at `mev0=2` and `mea0=2`. How do these increases in target-present means change maximum %*MSE*? What does this indicate about the relationship between the target-present and target-absent means and maximum %*MSE*?

9.4 Again, for the single sigmoidal unit trained using the delta rule to estimate target posterior probabilities, the original parameters were: all standard deviations set at 1, target-present and target-absent correlations set at 0, both the target-present and target-absent prior probabilities set at 0.5, the target-absent visual and auditory means set at 2, and the target-present visual and auditory means set at 4 and 3, respectively. With these settings we found a maximum %*MSE* of about 66%. What happens to maximum %*MSE* when, keeping the other parameters the same, all the standard deviations (target-present and target-absent, visual and auditory) are increased to 2? This can be done in script `bisensoryDeltaRule` using `sdv1=2`, `sdv0=2`, `sda1=2`, and `sda0=2`. What does this indicate about the relationship between the amount of overlap of the target-present and target-absent likelihood distributions and maximum %*MSE*?

References

Alvarado JC, Vaughan JW, Stanford TR, Stein BE (2007) Multisensory versus unisensory integration: Contrasting modes in the superior colliculus. *Journal of Neurophysiology* 97: 3193–3205.

Anastasio TJ, Patton PE (2004) Analysis and modeling of multisensory enhancement in the deep superior colliculus. In: Calvert G, Spence C, Stein B (eds) *The Handbook of Multisensory Processes*, Bradford Books/MIT Press, Cambridge, MA.

Anastasio TJ, Patton PE, Belkacem-Boussaid K (2000) Using Bayes' rule to model multisensory enhancement in the superior colliculus. *Neural Computation* 12: 997–1019.

Barlow HB (1969) Pattern recognition and the responses of sensory neurons. *Annals of the New York Academy of Sciences* 156: 872–881.

Behan M, Appell PP, Graper MJ (1988) Ultrastructural study of large efferent neurons in the superior colliculus of the cat after retrograde labeling with horseradish peroxidase. *The Journal of Comparative Neurology* 270: 171–184.

Bell AH, Meredith MA, VanOpstal AH, Munoz DP (2005) Crossmodal integration in the primate superior colliculus underlying the preparation and initiation of saccadic eye movements. *Journal of Neurophysiology* 93: 3659–3673.

Bishop CM (1995) *Neural Networks for Pattern Recognition*. Clarendon Press, Oxford.

Duda RO, Hart PE, Stork DG (2001) *Pattern Classification: Second Edition*. John Wiley and Sons, New York.

Knill DC, Richards W (1996) *Perception as Bayesian Inference*. Cambridge University Press, New York.

Marr D (1982) *Vision*. WH Freeman and Company, San Francisco.

Meredith MA, Stein BE (1986) Visual, auditory, and somatosensory convergence on cells in the superior colliculus results in multisensory integration. *Journal of Neurophysiology* 56: 640–662.

Oaksford M, Chater N (2001) The probabilistic approach to human reasoning. *TRENDS in Cognitive Sciences* 5: 349–357.

Papoulis A (1991) *Probability, Random Variables, and Stochastic Processes: Third Edition*. McGraw Hill, Boston.

Patton PE, Anastasio TJ (2003) Modeling cross-modal enhancement and modality-specific suppression in multisensory neurons. *Neural Computation* 15: 783–810.

Pouget A, Dayan P, Zemel RS (2003) Inference and computation with population codes. *Annual Review of Neuroscience* 26: 381–410.

Richard MD, Lippmann RP (1991) Neural network classifiers estimate Bayesian a-posteriori probabilities. *Neural Computation* 3: 461–483.

Stein BE, Meredith MA (1993) *The Merging of the Senses*. MIT Press, Cambridge MA.

Stich S (1985) Could man be an irrational animal? *Synthese* 64: 115–135.

Wurtz RL, Goldberg ME (1989) *The Neurobiology of Saccadic Eye Movements*. Elsevier, Amsterdam.

Zemel RS, Dayan P, Pouget A (1998) Probabilistic interpretation of population codes. *Neural Computation* 10: 403–430.

10

Time Series Learning and Nonlinear Signal Processing

Supervised learning through time can train neural networks to produce dynamic transformations and simulate certain forms of motor control and short-term memory

hinking, which is the quintessential cognitive function, involves a series of steps. Research supports what we would surmise through introspection: Thinking in humans involves an ordered sequence of operations. These include storage and updating of items in memory, mental manipulations that carry out logical and arithmetic processes, and attention that can be focused on specific memory items and processes (Smith and Jonides 2003). In its ordered storage, access, and manipulation of memory items, thinking as it is understood in humans resembles processing by digital computers. This resemblance lead Alan Turing, in 1950, to suggest that machines (specifically digital computers) could be constructed and programmed to think just as humans do. Whether or not a machine can "think" has been a matter of heated debate (Churchland and Churchland 1990; Epstein et al. 2008), but no one would dispute the fact that digital computers are powerful symbolic processors. Any computational paradigm equivalent to a digital computer would be powerful as well. In this chapter we will explore a neural systems modeling paradigm that is, in principle, as powerful as any digital computer, and we will use it to simulate certain forms of motor control and short-term memory.

Turing's confidence that computers could think may have derived in part from his proof that the functionality of all digital computers could be captured by a simple device that implements the apparent components of human thought. The "Turing machine" is an abstract computing device that consists of only three components: a memory, an executive unit, and a control unit. The memory is an array of locations in which symbols can be stored. The executive unit can move to any location in the memory array, can read from and write to memory, and can carry out simple commands. The control unit ensures that the executive unit carries out commands correctly. The symbols in the memory store correspond to numbers or to instructions. An example command might be "Add the number stored in location 4302 to the number stored in location 6809 and replace the number in the second location with the resulting sum." The command might be coded as 4302680917, where the first eight digits indicate the locations of the numbers to be added and the location of the sum, and 17 is the code for the adding instruction. Repeated application of this command recursively adds the number in location 4302 to the sum in 6809, so recursive computations are executable according to this simple scheme. This kind of recursive computation is essential because most computations of any significance cannot be computed in one step. Given certain assumptions, such as the infinite extent of the memory array, Turing proved that his simple "machine" is capable of performing any computation of which a conventional digital computer is capable (Turing 1936). Thus the Turing machine is a "universal computer."

The simplicity of the Turing machine lends itself well to formal description, and that facilitates the establishment of the equivalence between Turing machines and certain other computational paradigms. Because the Turing machine is a universal computer, any computational paradigm that is equivalent to a Turing machine is also a universal computer. Although real nervous systems are capable of processing that, in many ways, far exceeds the capability of current digital computers, most would agree that a neural systems modeling paradigm with Turing equivalence would be a powerful paradigm.

Two of the most powerful neural systems modeling paradigms we have explored so far in this book are dynamic networks and supervised learning. The dynamic networks we considered in Chapter 2 had recurrent (feedback) connections, and were therefore capable of producing dynamic input–output transformations, but they were composed of linear units. As such, they were capable of prolonging (or foreshortening) signals in time, and of oscillation, but their behavioral range was restricted in comparison with that of recurrent networks of nonlinear units. In Chapters 3 and 4 we studied recurrent networks of nonlinear units that simulated activity-bubble formation (see Chapter 3) or memory recall (see Chapter 4) by reaching stable states. The behavior of these attractor networks is useful for simulating some neural systems, but the inexorable pull of the activities of their units toward stable-states makes them poorly suited for simulating the kinds of continuous input–output transformations produced by other neural systems.

The networks we trained in Chapter 6 using supervised learning included those having multiple layers of nonlinear units. We explored the ability of multilayered networks of sigmoidal units, trained using back-propagation, to approximate a wide range of input–output transformations. Despite their flexibility, these networks were limited to static transformations because they lacked recurrent connections. In this chapter we will explore the use of an algorithm that enables supervised learning of dynamic input–output transformations by recurrent networks of nonlinear units (Williams and Zipser 1989). This is a very powerful paradigm. It has been proven mathematically that fully recurrent networks composed of sigmoidal units are equivalent to the Turning machine (Seigelmann and Sontag 1991). Therefore, in principle, recurrent networks composed of sigmoidal units are capable of any computation of which digital computers are capable. The learning algorithm we will explore essentially enables us to "program" these powerful processors.

In this chapter we will train recurrent networks of nonlinear units to perform dynamic input–output transformations, and we will compare the behavior of the units in these trained networks directly with that of real neurons. We will not attempt to simulate human "thinking" in this book, but we can touch on some of its apparent components. We will simulate "attention" (or a more well-defined quantity that may be analogous to attention) in Chapter 12. In Chapter 14 we will admit that mental manipulations such as the application of arbitrary rules so far eludes simulation using neural systems models. However, in this chapter we will train nonlinear, recurrent neural networks to simulate working (short-term) memory of the kind that appears to be involved in "thinking" (Goldman-Rakic 1987).

We will also revisit a topic we considered in detail in Chapter 2, that of velocity storage in the vestibulo-ocular reflex, which can be considered as a rudimentary form of memory. We will show how we can gain a deeper understanding of the neural mechanisms that underlie velocity storage when we simulate it using nonlinear recurrent neural networks. In particular, we will show how the trained network, and by analogy the brain as well, exploits the power of nonlinearity to enhance its ability to process signals in time. Our ability to use nonlinear recurrent neural networks to simulate these processes depends on our ability to train them to reproduce the kinds of dynamic input–output transformations that real neural systems produce. The algorithm we will use for this purpose is a direct extension of back-propagation to temporal patterns.

For a neural network to produce dynamic input–output transformations it needs to have recurrent, or feedback, connections between its units. In general, any unit in a recurrent network can be connected to any other unit, including itself. The back-propagation algorithm, which operates on static input–output patterns, can be used to train networks to produce dynamic input–output transformations through a process known as back-propagation through time (Rumelhart et al. 1986). Back-propagation through time is illustrated for a simple recurrent network in Figure 10.1.

The recurrent network shown in Figure 10.1A has two units, y_1 and y_2, which exert feedback on themselves directly over recurrent self-connections with weights w_{11} or w_{22}. They also exert feedback on themselves indirectly, each through the other, over recurrent connections with weights w_{12} and w_{21}. The responses in discrete time t of the units in this simple network are described by Equation 10.1:

$$\begin{bmatrix} y_1(t) \\ y_2(t) \end{bmatrix} = \begin{bmatrix} w_{11} & w_{12} \\ w_{21} & w_{22} \end{bmatrix} \begin{bmatrix} y_1(t-1) \\ y_2(t-1) \end{bmatrix} \qquad \textbf{10.1}$$

which is the same equation used to describe the responses of the two-unit networks we considered in Chapter 2, except that the input terms are absent. For this simple network without explicit input connections, we can imagine that the task to be learned is to transform the initial, nonzero states of y_1 and y_2 into some desired, time-varying signal.

Figure 10.1B shows this network "unfolded" in time, so that the states of the units y_k (k = 1, 2) on discrete time step $t-1$ are the inputs, while the states on

FIGURE 10.1   Back-propagation through time can be used to train neural networks with recurrent connections
(A) A simple recurrent neural network composed of units y_1 and y_2 that connect to each other and to themselves. (B) The network in (A) unfolded in time, where the states of the units at time $t-1$ ($y_{1,t-1}$ and $y_{2,t-1}$) serve as the inputs, and the states of the units at time t ($y_{1,t}$ and $y_{2,t}$) serve as the outputs. Given desired states for both units (y_1 and y_2) on each time step, the weights could be trained using the delta rule through time. Back-propagation through time could be used to train recurrent networks that have desired states for only some of the units on each time step. (After Rumelhart et al. 1986.)

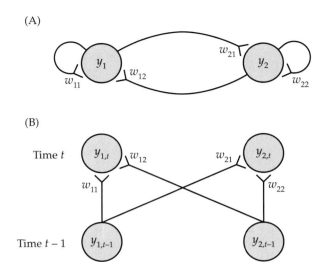

time step t are the outputs of a network in which the connections are purely feedforward. Because we know the desired output sequence, we can compute the error on each time step and can train the unfolded network on each time step using a conventional, static input–output supervised learning algorithm. For the special case in which we know the desired output on each time step of every unit in the network, the recurrent network unfolds into a two-layered feedforward network and we can use the delta rule for training (see Chapter 6). For the more general case in which the desired output is known only for some of the units, then the recurrent network would unfold into a multilayered feedforward network and would require back-propagation for training (Rumelhart et al. 1986).

Back-propagation through time can be used to train recurrent networks in principle, but it is cumbersome in practice. For this reason we will use an algorithm called real-time recurrent learning, developed by Williams and Zipser (1989), which treats weight updates as well as network unit states as dynamic variables. Real-time recurrent learning is more computationally complex than back-propagation through time (Haykin 1999), but its elegance and ease of use will more than compensate us. Because the weight updates produced by real-time recurrent learning are equivalent to those produced by back-propagation through time, we can refer to real-time recurrent learning as recurrent back-propagation. The derivation of the recurrent back-propagation algorithm is outlined in Math Box 10.1. The algorithm itself is described in the next section.

10.1 Training Connection Weights in Recurrent Neural Networks

Because of their structural flexibility, the units in recurrent neural networks cannot always be segregated into separate layers such as the input, hidden, and output layers of purely feedforward networks. Instead, certain units in recurrent networks are simply chosen to provide the input to, or to produce the desired output from, the network. All the other units can be considered as hidden units. A critically important factor distinguishing input from non-input (hidden and output) units is that input units in recurrent networks do not receive connections from other units. (In general, all units in recurrent networks, including input units, may send connections to non-input units.) The states of the hidden and output (non-input) units in a recurrent network

MATH BOX 10.1   DERIVATION OF REAL-TIME RECURRENT BACK-PROPAGATION

The derivation of real-time recurrent back-propagation (Williams and Zipser 1989) is similar to that of the delta rule and back-propagation (see Math Boxes 6.2 and 6.5) in that its goal is to determine how to compute weight changes that are proportional to the opposite of the gradient of network error with respect to the weights. The derivation is more complicated for recurrent back-propagation than for back-propagation or the delta rule and will only be sketched briefly here (see Williams and Zipser 1989 for details). The network error measure is defined in Equation B10.1.1:

$$E(t) = \frac{1}{2} \sum_{k \in U} \left[e_k(t) \right]^2 \qquad \text{B10.1.1}$$

where k indexes all of the non-input units U ($k \in U$) in the network (i.e., those units that receive potentially modifiable weights from other units) and t denotes discrete time. Error $e_k(t)$ is defined in Equation 10.5 of the main text but the definition is reproduced here in Equation B10.1.2 for convenience:

$$e_k(t) = \begin{cases} d_k(t) - y_k(t), & k \in D \\ 0, & k \notin D \end{cases} \qquad \text{B10.1.2}$$

where D is the subset of units $D \subseteq U$ that have desired values. Because all connection weights, including the input–hidden v, hidden–hidden w, and hidden–output u weights can be treated in the same way for this recurrent learning algorithm, we will include all of these weights as elements m_{ij} in connection weight matrix **M**. We seek weight changes $\Delta m_{ij}(t)$ that are proportional to the opposite of the gradient of $E(t)$ with respect to the weights, as shown in Equation B10.1.3:

$$\Delta m_{ij}(t) = -a \frac{\partial E(t)}{\partial m_{ij}} \qquad \text{B10.1.3}$$

The partial derivative $\partial E(t) / \partial m_{ij}$ in Equation B10.1.3 can be found by differentiating Equation B10.1.1 with respect to weight m_{ij}. Note that desired output $d_k(t)$ (see Equation B10.1.2) is not dependent on the network weights m_{ij} so that $\partial d_k(t)/\partial m_{ij} = 0$, and $\partial E(t)/\partial m_{ij}$ can be expressed as in Equation B10.1.4:

$$-\frac{\partial E(t)}{\partial m_{ij}} = \sum_{k \in U} e_k(t) \frac{\partial y_k(t)}{\partial m_{ij}} \qquad \text{B10.1.4}$$

where the $y_k(t)$ are the states of the non-input units on time step t. By reference to Equations 10.3 and 10.4 of the main text, which describe unit activation in the recurrent network, the value of each partial derivative $\partial y_k(t)/\partial m_{ij}$ can be computed in terms of the set of partial derivatives $\partial y_l(t)/\partial m_{ij}$ ($l \in U$) as shown in Equation B10.1.5:

$$\frac{\partial y_k(t)}{\partial m_{ij}} = f'\left(q_k(t)\right) \left[\sum_{l \in U} m_{kl} \frac{\partial y_l(t-1)}{\partial m_{ij}} + \delta_{ik} z_j(t-1) \right] \qquad \text{B10.1.5}$$

where $q_k(t)$ is the weighted input sum to the non-input unit y_k ($k \in U$) on time step t, $f'(\cdot)$ is the derivative of the squashing function (see Math Box 6.3), z_j ($j \in I \cup U$) is the state of any input or non-input unit, and δ_{ik} is the Kronecker delta where $\delta_{ik} = 1$ when $i = k$ but $\delta_{ik} = 0$ when $i \neq k$. Equation B10.1.5 is equivalent to the dynamic system defined in Equation B10.1.6:

$$h_{ij}^k(t) = f'\left(q_k(t)\right) \left[\sum_{l \in U} m_{kl} h_{ij}^l(t-1) + \delta_{ik} z_j(t-1) \right] \qquad \text{B10.1.6}$$

where the h_{ij}^k can be thought of as versions of every weight m_{ij} that belong to each unit y_k. Equation B10.1.6 is the same as Equation 10.7 of the main text. The correspondence between Equations B10.1.5 and B10.1.6 implies Equation B10.1.7:

$$h_{ij}^k(t) = \frac{\partial y_k(t)}{\partial m_{ij}} \qquad \text{B10.1.7}$$

In the text we refer to the h_{ij}^k as the elements of partial derivative matrices. More specifically, they are the partial derivatives of the state of each unit y_k with respect to each of the weights m_{ij}. Substituting Equation B10.1.7 into B10.1.4, and B10.1.4 into B10.1.3, we get Equation B10.1.8, which describes the weight updates for real-time recurrent back-propagation:

$$\Delta m_{ij}(t) = a \sum_{k \in U} e_k(t) h_{ij}^k(t) \qquad \text{B10.1.8}$$

Equation B10.1.8 is the same as Equation 10.6 of the main text.

at any time t are functions of the states of the input and non-input units at time $t-1$ (see Chapter 2). For computational convenience, the states of all the units are represented together in (column) vector $\mathbf{z}$, which has elements indexed by k as shown in Equation 10.2:

$$z_k(t) = \begin{cases} x_k(t), & k \in I \\ y_k(t), & k \in U \end{cases} \qquad \textbf{10.2}$$

where I is the set of input units, U is the set of all other (non-input) units, and the symbol $\in$ means "is an element of." Note that for the purposes of describing the state and weight updates in a recurrent network we have relaxed our erstwhile assignment of index j to states x, i to y, and k to z but will use i, j, k, and l more flexibly as state or weight subscripts as needed. All of the weights are contained in connectivity matrix $\mathbf{M}$, where m_{ij} represents the weight of the connection to non-input unit y_i ($i \in U$) from any input unit x_j or non-input unit y_j ($j \in U \cup I$). Using m_{ij} to represent any element of the connection weight matrix for the whole network will free us to use u, v, and w to label elements in distinct sub-matrices of the whole weight matrix. Use of these additional variable names to distinguish certain connection weights will be convenient for modeling purposes throughout this chapter.

The net input $q_k(t)$ to any unit $k \in U$ at time t is shown in Equation 10.3:

$$q_k(t) = \sum_{l \in U} m_{kl} y_l(t-1) + \sum_{l \in I} m_{kl} x_l(t-1) = \sum_{l \in U \cup I} m_{kl} z_l(t-1) \qquad \textbf{10.3}$$

and the output is computed as in Equation 10.4, where $f(\cdot)$ is the sigmoidal squashing function:

$$y_k(t) = f\big(q_k(t)\big) = \frac{1}{1 + \exp\big(-q_k(t)\big)} \qquad \textbf{10.4}$$

Thus, the dynamic networks we will consider in this chapter are like those we considered in Chapter 2, but in this case the activation functions of the units can be nonlinear, where the nonlinearity is the sigmoidal squashing function (see Chapter 6).

The goal of recurrent back-propagation, like that of many other supervised learning algorithms, is to adjust the weights in $\mathbf{M}$ to reduce the error between the desired and actual output of the network. As in the static form of back-propagation, this is done by computing the network error gradient in weight space, and using this gradient to find updates to the values of the weights (see Math Box 10.1). For dynamic input–output patterns, the gradient is also a function of time. The learning process begins as described in Equation 10.5 by finding the error between the desired and actual outputs:

$$e_k(t) = \begin{cases} d_k(t) - y_k(t), & k \in D \\ 0, & k \notin D \end{cases} \qquad \textbf{10.5}$$

In Equation 10.5, $D \subseteq U$ is the subset of units y_k in U ($k \in D$, $D \subseteq U$) for which desired values $d_k(t)$ exist. (The symbol $\subseteq$ means "is a subset of.") The weight changes are computed as shown in Equation 10.6:

$$\Delta m_{ij}(t) = a \sum_{k \in U} e_k(t) h_{ij}^k(t) \qquad \textbf{10.6}$$

where a is the fixed, positive learning rate. The h_{ij}^k values are computed iteratively for all $k \in U$, $i \in U$, and $j \in U \cup I$ as described in Equation 10.7:

$$h_{ij}^k(t) = f'\big(q_k(t)\big) \left[\sum_{l \in U} m_{kl} h_{ij}^l(t-1) + \delta_{ik} z_j(t-1) \right] \qquad \textbf{10.7}$$

where δ_{ik} is the Kronecker delta ($\delta_{ik} = 1$ if $i = k$, 0 otherwise), and $f'(q_k(t))$ is the derivative of the squashing function in Equation 10.4. Finally, each weight is updated by:

$$m_{ij}(t) = m_{ij}(t-1) + \Delta m_{ij}(t) \qquad \textbf{10.8}$$

The h_{ij}^k values in Equation 10.7 are equivalent to the partial derivatives of the non-input unit states y_k with respect to the connection weights m_{ij} (see Math Box 10.1). It is convenient to define the matrix containing the elements h_{ij}^k as $\mathbf{H}^k$. Then, in words, Equation 10.7 says that each unit y_k ($k \in U$) has its own matrix $\mathbf{H}^k$, with elements h_{ij}^k, which can be thought of as each unit's own, specific version of the whole network connection weight matrix $\mathbf{M}$ with elements corresponding to the m_{ij}. Note that input units x_j ($j \in I$) do not have $\mathbf{H}^k$ matrices. Equation 10.7 further specifies that the update of the $\mathbf{H}^k$ (partial derivative) matrix of each unit y_k is computed as the sum of the matrices $\mathbf{H}^l$ of all units y_l ($l \in U$) in the network (including y_k), where each matrix $\mathbf{H}^l$ is first scaled by the weight m_{kl} of the connection to y_k from y_l, and has state vector $\mathbf{z}^T$ added to its kth row. The sum is scaled by the derivative of the squashing function at the net input to unit y_k. Equation 10.6 specifies that the matrix $\Delta \mathbf{M}$ of connection weight updates is computed as the sum of the $\mathbf{H}^k$ matrices of each unit y_k that has a desired value d_k ($k \in D$) (see Equation 10.5), where each matrix $\mathbf{H}^k$ is first scaled by the error $e_k = d_k - y_k$. The sum is scaled by the learning rate a.

To take a specific example, consider the recurrent network in Figure 10.1A. Because all the connections occur between units y_k in the same layer, their weights would take variable names w_{ij} by the convention we have used previously for recurrent connections in this book. For consistency with Equations 10.2–10.8 describing the state and weight updates in recurrent networks, we can let these weights take variable names m_{ij}. Remember that the formula for the derivative of the squashing function (see Math Box 6.3) is $f'(q_k(t)) = y_k(t)[1 - y_k(t)]$. Then according to Equation 10.7, the update for $\mathbf{H}^1$ is described by Equation 10.9:

$$\mathbf{H}^1 = y_1(1-y_1)\left\{ m_{11}\left[\begin{array}{cc} h_{11}^1 & h_{12}^1 \\ h_{21}^1 & h_{22}^1 \end{array} \right] + \left[\begin{array}{cc} y_1 & y_2 \\ 0 & 0 \end{array} \right] + m_{12}\left[\begin{array}{cc} h_{11}^2 & h_{12}^2 \\ h_{21}^2 & h_{22}^2 \end{array} \right] + \left[\begin{array}{cc} y_1 & y_2 \\ 0 & 0 \end{array} \right] \right\} \qquad \textbf{10.9}$$

Similarly the update for $\mathbf{H}^2$ is described by Equation 10.10:

$$\mathbf{H}^2 = y_2(1-y_2)\left\{ m_{21}\left[\begin{array}{cc} h_{11}^1 & h_{12}^1 \\ h_{21}^1 & h_{22}^1 \end{array} \right] + \left[\begin{array}{cc} 0 & 0 \\ y_1 & y_2 \end{array} \right] + m_{22}\left[\begin{array}{cc} h_{11}^2 & h_{12}^2 \\ h_{21}^2 & h_{22}^2 \end{array} \right] + \left[\begin{array}{cc} 0 & 0 \\ y_1 & y_2 \end{array} \right] \right\} \qquad \textbf{10.10}$$

Note that all variables in Equations 10.9 and 10.10 are functions of time, but the time variable t is omitted for clarity. According to Equation 10.6, the weight update matrix $\Delta \mathbf{M}(t)$ for this simple network is as shown in Equation 10.11:

$$\Delta \mathbf{M}(t) = a\left[e_1(t)\mathbf{H}^1(t) + e_2(t)\mathbf{H}^2(t) \right] \qquad \textbf{10.11}$$

In numbers, suppose that on some time step t the elements of $\mathbf{H}^1$ and $\mathbf{H}^2$ are all 1s and that $y_1 = y_2 = 0.5$. Suppose also that the recurrent connection weights all have absolute value 1 but that the self-connection weights are positive while the reciprocal connection weights are negative, so $m_{11} = m_{22} = +1$, but $m_{12} = m_{21} = -1$, and $\mathbf{M}(t-1) = [+1\ -1; -1\ +1]$. (Here we use a semicolon, as in MATLAB®, to indicate a row break.) Through application of Equations 10.9 and 10.10 we find that $\mathbf{H}^1 = [0.25\ 0.25; 0\ 0]$ and $\mathbf{H}^2 = [0\ 0; 0.25\ 0.25]$. Now suppose that the desired outputs are both 1, so $e_1 = e_2 = 0.5$, and the learning rate a is 1. Then through application of Equation 10.11 we find that $\Delta \mathbf{M}(t) = [0.125\ 0.125;$

0.125 0.125]. Applying this update to the weights (see Equation 10.8) we find that $\mathbf{M}(t) = [+1.125\ -0.875;\ -0.875\ +1.125]$. This particular update using recurrent back-propagation causes the self-connection weights to increase but causes the reciprocal connection weights to decrease in absolute value.

The recurrent back-propagation procedure outlined above can be used to train any recurrent neural network to produce a desired output time series given some input time series (sequences of values). Before training, the modifiable weights in $\mathbf{M}$ are randomized by assigning to them random deviates drawn from a uniform distribution, over some range that encompasses both positive and negative values. All the h_{ij}^k values are initially set to 0. On each time step the input units are updated with the next values in the input sequence, and the response of the network to this new input, and to the previous states of the non-input units, is computed using Equations 10.3 and 10.4. The desired outputs are updated with the next values in the desired output sequence, and the errors, between the desired and actual outputs of the units that have desired outputs (y_k if $k \in D$), are computed using Equation 10.5. Then the h_{ij}^k values are updated using Equation 10.7, and the weight changes are computed according to Equation 10.6. Finally, the weights are modified using Equation 10.8, and the process is repeated for the next inputs and desired outputs in the series (sequence). Training can continue until the actual output matches the desired output to within a tolerance, or it can simply be continued for a set number of training iterations.

The recurrent back-propagation algorithm outlined above is not meant to simulate an adaptive process as it might occur in the real brain. In Chapter 14 we will discuss an algorithm based on perturbative reinforcement learning in the context of dynamic input–output transformations that is more plausible than recurrent back-propagation. In this chapter we will use recurrent back-propagation as a powerful tool with which to construct dynamic and non-linear network models of real neural systems, where the latter were presumably created through some combination of evolutionary, developmental, and adaptive processes. Recurrent back-propagation can be used to train recurrent networks to produce the same sorts of dynamic behaviors that are exhibited by the actual nervous system. As we will see, networks trained using recurrent back-propagation can reveal unexpected features that provide insight into the organization and function of real neural systems.

We will explore several different neural system behaviors in this chapter, but they all share in common an essential memory or storage ability. A model of short-term memory, as it has been studied for neurons in certain parts of cerebral cortex, will be developed in the last section. In the initial sections we will be concerned with simpler forms of signal processing that occur in the brainstem and that are involved in forming commands for moving the eyes. These commands generally consist of sustained or persistent signals, which are formed through reverberation of more transient signals. In the first problem we will train a simple recurrent network to act as a leaky integrator.

10.2 Training a Two-Unit Network to Simulate the Oculomotor Neural Integrator

For our first example we will train a simple neural network, having two linear output units, to produce a leaky integration of its inputs. The goal will be for the network to transform an input pulse into a much more slowly decaying output signal. In the extreme case, the network would transform the pulse input into a step output, which would never decay. The difficulty in learning to produce such a perfect integration (of the pulse to a step, with no leak) is the topic of Exercise 10.1. Here we will settle for a leaky integration of the inputs.

As you will recall from Chapter 1, the simplest integrator can be formed from one neural unit positively feeding back onto itself. If the unit feeds back with a self-connection weight of 1 it acts as a perfect integrator. If it feeds back with a weight between 0 and 1 it acts as a leaky integrator, where the leakiness depends on how close the feedback weight is to 0. The problem with building an integrator (leaky or not) from a single unit is that real input neurons often encode signals as modulations of a nonzero background firing rate. A single unit positively feeding back onto itself would integrate this nonzero background and would soon be driven into saturation. A neuron constantly firing at its saturation limit would be useless for signal processing.

The solution, which is the one apparently adopted by real neural systems that must produce integration (Robinson 1989), is to encode signals in pairs of inputs that operate in push–pull. Thus, a pulse would be encoded as an abrupt increase in the background rate of one member of the pair of inputs, and an abrupt decrease in the rate of the other member of the pair. This push–pull signal could be integrated by a pair of units that exert positive feedback on themselves not only via self-excitation, but also via mutual (reciprocal) inhibition. The beauty of reciprocal inhibition is that it cancels off the background rate (common signal component) of the inputs and only allows integration of the push–pull signal (differential component). This arrangement, which we explored in Chapter 2, was first described for the oculomotor neural integrator by Cannon, Robinson, and Shamma (1983).

The specific question we address in this example is whether the input and recurrent weight values needed to produce leaky integration in a reciprocally connected pair of units could be learned using recurrent back-propagation. We approach this problem by first setting the weights to desired values, and by using the network with those weights to compute a desired output. Then we will randomize the weights and see if recurrent back-propagation can learn the desired values. To make matters simpler we will modulate the inputs about background rates (states) of 0, even though the network could properly function with nonzero input background. We will also use linear units in this example. Linear units compute the weighted sum of their inputs but do not pass the result through the squashing function. The states of linear units are updated using Equation 10.3, after which $y_k(t) = q_k(t)$ for $k \in U$ (Equation 10.4 is not used with linear units). The derivative of this "identity activation function" is the number 1. Since the derivative of the activation function $f'(q_k(t))$ in the linear case is the multiplicative identity, it can simply be ignored in Equation 10.7, which updates the h_{ij}^k values. Note that we are using k to index the output unit states y. This is a departure from our convention of using i to index states y, but we use k in this chapter for consistency with Equations 10.2–10.8 for state and weight updating in recurrent networks.

The two-unit model of the oculomotor neural integrator is shown in Figure 10.2. This simple recurrent network is like the one in Figure 10.1A except that it has input units. If we assume for simplicity that the absolute values of the input (feedforward) weights v are equal, and separately that the absolute values of the recurrent weights w are equal, then Equation 10.12 describes the responses of the output units in the two-unit integrator network:

$$\begin{bmatrix} y_1(t) \\ y_2(t) \end{bmatrix} = \begin{bmatrix} +w & -w \\ -w & +w \end{bmatrix} \begin{bmatrix} y_1(t-1) \\ y_2(t-1) \end{bmatrix} + \begin{bmatrix} +v & -v \\ -v & +v \end{bmatrix} \begin{bmatrix} x_1(t-1) \\ x_2(t-1) \end{bmatrix} \qquad \textbf{10.12}$$

We set up the two-unit neural integrator this way in Chapter 2. Except for the condition that the absolute values are the same for all feedforward weights v, and separately the same for all recurrent weights w (v and w are not necessar-

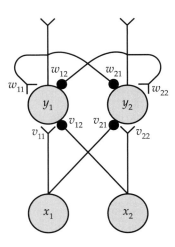

FIGURE 10.2   The two-unit model of the oc-ulomotor neural integrator The x_j ($j = 1, 2$) are input units and the y_i ($i = 1, 2$) are output units. Weights of connections from input to output units are designated as v_{ij}, while those between output units are designated as w_{kl}, ($k = 1, 2$ and $l = 1, 2$). The Y-shaped endings are excitatory (positive), while the ball-shaped endings are inhibitory (negative).

ily equal to each other), Equation 10.12 is equivalent to Equation 2.4. For the purposes of using recurrent back-propagation it is convenient to place all the weights (input and recurrent) into a connection weight matrix **M**, and to place all the states (input and output) into a state vector **z**, so that $\mathbf{y}(t) = \mathbf{Mz}(t - 1)$. Then Equation 10.12 can be rewritten as Equation 10.13:

$$\begin{bmatrix} y_1(t) \\ y_2(t) \end{bmatrix} = \begin{bmatrix} +v & -v & +w & -w \\ -v & +v & -w & +w \end{bmatrix} \begin{bmatrix} x_1(t-1) \\ x_2(t-1) \\ y_1(t-1) \\ y_2(t-1) \end{bmatrix} \qquad \textbf{10.13}$$

where $\mathbf{y} = [y_1\, y_2]^\mathrm{T}$, $\mathbf{z} = [x_1\, x_2\, y_1\, y_2]^\mathrm{T}$, and $\mathbf{M} = [+v\, -v\, +w\, -w; -v\, +v\, -w\, +w]$. Our specific task in this example is to set the values of v and w and use Equation 10.13 to find the desired outputs $d_1(t)$ and $d_2(t)$, then randomize the network connection weights and determine whether they can be learned using recurrent back-propagation. Script `rbpTwoUnitIntegrator`, listed in MATLAB Box 10.1, will do this.

Our goal throughout this chapter is to use recurrent back-propagation to train recurrent neural networks to produce dynamic input–output transformations. The inputs and desired outputs for dynamic transformations are sequences of values such as time series. In some of the examples we will consider in later sections we will set both the input and desired output time series according to formulas, but for the leaky integrator we will set the input time series only, and will use the responses of the network with desired weight values to find the desired outputs. Script `rbpTwoUnitIntegrator` sets an ending time step using `tEnd=500`, and then sets up a push–pull pulse input on time step `tEnd/10+1` using the commands `xHld=zeros(2,tEnd+1)`, `xHld(1,tEnd/10+1)=1`, and `xHld(2,tEnd/10+1)=-1`. (Note that array `xHld` has two rows, one for each input unit.) It also defines an array `dHld` to hold the desired outputs. It sets the absolute values of the input (feedforward) and recurrent weights at `vAb=0.5` and `wAb=0.495`. It then makes separate feedforward and recurrent weight matrices using the commands `V=[1 -1; -1 1]*vAb` and `W=[1 -1; -1 1]*wAb`, and it assembles connectivity matrix M using `M=[V W]`. It then finds the desired output in a loop where on each time step it sets the state vector using the command `z=[xHld(:,t-1);dHld(:,t-1)]`, and then computes the desired output using `dHld(:,t)=M*z`. This last command implements Equation 10.13. The result is the two-dimensional array `dHld` that holds the desired push–pull output.

MATLAB® BOX 10.1 **This script uses recurrent back-propagation to train a recurrent network with two linear output units to act as a leaky integrator.**

```
% rbpTwoUnitIntegrator.m

nOut=2; % set number of output units
a=0.005; % set learning rate
nIts=100; % set number of training cycles
vAb=0.5; % set desired input weight absolute value
wAb=0.495; % set desired recurrent weight absolute value
V=[1,-1;-1,1]*vAb; % set desired input weight matrix
W=[1,-1;-1,1]*wAb; % set desired recurrent weight matrix
M=[V W]; % assemble desired connectivity matrix
tEnd=500; % set end time
xHld=zeros(2,tEnd+1); % zero input hold vector
xHld(1,tEnd/10+1)=1; % set positive input
xHld(2,tEnd/10+1)=-1; % set negative input
dHld=zeros(nOut,tEnd+1); % zero desired output hold vector
for t=2:tEnd+1, % for each time step
    z=[xHld(:,t-1);dHld(:,t-1)]; % set the state vector
    dHld(:,t)=M*z; % find the desired output
end % end loop for computing desired output

M=(rand(nOut,2+nOut)-0.5)*0.02; % randomize connectivity matrix
H=zeros(nOut,2+nOut,nOut); % zero partial derivative matrices
for c=1:nIts, % for each training cycle
    if rand<0.5, x=xHld; d=dHld; % randomly choose direction of ...
    else x=xHld*(-1); d=dHld*(-1); end % input and desired output
    z=[x(:,1);0;0]; % initialize unit state vector
    for t=2:tEnd+1, % for each time step
        y=M*z; % find responses of output units
        e=d(:,t)-y; % find error vector
        Hpre=H; % save the partial matrices
        H=H-H; % zero the partial matrices
        for k=1:nOut, % for both output units
            for l=1:nOut, % for both output units
                hld=M(k,l+2)*Hpre(:,:,l); % weight each H matrix
                hld(k,:)=hld(k,:)+z'; % add state vector to row k
                H(:,:,k)=H(:,:,k)+hld; % find partial matrices
            end % end l loop
        end % end k loop
        deltaM=M-M; % zero weight-update matrix
        for k=1:nOut, % for both output units
            deltaM=deltaM+e(k)*H(:,:,k); % find weight-update matrix
        end % end k loop
        deltaM=a*deltaM; % scale weight changes by learning rate
        M=M+deltaM; % update the connectivity matrix
        z=[x(:,t);y]; % update unit state vector
    end % end t (time step) loop
end % end c (training) loop
```

Script `rbpTwoUnitIntegrator` then randomizes connectivity matrix `M` and trains it on inputs `xHld` and desired outputs `dHld` using recurrent back-propagation with learning rate `a=0.005` for `nIts=100` iterations. On each time step, indexed by `t`, we will both update the states of the units in the network and use recurrent back-propagation to update the connection weights (see Equations 10.2–10.8). On each training iteration (or training cycle, indexed by `c`) the script will train the network on an entire input/desired–output time series. Specifically, on each training cycle the script chooses at random whether to apply the inputs (array `x`) and desired outputs (array `d`) at their original polarity (`x=xHld` and `d=dHld`), in which the left-side response is positive and the right-side negative, or at the opposite polarity (`x=xHld*(-1)` and `d=dHld*(-1)`). Randomly swapping the polarity of the inputs and desired outputs improves learning. During training, the script updates the state vector using `z=[x(:,t);y]` on the previous time step. Then on the current time step it computes the output unit responses using `y=M*z` (note that the squashing function does not apply for linear units), and finds the error using `e=d(:,t)-y`, thereby implementing Equations 10.2–10.5 (skipping Equation 10.4).

The rest of script `rbpTwoUnitIntegrator` implements Equations 10.6–10.8, which describe connection weight adaptation using recurrent back-propagation as explained in detail in the previous section. In the script, `nOut=2` is the number of output units in the two-unit integrator. There are also two input units, so an offset of 2 is sometimes introduced for sizing and indexing purposes. For example, the whole network connection weight matrix `M` has dimensions (`nOut, 2+nOut`), with a row for each output unit and a column for each input and output unit. Note that `M` is a rectangular array (matrix). The $\mathbf{H}^k$ matrices for both output units are held in the cuboidal array `H` which is defined (and zeroed) using `H=zeros(nOut,2+nOut,nOut)`. A cuboidal matrix (array) can be thought of as a "book" whose "pages" are rectangular matrices. Array `H` has a row for each output unit, a column for each input and output unit, and a "page" (indexed along the third dimension) for each output unit. Note that $\mathbf{H}^1$ and $\mathbf{H}^2$ are held in the first and second pages of `H`, respectively. Each page of `H` has the same dimensions as `M`, and represents the version $\mathbf{H}^k$ of the whole weight matrix $\mathbf{M}$ that belongs to each unit. The array `Hpre`, of the same dimensions as `H`, holds the values of `H` from the previous update.

It should be possible, with the $\mathbf{H}^k$ matrices all held in cuboidal array `H`, to update the $\mathbf{H}^k$ matrices via matrix methods alone. To make their relationship with the update equations described in the previous section more obvious, we will update the $\mathbf{H}^k$ matrices in two nested loops. The loops have variables `k` and `l` (the letter "l") that both index the output units, and they process and sum up the $\mathbf{H}^l$ matrices to update the $\mathbf{H}^k$ matrices. The update for $\mathbf{H}^k$ begins by scaling $\mathbf{H}^l$ by weight m_{kl} using `hld=M(k,l+2)*Hpre(:,:,l)` where `hld` is an intermediate variable. Note that the offset of 2 in `M(k,l+2)` takes account of the two input units in indexing the weight corresponding to $\mathbf{H}^l$. The command `hld(k,:)=hld(k,:)+z'` adds state vector `z` to row `k` of (now scaled) $\mathbf{H}^l$, and `H(:,:,k)=H(:,:,k)+hld` adds this processed version of $\mathbf{H}^l$ to the sum that accumulates the updated version of $\mathbf{H}^k$.

After both $\mathbf{H}^k$ matrices are updated the matrix `deltaM`, which holds $\Delta\mathbf{M}$, is determined. This process begins by zeroing `deltaM` and then accumulating its value by scaling each $\mathbf{H}^k$ matrix by its corresponding error e_k and summing them up. This is done using `deltaM=deltaM+e(k)*H(:,:,k)` in a single loop with loop variable `k` over the output units. The matrix $\Delta\mathbf{M}$ is scaled by the learning rate using `deltaM=a*deltaM`, and the whole connection weight matrix is finally updated using `M=M+deltaM`. The computational procedures described here for implementing recurrent back-propagation weight updates in script `rbpTwoUnitIntegrator` are the same as those used in the other

TABLE 10.1   **Connection weights of the linear neural integrator model with two output units following training to produce leaky integration using recurrent back-propagation**

To	From			
	Input one (x_1)	Input two (x_2)	Output one (y_1)	Output two (y_2)
Output one (y_1)	+0.5036	−0.4981	+0.4955	−0.4945
Output two (y_2)	−0.4997	+0.4986	−0.4990	+0.4910

scripts in this chapter. The only differences are in numbers of units and, in nonlinear networks, in the use of the squashing function for unit activations and its derivative for scaling $\mathbf{H}^k$ matrices.

In learning to reproduce the output desired of the two-unit integrator, the algorithm must train the connection weights to take values close to those that we initially used to generate the desired output. The learned weights must not only match the desired weights in absolute value, but the signs of the learned weights must have the same pattern as the desired weights. This pattern is determined by the task that the two-unit leaky-integrator network must learn, which is to transform push–pull pulse inputs into slowly decaying push–pull outputs. In order for the outputs to be push–pull, the weights of the connections from the inputs should be positive to outputs on the same side, but negative to outputs on the opposite side. In order for the output units to produce leaky integration they must exert positive feedback on themselves, and for that to occur the weights of their self-connections must be positive, but the weights of their reciprocal connections must be negative. This pattern of excitatory (positive) and inhibitory (negative) weights is indicated in Figure 10.2 and in Equation 10.13.

The absolute values of the desired weights were 0.5 for the input–output (feedforward) weights v, and 0.495 for the recurrent (self-connection and reciprocal) weights w. Table 10.1 shows that the weights produced by the recurrent back-propagation algorithm do indeed come very close to the desired weights, both in absolute value and in their pattern of excitation and inhibition (see Figure 10.2 and Equation 10.13). Consequently, the actual output, shown in Figure 10.3, is indistinguishable from the desired output. The output in this

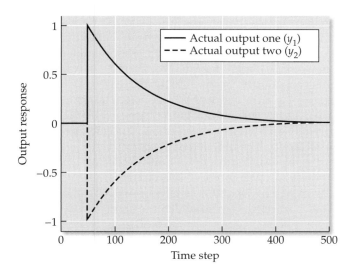

FIGURE 10.3   Responses in a recurrent network having two linear output units following training using recurrent back-propagation to produce leaky integration The push–pull input pulses are not shown. The actual outputs (y_1, solid line; y_2, dashed line) are push–pull decays. They almost perfectly match the desired outputs, which are not visible behind the actual output responses.

case is the leaky integral of a pulse input and, as such, it can be characterized as a decay with a sharp onset. Recall from Chapter 2 that if the input had itself been a decay with a sharp onset, then the leaky integrated output would be a rounded version of the input that could be characterized as a "lopsided bump." In this reciprocally connected network it would be a push–pull bump. We will refer frequently to this push–pull, lopsided bump type of response in later sections of this chapter.

The model neural integrator developed in this section is a simplified version of a model of the integrator of the oculomotor system that was proposed by Cannon, Robinson, and Shamma (1983). The job of the oculomotor system is, of course, to move the eyes. The oculomotor system needs an integrator because eye movement commands originate as velocity signals, but eye movement control requires signals proportional both to eye velocity and position (see Chapter 2). The oculomotor integrator is needed to transform velocity commands into position commands. The preponderance of evidence suggests that the oculomotor integrator, which is situated in the brainstem, does indeed integrate through the mechanism of reverberation of signals within a recurrent neural network (Robinson 1989; see also Chapter 2). In the next section we consider another form of oculomotor signal processing known as velocity storage, which seems to involve a similar mechanism at the brainstem level. Our recurrent neural network model of velocity storage, trained using recurrent back-propagation, will provide insight into the response properties of the brainstem neurons that mediate the vestibulo-ocular reflex.

10.3 Velocity Storage in the Vestibulo-Ocular Reflex

Velocity storage is a form of signal processing observed in the brainstem circuits that mediate the vestibulo-ocular reflex (VOR). The job of the VOR is to stabilize the retinal image during head movement. (See Chapters 2 and 6 for background on the VOR.) It does this by producing rotation of the eyes that is equal in velocity, but opposite in direction, to the rotation of the head. The VOR is a classic three-neuron reflex arc composed of primary afferent sensory neurons, from the vestibular semicircular canals, interneurons in the brainstem vestibular nuclei, and the motoneurons of the eye muscles (Wilson and Melvill Jones 1979). Vestibular primary afferents receive excitatory synaptic input from hair cell receptor cells, which are located within the semicircular canals. The semicircular canals and the hair cell receptor cells transduce head rotations into neural signals proportional to head rotational (angular) velocity, which are then carried to the vestibular nuclei by the canal afferent sensory neurons. Basically, velocity storage involves leaky integration to increase the persistence in time of the velocity signal provided by the canal afferents. The canal sensory signal, which constitutes the input to the VOR, already has some persistence in time, because the biophysics of the semicircular canals causes them to act as leaky integrators (Wilson and Melvill Jones 1979). Thus, the response of the canal afferents to a pulse of head angular acceleration can be described as an exponential decay. The function of the velocity-storage mechanism is to transform this input decay into a longer output decay.

What can loosely be called the "persistence" of an exponentially decaying signal is quantitatively described by its time constant τ, as in $x(t) = A \exp(-t/\tau)$ where t is time and A is the amplitude from which the signal decays. In the case of the VOR, vestibular nucleus neurons in the brainstem receive a canal afferent sensory signal with a time constant τ_C of about 5 seconds, and need to create a motoneuron command with a time constant τ_V of about 20 seconds

(Henn 1982). The velocity-storage mechanism lengthens the time constant of the canal afferent signal, from 5 to 20 seconds, and so prolongs the duration of the VOR response. It also preserves the sharp onset of the canal signal, so that the VOR will also have a sharp onset. The challenge in modeling velocity storage is to create a network that both lengthens the duration of the canal response and preserves its sharp onset.

A neural network model that represents the connectivity of the horizontal VOR in simplified form is shown in Figure 10.4. (For a review of VOR connectivity, see Anastasio 1994.) The horizontal VOR, as distinct from the vertical VOR, stabilizes the eye in the horizontal plane. (See Chapter 6 for a brief overview of the horizontal and vertical VOR.) The input to the horizontal VOR is provided by the sensory afferents of the left and right horizontal semicircular canals (LHC and RHC in Figure 10.4). These afferents project to vestibular nucleus neurons on the left and right sides of the brainstem (LVN1, LVN2, RVN1, and RVN2). The model represents the recurrent connections between vestibular nucleus neurons on either side of the brainstem (Wilson and Melvill Jones 1979) that are known to be required for the production of velocity storage (Blair and Gavin 1981). The vestibular nucleus neurons also project to the motoneurons of the lateral and medial rectus muscles (LR and MR), which work as an agonist/antagonist pair to rotate the eye in the horizontal plane. Many of the direct connections in the model actually occur through interneurons. Because those interneurons would act only as relays, they are not represented in the model for simplicity (see Anastasio 1994 for details).

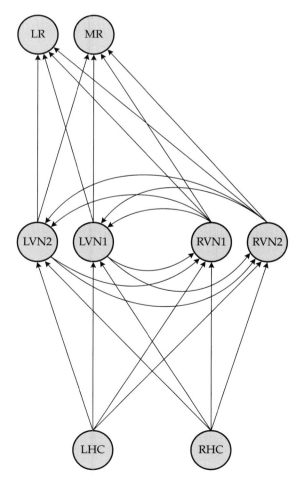

FIGURE 10.4   Recurrent neural network model of the vestibulo-ocular reflex The input units (LHC and RHC) represent sensory afferents from the left and right horizontal canals, the hidden units (LVN and RVN) represent neurons in the left and right vestibular nuclei, and the output units (LR and MR) represent the motoneurons of the lateral and medial rectus muscles of the left eye. Model structure is a simplification of actual vestibulo-ocular reflex connectivity. For example, canal afferents on one side project through interneurons to vestibular nucleus neurons on the other side, but these interneurons would act only as simple relays, so they are omitted from the model. The model respects the anatomical constraints that canal afferents do not project directly to motoneurons, and motoneurons neither project to each other nor project back to vestibular nucleus neurons or canal afferents. (After Anastasio 1991.)

FIGURE 10.5   The response of a semicircular canal primary afferent, and of the overall vestibulo-ocular reflex (VOR), to a step change in head angular velocity (A) Instantaneous firing rate, in impulses/s, of a horizontal semicircular canal primary afferent. (B) Eye angular velocity in degrees/s. (C) Eye angular position in degrees. (D) Head angular velocity in degrees/s. The eye position trace is extremely jagged, due to the fast, resetting eye movements that are made to reposition the eye when the VOR carries it to an eccentric position in the orbit. The velocities of these resetting eye movements are mostly clipped out of the eye velocity trace, the envelope of which shows eye velocity due to the VOR. Note that the duration of the VOR response is longer than that of the canal afferent response that drives it. Note also that the responses of the canal afferent, in both its on- and off-directions, are symmetric about its spontaneous (background) firing rate of about 150 impulses/s. (From Henn 1982.)

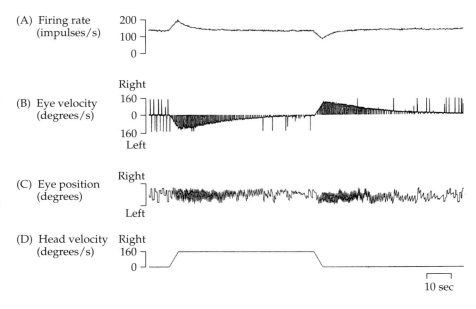

The series of simulations in Sections 10.4 and 10.5 will show how the network in Figure 10.4, following training using recurrent back-propagation to produce velocity storage, can provide insight into the response properties of real vestibular nucleus neurons. These properties are best appreciated through comparison with those of the canal sensory afferents. The responses of a representative primary canal afferent to a step change in horizontal head rotational (angular) velocity is shown in Figure 10.5. Note that a step change in head angular velocity is initiated by a pulse of head angular acceleration in one direction, and terminated by a pulse of head angular acceleration in the opposite direction. (The pulses of head angular acceleration and deceleration are not shown; only the step of head angular velocity that they produce is shown in Figure 10.5.) We will compare the responses of a canal afferent (see Figure 10.5) and of a vestibular nucleus neuron (Figure 10.6) to pulses of head angular acceleration.

The canal afferent in Figure 10.5 has a background firing rate of about 150 impulses/s. It increases this firing rate by about 50 impulses/s immediately following the pulse of head angular acceleration that brings the head to an angular velocity of 160 degrees/s. The amplitude of the response is the peak amount by which the firing rate changes from its background. Thus, the sensitivity, or gain, of this afferent, which is the ratio of its response amplitude in impulses/s to head velocity in degrees/s, is about 50/160 or 0.3 impulses/s/degree/s. Because canal afferents have relatively high background firing rates and low sensitivities, they can signal head rotations in both directions, either as increases (on-direction) or decreases (off-direction) in their background firing rates, and these on-direction and off-direction responses are symmetric. Figure 10.5 also shows the eye angular velocity produced by the VOR in response to the step change in head angular velocity. The VOR response, which is in the direction opposite to the head rotation, has a much longer duration than the canal afferent signal that drives it. As stated above, prolonging the duration of the canal afferent signal is the main function of the velocity-storage mechanism.

Vestibular nucleus neurons differ from canal afferents in having longer duration responses. They also differ in having lower background discharge rates, higher sensitivities, and pronounced response asymmetries. The responses of a representative vestibular nucleus neuron are shown in Figure 10.6. Note that the duration of the neural response is as long as the duration

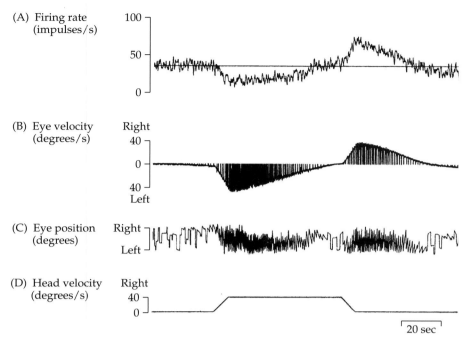

(A) Firing rate (impulses/s)

(B) Eye velocity (degrees/s)

(C) Eye position (degrees)

(D) Head velocity (degrees/s)

FIGURE 10.6   The response of a vestibular nucleus neuron, and of the overall vestibulo-ocular reflex (VOR), to a step change in head angular velocity (A) Instantaneous firing rate, in impulses/s, of a vestibular nucleus neuron. (B) Eye angular velocity in degrees/s. (C) Eye angular position in degrees. (D) Head angular velocity in degrees/s. As in Figure 10.5, the velocities of the resetting eye movements are clipped out of the eye velocity trace, the envelope of which shows eye velocity due to the VOR. Note that the vestibular nucleus neuron response has a sharp onset, but its duration is about the same as that of the VOR. Note also that the responses of the vestibular nucleus neuron in its on- and off-directions are not symmetric about its relatively low background firing rate of about 40 impulses/s. (From Henn 1982.)

of the VOR response. This indicates that velocity storage occurs at the level of the vestibular nuclei. The background firing rate of this vestibular nucleus neuron is less than 50 impulses/s, or less than one-third that of the canal afferent (see Figure 10.5). The on-direction response amplitude of the vestibular nucleus neuron is about 50 impulses/s. Since the size of the step change in head velocity is only 40 degrees/s in this case, the sensitivity of the vestibular nucleus neuron is about 1.3 impulses/s/degrees/s, or about four times that of the canal afferent. Because real neurons cannot have negative firing rates, the high sensitivity and low background rate of vestibular nucleus neurons cause their off-direction responses to cut-off (i.e., cause their firing rates to be driven to 0, or close to 0, in their off directions). This form of asymmetry is apparent for the vestibular nucleus neuron response shown in Figure 10.6.

As the data presented in this section illustrate, the phenomenon of velocity storage is puzzling in several respects. First is the velocity-storage mechanism itself, and the puzzle is how a recurrent neural network could both prolong the canal afferent response but also preserve its sharp initial peak. We already know, from the two-unit neural integrator example, that recurrent connections can be trained to produce leaky integration that could prolong the canal afferent response. The part of the puzzle that remains for us to solve is how a recurrent network can also preserve the sharp response onset. Second are the response properties of the vestibular nucleus neurons, and the puzzle is why they should have such low background rates, high sensitivities, and asymmetric responses as compared with the canal afferents that provide their input. Creating models of the VOR that can produce velocity storage, and that can provide insight into the response properties of vestibular nucleus neurons, are the goals of examples in the next two sections.

10.4 Training a Network of Linear Units to Produce Velocity Storage

We will approach the problem of modeling velocity storage in the VOR using a series of simulations of increasing complexity. All of the simulations will involve a neural network having the basic structure of the VOR model shown in Figure 10.4. This network is similar to the three-layered feedforward networks we considered in Chapter 6 (see Figure 6.4), except that it also has recurrent connections between its hidden units. Recall from Chapter 6 that we used x_j, y_i, and z_k to denote input, hidden, and output units, respectively, and weights were denoted by v_{ij} for connections to y_i from x_j, and by u_{ki} for connections to z_k from y_i. For recurrent connections (as in Chapters 2–4) we used w_{il} for connections to y_i from y_l. For convenience we will again use these variable names here but will also group sets of units into state vectors $\mathbf{y}$ or $\mathbf{z}$, and group sets of weights into submatrices of the whole network connection weight matrix $\mathbf{M}$.

All of the networks in the VOR velocity-storage simulations will have two input and two output units, and all velocity-storage simulations will involve the same set of inputs and desired outputs. The simulations will differ in the number of hidden units and in the activation functions of the hidden and output units. (Since the input values are specified directly, their activation functions are not relevant.) For the specific simulation in this section we will employ a network having two hidden units, and the hidden and output units will be linear. The linear unit responses can be described in matrix form as $\mathbf{y}(t) = \mathbf{Mz}(t-1)$, which is shown in Equation 10.14 in expanded form:

$$\begin{bmatrix} y_1(t) \\ y_2(t) \\ z_1(t) \\ z_2(t) \end{bmatrix} = \begin{bmatrix} +v & -v & 0 & -w & 0 & 0 \\ -v & +v & -w & 0 & 0 & 0 \\ 0 & 0 & -u & +u & 0 & 0 \\ 0 & 0 & +u & -u & 0 & 0 \end{bmatrix} \begin{bmatrix} x_1(t-1) \\ x_2(t-1) \\ y_1(t-1) \\ y_2(t-1) \\ z_1(t-1) \\ z_2(t-1) \end{bmatrix} \qquad \textbf{10.14}$$

where, for notational convenience, column vector $\mathbf{y}$ is $[y_1\, y_2\, z_1\, z_2]^{\mathrm{T}}$ and column vector $\mathbf{z}$ is $[x_1\, x_2\, y_1\, y_2\, z_1\, z_2]^{\mathrm{T}}$. Note also the grouping of weights of different types in weight matrix $\mathbf{M}$. Equation 10.14 describes the responses of the units in the VOR model shown in Figure 10.4 when input units x_1 and x_2 correspond to canal afferents LHC and RHC, hidden units y_1 and y_2 correspond to vestibular nucleus neurons LVN1 and RVN1, and output units z_1 and z_2 correspond to eye-muscle motoneurons LR and MR. Note that we exclude the second pair of hidden units in this section but will include them in the next section.

The connectivity matrix $\mathbf{M}$, shown in expanded form in Equation 10.14, is an abstraction of the known structure of the brainstem circuitry that mediates the VOR (Wilson and Melvill Jones 1979). The 2-by-2 submatrix of $\mathbf{M}$ containing the v weights shows that canal afferents on one side send excitatory projections to vestibular nucleus neurons on the same side of the brainstem, but send inhibitory projections to vestibular nucleus neurons on the opposite side. The 2-by-2 submatrix of $\mathbf{M}$ containing the u weights shows that vestibular nucleus neurons send excitatory and inhibitory projections to motoneurons in such a way that the canal signal is inverted. This ensures that eye rotations are made in the direction opposite to head rotations. The 2-by-2 submatrix of $\mathbf{M}$ containing the w weights shows that inhibitory recurrent connections between vestibular nucleus neurons on opposite sides of the brainstem are allowed, but that same side recurrent connections are not allowed. While same-side recurrent connections might exist in the brainstem, they are excluded from the model because their inclusion can result, after training, in responses with non-physiological (i.e., not experimentally observed) properties.

The 2-by-2 submatrix of 0s in the lower left of **M** (in Equation 10.14) represents the fact that canal afferents do not project directly to motoneurons in most vertebrates (Wilson and Melvill Jones 1979). Similarly, the 4-by-2 submatrix on the right side of **M** represents the fact that motoneurons do not project to themselves, nor do they send recurrent projections back to vestibular nucleus neurons. Matrix **M** has elements corresponding to all the weights onto non-input units that potentially could be modified by recurrent back-propagation. Connections that do not occur in the VOR are set to 0 for this example. This version of matrix **M** is thus highly constrained by neuroanatomy and does not allow all possible connections.

One further constraint involves modifiability of connections. It is generally believed that the only modifiable connections in the VOR are located on vestibular nucleus neurons (Wilson and Melvill Jones 1979). Thus, only the v and w connections should be modifiable in the model. This constraint is imposed by fixing the values of the u weights and by disallowing their modification during training. The constraints implied by the specific form of matrix **M** in Equation 10.14 are enforced by setting up a masking matrix, which has 1s at the positions of the v and w weights and 0s elsewhere, and by using this masking matrix to mask the weight changes computed by the algorithm before they are used to modify the weights in connection weight matrix **M**. With this further neurobiological constraint, the u weights are fixed, but the required values and signs of the v and w weights must be learned by the algorithm.

Our task in this section is to use recurrent back-propagation to try to train a neural network model of the VOR having two linear hidden units, and responses described by Equation 10.14, to produce velocity storage. Specifically, we want to convert a push–pull canal afferent input having a short time constant into an equal (in amplitude) but opposite motoneuron command having a long time constant. Script `rpbVelocityStorageLinear`, listed in MATLAB Box 10.2, will implement this simulation. The program will set up the inputs and desired outputs, randomize the modifiable connection weights in **M**, and set the unmodifiable weights u in **M**. The script will also make the masking matrix `Msk`, which will have a 1 wherever matrix **M** has a v or w (i.e., modifiable) element, and a 0 elsewhere (see Equation 10.14). In doing this the script will make use of the fact that the network has two input units and two output units, but can have a variable number of hidden units as stored in variable `nHid`, and will offset indices accordingly. The script will then activate and train the network according to Equations 10.2–10.8.

Neural firing rate, here as elsewhere in this book, is represented simply as the state of a unit. Push–pull signals are encoded by a pair of units as oppositely directed modulations of their background rates (states). The inputs and desired outputs for the velocity storage simulations are composed of sequences of 30 time steps, where each time step corresponds to 5 seconds. In `rpbVelocityStorageLinear` these time steps are stored in vector `tDK`. Each sequence begins with a stretch of background followed by an exponential decay. To match the responses of the canal afferents and of the overall VOR, this decay has a time constant of one time step (5 seconds) for the inputs and four time steps (20 seconds) for the desired outputs. In the script the canal and VOR time constants are set as `tauC=1` and `tauV=4`, and the decays are computed using `xdkC=exp(-tDK/tauC)` and `xdkV=exp(-tDK/tauV)`. The amplitude of the decay has the same absolute value for all inputs and desired outputs, but it modulates the background rate in different directions ("up" and "down"). The "up" canal input is set using the command `canUP=[zeros(1,5),+xdkC(1:tEndDK-5)]`, where `tEndDK=30` is the length of the decay

MATLAB® BOX 10.2   This script uses recurrent back-propagation to train a linear recurrent network to perform velocity storage.

```
% rbpVelocityStorageLinear.m

nHid=2; % set hidden unit number (there are two inputs and outputs)
a=0.01; % set learning rate
nIts=100; % set number of training cycles
tEndDK=30; % set end time for each decay
tDK=0:tEndDK-1; % set timebase for each decay
tEnd=tEndDK*2; % set end time for whole time course
tauC=1; % set canal time constant (in time steps)
tauV=4; % set VOR time constant (in time steps)
xdkC=exp(-tDK/tauC); % compute canal exponential decay
xdkV=exp(-tDK/tauV); % compute VOR exponential decay
canUP=[zeros(1,5),+xdkC(1:tEndDK-5)]; % set up input
canDN=[zeros(1,5),-xdkC(1:tEndDK-5)]; % set down input
vorUP=[zeros(1,7),+xdkV(1:tEndDK-7)]; % set up desired output
vorDN=[zeros(1,7),-xdkV(1:tEndDK-7)]; % set down desired output
xHld=[canUP,canDN;canDN,canUP]; % assemble input hold array
dHld=[vorDN,vorUP;vorUP,vorDN]; % assemble desired output array
M=(rand(nHid+2,nHid+4)-0.5)*0.02; % randomize and scale weight matrix
H=zeros(nHid+2,nHid+4,nHid+2); % zero partial derivative matrix
Msk=ones(nHid+2,nHid+2); % set masking matrix
Msk(nHid+1:nHid+2,1:2)=zeros(2); % zero input-output weights
Msk(1:nHid+2,3+nHid:3+nHid+1)=zeros(nHid+2,2); % weights from outputs
Msk(nHid+1:nHid+2,3:3+nHid-1)=zeros(2,nHid); % hidden-output weights
Msk(1:nHid/2,3:3+nHid/2-1)=zeros(nHid/2); % hidden same-side weights
Msk(nHid/2+1:nHid,3+nHid/2:3+nHid-1)=zeros(nHid/2); % hid same-side
M=M.*Msk; % mask connectivity matrix
uAb=2/nHid; % set hidden-output scale factor
U=ones(1,nHid/2)*uAb; % set and scale hidden-output weight submatrix
U=[-U,U;U,-U]; % set whole hidden-output matrix
M(nHid+1:nHid+2,3:nHid+2)=U; % insert hidden-output weights into M
```

(Continued on facing page)

time base tKD. Note that the five leading zeros constitute the canal response baseline. The "down" canal input canDN is set similarly, except that the sign on xdkC is negative. The "up" VOR desired output is set using the command vorUP=[zeros(1,7),+xdkV(1:tEndDK-7)], where the extra two time steps in the leading zero baseline account for the delay of two time steps in propagating the input to the output along the three-layered, feedforward backbone of the recurrent network (see Figure 10.4). The "down" VOR desired output is set similarly except that the sign on xdkV is negative.

The push–pull inputs and desired outputs must be arranged so that the VOR response is opposite to the canal response. For example, for a head rotation in one direction, x_1 would be up and x_2 would be down, while d_1 would be down and d_2 would be up. (Here d_1 and d_2 are the desired outputs for z_1 and z_2.) The opposite pattern pertains for head rotations in the opposite direction. The two-dimensional input and desired output arrays each consist of push–pull time series corresponding to the responses to head rotation in one direction followed by head rotation in the opposite direction. Specifically, the input array is set using xHld=[canUP,canDN;canDN,canUP] and the desired output array is set using dHld=[vorDN,vorUP;vorUP,vorDN]. To

MATLAB® BOX 10.2   (continued)

```
y=zeros(nHid+2,1); % initialize hidden and output state vector
for c=1:nIts, % for each training cycle
    sel=ceil(2*rand); % randomly set selector
    if sel==1, x=xHld; d=dHld; % if one then set first driven
    elseif sel==2,               % if selector is two then
        x=[xHld(2,:);xHld(1,:)];      % set second
        d=[dHld(2,:);dHld(1,:)]; end % driven pattern
    z=[x(:,1);y]; % initialize whole state vector
    for t=2:tEnd, % for each time step
        y=M*z; % find responses of hidden and output units
        e=d(:,t)-y(nHid+1:nHid+2); % compute error vector
        Hpre=H; H=H-H; % save and zero the partial matrices
        for k=1:nHid+2, % for all hidden and output units
            for l=1:nHid+2, % for all hidden and output units
                hld=M(k,l+2)*Hpre(:,:,l); % weight each H matrix
                hld(k,:)=hld(k,:)+z'; % add state vector to row k
                H(:,:,k)=H(:,:,k)+hld; % find partial matrices
            end % end l loop
        end % end k loop

        deltaM=M-M; % zero delta connectivity matrix
        for k=nHid+1:nHid+2, % for both output units
            deltaM=deltaM+e(k-nHid)*H(:,:,k); % find delta M
        end % end k loop
        deltaM=a*deltaM.*Msk; % apply learning rate and mask to changes
        M=M+deltaM; % update the connectivity matrix
        W=M(1:nHid,3:nHid+2); % extract hidden-hidden weights
        W=min(W,0); % eliminate positive weights
        M(1:nHid,3:nHid+2)=W; % replace hidden-hidden weights
        z=[x(:,t);y]; % update state vector
    end % end t (time step) loop
end % end c (training) loop
```

randomize the order of the head rotations the xHld and dHld arrays are both inverted on random training iterations.

The script rpbVelocityStorageLinear will set the absolute values of the hidden–output weights u according to the number of hidden units in the network using the command uAb=2/nHid, where nHid=2 is the number of hidden units used in this example. It sets the initial values of the modifiable weights onto the vestibular nucleus neurons (the v and w weights in matrix **M**) to uniformly distributed random deviates between –0.01 and +0.01 using M=(rand(nHid+2,nHid+4)-0.5)*0.02 followed by M=M.*Msk, where Msk is the masking matrix as set in the script, M is the weight matrix, and (.*) is element-by-element multiplication. The network is trained for nIts=100 iterations with a learning rate of a=0.01. The resulting connection weight values are shown in Table 10.2.

Following training, the modifiable weights, which are the v and w weights of **M** as expressed in Equation 10.14, have the correct reciprocal pattern. The weights of the connections from the inputs are positive to hidden units on the same side and negative to hidden units on the opposite side, and the reciprocal connections between the hidden units are negative. Despite the correct pattern

TABLE 10.2 Connection weights of the linear, recurrent vestibulo-ocular reflex model with two hidden units following training to produce velocity storage using recurrent back-propagation

To	From			
	LHC (x_1)	RHC (x_2)	LVN1 (y_1)	RVN1 (y_2)
LVN1 (y_1)	+0.1809	−0.1931	0	−0.6597
RVN1 (y_2)	−0.2280	+0.2260	−0.7039	0
LR (z_1)	0	0	−1.0000	+1.0000
MR (z_2)	0	0	+1.0000	−1.0000

The inputs (LHC and RHC) represent sensory afferents from the left and right horizontal canals, the hidden units (LVN1 and RVN1) represent neurons in the left and right vestibular nuclei, and the outputs (LR and MR) represent the motoneurons of the lateral and medial rectus muscles of the left eye.

of connection weights that results from training with recurrent back-propagation, the trained network fails to accurately produce the desired output. The inputs, desired outputs, and actual outputs for this network are shown in Figure 10.7A. The actual output is mushy. It does have a longer decay than

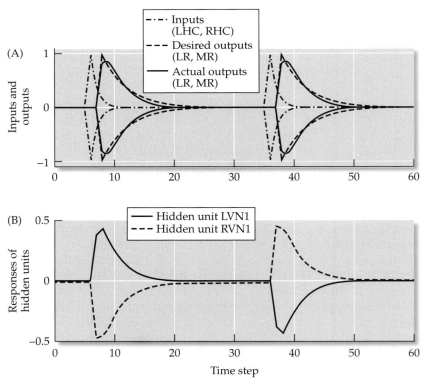

FIGURE 10.7   Responses in a linear recurrent network having two hidden units following training using recurrent back-propagation to produce velocity storage The simulated stimulus (not shown) is a pulse of head angular acceleration to the left on time step 6, followed by a pulse of head angular acceleration to the right on time step 36. (A) The push–pull input (dot-dashed lines; LHC, RHC) and desired (dashed lines) and actual (solid lines) output unit (LR, MR) responses. The actual output has a rounded initial response and otherwise fails to provide an accurate reproduction of the desired output. (B) The responses of the left (solid line) and right (dashed line) hidden units (LVN1, RVN1).

the input, but the actual output does not have a sharp onset. It appears that the network is acting as a simple leaky integrator, and is simply producing a leaky-integrated version of the input as the actual output. The output could be characterized as a push–pull, lopsided bump (see Section 10.2). It has not satisfactorily accomplished velocity storage.

Plots of the responses of the hidden units (i.e., model vestibular nucleus neurons) are shown in Figure 10.7B. Like the actual outputs they give rise to, the responses of the hidden units are mushy. They do show a longer decay than the inputs, but they lack the sharp onset of the inputs. They appear to be acting as simple leaky integrators. The hidden units have a background rate (state, or activity level) of 0, like the inputs. The amplitude of the hidden unit response can be measured in either direction as the maximal (minimal) amount by which hidden unit activity changes from its background activity. For these hidden units the response amplitude, symmetrically in both directions, is about 0.4. The sensitivity of the hidden units is defined as the ratio of their response amplitude to the input unit response amplitude. Given an amplitude of 1 for the inputs, by design, the sensitivity of the hidden units is also about 0.4. Thus, the hidden units in this simulation do have longer decays than the inputs, but they have the same background activity as the inputs, and less than half the sensitivity of the inputs. Real vestibular nucleus neurons are known to have longer decays, lower background rates, higher sensitivities, and more asymmetric responses than their canal afferent inputs. The model vestibular nucleus neurons in this simulation only account for one of the four salient properties of real vestibular nucleus neurons. The VOR neural network model with two linear hidden units neither produces velocity storage nor provides insight into the behavior of real vestibular nucleus neurons.

10.5 Training Networks of Nonlinear Units to Produce Velocity Storage

As discussed at the beginning of this chapter, nonlinear units offer a range of possibilities for signal processing that greatly exceeds that of linear units. The next possibility to explore in the case of the VOR is whether a network of the same configuration but composed of nonlinear units could learn the velocity-storage transformation. The script `rbpVelocityStorageNonlinear`, listed in MATLAB Box 10.3, will implement a nonlinear version of the model. We will use the sigmoidal squashing function as the nonlinear activation function (see Equation 10.4). As before, the network will have `nHid=2` hidden units. The responses of this network are described by $q(t) = Mz(t-1)$ and $y(t) = f(q(t))$, where $f(\cdot)$ is the sigmoidal squashing function. These equations are implemented using `q=M*z` followed by `y=1./(1+exp(-q))`. The vector and matrix variables have the same expanded form as in Equation 10.14. Script `rbpVelocityStorageNonlinear` will set up the input and desired output sequences as in the previous section, but will set the amplitudes to 0.1 and background rates to 0.5, which better suit the sigmoidal squashing function. As in the previous script `rbpVelocityStorageLinear` (see MATLAB Box 10.2), the absolute values of the hidden–output weights (the u weights in M) will be set to `uAb=2/nHid`, where `nHid=2` is the number of hidden units also used in this example.

Script `rbpVelocityStorageNonlinear` will set the initial values of the modifiable weights onto the vestibular nucleus neurons (the v and w weights in matrix M) to uniformly distributed random deviates between −1 and +1. The network is trained for `nIts=10000` iterations with a learning rate of `a=0.1`. Training using recurrent back-propagation is implemented in the same way as in the previous two scripts except that, after they are updated,

MATLAB® BOX 10.3 This script uses recurrent back-propagation to train a nonlinear recurrent network to perform velocity storage. (Training requires several minutes.)

```
% rbpVelocityStorageNonlinear.m

nHid=2; % set hidden unit number (there are two inputs and outputs)
a=0.1; % set learning rate (0.1 or 6)
nIts=10000; % set number of training cycles
tEndDK=30; % set end time for each decay
tDK=0:tEndDK-1; % set timebase for each decay
tEnd=tEndDK*2; % set end time for whole time course
tauC=1; % set canal time constant (in time steps)
tauV=4; % set VOR time constant (in time steps)
xdkC=exp(-tDK/tauC); % compute canal exponential decay
xdkV=exp(-tDK/tauV); % compute VOR exponential decay
canUP=[ones(1,5)*0.5,0.5+xdkC(1:tEndDK-5)*0.1]; % set up input
canDN=[ones(1,5)*0.5,0.5-xdkC(1:tEndDK-5)*0.1]; % set down input
vorUP=[ones(1,7)*0.5,0.5+xdkV(1:tEndDK-7)*0.1]; % set up desired out
vorDN=[ones(1,7)*0.5,0.5-xdkV(1:tEndDK-7)*0.1]; % set down desired out
xHld=[canUP,canDN;canDN,canUP]; % assemble input hold array
dHld=[vorDN,vorUP;vorUP,vorDN]; % assemble desired output array
M=(rand(nHid+2,nHid+4)-0.5)*2; % randomize and scale weight matrix
H=zeros(nHid+2,nHid+4,nHid+2); % zero partial derivative matrix
Msk=ones(nHid+2,nHid+4); % set masking matrix
Msk(nHid+1:nHid+2,1:2)=zeros(2); % zero input-output weights
Msk(1:nHid+2,3+nHid:3+nHid+1)=zeros(nHid+2,2); % weights from outputs
Msk(nHid+1:nHid+2,3:3+nHid-1)=zeros(2,nHid); % hidden-output weights
Msk(1:nHid/2,3:3+nHid/2-1)=zeros(nHid/2); % hidden same-side weights
Msk(nHid/2+1:nHid,3+nHid/2:3+nHid-1)=zeros(nHid/2); % hid same-side
M=M.*Msk; % mask connectivity matrix
uAb=2/nHid; % set hidden-output scale factor
U=ones(1,nHid/2)*uAb; % set and scale hidden-output weight submatrix
U=[-U,U;U,-U]; % set whole hidden-output matrix
M(nHid+1:nHid+2,3:nHid+2)=U; % insert hidden-output weights into M
```

(Continued on facing page)

TABLE 10.3 Connection weights of the nonlinear, recurrent vestibulo-ocular reflex model with two hidden units following training to produce velocity storage using recurrent back-propagation at a low learning rate

To	LHC (x_1)	RHC (x_2)	LVN1 (y_1)	RVN1 (y_2)
LVN1 (y_1)	+4.5543	−2.8576	0	−2.7389
RVN1 (y_2)	−2.5859	+4.4547	−2.9524	0
LR (z_1)	0	0	−1.0000	+1.0000
MR (z_2)	0	0	+1.0000	−1.0000

From (spanning LHC, RHC, LVN1, RVN1 columns)

Abbreviations designating model units are as listed in the captions to Table 10.2 and Figure 10.4.

MATLAB® BOX 10.3 (continued)

```
y=ones(nHid+2,1)*0.5; % initialize hidden and output state vector
for c=1:nIts, % for each training cycle
    sel=ceil(2*rand); % randomly set selector
    if sel==1, x=xHld; d=dHld; % if sel is one then set first driven
    elseif sel==2,             % if selector is two then
        x=[xHld(2,:);xHld(1,:)];    % set second
        d=[dHld(2,:);dHld(1,:)]; end % driven pattern
    z=[x(:,1);y]; % initialize whole state vector
    for t=2:tEnd, % for each time step
        q=M*z; % find weighted input sums to hiddens and outputs
        y=1./(1+exp(-q)); % squash weighted sums to hid and out
        e=d(:,t)-y(nHid+1:nHid+2); % compute error vector
        Hpre=H; H=H-H; % save and zero the partial matrices
        for k=1:nHid+2, % for all hidden and output units
            for l=1:nHid+2, % for all hidden and output units
                hld=M(k,l+2)*Hpre(:,:,l); % weight each H matrix
                hld(k,:)=hld(k,:)+z'; % add state vector to row k
                H(:,:,k)=H(:,:,k)+hld; % find partial matrices
            end % end l loop
            dSquash=y(k)*(1-y(k)); % derivative of squash
            H(:,:,k)=H(:,:,k)*dSquash; % scale by dSquash
        end % end k loop
        deltaM=M-M; % zero weight change matrix
        for k=nHid+1:nHid+2, % for both output units
            deltaM=deltaM+e(k-nHid)*H(:,:,k); % find delta M
        end % end k loop
        deltaM=a*deltaM.*Msk; % scale and mask weight changes
        M=M+deltaM; % update the connectivity matrix
        W=M(1:nHid,3:nHid+2); % extract hidden-hidden weights
        W=min(W,0); % eliminate positive weights
        M(1:nHid,3:nHid+2)=W; % replace hidden-hidden weights
        z=[x(:,t);y]; % update state vector
    end % end t (time step) loop
end % end c (training) loop
```

the $\mathbf{H}^k$ matrices are scaled by the derivative of the squashing function using `H(:,:,k)=H(:,:,k)*dSquash`, where `dSquash=y(k)*(1-y(k))`. The connection weight values resulting from training are shown in Table 10.3.

Following training, the modifiable weights, which are the v and w weights of $\mathbf{M}$ (see Equation 10.14), have the correct reciprocal pattern. The absolute values of the connectivity weights are larger in the nonlinear than in the linear network. This is due to the compressive nature of the squashing function. Recurrent weights with absolute values of this size would produce instability in the linear network (see Chapter 2). Like the linear network, the trained nonlinear network fails to accurately produce the desired output despite the correct pattern of connection weights that results from training. The inputs, desired outputs, and actual outputs for this network are shown in Figure 10.8A. As in the linear network, the actual output in the nonlinear network is mushy. It does have a longer decay than the input, but the actual output does not have a sharp onset. Consequently, the actual output, in the nonlinear as in the linear network, does not match the desired output. Again, it appears that the network is acting as a leaky integrator, and is simply producing a leaky-

FIGURE 10.8   Responses in a nonlinear recurrent network having two hidden units following training using recurrent back-propagation to produce velocity storage The learning rate was low. The stimuli (not shown) are simulated pulse head angular accelerations to the left and right that occur on time steps 6 and 36, respectively. (A) The push–pull input (dot-dashed lines; LHC, RHC) and desired (dashed lines) and actual (solid lines) output unit (LR, MR) responses. The actual output has a rounded initial response and otherwise fails to provide an accurate reproduction of the desired output. (B) The responses of the left (solid line) and right (dashed line) hidden units (LVN1, RVN1). They have a slightly lower background rate (state) and a higher gain (sensitivity) than the inputs, but like the inputs they also have symmetric on- and off-direction responses.

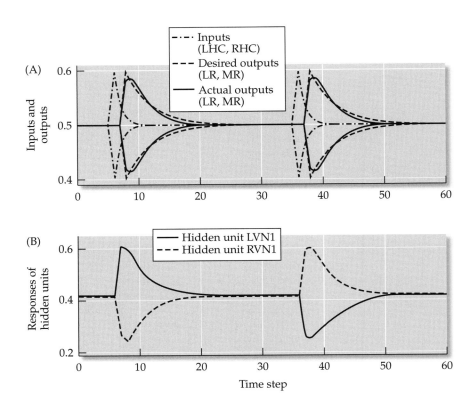

integrated version of the input (a push–pull, lopsided bump) as the actual output. It has not satisfactorily accomplished velocity storage.

Plots of the hidden unit (model vestibular nucleus neuron) responses in the nonlinear network are shown in Figure 10.8B. As in the linear network, the responses of the hidden units in the nonlinear network are mushy. They do show a longer decay than the inputs, but they lack the sharp onset of the inputs. They appear to be acting as simple leaky integrators. The hidden units have a background rate of about 0.4. This is slightly lower than the background rate of the inputs, which is set at 0.5 in the nonlinear network. The amplitude of the hidden unit response is about 0.2. Given an amplitude of 0.1 for the inputs, by design, the sensitivity of the hidden units in the nonlinear network is about 2. Thus, the hidden units in this simulation have longer decays than the inputs, slightly lower background rates, and about twice the sensitivity. The background rate is not low enough, nor the sensitivity high enough, for the model vestibular nucleus neurons (hidden units) to have asymmetric responses. They seem to account for three of the four salient properties of real vestibular nucleus neurons, but unconvincingly. The model vestibular nucleus neurons in this simulation have the mushy (lopsided bump) responses of a simple leaky integrator, and they do not adequately produce the velocity storage transformation.

It may be that the VOR network model with only two hidden units, whether linear or nonlinear, cannot produce the velocity-storage transformation. This conclusion seems valid. We know from the two-unit integrator example that two reciprocally connected units can leaky integrate a push–pull input, and the outputs of the VOR network models with two hidden units likewise seem to produce a leaky-integrated version of their push–pull inputs. In fact, the push–pull bumps produced by the two-hidden-unit VOR network models are simply push-pull versions of the single bump we produced in Chapter 2 when we followed one leaky integrator, which produced a decay with a sharp onset, with another leaky integrator, which produced a longer decay with a rounded onset (a bump).

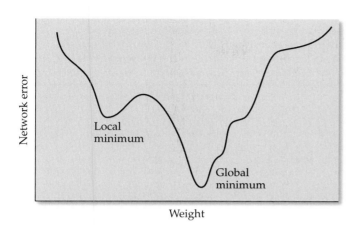

FIGURE 10.9   A one-dimensional abstraction providing an intuitive representation of the error of a neural network in weight space Supervised learning algorithms, including recurrent back-propagation, adjust connection weights so as to reduce network error. Sometimes the network gets trapped in a local error minimum in weight space but, in certain cases, training the weights with a higher learning rate can move network error out of a local minimum and into the global minimum.

Close inspection of the output unit responses of the linear and nonlinear, two-hidden-unit VOR networks we trained above (see Figures 10.7A and 10.8A) suggests an alternative interpretation. Although the actual outputs alternately undershoot and overshoot the desired outputs, the learning algorithm seems to be doing the best it can at fitting a bump to the desired decay with a sharp onset. It is possible that the bump is a local minimum of the network error in weight space. The poor performance of the two-hidden-unit VOR network models on the velocity storage task could be a sign that they are getting trapped in a local minimum.

Recurrent back-propagation (see Math Box 10.1), like conventional back-propagation (see Math Box 6.5) and the delta rule (see Math Box 6.2), is a gradient-descent procedure that adjusts network connection weights so as to minimize error. By adjusting the weights until the gradient is 0, the algorithm should ideally achieve the smallest possible error over the entire weight space, which is known as the global minimum. However, the gradient is also 0 at local minima, which correspond to errors that are low relative to nearby error values but still high relative to the global minimum. These minima can be visualized schematically. A two-dimensional projection representation of an error gradient for a simple network having only two weights is schematized in Figure 6.2. Figure 10.9 provides an alternative way to visualize the network error in weight space, in which all of the weights are hypothetically compressed into one value. Figure 10.9 depicts the global minimum as the lowest possible error. At the global minimum the gradient, which corresponds to the slope of the error curve in this one-dimensional illustration, is 0. The figure also depicts a local minimum as a point at which the gradient is likewise 0 but the error is higher than the global minimum.

In the case of the two-hidden-unit VOR network models we have studied so far, the global minimum might correspond to the small error that would be associated with a very close match between the actual and desired outputs, while the local minimum might correspond to the error between the desired outputs and the lopsided bumps that produce an imperfect match. The possibility that the networks are getting trapped in a local minimum suggests a strategy for improved learning. If the learning rate were increased, then it might be possible for the learning algorithm to "jump" out of the local minimum and reach the global minimum. There is the danger, with a higher learning rate, that the network could become unstable (see Chapter 2), or that the weight adjustments could become erratic (see Chapter 6), but it might be possible to avoid both those pitfalls and still reach the global minimum. To try this, we will re-randomize matrix **M**, and keep all the other parameters the same, but set the learning rate to a=6. The connection weights following nIts=10000 iterations are shown in Table 10.4.

TABLE 10.4 Connection weights of the nonlinear, recurrent vestibulo-ocular reflex model with two hidden units following training to produce velocity storage using recurrent back-propagation at a high learning rate

To	From			
	LHC (x_1)	RHC (x_2)	LVN1 (y_1)	RVN1 (y_2)
LVN1 (y_1)	+7.7900	−10.2765	0	−8.1984
RVN1 (y_2)	−10.2752	+7.7912	−8.1980	0
LR (z_1)	0	0	−1.0000	+1.0000
MR (z_2)	0	0	+1.0000	−1.0000

Abbreviations designating model units are as listed in the captions to Table 10.2 and Figure 10.4.

Following training, the modifiable weights, which are the v and w weights of **M** as configured in Equation 10.14, have the correct reciprocal pattern (see Table 10.4), and differ from the previous case (lower learning rate, see Table 10.3) mainly in having larger absolute values. Plots of the inputs and actual outputs of the nonlinear network trained using the higher learning rate are shown in Figure 10.10A. Unlike the two previous cases, the actual output in this case provides an excellent match to the desired output (the actual and desired outputs are indistinguisable). It appears that the network in this case is *not* acting as a simple leaky integrator. It is doing something extra, which must be related to the nonlinearity of the units.

Plots of the hidden unit (model vestibular nucleus neuron) responses in the nonlinear network, trained using the higher learning rate, are shown in Figure 10.10B. Unlike the previous two cases, but like real vestibular nucleus neurons, the hidden units in this network show markedly asymmetric responses. The responses are near 0 in their off-directions but sharply peaked in their on-directions. The responses show long decays in both directions. The marked asymmetry is caused by the low background rate and high sensitivity of the

FIGURE 10.10 Responses in a nonlinear recurrent network having two hidden units following training using recurrent back-propagation to produce velocity storage The learning rate was high. The stimuli (not shown) are simulated pulse head angular accelerations to the left and right that occur on time steps 6 and 36, respectively. (A) The push–pull input (dot-dashed lines; LHC, RHC) and actual output unit responses (solid lines; LR, MR). The actual output almost perfectly matches the desired output (not visible). (B) The responses of the left (solid line) and right (dashed line) hidden units (LVN1, RVN1). They have a lower background rate and a higher gain (sensitivity) than the inputs, and they have asymmetric on- and off-direction responses.

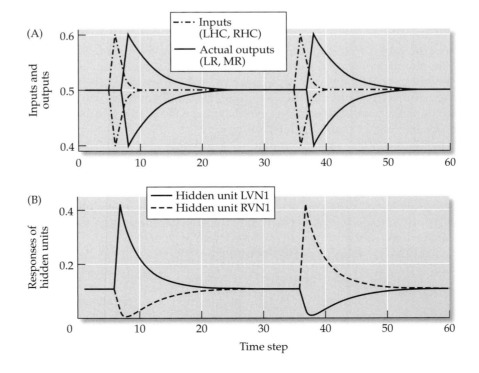

hidden units, which are about 0.1 and 3, respectively. The response properties of the hidden units in this case convincingly reproduce the salient properties of real vestibular nucleus neurons.

The response properties of the hidden units have functional consequences that contribute to their ability to produce the velocity storage transformation. The most striking features of the hidden unit responses in this case are that they have long decays but also have sharply peaked onsets in their on-directions. As in the previous two cases, the long decay is due to leaky integration, which is brought about by the reciprocal interaction between the hidden units. The question concerns how two neurons that act as leaky integrators could integrate the decaying tail of the input but not integrate its sharp initial peak. The answer is that the network has learned to exploit the nonlinearity of its units.

The peak in the on-direction response of the hidden unit on one side is a direct consequence of the simultaneous cut-off of the off-direction response of the hidden unit on the other side. When the unit on the other side cuts-off, it disrupts the reciprocal interaction between the units, and leaky integration is temporarily disabled. This allows the sharp peak of the input to pass unintegrated. As the hidden unit responses come back to their background rates, the reciprocal interaction between them is re-enabled, and leaky integration resumes and produces the long decay. In this way, the network exploits the nonlinearity of the units to pass the sharp peak of the input but integrate its tail and thereby produce velocity storage.

This example illustrates how a recurrent neural network can exploit the nonlinearity of its units to enhance signal processing. It also provides an account of how the response properties of real vestibular nucleus neurons may be related to their function, and suggests that the asymmetric responses of vestibular nucleus neurons allow them to preserve the initially sharp onset of their inputs while also prolonging their offset decays. It would seem that many secondary and higher-order sensory neurons throughout the brain would need to accomplish this same form of signal processing, and it is possible that mechanisms like the one created by recurrent back-propagation in the case of velocity storage in the VOR might also occur in many other neural systems.

Of course, the real VOR has more than two vestibular nucleus neurons, and it is of interest to see how velocity storage would be accomplished in a network having more than two model vestibular nucleus neurons. We explore this question by implementing the full VOR network model shown in Figure 10.4, complete with four hidden units, two per side. Network responses are again described by $\mathbf{q}(t) = \mathbf{M}\mathbf{z}(t-1)$ and $\mathbf{y}(t) = f(\mathbf{q}(t))$, where $f(\cdot)$ is the squashing function, or equivalently by $\mathbf{y}(t) = f(\mathbf{M}\mathbf{z}(t-1))$, but for the case of four hidden units the vector and matrix variables have the expanded form shown in Equation 10.15:

$$\begin{bmatrix} y_1(t) \\ y_2(t) \\ y_3(t) \\ y_4(t) \\ z_1(t) \\ z_2(t) \end{bmatrix} = f \left(\begin{bmatrix} +v & -v & 0 & 0 & -w & -w & 0 & 0 \\ +v & -v & 0 & 0 & -w & -w & 0 & 0 \\ -v & +v & -w & -w & 0 & 0 & 0 & 0 \\ -v & +v & -w & -w & 0 & 0 & 0 & 0 \\ 0 & 0 & -u & -u & +u & +u & 0 & 0 \\ 0 & 0 & +u & +u & -u & -u & 0 & 0 \end{bmatrix} \begin{bmatrix} x_1(t-1) \\ x_2(t-1) \\ y_1(t-1) \\ y_2(t-1) \\ y_3(t-1) \\ y_4(t-1) \\ z_1(t-1) \\ z_2(t-1) \end{bmatrix} \right) \qquad \textbf{10.15}$$

As in the smaller network, the u weights are fixed, but the values and signs of the v and w weights must be learned by the algorithm. To use script

FIGURE 10.11 **Responses in a nonlinear recurrent network having four hidden units following training using recurrent back-propagation to produce velocity storage** The learning rate was high. The stimuli, push–pull inputs, and desired outputs are the same as in the previous velocity storage simulations (see Figures 10.7, 10.8, and 10.10), and the actual output almost perfectly matches the desired output (not shown). (A, B) The responses of the two left (solid lines; LVN1, LVN2) and the two right (dashed lines; RVN1, RVN2) hidden units. All four hidden units have lower background rates and higher gains than the inputs, and they have asymmetric on- and off-direction responses. However, the responses of the two units on each side are distinct. One hidden unit on each side has a rounded initial response (A), while the other hidden unit on each side has a sharp initial response (B). All of the hidden units have longer decay times than the inputs.

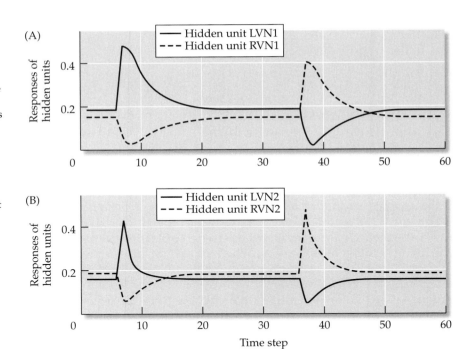

rbpVelocityStorageNonlinear to train this network, simply change the number of hidden units to nHid=4. The script will set the absolute values of the fixed, hidden–output weights u of **M**, will randomize the modifiable weights v and w of **M**, and will set masking matrix Msk for the case of four hidden units so that only the v and w weights of **M** (M in the script) are adjusted by the algorithm. The network is trained as before for nIts=10000 iterations at the higher learning rate of a=6.

Following training of the four-hidden-unit VOR network model, the actual output provides an excellent match to the desired output (not shown), as in the previous case. Plots of the responses of the four vestibular nucleus neurons in this simulation are shown in Figure 10.11. Note that, due to the randomness inherent in the training procedure (i.e., the initially random connection weights and the random input polarity) the hidden unit responses you observe on any particular simulation are likely to differ from the responses shown in Figure 10.11, but these responses are representative. They have longer decays, lower background rates (about 0.2), higher sensitivities (about 3), and more asymmetric responses than the inputs. In their response patterns they repro-

TABLE 10.5 **Connection weights of the nonlinear, recurrent vestibulo-ocular reflex model with four hidden units following training to produce velocity storage using recurrent back-propagation at a high learning rate**

To	From					
	LHC	**RHC**	**LVN1**	**LVN2**	**RVN1**	**RVN2**
LVN1	+6.6102	−7.2774	0	0	−4.8810	−2.1789
LVN2	+5.5281	−8.5033	0	0	−1.3306	−0.0003
RVN1	−7.3450	+6.0682	−5.0386	−0.9527	0	0
RVN2	−8.3180	+6.1415	−2.2061	−0.0029	0	0
LR	0	0	−0.5000	−0.5000	+0.5000	+0.5000
MR	0	0	+0.5000	+0.5000	−0.5000	−0.5000

Abbreviations designating model units are as listed in the captions to Table 10.2 and Figure 10.4.

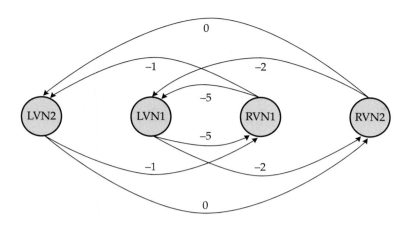

FIGURE 10.12 **Recurrent connection weight values for the model of the vestibulo-ocular reflex with four nonlinear hidden units, trained using recurrent back-propagation to produce velocity storage** The learning rate was high. The trained weight values for the recurrent connections are those shown in Table 10.5 but rounded to the nearest integer. Hidden units LVN1 and RVN1 exert strong reciprocal inhibition on each other. Hidden units LVN2 and RVN2 exert essentially zero reciprocal inhibition on each other, but the LVN2-RVN2 pair is coupled to the LVN1-RVN1 pair through moderately strong connections.

duce the salient properties of real vestibular nucleus neurons. Due to their asymmetric responses they also exploit nonlinearity in producing velocity storage. The four hidden units also seem to be organized in pairs composed of one hidden unit on either side. The hidden units in one pair have a more rounded initial response and a more pronounced decay (see Figure 10.11A), while those in the other pair have a more peaked initial response and a less pronounced decay (see Figure 10.11B). These responses can be explained on the basis of the reciprocal connection weights.

The connection weights in the four-hidden-unit VOR network model following training with recurrent back-propagation are listed in Table 10.5. The weights have adopted a reciprocal pattern as in the previous simulations and as detailed specifically for the four-hidden-unit case in Equation 10.15. As an aid to visualization, Figure 10.12 shows the sub-network of the VOR model that is composed only of the hidden units and their recurrent connections. The approximate values of the weights in the corresponding submatrix will allow us to explore the issue we raised in Chapter 2 concerning the neural mechanism of velocity storage, and whether it involves parallel leaky-integrated and direct pathways to the motoneurons (Raphan et al. 1979), or feedback through a leaky integrator (Robinson 1981). The parallel-pathway and feedback models of velocity storage are reproduced from Chapter 2 in Figure 10.13.

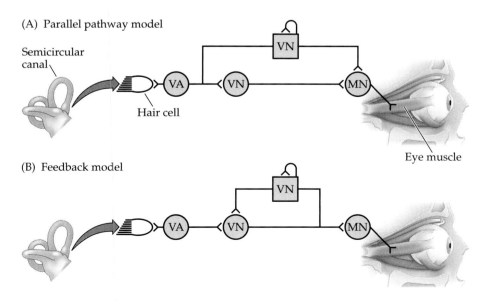

FIGURE 10.13 **Two models of velocity storage in the mammalian vestibulo-ocular reflex** (A) In the parallel pathway model, vestibular nucleus neurons pass the vestibular afferent signal to the motoneuron both directly and indirectly through a leaky integrator. (B) In the feedback model, the vestibular nucleus neuron that receives the vestibular afferent signal sends its output to the motoneuron and also feeds back onto itself through a leaky integrator. The leaky integrator is drawn as a box to distinguish it from the other neural elements, which are drawn as circles. (VA, vestibular afferent; VN, vestibular nucleus neuron; MN, motoneuron.) (A after Raphan et al. 1979; B after Robinson 1981.)

The hidden units corresponding to LVN1 and RVN1 are strongly reciprocally connected and produce leaky integration. They are the hidden units that have the rounded initial responses and more pronounced decays (see Figure 10.11A). The hidden units corresponding to LVN2 and RVN2 are essentially unconnected. They do not integrate by themselves and would pass the input signal unintegrated. Their weak reciprocal connections in part allow them to preserve the sharp initial onset of the input signal (see Figure 10.11B). Considering these reciprocal connections, it seems that the network has developed parallel, direct and leaky-integrated pathways to the outputs. This architecture was originally suggested for velocity storage by Raphan and co-workers (1979). A schematic of the parallel pathway model of velocity storage is shown in Figure 10.13A.

Further scrutiny of the reciprocal connection weights suggests that the configuration developed by recurrent back-propagation in this example is not quite that simple. Although units LVN2 and RVN2 are not coupled to each other, they are coupled to the integrating pair (LVN1 and RVN1) through moderately strong connections. Thus, LVN2 and RVN2 essentially feed back onto themselves through the leaky integrator formed by the strong reciprocal connections between LVN1 and RVN1. This provides units LVN2 and RVN2 with their less pronounced but definitely long decays (see Figure 10.11B). Considering these recurrent connections, it seems that the network has also developed the mechanism of feedback through a leaky integrator that was suggested for velocity storage by Robinson (1981). A schematic of the feedback model of velocity storage is shown in Figure 10.13B.

Considering the whole set of recurrent connections together, it seems that recurrent back-propagation has created a structure for producing velocity storage that combines the mechanisms of parallel pathways and feedback (Anastasio 1991). Because all of the hidden units in the four-hidden-unit model have low background rates, high sensitivities, and asymmetric responses, they also exploit nonlinear mechanisms in producing the velocity storage transformation. Thus, recurrent back-propagation has constructed a network that produces velocity storage by gracefully melding several different mechanisms together, each of which could produce the transformation by itself (Anastasio 1993). The "brain-like" structure created by recurrent back-propagation is strikingly different from those that were designed by human modelers (e.g., Raphan et al. 1979; Robinson 1981). While the recurrent back-propagation algorithm is admittedly non-physiological as an adaptive mechanism, it is nevertheless successful in constructing recurrent, nonlinear neural network models that capture the salient properties of real neural systems. Recurrent back-propagation has created a model for the VOR that provides deep insight into the subtle complexity of the solutions to signal processing problems that are implemented by the nervous system.

Like all of the models we consider in this book, the recurrent neural network model of the VOR is a hypothesis that must be verified experimentally. Many properties of the recurrent neural network model of the VOR are already consistent with experimental findings (Anastasio 1991, 1993, 1994). Some of these involve the consequences for the response properties of the output units in the network following simulated transection of the commissural connections, through which the recurrent interactions between the vestibular nucleus neurons (hidden units) take place (Wilson and Melvill Jones 1979). Changes in the response properties of the output units in the model should correspond to changes in the overall VOR in experimental animals. One such correspondence offers an explanation for a paradoxical finding.

Simulated commissurotomy, which is achieved in the network by setting all of the recurrent connection weights w to 0, not only decreases the time constant of the output units to that of the inputs but also increases output unit gain. This finding is somewhat surprising, since positive feedback is generally associated with signal amplification (notably when it results in instability), so that loss of positive feedback is not expected to produce a gain increase. In the network, removal of the recurrent connections makes the responses of the hidden units more symmetric. Because their off-direction gain (sensitivity) is higher, increased hidden unit response symmetry increases the push–pull drive of the output units by the hidden units and so increases output unit gain (Anastasio 1994). This modeling result is consistent with observation. Vestibular commissurotomy in monkeys also results in a decrease in VOR time constant but an increase in VOR gain (Blair and Gavin 1981).

The recurrent network model of the VOR has also been used to derive experimentally testable predictions (Anastasio 1994). These involve the consequences for the response properties of real vestibular nucleus neurons of actual commissurotomy, which are predicted by the effects on hidden unit responses of simulated commissurotomy in the model. They include an increase in background firing rate, increase in response symmetry, and decrease in response time constant. These predictions await experimental verification.

The predicted consequences of commissurotomy also include a decrease in the diversity of response properties over the population of vestibular nucleus neurons. We see a small-scale example of this diversity in the four-hidden-unit model, in which one pair of hidden units (see Figure 10.11A) carries some of the peak but most of the prolonged decay, while the other pair (see Figure 10.11B) carries most of the sharp initial peak but also carries some of the prolonged decay. In recurrent neural network models of the VOR with many hidden units, response components such as gain, peaked onsets, and prolonged decays are divided up and distributed even more non-uniformly, in a dynamic form of non-uniform distributed representation (Anastasio 1993; see also Exercise 10.2).

We have explored population coding and non-uniform distributed representations in previous chapters. In Chapter 8 we saw how the inherent randomness (stochasticity) of neurons requires that even relatively few signal components must be represented by an abundance of neurons. In Chapters 6 and 7 we saw how static signal components could be divided up and distributed non-uniformly over populations of neural units, and in this chapter we see that concept extended to dynamic signals. The tool that made this possible is recurrent back-propagation, which enables us to train recurrent, distributed, and nonlinear neural systems models on dynamic input–output transformations.

The extensive series of simulations just completed demonstrates many important issues concerning learning in recurrent neural networks. These include issues of stability, diversity, and the functional benefits of nonlinearity. They also include the pitfalls of local minima and the possibility of sometimes avoiding them. The simulations show that the types of solutions to problems found by adaptive algorithms are often different from those that human designers would propose. The neural integrator and velocity storage simulations just completed were focused on the brainstem, but this is certainly not the only region of the brain where recurrent interactions are thought to occur. They probably occur in most brain regions. In some sense, the leaky integration we studied in the brainstem may be similar to mechanisms of short-term memory that operate at the cortical level. Recurrent back-propagation has been used to model short-term memory in cortex by Zipser (1991). The last example in this chapter concerns that topic.

FIGURE 10.14 A recurrent neural network model of short-term memory, and methods for training and testing it The analog inputs, drawn at random from a uniform distribution of values between 0 and 1, are the items to be remembered. The desired output takes the value of the item that coincides in time with a gating input. It transitions to that value when the gating input is terminated, and remains at that value until the next item is gated in and replaces it. An item at a particular analog level is gated in and then out again to test the network after training. (After Zipser 1991.)

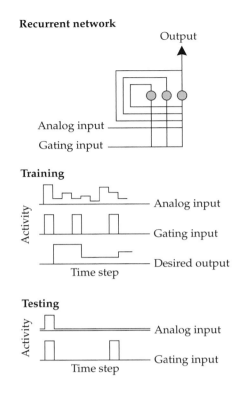

10.6 Training a Recurrent Neural Network to Simulate Short-Term Memory

The goal of this example is to reproduce the Zipser (1991) model of short-term memory. This model is schematized in Figure 10.14. It is a recurrent neural network that has two inputs (plus a bias) and eight nonlinear (sigmoidal) units. For simplicity, the inputs are not represented explicitly as input units, so all eight units are non-input units. The eighth unit is the output unit, and the network will be trained so that the state of the output unit is maintained over the short-term memory interval, at some level that is equal to the value of the item to be remembered. The first input (called the analog input in Figure 10.14) consists of "items," which are simply a series of random deviates distributed uniformly between 0 and 1. A new item, with a different value, appears on every time step. The second input constitutes a "gate," which indicates which item is to be remembered (i.e., stored in short-term memory). The gate comes on at random times, on average every few time steps, and goes off again after one time step. The network must "remember" the value of the item that appeared when the gate came on. Operationally, when the gate goes off, the value of the desired output transitions to the value of the item that appeared when the gate came on. The desired output maintains this value until a new item is gated in. Following training, the network is tested by gating an item in and out again and observing the state of the output unit over the short-term memory interval, which is the interval between the gating signals.

The focus of the tests is on the responses of unit eight, which is the designated output of the network, but the behavior of the other units, which are the hidden units, is also of considerable interest. The hidden units participate in producing the output, and the hope in this modeling is that their properties will be similar to those of the real neurons in cortex that mediate short-term memory. If they are, then it is possible that the mechanism, constructed by the

(A)

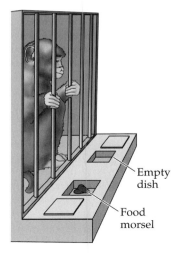 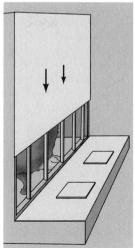 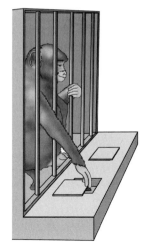

Empty
dish

Food
morsel

Cue:
Food is placed
in randomly
selected well
visible to monkey

Delay:
Screen is lowered
and food covered
for a standard time

Response:
Screen is raised
and monkey
uncovers well
containing food

(B)

Dorsolateral prefrontal cortex

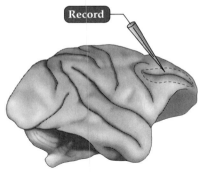

Record

(C)

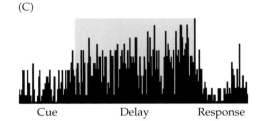

Cue   Delay   Response

FIGURE 10.15 Illustration of the delayed response task (A) A cue, in this case a morsel of food, is placed in one of two wells in view of a monkey. Then a screen is lowered during a delay period in which the food wells are covered. After the delay the screen is raised again and the monkey, in response, is allowed to uncover only one well. If it chooses correctly it can keep the food morsel as a reward. (B) Some neurons in the dorsolateral prefrontal cortex show increased activity during the delay period. (C) Histogram showing the number of action potentials per time bin of a neuron in the dorsolateral prefrontal cortex during the cue, delay, and response periods. (After Goldman-Rakic 1987.)

recurrent back-propagation learning algorithm to produce the desired output, can provide insight into the mechanism of real short-term memory.

In the experimental situation the neural responses are recorded while an animal performs a delayed response task. A diagram illustrating the delayed response task is shown in Figure 10.15. The task begins with a cue in which the animal (usually a monkey) is shown a sample stimulus (such as an object, an image, or a morsel of food). After an interval in which the sample is absent, the animal must choose the sample over one or more alternative stimuli. The correct choice elicits a reward, and the cue and reward in the experimental situation correspond to the first and second gating signals in the model.

In order to successfully accomplish the delayed response task, the animal must store neural activity related to the sample stimulus, during the delay interval, in short-term memory. The activities of some real cortical neurons during short-term memory tasks, along with the responses of some of the hidden units in the original Zipser (1991) model, are shown in Figure 10.16. Some real cortical neurons show activity between gating signals that can be characterized as sustained or changing increases or decreases in firing rate. Other cortical neurons respond to the onset and/or offset of gating signals. Still others show responses to the gating

FIGURE 10.16   Comparison of the activities of real neurons in delayed-response tasks and of units in the short-term memory model To accomplish the task both the real and the simulated neural systems must maintain, over the short-term memory interval, activity that is related to the item to be remembered. For the experimental data (left column) the neural activity related to the memory item is bracketed by a sensory cue and the receipt of reward, which are shown as bars and arrows underneath the response histograms. The reward is delivered after successful completion of the delayed-response task. The cue and reward in the experimental situation correspond to gating signals in the model (right column). Both the real and simulated responses consist of item-related and gate-related activity, and both the real neurons and model units show considerable diversity with regard to the manner in which they represent the item and gate-related signals. The diverse responses can be characterized as sustained or changing increases or decreases in activity between gating signals, transient increases or decreases associated with the gating signals, or various combinations of item and gate-related activity. The diversity of the responses of the units in the network (right column, A–F after Zipser 1991) matches that observed for real neurons from various cortical regions (left column): lateral intraparietal cortex (A after Gnadt and Anderson 1988), inferotemporal cortex (B after Furster et al. 1985), and frontal cortex (C and F after Fuster 1984; D after Quintana et al. 1989; E after Shintaro et al. 1990).

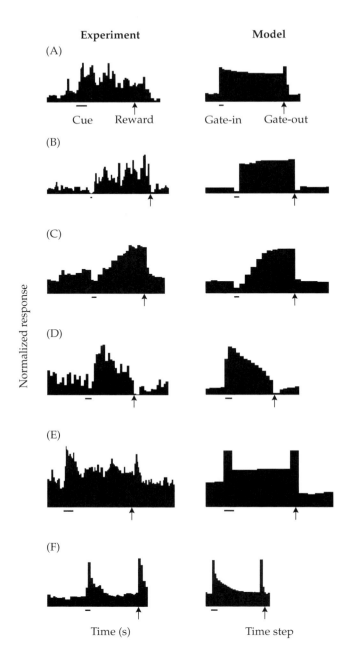

signals as well as activity between the gating signals. It appears that gating and memory signals are divided up and distributed non-uniformly over the population of cortical neurons. Hidden units in the recurrent neural network model of short-term memory also show these types of responses and simulate the observed response diversity. Our goal is to reproduce these modeling results.

In addition to the item and gate inputs, the recurrent network model of short-term memory requires a bias input. To train the network, all of the connection weights are modified by the recurrent back-propagation algorithm except the weights of the bias connections. Script rbpShortTermMemTrain, listed in MATLAB Box 10.4, will train a recurrent network of nonlinear (sigmoidal) units on the short-term memory task. The **M** matrix for this recurrent network has eight rows, one for each of the units, and eleven columns, one for each unit plus one column each for the bias, item, and gate inputs. The elements of the first column, which is the column of bias weights, are fixed

MATLAB® BOX 10.4   **This script uses recurrent back-propagation to train a nonlinear recurrent network to simulate short-term memory. (Training requires several minutes.)**

```
% rbpShortTermMemTrain.m

nUnits=8; % set number of units
b=1; % set bias
commonBwt=-2.5; % set common bias weight value
a=0.1; % set learning rate
nIts=100000; % set number of training iterations
pGate=0.5;% set proportion of gates
M=(rand(nUnits,nUnits+3)-0.5)*2; % randomize connectivity matrix
M(:,1)=ones(nUnits,1)*commonBwt; % set common bias weights
H=zeros(nUnits,nUnits+3,nUnits); % zero partial derivative matrix
Msk=ones(nUnits,nUnits+3); % set masking matrix to all ones
Msk(:,1)=zeros(nUnits,1); % mask out bias weights

item=0.01; itemPre=item; % set initial and previous item
gate=0.00; gatePre=gate; % set initial and previous gate
dout=0.01; doutPre=dout; % set initial and previous desired output
y=ones(nUnits,1)*itemPre; % set initial y value
z=[b;item;gate;y]; % initialize state vector
for c=2:nIts, % for each training cycle
    q=M*z; % find weighted input sums to hidden and output units
    y=1./(1+exp(-q)); % squash weighted sums to hid and out
    e=dout-y(nUnits); % compute error vector
    Hpre=H; H=H-H; % save then zero the partial matrices
    for k=1:nUnits, % for all hidden and output units
        for l=1:nUnits, % for all hidden and output units
            hld=M(k,l+3)*Hpre(:,:,l); % weight each H matrix
            hld(k,:)=hld(k,:)+z'; % add state vector to row k
            H(:,:,k)=H(:,:,k)+hld; % find partial matrices
        end % end l loop
        dSquash=y(k)*(1-y(k)); % derivative of squash
        H(:,:,k)=H(:,:,k)*dSquash; % scale by dSquash
    end % end k loop
    deltaM=e*H(:,:,nUnits); % find delta M
    deltaM=a*deltaM.*Msk; % apply learning rate and mask delta M
    M=M+deltaM; % update the connectivity matrix
    item=rand; % set new item at a random value
    if gatePre==1, % if the gate had been open...
        dout=itemPre; % then set desired output to previous item...
        gate=0; % and zero the gate
    elseif gatePre==0; % if the gate had not been open...
        dout=doutPre; % then keep the previous desired output
        gate=rand<pGate; % probabilistically open the gate
    end % end item gating procedure
    z=[b;item;gate;y]; % update state vector
    itemPre=item; gatePre=gate; doutPre=dout; % store previous values
end % end c (training) loop
```

at –2.5. The modifiable weights in the remaining columns (2 through 11) are initially set to random deviates, uniformly distributed between –1 and +1. To prevent the bias weights from being modified during learning, the script sets up an 8-by-11 masking matrix Msk with the first column all of 0s and the remaining columns all of 1s. Element-by-element multiplication of the

---

MATLAB® BOX 10.5 **This script tests the ability of recurrent neural networks to simulate short-term memory.**

```
% rbpShortTermMemTest.m
% script rpbShortTermMemTrain.m must be run first

b=1; % set bias
bg=0.01; % set background
sl=60; % set segment length
level=0.1:0.1:1; % set desired input item levels
Out=zeros(nUnits,sl,10); % zero actual output array
DesOut=zeros(10,sl); % zero desired output array
gate=zeros(1,sl); % set gate input to zero
gate(sl/3)=1; % set the "in" gate
gate(2*(sl/3))=1; % set the "out" gate

for l=1:10, % for each level
    item=ones(1,sl)*bg; % set background of item input
    DesOut(l,:)=ones(1,sl)*bg; % set background of desired output
    item(sl/3)=level(l); % set item level
    DesOut(l,sl/3+2:2*(sl/3)+1)=ones(1,sl/3)*level(l); % desired out
    y=ones(nUnits,1)*bg; % set initial y value
    Out(:,1,l)=y; % set first y output value
    z=[b;item(1);gate(1);y]; % set initial state
    for t=2:sl, % for each time step
        q=M*z; % compute weighted input sum
        y=1./(1+exp(-q)); % squash weighted sum
        Out(:,t,l)=y; % store y output
        z=[b;item(t);gate(t);y]; % reset state
    end % end t (time step) loop
end % end l (level) loop
```

masking matrix and the weight-change matrix, before the weight changes are applied to the weights, will prevent modification of the bias weights. (A similar weight update masking procedure was used for the velocity storage simulations.) In this script the number of (non-input) units is held in variable nUnits. The variable nUnits, and the number 3 of inputs, are used to set up the masking matrix Msk and as offsets for other indexing purposes in script rbpShortTermMemTrain.

As for the nonlinear VOR models, the responses of the units in the non-linear short-term memory model are described by $y(t) = f(\mathbf{M}z(t-1))$, where $f(\cdot)$ is the sigmoidal squashing function. This equation essentially implements Equations 10.2–10.4. As in previous examples, the weight changes are computed according to Equations 10.5–10.7 and applied according to Equation 10.8. (Implementation of the weight update equations for recurrent back-propagation is explained in detail in Section 10.1.)

Time steps are the same as learning iterations in the short-term memory simulation. Thus, learning occurs on each time step, and a new item also appears on each time step, but the desired output transitions to a new, sustained value only when the gate opens and then closes again. The gate stays open for only one time step. A set of conditionals in script rbpShortTermMemTrain determines the desired output (dout) on each time step (learning cycle). If the gate had been open on the previous time step then it closes on the current time step, and the desired output on the current time step transitions to the value of the item on the previous time step (i.e., the time step on which the gate had been open). If the gate had been closed on the previous time step, then the desired output on the current time step is the same as it was on the previous time step. The closed gate will open on any time step with a probability of pGate=0.5. The previous values of the variables item, gate, and dout are held in itemPre, gatePre, and doutPre, respectively.

Training with recurrent back-propagation occurs for nIts=100000 iterations at a learning rate of a=0.1. Following training, the recurrent, nonlinear neural network model of short-term memory is tested using script rbpShortTermMemTest, listed in MATLAB Box 10.5. This script will compute the responses of all the units in the network (hidden as well as output) according to $\mathbf{y}(t) = f(\mathbf{Mz}(t-1))$ (i.e., Equations 10.2–10.4) for items with values set at ten discrete levels (held in array level) that span the range of item values from 0.1 to 1.0. For each level, the network is tested over a segment of sl=60 time steps, and each item is gated in and gated out again over a short-term memory interval of 20 time steps (sl/3) in the middle of this segment. The desired outputs are stored in rectangular array DesOut, which has a row for each level and a column for each time step. The unit responses are held in cuboidal array Out, which has a row for each unit (hidden or output), a column for each time step, and a "page" for each memory item level.

The responses of the output unit (unit eight) for items at each of ten levels are shown in Figure 10.17. Note that, due to the randomness inherent in the training procedure (i.e., the initially random connection weights, the random

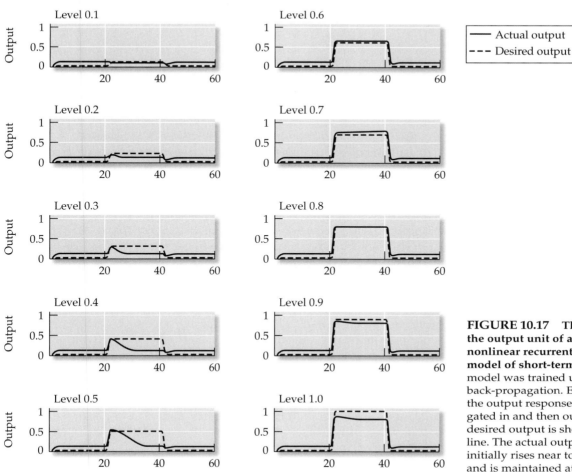

FIGURE 10.17   The responses of the output unit of an eight-unit, nonlinear recurrent neural network model of short-term memory The model was trained using recurrent back-propagation. Each panel shows the output response as an item is gated in and then out again. The desired output is shown as a dashed line. The actual output (solid line) initially rises near to the desired level and is maintained at that level for a duration that depends on its value.

Initial value

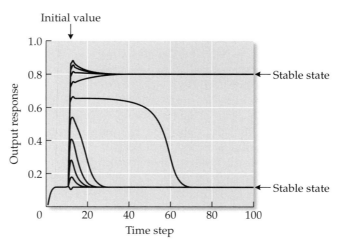

FIGURE 10.18 **Recurrent back-propagation trains the nonlinear recurrent network to simulate short-term memory essentially by causing it to develop two stable states** To reveal a stable state, an item at some test value is gated into the trained network and *not* replaced by gating in a different item until a stable state is reached. The output initially rises near to the value of the test item and then drifts to whichever of the two stable states is closer to that value. The two stable states for this model are at approximately 0.1 and 0.8. The lower six initial values seek the lower state, while the higher four initial values seek the higher state.

gate times, and the random item values) the responses you observe on any particular simulation are likely to differ from the responses shown in Figure 10.17, but these responses are representative. The output initially rises near to the value of the item at each level, and maintains that response value, but for a variable amount of time that depends on the value. For example, the output unit response in this particular run maintains the value of the item at levels 0.1, 0.6, and 0.8 for the entire short-term memory interval, but drifts away from the value at the other levels. This behavior is a consequence of the dynamics that recurrent back-propagation has trained the network to produce.

To explore network dynamics the network is subjected to a different test, in which items with values that span the range are gated in but are *not* gated out again. A modified version of `rbpShortTermMemTest` implements this test (see Exercise 10.3), which explores the longer-term behavior of the network. The results are shown in Figure 10.18, in which the output responses to the items with values at each of the ten levels are plotted together on the same graph. The figure shows the mechanism that recurrent back-propagation has created in order to simulate short-term memory. In this specific instance, recurrent back-propagation has trained the nonlinear, recurrent neural network to develop two stable states, and the mode of operation of the network involves movement toward those states. Specifically, the trained network maintains output activity at (or near) a specific level as the initial output response rises to (or near to) the value of the item to be remembered and then slowly drifts to whichever of the two stable states is closer to the initial output unit response. Thus, recurrent back-propagation has learned to exploit the ability of nonlinear, recurrent neural networks to possess multiple stable states.

We studied multiple stable states in the context of winners-take-all networks in Chapter 3, and of auto-associative networks in Chapter 4 (both of these recurrent network types are composed of nonlinear units). In the case of winners-take-all networks we set the recurrent connection weights according to a pre-defined (difference of Gaussians) profile. In the case of auto-associative networks we trained the recurrent weights using Hebbian rules accord-

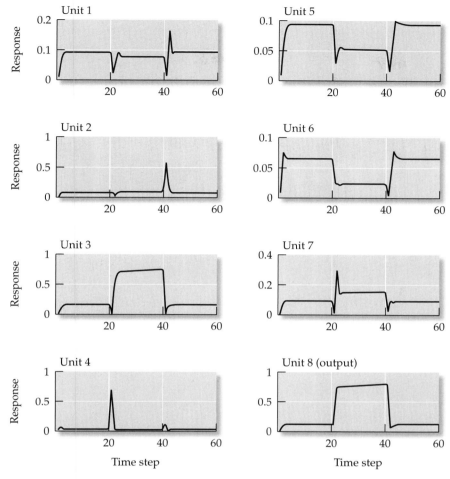

**FIGURE 10.19   Sustained and gate-associated responses of the eight units in
the nonlinear recurrent neural network model of short-term memory** An item
of value 0.8 is gated in and then out again. The bottom right panel represents the
output unit.

ing to training-pattern covariation. In the short-term memory example we
consider here, recurrent back-propagation uses error-driven learning through
time to train the recurrent, nonlinear network to develop stable states at two
specific values. (Training on the short-term memory problem does not always
produce two stable states; see Exercises 10.3 and 10.4.) The two stable states
developed by the network in this particular instance are near 0.1 and 0.8, and
that explains why simulated short-term memory is so good for items with
those values. Interestingly, the network can hold a value near 0.6 for a longer
duration than for other non-stable values before it drifts to a stable state, and
this accounts for the good performance of the model for items with values
near 0.6. You will observe a different performance each time you rerun the
simulation. The responses presented here are representative of a good run.

Since the actual neural mechanism of short-term memory is unknown, the
principle means for evaluating whether this model is a good model of short-
term memory is to compare the behavior of the units with that of real cortical
neurons during short-term memory tasks. Plots of the actual responses of all
eight of the units in the short-term memory network for an item value of 0.8
are shown separately in Figure 10.19. The units show sustained increases or
decreases in activation, or activity associated with the gate signals, or combi-

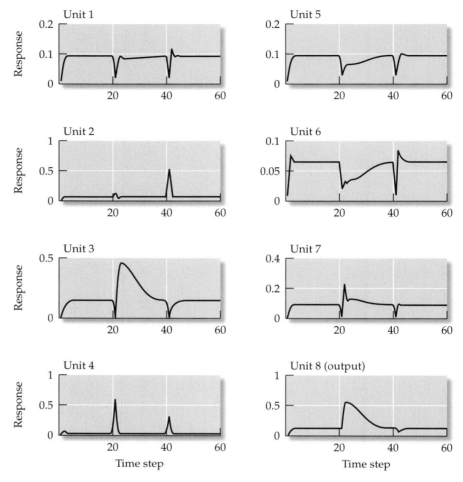

FIGURE 10.20 Changing and gate-associated responses of the eight units in the nonlinear recurrent neural network model of short-term memory An item of value 0.5 is gated in and then out again. The bottom-right panel represents the output unit.

nations of the two. These responses are consistent with those that have been reported for neurons in cortex that show sustained and/or gate-related activity during short-term memory tasks (see Figure 10.16). Plots of the actual responses of all eight of the units in the short-term memory network for an item value of 0.5 are shown separately in Figure 10.20. The units show changing increases or decreases in activation, or activity associated with the gate signals, or combinations of the two. These responses are consistent with those of other neurons in cortex that show changing rather than sustained activity between gates during short-term memory tasks (see Figure 10.16). Together the unit responses form a non-uniform, distributed representation of gate and item-related signals, and capture the diversity of responses of real cortical neurons in short-term memory tasks.

Our version of the recurrent neural network model of short-term memory, like the original model (Zipser 1991), provides a nice agreement with the data. It suggests that the brain may represent the value of an item held in short-term memory in terms of the sustained (or slowly changing) firing rate of certain cortical neurons. The fact that the short-duration responses of the units in the network resemble those of real cortical neurons suggests that something like the stable-state mechanism developed by the recurrent back-propagation algorithm in this model may be operating in the cortex as well. It might be possible to test this hypothesis by recording the long-duration responses of the cortical neurons that show sustained activity during delayed response tasks. Specifically, the model predicts that, in the long term, the responses of neurons mediating short-term memory should drift to one of a relatively small number of stable states. This prediction remains untested.

Although the precise mechanism of short-term memory is still not known, most current models of short-term and working memory rely on recurrent connections to produce persistent responses (e.g., O'Reilly and Frank 2006). Like Hebbian plasticity (see Chapter 4) the idea that short-term memory is mediated by recurrent networks also goes back to Donald Hebb (1949). Hebb suggested that neural activity could be sustained as it passes from one neuron to another around closed loops that he called "reverberatory circuits." That seminal idea has persisted to this day in the form of the recurrent, nonlinear neural network models that stand as hypotheses concerning the neural mechanisms that underlie short-term memory.

Exercises

10.1 We used script `rbpTwoUnitIntegrator` (see MATLAB Box 10.1) to train two recurrently connected output units to leaky integrate their push–pull inputs. Specifically, we trained them to develop excitatory self-connections, and mutually inhibitory reciprocal connections, of absolute value near 0.495. The integrator would be perfect (not leaky) if the absolute value of all of these weights (its recurrent weights) was equal to 0.5. Keeping the learning rate at 0.005 (`a=0.005`), and the absolute value of the input–output (feedforward) weights at `vAb=0.5`, try to train the integrator to be less leaky by setting its desired recurrent weight absolute value to `wAb=0.499`. Can it accomplish this training? What happens? Try decreasing the learning rate and increasing the number of iterations (`nIts`). Can you get the integrator to learn to develop recurrent weights with absolute values near 0.499? Like the model, the synaptic weights of the real oculomotor neural integrator are probably also adjusted through a plastic mechanism (Robinson 1989). Does this exercise give you insight into why the real neural integrator is leaky?

10.2 We used script `rbpVelocityStorageNonlinear` (see MATLAB Box 10.3) to train a recurrent network with four nonlinear (sigmoidal) hidden units to produce velocity storage. The recurrent back-propagation algorithm produced a network with two functionally distinct pairs of hidden units. One pair was strongly recurrently connected and the units had rounded initial responses, while the other pair was weakly recurrently connected and had sharp initial responses. Try increasing the number of hidden units in the network to eight (`nHid=8`). How do the responses of the units in the eight-hidden-unit network compare with those in the four-hidden-unit network? The increased variability you should observe corresponds to the variability in spontaneous (background) firing rate, gain (sensitivity), and the temporal response properties of real vestibular nucleus neurons (Fuchs and Kimm 1975).

10.3 The script `rbpShortTermMemTrain` (listed in MATLAB Box 10.4) uses recurrent back-propagation to train recurrent networks to produce sustained outputs at various levels, which simulates a simple form of short-term memory. A successfully trained network produces short-term memory by causing its output to drift slowly to whichever of two stable states is closer to the level (numerical value) of the item to be remembered. The script `rbpShortTermMemTest` (see MATLAB Box 10.5) will test the ability of recurrent networks to simulate short-term memory by gating in an item and then gating it out again after a short time interval. Modify this script so that it can reproduce the stable-state test in Figure 10.18. This change mainly involves removing the second ("out") gate and extending the segment length `sl`. Then retrain the network several times, and each time observe its stable-state output behavior. Does the recurrent back-propagation algorithm always train the network to have two stable states? Does it ever cause the network to develop more than two stable states?

10.4 For our simulation of short-term memory we employed a neural network that had eight recurrently connected units, and in which the eighth (last) unit was designated as the output. The script `rbpShortTermMemTrain` (listed in MATLAB Box 10.4) uses recurrent back-propagation to train recurrent networks to simulate short-term memory, essentially by causing them to develop two stable states. Are eight units necessary for the development of two stable states? Reduce the number of units and retrain the network several times on the short-term memory task. Can you train a network having fewer than eight units to develop two stable states? How many units are sufficient? Now increase the number of units and retrain the network. Can you get more than two stable states?

References

Anastasio TJ (1991) Neural network models of velocity storage in the horizontal vestibulo-ocular reflex. *Biological Cybernetics* 64: 187–196.

Anastasio TJ (1993) Modeling vestibulo-ocular reflex dynamics: From classical analysis to neural networks. In: Eeckman FH (ed) *Neural Systems: Analysis and Modeling*. Kluwer Academic Publishers, Norwell, MA.

Anastasio TJ (1994) Testable predictions from recurrent back-propagation models of the vestibulo-ocular reflex. *Neurocomputing* 6: 237–255.

Blair SM, Gavin M (1981) Brainstem commissures and control of the time constant of vestibular nystagmus. *Acta Otolaryngology* 91: 1–8.

Cannon SC, Robinson DA, Shamma S (1983) A proposed neural network for the integrator of the oculomotor system. *Biological Cybernetics* 49: 127–136.

Churchland PM, Churchland PS (1990) Could a machine think? *Scientific American* 262: 32–37.

Epstein R, Roberts G, Beber G (eds) (2008) *Parsing the Turing Test: Philosophical and Methodological Issues in the Quest for the Thinking Computer*. Springer, The Netherlands.

Fuchs AF, Kimm J (1975) Unit activity in vestibular nucleus of the alert monkey during horizontal angular acceleration and eye movement. *Journal of Neurophysiology* 38: 1140–1161.

Fuster JM (1984) Behavioral electrophysiology of the prefrontal cortex. *Trends in Neuroscience* 7: 408–414.

Fuster JM, Bauer RH, Jervey JP (1985) Functional interactions between inferotemporal and prefrontal cortex in a cognitive task. *Brain Research* 30: 299–307.

Gnadt JW, Andersen RA (1988) Memory related motor planning activity in posterior parietal cortex of macaque. *Experimental Brain Research* 70: 216–220.

Goldman-Rakic PS (1987) Circuitry of the prefrontal cortex and the regulation of behavior by representational memory. In: Plum F (ed) *Handbook of Physiology. Section 1, The Nervous System. vol 5, Higher Functions of the Brain, Part I.* American Physiological Society, Bethesda, MD, pp 373–417.

Haykin S (1999) *Neural Networks: A Comprehensive Foundation. Second Edition.* Prentice Hall, Upper Saddle River, NJ, pp 732–789.

Hebb DO (1949) *The Organization of Behavior.* Wiley, New York.

Henn V (1982) The correlation between motion sensation, nystagmus, and activity in the vestibular nerve and nuclei. In: Honrubia V, Brazier MAB (eds) *Nystagmus and Vertigo: Clinical Approaches to the Patient with Dizziness.* Academic Press, New York, pp 115–124.

O'Reilly RC, Frank MJ (2006) Making working memory work: A computational model of learning in the prefrontal cortex and basal ganglia. *Neural Computation* 18: 283–328.

Quintana J, Fuster JM, Yajeya J (1989) Effects of cooling parietal cortex on prefrontal units in delay tasks. *Brain Research* 503: 100–110.

Raphan T, Matsuo V, Cohen B (1979) Velocity storage in the vestibuloocular reflex arc (VOR). *Experimental Brain Research* 35: 229–248.

Robinson DA (1981) The use of control systems analysis in the neurophysiology of eye movements. *Annual Review of Neuroscience* 4: 463–503.

Robinson DA (1989) Integrating with neurons. *Annual Review of Neuroscience* 12: 33–45.

Rumelhart DE, Hinton GE, Williams RJ (1986) Learning internal representations by error propagation. In: Rumelhart DE, McClelland JL, PDP Research Group (eds) *Parallel Distributed Processing: Explorations in the Microstructure of Cognition, vol 1: Foundations.* MIT Press, Cambridge, MA, pp 318–362.

Shintaro F, Bruce CJ, Goldman-Rakic PS (1990) Visuospatial coding in primate prefrontal neurons revealed by oculomotor paradigms. *Journal of Neurophysiology* 63: 814–831.

Siegelmann HT, Sontag ED (1991) Turing computability with neural nets. *Applied Mathematics Letters* 4: 77–80.

Smith EE, Jonides J (2003) Executive control and thought. In: Squire LR, Bloom FE, McConnell SK, Roberts JL, Spitzer NC, Zigmond MJ (eds) *Fundamental Neuroscience. Second Edition.* Academic Press, San Diego, CA, pp 1377–1394.

Turing AM (1936) On computable numbers with an application to the Entscheidungs problem. *Proceedings of the London Mathematical Society, Series 2*, 42: 230–265; Correction (*Ibid.*) 43: 544–546.

Turing AM (1950) Computing machinery and intelligence. *Mind* 59: 433–460.

Williams RJ, Zipser D (1989) A learning algorithm for continually running fully recurrent neural networks. *Neural Computation* 1: 270–280.

Wilson VJ, Melvill Jones G (1979) *Mammalian Vestibular Physiology*. Plenum Press, New York.

Zipser D (1991) Recurrent network model of the neural mechanism of short-term active memory. *Neural Computation* 3: 179–193.

Temporal-Difference Learning and Reward Prediction

Temporal-difference learning can train neural networks to estimate the future value of a current state and simulate the responses of neurons involved in reward processing

As Yogi Berra is famously purported to have said, "Prediction is very hard, especially about the future." However you express it, the unavoidable uncertainly associated with the future often leaves us no choice but to make our best bet. Economically, the best bet is the one with the highest expected value. In a typical bet, you risk some amount of money on an uncertain event (for example, that the Yankees will win the World Series), and the expected value of the bet is the amount you expect to win minus the amount you expect to lose. The amount you expect to win is the amount of the wager multiplied by the probability that the event will occur (e.g., that the Yankees will win), while the amount you expect to lose is the amount of the wager multiplied by the probability that the event will not occur (e.g., that the Yankees will lose). In baseball, as in life generally, we often get to choose among bets (you could bet instead for the Cubs). You might choose a particular team for an idiosyncratic reason (your home team, perhaps), but in monetary terms your best bet is the one with the highest expected value.

Of course, the payoff from winning a bet, or from winning any gamble, is more than strictly monetary. There is something intrinsically rewarding about it. We will not consider the motivations that underlie gambling in this chapter, but we will simulate the responses of certain neurons that are part of the "reward" system of the brain. These neurons appear to be involved in learning the expected values of sensory events and behavioral options.

When discussing expected value it is useful to distinguish between states and actions. We can think of a "state" as some configuration of the world, and an "action" as something that changes the configuration of the world. For example, Yankee fans assigned a high expected value to the state of the world in which Joe DiMaggio was at bat. They also assigned a high expected value to the action that Joe took a swing, because both the state and the action were likely to lead to an increase in the score for the Yankees. We can also think in terms of state-action pairs, such as Joe taking a swing at a favorable pitch with the bases loaded. As this baseball example illustrates, the expected value is the value we expect to receive in going forward from a state, action, or state-action pair. In general, there are potential gains and losses in proceeding from any situation or act, and the expected value is precisely the sum of the potential gains (positive values) and losses (negative values) weighted by their associated probabilities (see Section 11.1). We often get to choose among options, whether they are states, actions, or state-action pairs, and knowing the expected values associated with the various options enables us to decide effectively among them. According to decision theory, and assuming we know the expected values of the available options, the optimal decision is made by choosing whichever option has the highest expected value (Berger 1985).

Not only do primates (human and nonhuman) appear to make optimal decisions, but the activities of neurons in many regions of the forebrain, including the frontal and parietal cortices and the striatum, are correlated with the expected values of various sensory cues and behavioral alternatives (Platt and Glimcher 1999; Schultz 2004; Lee and Seo 2007; Lau and Glimcher 2008). In nonhumans, and usually in humans as well, expected values are not known precisely but could be estimated though experience, according to discrepancies between the expected values and the actual values that are ultimately realized (Lee and Seo 2007). Because an expectation can be considered as a prediction, the difference between the expected and actual values can be thought of as a prediction error. Evidence indicates that the brain may actually learn to estimate expected value on the basis of experience. Experiments show that the activities of neurons in certain regions of the midbrain (ventral tegmentum) and the forebrain (striatum) are correlated with prediction error (Montague et al. 1996; King-Casas et al. 2005). We will simulate the activities of midbrain neurons as carriers of prediction error signals in this chapter.

In very loose terms, the trick in learning expected value is in learning to predict the future. More precisely, the goal in learning the expected value of some state of affairs is in learning the value that you will obtain on average in progressing from that state. As prediction problems, many games of chance are relatively simple, because we realize the actual value in one step, like a roll of the dice or a spin of the roulette wheel. Because the outcomes of a game of chance are random, we would need many plays (trials) of a particular game before we could accurately estimate its expected values, but on each trial we would know the outcome in one step. In contrast, some games, and many real-world situations, are not that simple.

Rather than happening in one step, many real-world situations are sequential processes in which the outcome is not known until the end of the sequence. A common example is finding your way from a start location to a destination in a new environment. Ultimately, you will develop a map-like mental representation of the environment, but before that happens you will learn to progress from landmark to landmark. At first, you do not know until you reach your destination whether the steps you took along the way were correct. But as you experience many trips, both successful and unsuccessful, you learn the expected values of various landmarks as steps toward your desired destination. (You also learn, by experience, the expected values of various landmarks as steps toward undesirable locations.)

Temporal-difference learning is a parsimonious method for learning the expected values of states in a sequential process in which the outcome may not be known until the end of the sequence (Sutton and Barto 1998). The power of temporal-difference learning is well illustrated by a classic example in which the algorithm was used to train a computer to play the game of backgammon (Tesauro 2002). This popular board game for two players involves a sequence of moves of game pieces between board locations. The game ends when the winning player has moved all her pieces off the board. The number of moves per turn is determined by rolling two dice, introducing a random element to the game that greatly increases its complexity. The rules of the game allow some strategy, but backgammon is so complex that human players most likely rely on judgment derived from experience when playing it. Guided by a general backgammon strategy, human players simply choose the specific move they feel will be the most valuable given the current configuration of the various pieces on the board (i.e., its current state).

The computer program, known as TD-gammon, is actually a collection of processes, some of which were programmed explicitly while others were learned via the temporal-difference algorithm as the program played many rounds of backgammon against itself. The explicitly programmed components imitate the kinds of general strategies that humans might deploy, while temporal-difference learning is used to teach TD-gammon to estimate the expected values of various states (configurations) of the board. Temporal-difference learning can be appropriately applied in the context of a game like backgammon because the outcome of the sequence of moves (sequence of states, or board configurations) cannot be known until after the game is over and the winner and loser have been determined. Following training, the moves made by TD-gammon are to states (board configurations) that have the highest estimated expected values. Learning expected state values endows TD-gammon with "judgment," and it is in this latter attribute that TD-gammon most decisively outperforms human experts (Tesauro 2002).

Temporal-difference learning can be used to estimate the expected values of states in any terms (such as monetary, geographic, or competitive), but it is most often used in the context of reinforcement learning (Sutton and Barto 1998). Reinforcement can be regarded as anything that motivates behavior, including learning (Robbins and Everitt 2003). In Chapter 7 we used reinforcement learning to model simple forms of associative conditioning, in which learned weight changes occurred so as to increase the amount of positive reinforcement, and decrease the amount of negative reinforcement, received by the learner. (In that case, the learner was a schema-based model of a rabbit.) In this chapter we will consider both positive and negative reinforcement in the context of temporal-difference learning. We can think of positive reinforcement as "reward" and negative reinforcement as "punishment." This would be consistent with conditioning experiments showing that animals behave so as to increase positive and decrease negative reinforcement, but we can only assume that animals subjectively experience positive or negative reinforcement as "reward" or "punishment," respectively (Robbins and Everitt 2003; see Chapter 7 for a fuller discussion of reinforcement learning).

In Chapter 7, we studied neural systems (including schema-based models) that learned the values of specific connection weights over many single-step learning trials, in which reinforcement was received immediately following each single step. Temporal-difference learning will enable agents (including neural networks) to learn to estimate the values of states from state sequences, regardless of where and when in the sequence reinforcement is available. Most of the learning algorithms we have considered so far were specific to neural networks. Here we will use temporal-difference learning to adjust the weights in a neural network, or to adjust the state value estimates of a more abstract learning agent. In cases where reinforcement is delivered only in selected states, the learner (agent or neural network) needs to work backward from the reinforcing event in order to update the estimated values of the states that led up to it. For that to work, the states must have some temporal or sequential relationship with one another. Because of its analytical tractability, temporal-difference learning is often studied in the context of Markov processes.

A Markov process is a stochastic (i.e., random) process in which the current state depends probabilistically on the previous state, but only on the previous state and not on any states further back in the sequence. In an environment that exhibits the Markov property, random transitions between allowed states occur with some probability until a terminal state is reached. Terminal states (and sometimes non-terminal states) can be associated with reinforcement (positive, reward; negative, punishment). Temporal-difference learning can be used to estimate the expected values of the various, non-terminal states through exposure to the Markov environment. The problem is best illustrated with a simple, concrete example. This example is adapted from Russell and Norvig (1995).

Consider the gridworld shown in Figure 11.1. This gridworld has three rows and four columns of cells that represent its states. Their coordinates as row, column pairs specify the states, or they can be numbered consecutively from state 1 (coordinates 1, 1) to state 12 (coordinates 3, 4) (see Figure 11.2). Certain states have a special purpose. Each state sequence begins at (1, 1), the start state. State (2, 2) is a disallowed state (no transition leads to it). States (2, 4) and (3, 4) are terminal states, and the state sequence ends when the agent reaches either of those. In this simple gridworld the agent receives its only reinforcement in the terminal states: either reward (+1 in state 3, 4) or punishment (−1 in state 2, 4). (In general, reinforcement can be received in any state.) A sequence (or trajectory) through the gridworld is often referred to as an epoch.

The arrows (shown in Figure 11.1) indicate the allowed transitions between states. The problem for the agent is to learn the expected values of all allowed,

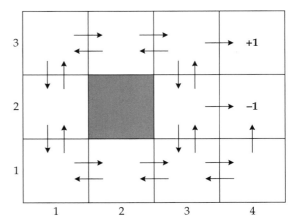

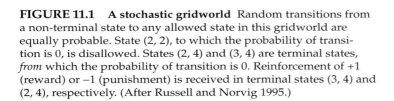

FIGURE 11.1   A stochastic gridworld Random transitions from a non-terminal state to any allowed state in this gridworld are equally probable. State (2, 2), to which the probability of transition is 0, is disallowed. States (2, 4) and (3, 4) are terminal states, *from* which the probability of transition is 0. Reinforcement of +1 (reward) or −1 (punishment) is received in terminal states (3, 4) and (2, 4), respectively. (After Russell and Norvig 1995.)

MATLAB® BOX 11.1   This script sets up a stochastic gridworld.

```
% gridWorldSetUp.m

nStates=12; % set number of states
stateVec=(1:12)'; % set a state number vector
r=zeros(nStates,1); % set a reinforcement vector
ProbMat=zeros(nStates); % define a probability matrix

tsr=12; % designate the terminal state of reward
tsp=8; % designate the terminal state of punishment
intReSt=7; % designate an intermediate state for reinforcement
r(tsr)=+1; % set reinforcement of reward terminal state
r(tsp)=-1; % set reinforcement of punishment terminal state
r(intReSt)=0; % set intermediate reinforcement if desired

% enter the transition matrix
TM = ...
[0  1  0  0  1  0  0  0  0  0  0  0
 1  0  1  0  0  0  0  0  0  0  0  0
 0  1  0  1  0  0  1  0  0  0  0  0
 0  0  1  0  0  0  0  0  0  0  0  0
 1  0  0  0  0  0  0  0  1  0  0  0
 0  0  0  0  0  0  0  0  0  0  0  0
 0  0  1  0  0  0  0  0  0  0  1  0
 0  0  0  1  0  0  1  0  0  0  0  0
 0  0  0  0  1  0  0  0  0  1  0  0
 0  0  0  0  0  0  0  0  1  0  1  0
 0  0  0  0  0  0  1  0  0  1  0  0
 0  0  0  0  0  0  0  0  0  0  1  0];

% use the transition matrix to find the probability matrix
for j=1:nStates, % for each state
    indx=find(TM(:,j)~=0); % find indices of allowed next states
    if isempty(indx), prob=0; % if no next state assign zero prob
    else prob=1/sum(TM(:,j)); end % else compute probability
    ProbMat(indx,j)=prob; % enter probability into prob matrix
end % end probability matrix loop

% solve for the exact state values
exVals=inv(ProbMat'-eye(nStates))*(-r);
```

non-terminal states. Were the gridworld deterministic, the problem would be easy to solve. In a deterministic gridworld, the start state would lead inexorably to either one of the two terminal states, and the expected values of the start state and all other non-terminal states along the trajectory would equal the value of that terminal state. (States not visited along the deterministic trajectory would have expected value 0). To make the problem more interesting (and more realistic) we consider a stochastic gridworld in which the current state will always make a random transition to another state, with each of the allowed transitions from the current state being equally probable. For example, three arrows lead out of state (3, 3). Thus, if the agent were positioned at (3, 3), then it would randomly transition either to (3, 2), (2, 3), or the reward state (3, 4), and the probability of each of those transitions is 1/3.

This stochastic gridworld is set up using the script `gridworldSetUp`, which is listed in MATLAB® Box 11.1. The states are designated in the script not according to their coordinates but according to their consecutive number-

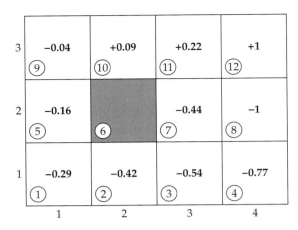

FIGURE 11.2   The exact values of the states in the stochastic gridworld
The exact state values are computed using Equation 11.1 (see also Math Box 11.1). The states, which can be designated by their (row, column) coordinates, are also numbered (encircled) from 1 to 12 for convenience. (After Russell and Norvig 1995.)

ing, as shown in Figure 11.2. This script sets parameters such as the number of states (nStates=12), and the identity of the terminal states (tsr=12 sets the terminal state of reward to state number 12, while tsp=8 sets the terminal state of punishment to state number 8). Script gridworldSetUp defines a reinforcement vector r with one element for each state of the gridworld (r=zeros(nStates,1)), and then sets the reinforcements associated with the terminal states (r(tsr)=+1 and r(tsp)=−1). The script also offers the option of assigning reinforcement to one non-terminal state (see Exercise 11.1).

The script gridworldSetUp sets up the state transition matrix (matrix TM) in which each allowed or disallowed transition takes the value of 1 or 0, respectively. Element (i, j) of matrix TM is a 1 if the transition to state i from state j is allowed. (Note that this "to–from" ordering, respectively for the row and column indices, matches the ordering we have been using for network connection weights.) The matrix TM is constructed to facilitate the computations associated with movement through, and learning in, this particular stochastic (random) gridworld, in which all transitions allowed from any state are equally probable. For example, column 11, which specifies the three transitions allowed from state 11 (which are 7, 10, and 12) has three 1s in it. The row indices of the 1s (which are 7, 10, and 12 in column 11) identify the states to which the agent is allowed to transition from state 11. The reciprocal of the sum over column 11, which is 1/3, is the probability of transitioning to any one of those three states. For example, the transition probability from state j = 11 could be found using prob=1/sum(TM(:,j)).

Expected values, as explained above, are generally used in the context of decision-making, but once the expected values are known, the decision to choose the option with the highest expected value is easy. The hard part is in learning the expected values in the first place, and it is to that learning problem that we devote our attention in this chapter. Because our agent needs to learn the actual characteristics of its environment, it will not "decide" to which state to move but will undergo random state transitions according to the transition probabilities specified for the gridworld. In our case, the agent's job is to learn the expected values of the states. Note that, for simplicity in this chapter, we will be concerned only with the expected values of states, not of actions or of state-action pairs (see Sutton and Barto 1998 for a full range of examples and applications).

Due to the stochasticity of the gridworld, the agent can never be "sure" as to which of the allowed state transitions it will randomly undergo (unless it is in a terminal state), but some states are clearly better to be in than others. For example, state 11 has a 1/3 chance of transitioning to the reward state 12. In contrast, state 4 has a 1/2 chance of transitioning to the punishment state 8. Clearly, it is more valuable for the agent to be in state 11 than in state 4. Determining, in a rigorous way, the exact expected value of each state is the goal of learning in a Markov environment.

Precisely stated, the expected value of a state is the reinforcement that the agent can *expect* to receive in progressing from that state. As far as the agent is concerned, the "expected" value of a state is the "real" value of that state, even though the agent may not receive actual reinforcement until it progresses from that state. For this reason we can consider "value" as synonymous with "expected value." Despite its stochastic nature, the structure inherent in the Markov environment constrains the agent's movement within it (transitions are allowed only between adjacent states, for example). This structure also determines the values that the states can take, given their relative locations and the locations of the reinforcements in the environment. Due to structural constraints, the value of a state in a Markov environment is the average (probability-weighted sum) of the values of its successor states plus its own reinforcement (Bellman 1957; Sutton and Barto 1998). It follows that the values v_j (same as expected values) can be computed on the basis of the state transition probabilities and the reinforcement associated with each state by solving the set of simultaneous equations implied by Equation 11.1:

$$v_j = r_j + \sum_i p_{ij} v_i \qquad\qquad \textbf{11.1}$$

where j designates the current state and i indexes each of its successor states. Each state (equivalently indexed by i or j) has value v and could have reinforcement r. (In the examples we explore in this chapter, only the terminal states are reinforcing, but any state could be reinforcing in general; see Exercise 11.1.) The variable p_{ij} designates the transition probability to state i from state j. The "to–from" subscript ordering is the same as the one we have been using to designate connection weights.

Because we have constructed the gridworld, we know the r_j and p_{ij} and can use Equation 11.1 to compute the exact values v_j for all the states. The script gridworldSetUp will solve Equation 11.1 and find these state values (see MATLAB Box 11.1). The script converts transition matrix TM into the matrix ProbMat of transition probabilities (with elements p_{ij}). It solves for the state values v_j by first transposing ProbMat and then using the methods of linear algebra (see Math Box 11.1). The exact state values, which are shown in Figure 11.2, make qualitative sense. The values of the states along the top row are greater than those along the bottom row, because the states along the top row have a higher expected reinforcement. The exact values of the states reflect the fact that an agent undergoing random transitions between adjacent states in the gridworld is more likely to reach a reward of +1 from the states along the top row, and is more likely to reach a punishment of –1 from the states along the bottom row.

Although we have complete knowledge of the gridworld we have constructed, an agent, in general, does not have access to complete knowledge of an environment, so it must learn about the environment through experience. We will provide experience in the gridworld to a learning agent by starting it at the start state and allowing it to make transitions randomly, according to the transition probabilities, until either of the terminal states is reached. Such a journey through the gridworld, during which the agent learns, constitutes a

MATH BOX 11.1   FINDING STATE VALUES BY SOLVING A SET OF SIMULTANEOUS LINEAR EQUATIONS

The values of the states in the stochastic gridworld can be computed on the basis of the state transition probabilities and the reinforcement associated with each state by solving the set of simultaneous equations implied by Equation B11.1.1 (which is the same as Equation 11.1 of the main text):

$$v_j = r_j + \sum_i p_{ij} v_i \qquad \text{B11.1.1}$$

where the v_j (equivalently v_i) are the state values and p_{ij} is the probability of transitioning to state i from state j ($i = 1,\ldots, n$ and $j = 1,\ldots, n$). We use this "to–from" subscript designation because it is consistent with the connection weight subscripting we use throughout this book. In the context of dynamic programming problems, the "to–from" subscript designation when assigned to transition probabilities could be considered "backward," but this is a minor problem. If we express our transition probabilities p_{ij} using the "to–from" subscript designation, and we insert them as the elements of transition probability matrix $\mathbf{P}$, then we need only transpose $\mathbf{P}$ in computations involving the matrix form of Equation B11.1.1, to which we now turn our attention.

The matrix form of Equation B11.1.1 can be written as in Equation B11.1.2:

$$\mathbf{v} = \mathbf{r} + \mathbf{P}^{\mathrm{T}} \mathbf{v} \qquad \text{B11.1.2}$$

where vector $\mathbf{v}$ has elements v_j (equivalently v_i), vector $\mathbf{r}$ has elements r_j, and $\mathbf{P}^{\mathrm{T}}$ is the matrix transpose of $\mathbf{P}$, as shown in expanded form in Equation B11.1.3:

$$\mathbf{P}^{\mathrm{T}} = \begin{bmatrix} 0 & p_{21} & \cdots & p_{n1} \\ p_{12} & 0 & & \\ \vdots & & \ddots & \\ p_{1n} & p_{2n} & \cdots & 0 \end{bmatrix} \qquad \text{B11.1.3}$$

Since the probability of a state transitioning to itself is 0 ($p_{ij} = 0$ when $i = j$), the diagonal of $\mathbf{P}^{\mathrm{T}}$ (and of $\mathbf{P}$) is 0. We can manipulate Equation B11.1.2 via the methods of linear algebra to solve the set of simultaneous equations implied by Equation B11.1.1.

If $\mathbf{I}$ is the n-by-n identity matrix, then $\mathbf{Iv} = \mathbf{v}$ and Equation B11.1.2 can be rewritten as in Equation B11.1.4:

$$-\mathbf{r} = \left(\mathbf{P}^{\mathrm{T}} - \mathbf{I} \right) \mathbf{v} \qquad \text{B11.1.4}$$

Equation B11.1.4 can be solved for $\mathbf{v}$ using matrix inversion. If $\mathbf{b} = \mathbf{Ac}$, where $\mathbf{A}$ is a (square) matrix, $\mathbf{b}$ is a vector of know quantities, and $\mathbf{c}$ is a vector of unknowns, then $\mathbf{c} = \mathbf{A}^{-1}\mathbf{b}$, where $\mathbf{A}^{-1}$ is the matrix inverse of $\mathbf{A}$ and $\mathbf{AA}^{-1} = \mathbf{A}^{-1}\mathbf{A} = \mathbf{I}$ (Noble and Daniel 1977). By analogy, we can solve Equation B11.1.4 using Equation B11.1.5:

$$\mathbf{v} = \left(\mathbf{P}^{\mathrm{T}} - \mathbf{I} \right)^{-1} (-\mathbf{r}) \qquad \text{B11.1.5}$$

where we substitute $\mathbf{v}$ for $\mathbf{c}$, $(\mathbf{P}^{\mathrm{T}} - \mathbf{I})$ for $\mathbf{A}$, and $-\mathbf{r}$ for $\mathbf{b}$. We use this method in script `gridworldSetUp` (see MATLAB Box 11.1) to find the exact state values $\mathbf{v}$, given a vector of reinforcements $\mathbf{r}$ and a (square) transition probability matrix $\mathbf{P}$.

training epoch. The agent is permitted a large number of training epochs. During this experience, we assume that the agent can know two things concerning its current state in the gridworld: the identity (i.e., the number) of the state and any reinforcement associated with that state. The agent will represent the gridworld in terms of a vector $\mathbf{v}$ of values (same as expected values), one for each state in the gridworld. Its goal is to learn the values of the states from experience in the gridworld.

Our ultimate goal in this chapter is to use the temporal-difference learning paradigm to simulate the behavior of midbrain neurons, specifically those that encode a signal that could be used to learn the expected values of certain events. Before we do that we will explore the temporal-difference learning algorithm itself, using the simple gridworld. By way of building up to temporal-difference learning, we will first explore two other methods for learning expected values. These methods assume more processing power than temporal-difference learning but they help to illustrate how temporal-difference learning actually works. The first two methods we will explore are called iterative dynamic programming and least-mean-squares learning. (Sections 11.1, 11.2, and 11.3 are adapted from Russell and Norvig 1995; see also Sutton and Barto 1998 for a more in-depth treatment of these methods.)

11.1 Learning State Values Using Iterative Dynamic Programming

Dynamic programming is a collection of methods for solving systems of equations like that implied by Equation 11.1 (Bellman 1957). Iterative dynamic programming is an iterative version of Equation 11.1. It is a rapid and effective way to learn expected state values, but it requires knowledge of the state transition probabilities. In principle, and if the agent had enough memory, it could record the states and the transitions between them as it moved randomly through the gridworld over many epochs, and could accurately estimate the transition probabilities based on the number of times it makes each transition. It could then use these (presumably accurate) transition probability estimates to iteratively estimate state values according to Equation 11.2:

$$v_j(c_j + 1) = r_j + \sum_i p_{ij} v_i(c_i) \qquad \textbf{11.2}$$

where c_i and c_j count the updates to the estimated values of states i and j, respectively (each value estimate has its own counter). Both i and j can index the states from 1 to n where $n = 12$ for the simple gridworld (see Figure 11.2). Using Equation 11.2 the estimated value v_j of state j can change with each update. Note that the term $v_i(c_i)$ stands for the estimated value of state i after it has been updated c_i times. Similarly, the term $v_j(c_j + 1)$ stands for the estimated value of state j for update $c_j + 1$. In general, terms of the form $v_i(c_i)$ and $v_j(c_j + 1)$ simply mean that the value estimates are functions of the updates. The update counts themselves are not used in the formula for iterative dynamic programming, but they are used explicitly in the formulas for the other forms of learning we will consider in this chapter. According to Equation 11.2, when the agent transitions to a state, it updates its estimate of the value of that state by weighting the value estimates of all its successor states by the probability of transition to each state, and then it sums them up. Recall that in our simple gridworld the probabilities of transition from state j to all allowed states i (p_{ij}) are equal to each other. (This is not the case in general.) To complete the update the learning agent adds any reinforcement received in that state.

To take a simple numerical example, suppose the agent arrives in state 2, and its current value estimate for that state is $v_2(c_2) = 0.1$. Reinforcement in state 2 is $r_2 = 0$. Its allowed successor states are 1 and 3 (see Figures 11.1 and 11.2). Suppose that the current value estimates of states 1 and 3 are $v_1(c_1) = -0.2$ and $v_3(c_3) = -0.4$. The probabilities of transitioning to them are both 1/2. The successor state probabilities are designated as p_{12} and p_{32}, where p_{12} is the probability of transitioning to state 1 from state 2, while p_{32} is the probability of transitioning to state 3 from state 2. Then, by Equation 11.2, the agent's updated value estimate for state 2 would be $v_2(c_2 + 1) = r_2 + p_{12}v_1(c_1) + p_{32}v_3(c_3) = 0 + (1/2)(-0.2) + (1/2)(-0.4) = -0.3$.

Iterative dynamic programming involves repeated application of Equation 11.2 as the agent undergoes further transitions, through multiple epochs, and updates its state value estimate on each transition. The estimates will converge to the exact state values, given the exact transition probabilities. To demonstrate this, we will use the iterative-dynamic-programming method to learn the values of the states in the gridworld (see Figures 11.1 and 11.2). This method is implemented by script `iterativeDynamicProg`, which is listed in MATLAB Box 11.2. We will assume that the agent has already experienced many state sequences and has accurately estimated the transition probabilities. Because the script will use transition matrix `TM` and reinforcement vector `r`, it will be necessary to run script `gridworldSetUp` before running `iterativeDynamicProg`. Although `gridworldSetUp` offers the option of assigning reinforcement to a non-termi-

MATLAB® BOX 11.2 This script updates state value estimates for the stochastic gridworld using iterative dynamic programming.

```
% iterativeDynamicProg.m
% script gridWorldSetUp must be run first

nEpo=100; % set number of epochs

v=zeros(nStates,1); % define estimated state value vector
v(tsr)=r(tsr); v(tsp)=r(tsp); % set terminal state values
vEst=zeros(ceil(nEpo/10+1),nStates); % define value hold array
rms=zeros(ceil(nEpo/10+1),1); % define RMS error hold array
vEst(1,:)=v'; % save initial state values
rms(1)=sqrt(mean((exVals-v).^2)); % save initial RMS error

for epo=1:nEpo, % do for all epochs
    tsf=0; % zero terminal state flag
    st=1; % start epoch at state one
    while tsf==0, % while terminal state flag equals zero
        indx=find(TM(:,st)~=0); % find indices of allowed next states
        prob=1/sum(TM(:,st)); % prob of transitions to each next state
        v(st)=r(st)+sum(prob*v(indx)); % update state value
        nIndx=length(indx); % find the number of allowed next states
        choose=ceil(rand*nIndx); % choose an index at random
        nextSt=indx(choose); % choose the next state at random
        if nextSt==tsr | nextSt==tsp, tsf=1; end % check if terminal
        st=nextSt; % set current state to next state
    end % end of while loop, end of one epoch

    if rem(epo,10)==0, % every ten epochs
        vEst(epo/10+1,:)=v'; % save value estimates
        rms(epo/10+1)=sqrt(mean((exVals-v).^2)); % save rms error
    end % end conditional
end % end of nEpo epochs
```

nal state, we will forgo this option for these simulations and assign reinforcement only to the terminal states (but see Exercise 11.1).

The script `iterativeDynamicProg` begins by setting the estimated values of all non-terminal states in vector v to 0, but it directly assigns the values of the terminal states to their reinforcements. Recall that transitions from terminal states are not allowed, so that the probability p_{ij} of transitioning to any state i from either terminal state j ($j = 8$ or $j = 12$) is 0. For the terminal states, where all the $p_{ij} = 0$, Equation 11.2 specifies that the state value v_j is simply equal to its reinforcement r_j. Thus, for efficiency, the script assigns the values of the terminal states to their reinforcements at the beginning, rather than reassign them every time using Equation 11.2. It makes these terminal state value assignments using `v(tsr)=r(tsr)` and `v(tsp)=r(tsp)`. Not updating the values of the terminal states, which are simply equal to their known reinforcements, affords several other programming simplifications. For this reason we will also directly assign the values of the terminal states to their reinforcements at the beginning of the scripts that implement least-mean-squares and temporal-difference learning (see Sections 11.2 and 11.3). Script `iterativeDynamicProg` allows the agent to undergo random state transitions over many epochs, and it applies Equation 11.2 in each new (non-terminal) state to iteratively compute its value.

To make a transition from state `st` in the gridworld, the script first finds the indices of all allowed successor states and stores them in vector `indx` using the command `indx=find(TM(:,st)~=0)`. It finds the length (number of elements) of this vector using `nIndx=length(indx)`, and it draws a random number from 1 to the number of allowed successor states using `choose=ceil(rand*nIndx)`. Because transitions to all allowed successor states are equally probable in this simple gridworld, the script chooses the next state simply using `nextSt=indx(choose)`. This method of making state transitions is also employed by the least-mean-squares and temporal-difference learning procedures we will study in Sections 11.2 and 11.3.

To apply Equation 11.2 to estimate the value of any current state `v(st)`, the script computes the transition probability `prob` for all allowed transitions from state `st` using the transition matrix `TM` and the command `prob=1/sum(TM(:,st))`. It then weights the value estimates of its possible successor states `v(indx)` by `prob` and sums them up. It completes the update of the value estimate for the current state by adding this sum to any reinforcement associated with the current state. The full update command is `v(st)=r(st)+sum(prob*v(indx))`. Note that in these simulations all non-terminal states have zero reinforcement, but vector `r` has one element for each state and could be used to hold non-terminal state reinforcements if desired. Note also that the script uses `st` and `nextSt`, rather than j and i, to designate the current state and the next state, because these variable names facilitate the readability of the code. After making an update to the current state `st`, the script allows the agent to undergo a random transition to the next state `nextSt` and the process is repeated.

Initially, the learning agent will have nonzero value estimates only for the terminal states, because they are the only ones that have nonzero reinforcement. The first time that the iterative-dynamic-programming agent arrives at a next-to-terminal state, it can assign a nonzero value estimate to it, because it can use the nonzero value of the terminal state in its computation. On subsequent epochs, the agent can update the estimates of states at further remove from the terminal states, because it can use its nonzero estimates of the values of the states bordering the terminal states in its computations. In this way, the value estimates made by the agent gradually spread backward from the terminal states. This idea of spreading backward from reinforcement signals is central to the temporal-difference learning paradigm.

To see this spreading backward, run `iterativeDynamicProg` for only one epoch (set `nEpo=1`). If the sequence by chance was short, then you will observe that some of the estimated state values are still 0. A representative example of a first epoch of iterative dynamic programming is shown in Figure 11.3. In this figure the elements of the vector `v`, which the agent uses to hold its estimates of the state values, are entered into a replica of the gridworld for ease of illustration.

Initially, all but the terminal states have value estimates of 0. When the agent arrives at a state that does not boarder a terminal state, it finds value estimates of 0 in all subsequent states. In this case the iterative-dynamic-programming algorithm would assign an update of 0 to the current state (see Equation 11.2). When the agent first arrives at a state that immediately precedes a terminal state, the iterative-dynamic-programming algorithm can produce a nonzero update for that state because it has a nonzero value estimate for one of its successor states (i.e., the reinforcement assigned to the terminal state). On the sequence shown in Figure 11.3, the agent visited states adjacent to the punishment state and was able to update its value estimates for those

FIGURE 11.3 **Estimated state values for the gridworld after one epoch of iterative dynamic programming** On this epoch, the agent visited states near the punishment state and was able to make nonzero updates to the estimated values of those states.

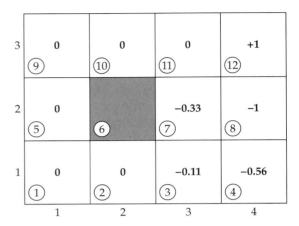

states. On subsequent epochs the algorithm will be able to update its value estimates for states at further remove from the terminal states, because it will now have nonzero value estimates for the states adjacent to the terminal states. In this way, nonzero value estimates spread backward from terminal states to preceding states.

Many updates are required for the iterative-dynamic-programming agent to determine precise state value estimates. To see this, we will allow the iterative-dynamic-programming agent to learn for 100 epochs (set `nEpo=100`). After every ten epochs, the script will save the state value estimates in array `vEst`, and save the root-mean-square differences between the estimated and exact state values in vector `rms`. The state value estimates and the root-mean-square errors over the 100 epochs, or training sequences through the stochastic grid-world, using iterative dynamic programming are shown in Figure 11.4. The final state value estimates are compared with the exact values in Table 11.1. Because the state transition probabilities are known, the iterative-dynamic-programming algorithm works fast. The figure shows that the estimated state values converge to the exact values in less than 50 epochs. Other methods for estimating state values can operate without knowing the state transition

FIGURE 11.4 **Estimated state values and root-mean-square error over 100 epochs of iterative dynamic programming in the gridworld** (A) The state values estimated by iterative dynamic programming are shown as solid curves, while the exact state values are shown as dashed lines. (B) The root-mean-square (RMS) error. Results are reported after every ten epochs.

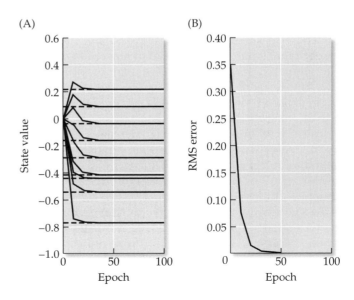

TABLE 11.1 Exact gridworld state values compared with values estimated following 100 epochs of iterative dynamic programming

State number	Exact value	Estimated value
1	−0.29	−0.29
2	−0.42	−0.42
3	−0.54	−0.54
4	−0.77	−0.77
5	−0.16	−0.16
6	0.00	0.00
7	−0.44	−0.44
8	−1.00	−1.00
9	−0.04	−0.04
10	+0.09	+0.09
11	+0.22	+0.22
12	+1.00	+1.00

State 6 is a disallowed state, and states 8 and 12 are terminal states of punishment and reward, respectively. Estimated state values match the exact values.

probabilities, but they are slower and less accurate than iterative dynamic programming, as we will see.

11.2 Learning State Values Using Least Mean Squares

In actually using the iterative-dynamic-programming algorithm from scratch, many state sequences would be required before the agent could obtain accurate estimates for the state transition probabilities, and these estimates would be needed before the algorithm could start updating its state value estimates. The least-mean-squares method provides an alternative that allows a learning agent to update its state value estimates without knowing the state transition probabilities. Basically, the least-mean-squares algorithm works by taking whole state sequences from (or trajectories through) the environment. Note that a sequence is an ordered list of states, while a trajectory is an actual path through the gridworld, but we can use "sequence" and " trajectory" synonymously. The least-mean-squares algorithm assumes that the agent can remember all of the states that it has passed through on a given trajectory. It also assumes that it can keep a tally, over all subsequent sequences, of the number of times it has visited each state.

Remember that the exact value of a state is the reinforcement we can expect to receive in proceeding from that state. The least-mean-squares algorithm essentially estimates a state value by averaging the reinforcements that were received, over a number of trajectories, each time the agent passes through that state. In general, reinforcement can be received in any state but, for the examples we consider, reinforcement is received only in the terminal states, and this simplifies the calculations. For example, imagine that the agent completes two sequences. On the first sequence it passes through state 2 once, and the sequence terminates with reinforcement +1. On the second sequence it passes through state 2 twice, and the sequence terminates with reinforcement −1. The least-mean-squares method would then estimate the value of state 2 as $(+1-1-1)/3$ or −0.3.

Rather than wait until all sequences are over, the least-mean-squares algorithm can update its state value estimates after each sequence by computing a running average. In general, if some average value $v(n)$ has currently been computed over n observations, and we obtain a new observation o, then the new average value $v(n + 1)$ can be computed using Equation 11.3:

$$v(n+1) = v(n) + \frac{o - v(n)}{n+1}$$ **11.3**

where, in the second term on the right, the difference $[o - v(n)]$ is divided by the current number of observations plus 1 $(n + 1)$. The running average is interesting in its own right, and we will consider it further as a simple example of a predictor-corrector model in the next chapter. Here we note the equivalence between the running average and the least-mean-squares learning method.

The least-mean-squares algorithm works with a quantity called reinforcement to go (r_{tg}), which is the reinforcement left to be obtained in progressing from the current state to the terminal state in a sequence. In the simple gridworld we consider, r_{tg} is always just the reward of +1 or the punishment of –1 that is received in the terminal state of each sequence. In the context of the least-mean-squares algorithm, the running average equation is applied as shown in Equation 11.4:

$$v_j(c_j + 1) = v_j(c_j) + \frac{r_{tg} - v_j(c_j)}{c_j + 1}$$ **11.4**

where the counter c_j counts the updates to the value estimate for state j. Note that, in the second term on the right, the difference $[r_{tg} - v_j(c_j)]$ is divided by the number of times v_j has already been updated, plus 1 $(c_j + 1)$. Equation 11.4 shows that, for the least–mean-squares algorithm, it is necessary to keep track of the number of times each state value estimate has been updated. The reward-to-go r_{tg} in Equation 11.4 is analogous to the observation o in Equation 11.3, and comparison between Equations 11.3 and 11.4 makes clear that the least-mean-squares algorithm basically estimates the value v_j of each state as a running average of r_{tg}. In this way, the least-mean-squares algorithm can estimate state values without knowing the state transition probabilities. The algorithm will converge to the correct state values after many training epochs (see Sutton and Barto 1998 for details).

To take a simple numerical example (in numbers rounded to the nearest tenth), suppose that the agent arrives in state 2, and its current value estimate for state 2 is $v_2(c_2) = -0.1$ but its reinforcement is 0. Suppose its current trajectory ends in the punishment state with reinforcement –1. Because all non-terminal reinforcements are 0 in our example, r_{tg} is just –1. Suppose that the agent has already visited this state 9 times, so $c_2 = 9$. Then, by Equation 11.4, its updated state value estimate is $v_2(c_2 + 1) = v_2(c_2) + [r_{tg} - v_2(c_2)] / (c_2 + 1) = -0.1 + [-1 - (-0.1)] / (9 + 1)$ $= -0.2$. The least-mean-squares method involves repeated applications of Equation 11.4, as the agent undergoes many epochs and updates its estimated values for all the states visited on each trajectory. The estimates should come reasonably close to the exact state values, given sufficiently many epochs.

To demonstrate this, we will use the least-mean-squares algorithm to estimate the values of the states in the simple, stochastic gridworld. The script `leastMeanSquares`, listed in MATLAB Box 11.3, will implement this method. (Note that `gridworldSetUp` must be run first.) Although we consider reinforcement only in terminal states, the script can manage reinforcement in a non-terminal state also. To do this, the script generates and saves a state sequence (trajectory) `trj` and then flips it using `trj=fliplr(trj)`, so that the terminal state is first and the start state is last. It sets the reinforcement received in the terminal state (`tsr` or `tsp`), and also sets the reinforcement for non-terminal

MATLAB® BOX 11.3   This script updates state value estimates for the stochastic gridworld using least-mean-squares learning.

```
% leastMeanSquares.m
% script gridWorldSetUp must be run first

nEpo=1000; % set number of epochs

v=zeros(nStates,1); % define estimated state value vector
v(tsr)=r(tsr); v(tsp)=r(tsp); % set terminal state values
count=zeros(nStates,1); % define update count holding vector
vEst=zeros(ceil(nEpo/10+1),nStates); % define value hold array
rms=zeros(ceil(nEpo/10+1),1); % define RMS error hold array
vEst(1,:)=v'; % save initial state values
rms(1)=sqrt(mean((exVals-v).^2)); % save initial RMS error

for epo=1:nEpo, % do for all epochs
    tsf=0; % zero terminal state flag
    st=1; % start epoch at state one
    trj=st; % set the first state of the trajectory
    while tsf==0, % while terminal state flag equals zero
        indx=find(TM(:,st)~=0); % find indices of allowed next states
        nIndx=length(indx); % find the number of allowed next states
        choose=ceil(rand*nIndx); % choose an index at random
        nextSt=indx(choose); % choose the next state at random
        if nextSt==tsr | nextSt==tsp, tsf=1; end % check if terminal
        st=nextSt; % set current state to next state
        trj=[trj st]; % add new state to the state trajectory
    end % end of trajectory
    lTrj=length(trj); % find the length (in states) of trajectory
    rTrj=zeros(lTrj,1); % set up the reinforcement trajectory
    trj=fliplr(trj); % reverse the order of the state trajectory
    if trj(1)==tsr, rTrj(1)=r(tsr); % set end-state reward ...
    elseif trj(1)==tsp, rTrj(1)=r(tsp); end % or punishment
    rTrj(find(trj==intReSt))=r(intReSt); % intermediate reinforcement
    rtg=0; % zero the reward-to-go
    for tr=1:lTrj, % for each transition on (reversed) trajectory
        rtg=rtg+rTrj(tr); % increment the reward to go
        v(trj(tr))=v(trj(tr))+... % update the state values ...
            (rtg-v(trj(tr)))/(count(trj(tr))+1); % via LMS
        count(trj(tr))=count(trj(tr))+1; % increment the counter
    end % end trajectory update loop
    if rem(epo,10)==0, % every ten epochs
        vEst(epo/10+1,:)=v'; % save value estimates
        rms(epo/10+1)=sqrt(mean((exVals-v).^2)); % save rms error
    end % end conditional
end % end of nEpo epochs
```

state intReSt (if non-terminal reinforcement was set in gridworldSetUp), and holds these in vector rTrj of reinforcements for each state on the trajectory. It then updates r_{tg} using rtg=rtg+rTrj(tr) for every transition tr as it progresses through the reversed sequence, so that r_{tg} reflects the reinforcement left to go from any point along the sequence. Because reinforcement in general can be received in any state, the least-mean-squares learning method involves trajectory reversal.

FIGURE 11.5   Estimated state values for the gridworld after one epoch of least-mean-squares learning On this epoch the agent visited states along trajectory (1) (2) (3) (7) (8), ending in the punishment state, and made nonzero updates to the estimated values of all states along the trajectory.

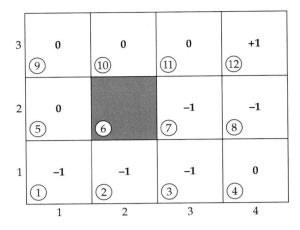

The script updates the estimate of the value of each state it encounters as it progresses through the reversed trajectory by implementing Equation 11.4 using the command `v(trj(tr))=v(trj(tr))+(rtg-v(trj(tr)))/(count(trj(tr))+1)`. Note that the term `trj(tr)` is the state along trajectory `trj` at transition `tr`. These more descriptive variable names are used in place of *j* to facilitate the readability of the code. The script also increments the update counter for each state value each time it encounters the state along the reversed trajectory using `count(trj(tr))=count(trj(tr))+1`. For consistency with the other scripts `leastMeanSquares` also directly assigns the values of the terminal states to their reinforcements, but this is not necessary when using the least-mean-squares algorithm because Equation 11.4 automatically makes these assignments the first time it updates each terminal state. (Note that the update counter for all states is zero on their first update.) To examine the behavior of the least-mean-squares algorithm, we will first apply it on a single training epoch (set `nEpo=1`).

The state values estimated using least-mean-squares after a single epoch are shown in Figure 11.5. On this particular (short) trajectory, the learning agent went along the bottom row from the start state, then up to the second row, and then over to the terminal state of punishment. This trajectory is a bit unusual in that no state was visited more than once. (Bouncing back and forth between states happens often in this stochastic gridworld.) The algorithm has assigned nonzero value estimates to all the states visited in this single sequence. This illustrates that the least-mean-squares method can make nonzero updates to the value estimates of all the states encountered along a trajectory, even when the only nonzero value available to the algorithm is the reinforcement belonging to a terminal state. States not visited in this single sequence still have estimated values of 0. The r_{tg} was −1 for every state along the trajectory, so the least-mean-squares formula (see Equation 11.4) stipulates that each state visited along this trajectory should have a state value estimate of −1.

All the state value estimates approach their exact values as more state sequences are generated and the least-mean-squares algorithm is able to compute more accurate estimates of the reinforcement to be expected in proceeding from each state in the gridworld. Figure 11.6 shows the state value estimates, and the root-mean-square error between the exact and estimated state values, after 1000 epochs (`nEpo=1000`) using the least-mean-squares algorithm. The figure shows that the state value estimates have roughly converged to the exact values. Variability in the state value estimates is due to the stochastic nature of the sequences that the least-mean-squares algorithm must relay on in order to learn from experience in the gridworld. The final state values estimated after 1000 epochs of least–mean-squares learning are

(A)

(B)

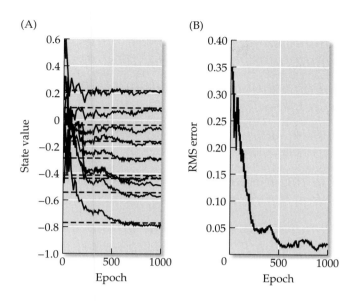

FIGURE 11.6 **Estimated state values and root-mean-square error over 1000 epochs of least-mean-squares learning in the gridworld** (A) The state values estimated by least-mean-squares learning are shown as solid curves, while the exact state values are shown as dashed lines. (B) The root-mean-square (RMS) error. Results are reported after every ten epochs.

compared with the exact state values in Table 11.2. Due to the stochastic nature of the gridworld, the results you obtain on any particular run of least-mean-squares learning are likely to differ from the results reported in Table 11.2 and Figure 11.6, but these results are representative.

11.3 Learning State Values Using the Method of Temporal Differences

Compared with least-mean-squares learning and iterative dynamic programming, the temporal-difference method has the least demanding requirements. The least-mean-squares algorithm can provide reasonable estimates of state values, but it cannot update a state value until after the sequence containing the state has terminated. Least-mean-squares also requires that the entire tra-

TABLE 11.2 **Exact gridworld state values compared with values estimated following 1000 epochs of least-mean-squares learning**

State number	Exact value	Estimated value
1	−0.29	−0.30
2	−0.42	−0.43
3	−0.54	−0.57
4	−0.77	−0.79
5	−0.16	−0.18
6	0.00	0.00
7	−0.44	−0.49
8	−1.00	−1.00
9	−0.04	−0.07
10	+0.09	+0.07
11	+0.22	+0.20
12	+1.00	+1.00

State 6 is a disallowed state, and states 8 and 12 are terminal states of punishment and reward, respectively. Estimated state values are in good agreement with exact values.

jectory (state sequence) be made available in memory. The iterative-dynamic-programming algorithm can update a state value estimate immediately, but it requires the value estimates of all possible successor states, and accurate estimates of their transition probabilities. When these requirements cannot be met, state value estimates can still be updated immediately using the method of temporal differences (Sutton and Barto 1998).

The temporal-difference method updates the estimated value of a state after the agent has transitioned to the next state in the sequence. Thus the temporal-difference algorithm does not update the value v_i of the state i it is currently in. Instead it updates the value v_j of the state j from which it has just transitioned. The update to v_j is based on the reinforcement r_j associated with the previous state j, if any, and on the estimated values of both the previous state v_j and the current state v_i. It works on the principle that the value of a state should reflect the values of its successor states, because they lie between that state and reinforcement. For example, if state j currently has a value estimate of –0.5, then the expected reinforcement of a trajectory through state j is negative. But suppose that state j transitions to state i with a value estimate of +0.5, which indicates a positive expected reinforcement. It would seem that the value of state j has been underestimated and should be increased. The temporal-difference algorithm will make state value updates based on the difference between the estimated values of a state and the next state in a sequence.

The temporal-difference algorithm essentially solves the dynamic programming problem through updates on each state transition, but without knowing the state transition probabilities, by trying to match the value estimate of each state to that of its successor. The basic temporal-difference update rule is shown in Equation 11.5:

$$v_j(c_j + 1) = v_j(c_j) + a\left[r_j + v_i(c_i) - v_j(c_j)\right] \qquad \textbf{11.5}$$

where c_j counts the updates to v_j and c_i counts the updates to v_i. The heart of the temporal-difference algorithm lies in computing the difference between the estimated values v_j and v_i, which are those for the state and for its immediate successor in the sequence. Another way to understand temporal-difference learning is to view the term $r_j + v_i$, which is the sum of the reinforcement r_j (if any) associated with state j and the value v_i of the successor state i, as the "target" value that the algorithm "tracks" as it updates value estimate v_j. (This target tracking idea is discussed in Section 1.5.) Note that temporal-difference updates are 0 when a state value equals its target value ($v_j = r_j + v_i$). The last term in brackets in Equation 11.5, which is $[r_j + v_i - v_j]$ (we have omitted the update count variables for clarity), is the temporal-difference error, or prediction error, that will figure prominently in the model of the behavior of neurons in the midbrain that we will consider in Section 11.4. The temporal-difference error $[r_j + v_i - v_j]$ is scaled by learning rate a and added to the current state estimate v_j to yield the updated estimate.

To take a numerical example (in numbers rounded to the nearest tenth), suppose that the agent arrives in state 2, and its current value estimate $v_2(c_2)$ for state 2 is –0.1. The reinforcement r_2 associated with state 2 is 0. Now suppose the agent transitions from state 2 to state 3, and its value estimate $v_3(c_3)$ for state 3 is –0.9. Assume that both states have already been updated 5 times, and that the learning rate a is 0.1. By Equation 11.5, the temporal-difference update would be: $v_2(c_2 + 1) = v_2(c_2) + a[r_2 + v_3(c_3) - v_2(c_2)] = (-0.1) + 0.1[0 + (-0.9) - (-0.1)] = -0.2$. For this update we have ignored the number of times each state value estimate has been updated. To improve the performance of the temporal-difference algorithm, we can use the update count for each state value estimate to reduce its learning rate as its number of updates increases.

MATLAB® BOX 11.4   This script updates state value estimates for the stochastic gridworld using temporal-difference learning.

```
% temporalDifference.m
% script gridWorldSetUp must be run first

nEpo=1000; % set number of epochs
a=0.1; % set learning rate
dec=0.999; % set learning rate decrement

v=zeros(nStates,1); % define estimated state value vector
v(tsr)=r(tsr); v(tsp)=r(tsp); % set terminal state values
count=zeros(nStates,1); % define update count holding vector
vEst=zeros(ceil(nEpo/10+1),nStates); % define value hold array
rms=zeros(ceil(nEpo/10+1),1); % define RMS error hold array
vEst(1,:)=v'; % save initial state values
rms(1)=sqrt(mean((exVals-v).^2)); % save initial RMS error

for epo=1:nEpo, % do for all epochs
    tsf=0; % zero terminal state flag
    st=1; % start epoch at state one
    while tsf==0, % while terminal state flag equals zero
        count(st)=count(st)+1; % increment counter
        indx=find(TM(:,st)~=0); % find indices of allowed next states
        nIndx=length(indx); % find the number of allowed next states
        choose=ceil(rand*nIndx); % choose an index at random
        nextSt=indx(choose); % choose the next state at random
        v(st)=v(st)+(a*dec^count(st))*... % update value of ...
            (r(st)+v(nextSt)-v(st)); % current state using TD
        if nextSt==tsr | nextSt==tsp, tsf=1; end % check if terminal
        st=nextSt; % set current state to next state
    end % end of while loop, end of one epoch

    if rem(epo,10)==0, % every ten epochs
        vEst(epo/10+1,:)=v'; % save value estimates
        rms(epo/10+1)=sqrt(mean((exVals-v).^2)); % save rms error
    end % end conditional
end % end of nEpo epochs
```

It is clear that, in the absence of reinforcing events, the temporal-difference update rule will cause the estimated state values to be closer to those of their successors. Thus, in temporal-difference learning, each state value estimate tracks the value estimates for the successor states. In a sense, the temporal-difference algorithm combines the best of the iterative-dynamic-programming and least-mean-squares algorithms. It can update the value of a state immediately (without storing the sequence and waiting for the end of the trajectory as in least-mean-squares learning), yet it does not require that the transition probabilities be known (as in iterative dynamic programming). There are many variations on the temporal-difference theme expressed in Equation 11.5, but even the basic temporal-difference algorithm will produce average state value estimates that will converge to the exact values (for details see Sutton and Barto 1998).

To demonstrate this, we will use the temporal-difference algorithm to estimate the values of the states in the stochastic gridworld. The script temporalDifference, listed in MATLAB Box 11.4, will implement this

FIGURE 11.7   Estimated state values for the gridworld after one epoch of temporal-difference learning The trajectory ended with a transition from state (11) to the terminal reward state (12). Only the estimated value of the one, immediately pre-terminal state received a nonzero update.

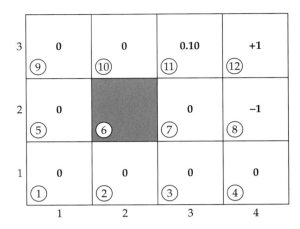

algorithm. (Note that `gridworldSetUp` must be run first.) Although we consider reinforcement only in terminal states, the script can manage reinforcement received in non-terminal states also. Because a terminal state has no successor state, by definition, its value is simply its reinforcement, and we could actually use Equation 11.5 to learn the values of the terminal states. To do this for the terminal states we could set the values of their nonexistent successor states v_i to 0 in Equation 11.5. Then the target value that the algorithm would track in updating either terminal state value v_j ($j = 8$ or $j = 12$) would be ($r_j - v_j$), which is just the difference between the current value estimate for the terminal state and its reinforcement. By this procedure the terminal state values could gradually be learned, according to learning rata a, but this is inefficient. As in the previous two scripts, `temporalDifference` sets the values of the terminal states to their respective reinforcements, rather than updating them from scratch.

The temporal-difference algorithm, based on Equation 11.5, updates a state value estimate each time it makes a state transition. In this sense it is more like iterative dynamic programming than least-mean-squares. After each transition to a new state `nextSt`, script `temporalDifference` updates the learning agent's value estimate for the previous state `v(st)` using the command `v(st)=v(st)+ (a*dec^count(st))*(r(st)+v(nextSt)-v(st))`, where `st` is the index of the state being updated, `a` is the learning rate, and `dec` is a decrement factor close to 1. (Again we use `nextSt` and `st` rather than i and j for readability.) The script keeps track of the number of times the agent's value estimate for each state has been updated, and it uses this count to reduce the learning rate on each update using the sub-command `a*dec^count(st)`, where `count` is the vector of counts.

The temporal-difference algorithm works backward from reinforcing events through successor states to influence the value estimates for previous states. To see this, run the script `temporalDifference` for one epoch (set `nEpo=1`). The state values estimated by the temporal-difference algorithm after one trajectory through the gridworld are shown in Figure 11.7. Note that only one non-terminal state has been assigned a nonzero value estimate. This non-terminal state is the one immediately preceding the reward state, which was the terminal state reached on this single trajectory. The temporal-difference algorithm made a nonzero update to the agent's value estimate for this state only, because it was the only state during this single epoch that had a successor with a nonzero value.

The basic temporal-difference algorithm (see Equation 11.5) computes an update to a state value estimate based only on the reinforcement associated with

(A)

(B)

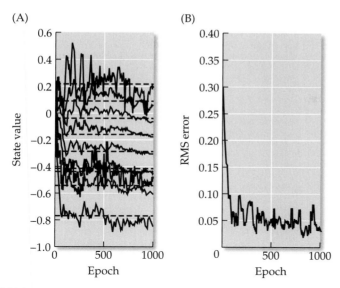

FIGURE 11.8   **Estimated state values and root-mean-square error over 1000 epochs of temporal-difference learning in the gridworld** (A) The state values estimated by temporal-difference learning are shown as solid curves, while the exact state values are shown as dashed lines. (B) The root-mean-square (RMS) error. Results are reported after every ten epochs.

that state (if any) and its estimated value for the actual successor of that state in a sequence. In contrast, the iterative-dynamic-programming algorithm updates a state value estimate on the basis of its value estimates for all allowable successor states. The least-mean-squares algorithm updates its value estimates for all states in a sequence based on the reward-to-go of that sequence. Thus, the iterative-dynamic-programming and least-mean-squares algorithms will generally update their value estimates for more states on the first epoch than will the basic temporal-difference algorithm. (Versions of temporal-difference learning will update their value estimates for a series of previous states; for details see Sutton and Barto 1998.) Of the three, the basic temporal-difference algorithm represents the most restrictive form of learning backward from a reinforcement event, but it is also the least computationally complex, because it requires neither knowledge of the transition probabilities nor storage of entire state sequences. These properties of temporal-difference learning have made it attractive as a model of learning in certain regions of the brain (see next section).

The state value estimates and the root-mean-square differences between the estimated and the exact values for the states over 1000 epochs (nEpo=1000) of temporal-difference learning are shown in Figure 11.8, and the final state value estimates are compared with the exact values in Table 11.3. As for the least-mean-squares algorithm, state value estimates for the temporal-difference algorithm also roughly converge to the exact values after 1000 epochs. The curves look a bit more ragged for temporal difference than for least-mean-squares, but the state value estimates reached and the time course of learning are about the same for both. In any case, what has made the temporal-difference learning algorithm an appropriate tool for building neural systems models is not its accuracy as compared with iterative dynamic programming or the least-mean-squares algorithm. Instead, the low computational complexity of temporal-difference learning facilitates its transfer from the general adaptive agent context to the neural network context. We will consider one such neural systems model in detail in the next section.

TABLE 11.3 Exact gridworld state values compared with values estimated following 1000 epochs of temporal-difference learning

State number	Exact value	Estimated value
1	−0.29	−0.31
2	−0.42	−0.45
3	−0.54	−0.62
4	−0.77	−0.86
5	−0.16	−0.18
6	0.00	0.00
7	−0.44	−0.47
8	−1.00	−1.00
9	−0.04	−0.06
10	+0.09	+0.05
11	+0.22	+0.25
12	+1.00	+1.00

State 6 is a disallowed state, and states 8 and 12 are terminal states of punishment and reward, respectively. Estimated state values are in good agreement with exact values.

11.4 Simulating Dopamine Neuron Responses Using Temporal-Difference Learning

Part of the inspiration for the development of the temporal-difference algorithm actually came from studies of animal learning (Sutton and Barto 1998). Fittingly, the temporal-difference algorithm is now used to simulate the responses of neurons in certain regions of the brain that may actually carry the temporal-difference learning signal. In the example in this section we will use the temporal-difference algorithm to train a neural network to associate a sensory cue with a reward that follows it in time. Changes in timing of the temporal-difference learning signal will be expressed as changes in timing of the responses of a model neuron, and these will correspond well with changes in timing of the responses of real neurons in the midbrain dopamine system. The simulations will provide insight into the behavior of dopamine neurons, which were revealed in experiments involving sensory cues and rewards. The results were surprising.

The midbrain dopamine system is schematized in Figure 11.9. Dopamine is a neurotransmitter that is associated with the "reward" system of the brain (Stahl 1996; Schultz 2007). Most of the neurons that synthesize and secrete dopamine are located in the midbrain (mesencephalon) and send projections to many cortical and sub-cortical regions throughout the brain that are involved, among other things, in determining and initiating behavior. Activation of the midbrain (mesencephalic) dopamine system seems to produce a sensation of pleasure. For example, experimental animals will voluntarily (and vigorously) perform actions that result in activation of this system (Olds and Milner 1954; Robbins and Everitt 2003; see Chapter 7 for further discussion). Also certain drugs of abuse, such as the amphetamines and cocaine, achieve their addictive effects by potentiating the midbrain dopamine system (Stahl 1996).

The receipt of a reward also activates the midbrain dopamine system, suggesting that the latter is what endows the former with its subjectively pleasurable qualities. The activation of a dopamine neuron upon receipt of a food reward is illustrated in Figure 11.10A. These data were obtained during a study of the

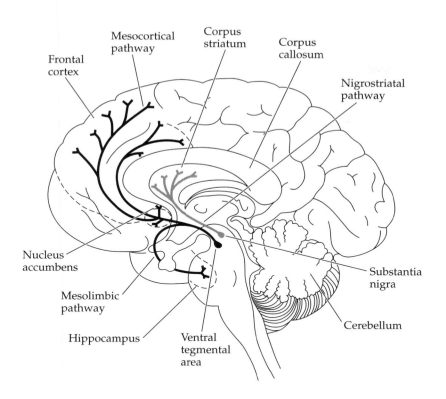

FIGURE 11.9 The midbrain dopamine pathways Each pathway is composed of dopamine-secreting neurons that originate either in the substantia nigra or the ventral tegmental area of the midbrain (mesencephalon), and project from there to various cortical or subcortical regions. The nigrostriatal dopamine pathway projects from the substantia nigra to the striatum and is involved in movement control. The mesolimbic dopamine pathway projects from the ventral tegmental area to the nucleus accumbens and hippocampus, while the mesocortical dopamine pathway projects from the ventral tegmental area to the limbic cortex. The mesolimbic and meso-cortical pathways are involved in reward processing.

relationship between the activity of dopamine neurons and arm movements in monkeys (Romo and Schultz 1993). The experimenters induced hungry monkeys to make arm movements by opening the door to a food box. As shown in Figure 11.10A, a dopamine neuron is activated when a monkey touches the food and thereby receives the reward. It is possible that activation of the dopamine neuron mediates the sensation of pleasure that the hungry monkey experiences upon grasping the food. It is also possible that the dopamine neuron is providing a signal indicating that reward has been received, and that the behavioral state in which the monkey is grasping food is a valuable state.

Serendipitously, it seems, these experiments led to the discovery that dopamine neurons carry what may be a temporal-difference learning signal. Over many trials, the response of the dopamine neuron transfers from the time of

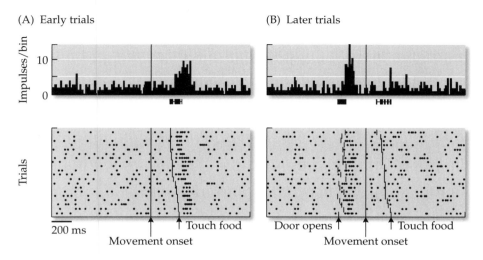

FIGURE 11.10 The activity of a midbrain dopamine neuron transfers from a reward to a cue that predicts the reward Each panel shows the discharge of a single dopamine neuron during many trials, both as rasters for each trial and as a histogram over all trials. On each trial, the door to a food box opens and a monkey reaches through the door for a food reward. Initially (A) the dopamine neuron is activated upon receipt of the reward. After many trials (B), the dopamine neuron is no longer activated by the reward but by the cue (door opens) that predicts the reward. (After Romo and Schultz 1990.)

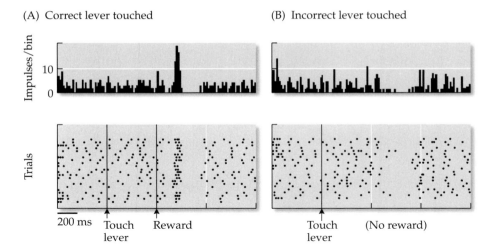

(A) Correct lever touched

(B) Incorrect lever touched

Impulses/bin — 10 — 0

Trials

200 ms   Touch lever   Reward   Touch lever   (No reward)

FIGURE 11.11   The activity of a midbrain dopamine neuron is enhanced if a reward is received, and is suppressed if an expected reward is not received
Each panel shows the discharge of a single dopamine neuron during many trials, both as rasters for each trial and as a histogram over all trials. On each trial, a monkey reaches toward one of two levers, and it receives a reward if it touches the correct lever, but receives nothing if it touches the incorrect lever. Early in training (A), the activity of the neuron is enhanced by receipt of the reward following correct responses. Following incorrect responses (B), the activity of the neuron is suppressed at the time at which a reward would have been received if a correct response had been made. (After Schultz et al. 1993.)

the reward to the time at which the door to the food box is opened (Figure 11.10B). This result was completely unexpected. One possible interpretation is that the dopamine neuron response has now shifted to provide a signal indicating that the cue that reliably predicts the reward is valuable. These observations were elaborated in further experiments (Schultz et al. 1993). For example, if the interval between the cue and the reward is variable, so that the cue unreliably predicts the reward, then the dopamine neuron response does not fully shift (transfer) from the reward to the cue but shows some response to both. Also, whether early or late in training (before or after transfer), the activity of the dopamine neuron is suppressed when an expected (predicted) reward is not received, as shown in Figure 11.11.

These phenomena are consistent with the hypothesis that midbrain dopamine neurons carry a temporal-difference learning signal. More specifically, they are consistent with the hypothesis that they carry the temporal-difference, or prediction, error signal. As we saw in the previous section, the temporal-difference algorithm estimates the values of the states in a sequence by minimizing the differences in its value estimates for successive states that lead to reinforcement. Thus, the state values predict the amount of reinforcement that ultimately will be received, and the temporal-difference learning signal essentially indicates the error in that prediction. For this reason the temporal-difference learning signal is often called a prediction error signal. The ability to predict the outcome of a sequence of states is of obvious importance to an animal. It is reasonable to suppose that there are some neurons in the brain that carry a prediction error signal, and midbrain dopamine neurons are likely candidates.

Dopamine neuron responses were simulated by Montague, Dayan, and Sejnowski (1996), using a neural network model that was configured specifically to implement temporal-difference learning. The model learns the value of a sensory cue that predicts a reward. One of the units in the network carries the prediction error signal, and the behavior of this model neuron is similar

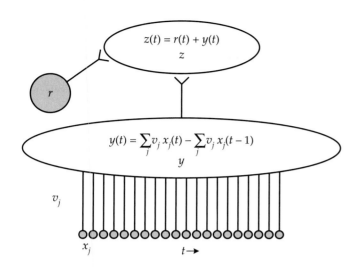

FIGURE 11.12   Temporal-difference learning implemented in a neural network model of the midbrain dopamine system The input units x_j project to the difference unit y over connections with weights (values) v_j ($j = 1,...,$ 20). The response of the difference unit $y(t)$ is the difference between its weighted input sums at times t and $t - 1$ (the equation shown within unit y is the same as Equation 11.6). The difference unit y and the reward unit r project to the prediction error unit z over connections that both have weight 1. The response of the prediction error unit $z(t)$ is the sum of its inputs from y and r at time t (the equation shown within unit z is the same as Equation 11.7). The prediction error unit z represents a dopamine neuron.

to that of real dopamine neurons. We will study a simplified version of this model, which is depicted in Figure 11.12.

The model will be trained for 200 trials, and each trial will consist of 50 time steps. A stimulus cue will come on at time step 10, and will be followed by reward at time step 30. The network has 20 binary input units x_j ($j = 1, ...,$ 20) that respond to the stimulus cue in an unusual way. When the cue comes on, it activates the first input unit. (Its response goes from 0 to 1.) At the next time step the cue goes off, and the response of the first input unit returns to 0, but the response of the second input unit goes to 1. At the next time step the second input unit goes off but the third comes on, and this continues for 17 more time steps, until all 20 input units have come on and gone off again. Each input unit x_j provides a weighted connection v_j to a differencing unit y. The differencing unit computes the weighted input sum on two consecutive time steps ($t - 1$ and t) and subtracts them as shown in Equation 11.6:

$$y(t) = \sum_j v_j \, x_j(t) - \sum_j v_j \, x_j(t - 1) \qquad \textbf{11.6}$$

Note that each input unit goes to 1 on only one time step during each trial, and stays at 0 for the other time steps. Thus, the weights v_j from inputs x_j to unit y can be interpreted as the values associated with the states in which each x_j is the only active input unit. In other words, the model represents the values of the states of the neural system in terms of the values of the connection weights v_j. Because of the binary and serially active nature of the input units, the weighted input sum at any time t reduces to the value of weight of the input unit that is active at that time.

The output of the differencing unit is sent to a unit z that adds a reinforcement signal r to the difference signal as described in Equation 11.7:

$$z(t) = r(t) + y(t) \qquad \textbf{11.7}$$

Output unit z carries the prediction error signal, which is also the temporal-difference learning signal. The z signal is used to update the weights according to the relationship shown in Equation 11.8:

$$v_j(c + 1) = v_j(c) + ax_j(t - 1, c)z(t, c) \qquad \textbf{11.8}$$

where a is the learning rate, c indexes the trials (update cycles), and t indexes the time steps within each trial. The unconventional mixing of update cycles c and time steps t in Equation 11.8 facilitates the description of learning in this model. Because this is a temporal-difference model, the value of a previous state is updated after the transition to the current state. In this model, the weight v_j of the input unit $x_j(t-1)$ that is active (state of 1) at time $t-1$ is updated by the prediction error signal $z(t)$ at time t. This implies that the learning system can "remember" which input unit was active at time $t-1$. Such "memory" by neurons or even by individual synapses is not implausible (see Chapter 14). The issue that concerns us here is that $z(t)$, which was computed in part from v_j and $x_j(t-1)$ (see Equations 11.6 and 11.7) obviously does not violate causality and go back in time to modify v_j during the same trial c. Instead, the $z(t, c)$ signal is computed according to the weight values $v_j(c)$ on current trial c, and the update (see Equation 11.8) is applied to weights $v_j(c)$ producing the updated weights $v_j(c+1)$, which are then used to compute a new $z(t, c+1)$ signal on trial $c+1$. The set of Equations 11.6, 11.7, and 11.8, with binary input unit activations as defined, is equivalent to Equation 11.5, which is the equation for temporal-difference learning.

The application of Equations 11.6–11.8 is illustrated using a simple numerical example in Table 11.4. Each sub-table corresponds to a different trial (as would be indexed by c). Assume that the network only has five input units, and that each trial comprises only seven time steps. The first column t lists the time steps, 0 through 6. The cue comes on at time step 1 and the reward is delivered at time step 6. The second column lists the index j of the input unit x_j that is active at the corresponding time, starting at time step 1, and the third column v_j lists the weights. The fourth column y is the output of the differencing unit, the fifth column r is the reinforcement (reward in this case), and the sixth column z is the prediction error signal. On the first trial (see Table 11.4A) all the weights v_j are 0, so the inputs to the differencing unit are all 0 and the responses of the differencing unit y are all 0 (see Equation 11.6). The temporal-difference learning signal z is the sum of the differencing unit responses y and the reward r (see Equation 11.7), so z takes value +1 on time step 6 (when the reward is received) and is 0 otherwise. Output unit x_5 was active (state 1) on time step 5, and this is one time step before that on which z takes its only nonzero value, so the weight v_5 of input x_5 receives a nonzero update (see Equation 11.8). We assume for simplicity in this numerical example that the learning rate a is 1, so that weight v_5 is updated to 1.

At the start of the second trial (see Table 11.4B), the value of v_5 is 1, but all other weights v_j are 0. The differencing unit y gets an input of 1 on time step 5, and 0 on all other time steps. Now the difference (the output of y) between the current and the previous inputs to y is +1 on time step 5, −1 on time step 6, and 0 on all other time steps. These responses of y have an interesting effect on the response of z, which is the sum of y and r. The z unit responds to its input from y of +1 on time step 5, but the −1 response of y on time step 6 cancels the reward r on time step 6, so the response of z to the reward vanishes. Thus, the response of the simulated dopamine neuron is already starting to transfer backward in the sequence from the reinforcing event. The z response of +1 on time step 5 then makes a nonzero update to 1 of the weight v_4 of input x_4.

By the sixth trial (see Table 11.4C), all of the weights v_j have been updated to 1. The response of the difference unit y is +1 on time step 1, −1 on time step 6, and 0 on all other time steps. The −1 response of y and the reward r of +1 on time step 6 again cancel each other, so the response of z to the reward is still 0. The z unit responds to y on time step 1, and the simulated dopamine neuron response has backed up all the way to the cue on time step 1. Since there are no other stimulus cues that precede this cue, the response of z to this cue will remain, but only as long as the reward remains.

In Table 11.4D the reward is removed. Now reward r of +1 on time step 6 is not available to cancel the −1 response of y on time step 6, and the response of z on time step 6 goes negative. This simulates the suppression of the responses of dopamine neurons when an expected (predicted) reward is not received.

TABLE 11.4   Some steps in the operation of a smaller version of the temporal-difference learning model of midbrain dopamine neurons

(A) First trial, dopamine unit responds to reward and updates the value of input 5

	Time step t	Index j of input x_j	Value or input weight v_j	Difference unit y	Reward unit r	Dopamine unit z
	0		0	0	0	0
Cue	1	1	0	0	0	0
	2	2	0	0	0	0
	3	3	0	0	0	0
	4	4	0	0	0	0
	5	5	0 (goes to 1)	0	0	0
Reward	6		0	0	+1	+1

(B) Second trial, dopamine unit responds to input 5 and updates the value of input 4

	t	j of x_j	v_j	y	r	z
	0		0	0	0	0
Cue	1	1	0	0	0	0
	2	2	0	0	0	0
	3	3	0	0	0	0
	4	4	0 (goes to 1)	0	0	0
	5	5	1	+1	0	+1
Reward	6		0	−1	+1	0

(C) Sixth trial, dopamine unit responds to input 1, all input values have been updated

	t	j of x_j	v_j	y	r	z
	0		0	0	0	0
Cue	1	1	1	+1	0	+1
	2	2	1	0	0	0
	3	3	1	0	0	0
	4	4	1	0	0	0
	5	5	1	0	0	0
Reward	6		0	−1	+1	0

(D) Remove reward, dopamine unit responds to input 1, but goes negative on time step 6

	t	j of x_j	v_j	y	r	z
	0		0	0	0	0
Cue	1	1	1	+1	0	+1
	2	2	1	0	0	0
	3	3	1	0	0	0
	4	4	1	0	0	0
	5	5	1	0	0	0
	6		0	−1	0	−1

This smaller version of the midbrain dopamine model has only five input units. *Abbreviations*: t, time step ($t = 0,\ldots, 6$); j, index of active input unit x_j ($j = 1,\ldots, 5$); v_j, value (or weight of connection from input unit x_j to the difference unit y); y, difference unit; r, reinforcement unit; z, prediction error (dopamine) unit (see also Figure 11.12).

The z response of −1 on time step 6 would make an update of −1 to the weight v_5 of input x_5 and set it to 0. In the continued absence of reward this negative prediction error signal would back up until all the weights v_j had been set to 0. Reinstatement of reward would restart the whole process.

The simple numerical example in Table 11.4 simulates some of the salient properties of midbrain dopamine neurons. It also captures the essential features of the neural network simulation (as we shall see), and suggests a vectorial approach for implementing temporal-difference learning in the model. Because the inputs are serially active in a strict sequence on each trial, all of the weights can be updated simultaneously. In other words, the responses of the differencing unit y and the prediction error unit z on each trial can be found for all time steps in one vectorial operation. In implementing the simulation it is only necessary to loop through the trials.

This vectorial approach is taken in script midbrainDopamine, which is listed in MATLAB Box 11.5. Each of the vector variables x, y, v, r, and z have one element for each of the 50 time steps (nTimes=50). The cue appears on time step 10 (qTime=10), so elements 10 through 29 of vector x take value 1, to represent the activity of the 20 input units as they come on and go off again over the course of the trial (temporal sequence). The other elements of x are 0. All elements of reinforcement vector r are 0 except for element 30, which takes value +1 to represent the reward that is (usually) provided at time step 30 (rTime=30). The reward is present on all 200 trials (nTrials=200) except trial 100 (nTrials/2). All the elements of weight (state value estimate) vector v are initially set to 0.

On each trial, the vector of weighted inputs to the y (differencing) unit are computed using v.*x, where the (.*) operator is element-by-element multiplication rather than the inner (dot) product. The vector of the actual responses of the differencing unit is computed using y=[0;diff(v.*x)]

MATLAB® BOX 11.5   This script simulates the responses of midbrain dopamine neurons using temporal-difference learning.

```
% midbrainDopamine.m

a=0.3; % set learning rate
nTrials=200; % set number of trials
nTimes=50; % set number of time steps per trial

x=zeros(nTimes,1); % define input unit vector
y=zeros(nTimes,1); % define difference unit vector
v=zeros(nTimes,1); % define weight (value estimate) vector
r=zeros(nTimes,1); % define reward vector
z=zeros(nTimes,1); % define prediction unit vector
Tcourse=zeros(nTrials,nTimes); % define time course hold array

qTime=10; % set time of cue
rTime=30; % set time of reward

x(qTime:rTime-1)=1; % set input responses

for c=1:nTrials, % for each learning trial
    r(rTime)=1; % set the reward at reward time
    if c==nTrials/2, r(rTime)=0; end % withhold reward once
    y=[0; diff(v.*x)]; % find the response of difference unit
    z=y+r; % find the response of prediction error unit
    v=v+a*x.*[z(2:nTimes);0]; % update the weights (values)
    Tcourse(c,:)=z'; % save the prediction unit time course
end % end learning trial loop
```

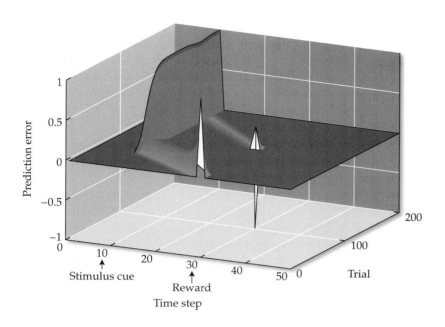

FIGURE 11.13   Simulating the responses of midbrain dopamine neurons using temporal-difference learning A stimulus cue occurs on time step 10 on all trials. A reward is presented on time step 30 on all trials except trial 100, on which the reward is withheld. The positive prediction error signal backs up from the reward to the stimulus cue. Absence of reward on trial 100 causes the prediction error signal to go negative. The prediction error signal simulates the responses of dopamine neurons.

where the `diff` command (function) computes the first difference of the elements in its vector argument. (The leading 0 is needed to ensure that `y` is `nTimes` elements long, because the vector produced by `diff` is one element shorter than its vector argument.) The response of the z (prediction error) unit is computed using `z=y+r`, and the weights are updated using the command `v=v+a*x.*[z(2:nTimes);0]`, where a is the learning rate, set to 0.3, and where vector z is shifted to line up with vector x at the previous time step. Vector z is saved after every trial in array `Tcourse`.

Figure 11.13 shows the response of output unit z on every time step for all 200 trials. The z unit carries the prediction error signal. On the first trial, the z unit responds only to the reinforcement (reward). The z unit response gradually transfers from the reward to the stimulus cue on subsequent trials, and has fully transferred to the cue after about 50 trials. Once it has transferred back from the reward, the full response to the stimulus cue requires several trials to build up, because the learning rate is less than 1. Reinforcement was withheld on trial 100, and the z unit response goes negative. The model z unit is similar to real midbrain dopamine neurons in that its response transfers from the reward to the cue and is suppressed by the absence of an expected reward. (Compare Figure 11.13 with Figures 11.10 and 11.11.)

The z unit computes the prediction error signal used in temporal-difference learning. The correspondence between the behavior of the prediction error unit in the model and the responses of real midbrain dopamine neurons suggests that these neurons carry something like a prediction error signal, and that learning driven by the midbrain dopamine system may involve something like temporal-difference learning. Experimentally testable predictions, in terms of changes in the sizes of the responses of midbrain dopamine neurons due to changes in the timing of the reward relative to the cue, have been derived from this model (Montague et al. 1996). Neural activity related to prediction error has also been observed in parts of the brain other than the midbrain. For example, functional imaging in humans shows that activity in the caudate nucleus (part of the basal ganglia) is related to the reward a subject receives in an economic exchange (King-Casas et al. 2005). Over repeated exchanges, the caudate activity transfers backward from the end of the exchange, when money is received, to the beginning, when the exchange is initiated.

11.5 Temporal-Difference Learning as a Form of Supervised Learning

The nature of temporal-diffference learning is rather subtle, but can be brought out by comparing the algorithm with others that we have studied in previous chapters. Because temporal-difference learning is driven by the prediction error signal it can be considered as a form of error driven, or supervised, learning (Sutton and Barto 1998). We considered supervised learning previously in the contexts of the delta rule and back-propagation (see Chapter 6), and recurrent back-propagation (see Chapter 10). In those forms of supervised learning the error is computed as the difference between the desired and actual activities of the output units. By making weight changes that reduce the error the supervised algorithms match the actual output to the desired output. According to the analogy with feedback, error-driven processes that we made in Chapter 6, we could consider the desired output as a "reference" or a "target" that supervised algorithms "track" by making weight changes.

The algorithms we studied in this chapter can also be seen as tracking a target. For temporal-difference learning the (prediction) error signal is $(r_j + v_i - v_j)$, and the algorithm makes changes in v_j that track $(r_j + v_i)$ as a target (where v_i and v_j are the values of states i and j, r_j is any reinforcement associated with state j, and we omit the c_i and c_j counters for clarity; see Equation 11.5). Similarly, $(r_{tg} - v_j)$ is the error signal for the least-mean-squares algorithm, which makes changes in v_j that track the reward-to-go r_{tg} as a target (see Equation 11.4). In Chapter 9 we saw how the delta rule and back-propagation could train neural units or networks to estimate posterior probabilities (we will take this up again in Chapter 12). In this chapter we see how temporal difference and least-mean-squares can train a neural network to estimate expected values, which are future values weighted by their probabilities (see Equation 11.1).

The update rules we used in Chapter 7 for the schema-based model of reinforcement learning can also be considered within the framework of targets and tracking. The schema model weight updates, described by Equations 7.5, 7.6, and 7.7 (see Chapter 7), take the general form shown in Equation 11.9:

$$v_j(c_j + 1) = v_j(c_j) + a\left[r - v_j(c_j)\right] \qquad \textbf{11.9}$$

where r is a generic reinforcement signal, v_j is the value of the input connection weight onto schema j, c_j is the update counter for weight v_j, and a is the learning rate, as before. Note that Equation 11.9 is the same as Equation 11.5 for the temporal-difference update, with one notable exception that we will discuss below in this section. Here we point out that Equation 11.9, which we used to train a reinforcement learning model, can be seen in the target-tracking framework as a form of supervised learning in which changes in input weight v_j track reinforcement r as a target. Thus, we make a distinction between supervised and reinforcement learning that involves both the mechanism and the goal of the adaptive process.

Like the models we studied in this chapter, the schema model in Chapter 7 was trained on reinforcement signals that could be considered as rewards or punishments. Because the overall schema model learns to increase the amount of reward (and decrease the amount of punishment) it receives it is, strictly speaking, a reinforcement learning model (see Chapter 7 for further details). However, it accomplishes reinforcement learning using the rule described in Equation 11.9 which is, strictly speaking, a supervised learning rule. The rule in Equation 11.9 is a supervised learning rule that happens to track reinforcement as a target. This supervised learning rule enables the schema model to learn the values of specific actions, and the overall model uses those learned values to choose actions that increase the amount of reward (and decrease the amount of punishment) it receives from the environment. The same distinction applies to the models and algorithms we studied in this chapter. Temporal difference and least-mean-squares are supervised learning algorithms that can train a learning agent to estimate the values of the states of an environment. If the agent then uses those expected value estimates to make decisions that increase the net reinforcement it receives from the environment, then it has accomplished reinforcement learning.

The model by Montague and colleagues (1996) that we studied in Section 11.4 is an adaptation of the temporal-difference learning procedure in a neural network context. It learns state values that it represents as the weights of the connections from input units, and it represents the states themselves as the activation levels of those input units. The input units x_j in the model come on and go off again in a strict sequence starting at the stimulus cue and ending just before the reward. This complete (continuous) serial response ordering serves to bridge the temporal gap between the cue and the reinforcement. Other neurobiologically plausible mechanisms are possible. Consider, for example, a unit s that produces a sustained activation that begins at the stimulus cue and terminates just before the reinforcement is received. Such a neuron s, by virtue of its sustained activity, would by itself bridge the temporal gap between the cue and the reward. A "phasic" unit receiving input from s could be proposed that would produce a positive response when s comes on and a negative response when s goes off, and in this behavior would resemble the differencing unit y in the model of midbrain dopamine neurons.

Neurons with sustained activity after a cue have been observed in many parts of the brain. As we observed in Chapter 7, neurons in the cingulate cortex and other areas of the limbic system show sustained responses to an auditory cue that persist at least until the behavioral response is made, and probably until the reinforcement associated with the outcome of the response has been received. We took advantage of this sustained response in the schema-based model we studied in Chapter 7 (which we also compared earlier in this section with temporal-difference learning). The schema model simulates a rabbit that learns to associate an auditory cue with reinforcement. The behavior of the simulated rabbit depends on the relative sizes of the responses to the cue of various schemata, which are functional elements representing groups of neurons. The response sizes of the schemata depend, in turn, on the values of the weights of the connections they receive from their auditory inputs. The sustained responses we assume for the schemata are instrumental in using supervised learning to adjust the values of their weights from the auditory inputs. Comparing the schema model weight update (see Equation 11.9) with the temporal-difference update (see Equation 11.5) reveals what may be a functional benefit of sustained responses to adaptive processes in the real brain.

The difference between the temporal-difference and schema model updates is best appreciated within the supervised learning as target tracking framework we introduced earlier in this section. For temporal-difference learning (see Equation 11.5) the target, which is the quantity tracked by the state value estimate v_j, comprises not only the reinforcement r_j of the state but also the value estimate v_i of the next state in the sequence ($r_j + v_i$). In contrast, the target for the schema model update (see Equation 11.9) is simply the reinforcement r by itself. Because the sustained response we assume for a schema bridges the temporal gap between the cue and the reinforcement, the reinforcing event can be associated with the sustained response without the need to propagate it backward through any intervening states. After learning, the size of the sustained response to the cue can "predict" the amount of reinforcement that will follow from it. It is possible that neurons with sustained responses, such

FIGURE 11.14 Reverse replay of rat hippocampal place cell activity (A) The position of the rat as a function of time as it runs from side to side along a track for 13 laps. The dark areas at the end of each lap represent rest periods, which could exceed one minute. (B) The averaged activity of a set of hippocampal place cells *during* a run. Each histogram shows the activity of a different cell. Each cell responds in turn as the rat runs through the cell's preferred place along the track. (C) The activity of the same set of place cells *after* running, during the rest periods at the ends of laps 1 through 4. (Similar activity is observed after every lap but is not shown.) Each panel in C shows a separate temporal segment of about one-third of a second that is laid out as in B, but with a raster scan line of action potentials (rather than a histogram) for each place cell. During the rest periods, the place cells become active repeatedly but in reverse order, as though replaying the run backwards. (From Foster and Wilson 2006.)

as those in the cingulate cortex and other limbic areas, can learn to represent the expected values of certain cues without the need for explicit temporal-difference learning (see Chapter 7 for data on these neurons).

We also observed in Chapter 10 that neurons with sustained activity during delayed response tasks are found in various parts of the cortex. We simulated these sustained responses using a recurrent neural network model, trained using recurrent back-propagation, to simulate working memory. Sustained responses may be one way in which the brain assigns value to cue events (including sensory responses), which precede reinforcing events (such as rewards or punishments). Of course, there is a limit to the duration of sustained responses. Also, as we discussed at the beginning of this chapter, many tasks are more complex than simple cue–response tasks and involve a sequence of steps. For estimating the values of the states in a sequence, learning mechanisms other than the simple update described in Equation 11.9 (and Chapter 7) must be employed.

Temporal-difference learning is a form of learning that enables agents, such as neural networks and, quite likely, real brains also, to learn the values of states from state sequences, and so to predict the amount of some quantity (such as reinforcement) to be obtained in progressing from a given state. As we have seen in this chapter, temporal-difference learning is not the only way to achieve such learning. In its most basic form, temporal-difference learning assumes that the learning agent has access only to the values of two states immediately adjacent in time. It is possible that, in some parts of the brain, whole sequences (trajectories) of states are stored, in proper order, and are made available for learning.

Place cells are neurons in the hippocampus that are activated when an animal is located in a particular place in an environment (Wilson and McNaughton 1993). Individual place cells are specialized for specific locations. Place cells, for example, could encode the location of an animal in an environment such as the simple gridworld we considered in the earlier sections of this

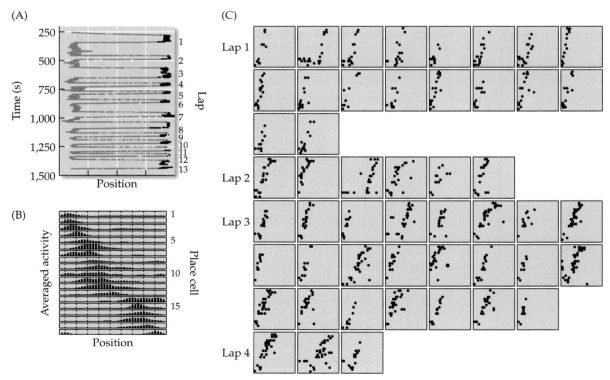

chapter (see Figure 11.1). Multiunit recordings from the rat hippocampus show that the sequences of place cells that are activated while a rat moves along a trajectory are replayed, repeatedly and in reverse order, during rest periods (Foster and Wilson 2006). Some actual data from a behaving, moving rat are shown in Figure 11.14. It seems that the hippocampus stores entire state sequences (trajectories), and it is possible that it makes them available for use by learning mechanisms. These mechanisms may be similar to those forms of temporal- difference learning that will update the values of a series of previous states (Sutton and Barto 1998). It is also possible that learning mechanisms akin to the least-mean-squares algorithm (see Section 11.2), which work on entire state sequences replayed in reverse, also occur in certain parts of the brain (see Exercise 11.4). Considering the behavioral importance of the ability to predict the outcome of a sequence of states, it is likely that many mechanisms for learning to predict occur in the brain.

Exercises

11.1 The simple stochastic gridworld has reinforcements only in the terminal states, but the option to set an intermediate reinforcement is available in `gridWorldSetUp` (see MATLAB Box 11.1). Set the reinforcement of non-terminal state 7 to +1. This is done using `intReSt=7` and `r(intReSt)=+1`. Also, change the reinforcements of terminal states 8 and 12 to −2 and +2, respectively, using `tsp=8`, `tsr=12`, `r(tsp)=-2`, and `r(tsr)=+2`. How do these changes affect the state values? Are the three methods (iterative dynamic programming, least-mean-squares, and temporal difference) able to learn the new state values with an intermediate reinforcement?

11.2 In the midbrain dopamine neuron simulation (script `midbrainDopamine`, see MATLAB Box 11.5), temporal-difference learning takes place over 200 trials (`nTrials=200`), and reinforcement was withheld on trial 100 (`nTrials/2`), after the simulated response had already backed up from the reward to the stimulus cue. What happens if reinforcement is withheld on trial 20 (`nTrials/10`), well before the response has fully backed up? Is the response still suppressed by the missing reward?

11.3 In the midbrain dopamine neuron simulation (script `midbrainDopamine`, see MATLAB Box 11.5), the reward occurred at the same time (`rTime=30`) on each trial (except that it was withheld on trial 100). The simulated response backed up from the reward to the cue, and the estimated state values (weights `v`) fully predicted the time of reward (except, of course, on trial 100). Rerun this simulation, but have the reward occur at a variable time. This is equivalent to random variation between trials in the position of the reward value of 1 in reward vector `r`. If the trial is `nTimes` time steps long, then a reward of 1 can be delivered at a time that varies randomly over a range of three time steps before `rTime` using `r=zeros(nTimes,1)`, `rJitter=rTime-ceil(3*rand)`, and `r(rJitter)=1` on each trial. Do not withhold reward on any trial. Does the response completely back up from the reward to the cue in this case, in which the reward time is not fully predictable?

11.4 The script `midbrainDopamine` (see MATLAB Box 11.5) simulates the responses of midbrain dopamine neurons in the cue–reward example using temporal-difference learning. In so doing, it learns the values of the weights of a set of input units that are activated in sequence by a stimulus cue. Experimental findings from the hippocampus show that the entire sequence of activation of place cells during behavior is replayed in reverse order during periods of rest (Foster and Wilson 2006; see also Figure 11.14). These findings suggest that learning may occur off-line during the replays, in a manner reminiscent of least-mean-squares learning (see script `leastMeanSquares` in MATLAB Box 11.3). Modify `midbrainDopamine` to use the least-mean-squares method to learn the values of the weights in the cue–reward example. Because each unit is activated in a strict sequence on each trial, all the weights can be updated synchronously. Also, each weight is updated only once per trial, so you can use scalar variable `count` to count the number of trials, which is the same as the number of updates for each weight. Because reward is presented only at the end of the sequence, the reward-to-go `rtg` over each sequence is equal to the reward received at the end. Because of synchronous weight (value) updates and absence of intermediate reward, state-by-state updating and sequence reversal for least-mean-squares learning are not needed in this exercise, although evidence indicates that sequence reversal actually does occur in the hippocampus (see Figure 11.14). This is consistent with least-mean-squares learning in general, which can account for intermediate reward (see MATLAB Box 11.3). With the simplifications we employ in this exercise, the update command using least-mean-squares learning for the whole weight vector `v` on each trial is `v=v+(rtg–v)/(count+1)`. Try 20 trials of least-mean-squares learning. Set the reward to 1 on all trials (`rtg=1`) except on trial 10, in which you can set the reward to 0 (`rtg=0`). What happens during the first nine trials? What happens on trial 10? Do the values fully recover by trial 20? How does least-mean-squares learning compare with temporal-difference learning in this exercise?

References

Bellman RE (1957) *Dynamic Programming*. Princeton University Press, Princeton. NJ.

Berger JO (1985) *Statistical Decision Theory and Bayesian Analysis. Second Edition*. Springer, New York.

Foster DJ, Wilson MA (2006) Reverse replay of behavioral sequences in hippocampal place cells during the awake state. *Nature* 440: 680–683.

King-Casas B, Tomlin D, Anen C, Camerer CF, Quartz SR, Montague PR (2005) Getting to know you: Reputation and trust in a two-person economic exchange. *Science* 308: 78–83.

Lau B, Glimcher PW (2008) Value representations in the primate striatum during matching behavior. *Neuron* 58: 451–463.

Lee D, Seo J (2007) Mechanisms of reinforcement learning and decision making in the primate dorsolateral prefrontal cortex. *Annals of the New York Academy of Science* 1104: 108–122.

Montague PR, Dayan P, Sejnowski TJ (1996) A framework for mesencephalic dopamine systems based on predictive Hebbian learning. *Journal of Neuroscience* 16: 1936–1947.

Noble B, Daniel JW (1988) *Applied Linear Algebra, Third Edition.* Prentice Hall, Englewood Cliffs, NJ.

Olds J, Milner P (1954) Positive reinforcement produced by electrical stimulation of septal area and other regions of rat brain. *Journal of Comparative and Physiological Psychology* 47: 419–427.

Platt ML, Glimcher PW (1999) Neural correlates of decision variables in parietal cortex. *Nature* 400: 233–238.

Robbins TW, Everitt BJ (2003) Motivation and reward. In: Squire LR, Bloom FE, McConnell SK, Roberts JL, Spitzer NC, Zigmond MJ (eds) *Fundamental Neuroscience. Second Edition.* Academic Press, Orlando, FL, pp 1109–1126.

Romo R, Schultz W (1990) Dopamine neurons of the monkey midbrain: Contingencies of responses to active touch during self-initiated arm movements. *Journal of Neurophysiology* 63: 592–606.

Russell S, Norvig P (1995) *Artificial Intelligence: A Modern Approach.* Prentice-Hall, Upper Saddle River, NJ, pp 598–607.

Schultz W (2004) Neural coding of basic reward terms of animal learning theory, game theory, microeconomics and behavioral ecology. *Current Opinion in Neurobiology* 14: 139–147.

Schultz W (2007) Multiple dopamine functions at different time courses. *Annual Review of Neuroscience* 30: 259–288.

Schultz W, Apicella P, Ljungberg T (1993) Responses of monkey dopamine neurons to reward and conditioned stimuli during successive steps of learning a delayed response task. *Journal of Neuroscience* 13: 900–913.

Stahl SM (1996) *Essential Psychopharmacology: Neuroscientific Basis and Clinical Application.* Cambridge University Press, Cambridge.

Sutton RS, Barto AG (1998) *Reinforcement Learning: An Introduction.* MIT Press, Cambridge, MA.

Tesauro G (2002) Programming backgammon using self-teaching neural nets. *Artificial Intelligence* 134: 181–199.

Wilson MA, McNaughton BL (1993) Dynamics of the hippocampal ensemble code for space. *Science* 261: 1055–1058.

12

Predictor–Corrector Models and Probabilistic Inference

Predictor–corrector models accomplish inference by combining internal expectations with external observations and can simulate the responses of certain sensory neurons

ost of us experience annoyance when an interlocutor finishes a sentence that we are in the process of uttering. What is most annoying about it is that the interlocutor usually finishes our sentence correctly. This success can be attributed to the ability of humans to anticipate what other humans are about to say. The ability to anticipate speech may have evolved partly to enhance our capacity to annoy one another, but mostly as an essential component of speech comprehension. It is likely that our ability to anticipate words during conversation is important for understanding speech in real time, and even for understanding language in general. Studies based on event-related potentials (ERPs), which are recordings of large-scale brain activity measured using arrays of scalp electrodes, suggest that humans anticipate upcoming words in discourse and in reading, and that this anticipation contributes to the comprehension of speech and written text (Van Berkum et al. 2005). Far from being confined to language understanding, the ability to anticipate seems to be essential to perception in all modalities and on all levels.

New research findings continue to support the conclusion that perception is not a function of bottom-up sensory input alone, but involves an interaction between bottom-up signals from the sensory organs and top-down signals from higher brain regions (Lee and Mumford 2003; Gilbert and Sigman 2007). Top-down connections might carry signals indicating the features that higher centers "anticipate" will be present in the bottom-up sensory signals arriving from lower centers. Actual top-down effects include enhancement or suppression of responses, sharpening of tuning curves, and altering the adaptability of sensory neurons (Gilbert and Sigman 2007). Top-down influence is sometimes attributed to "attention," and some of the clearest neurophysiological evidence for top-down effects involves the modulation of the responses of visual cortical neurons by shifts in attention, either toward or away from the region of the stimulus (Motter 1993; McAdams and Maunsell 1999; Reynolds et al. 1999). Hierarchical Bayesian inference, which involves probabilistic inference using directed graphs that describe the statistical dependencies among an ordered set of random variables, is emerging as the predominant conceptual paradigm for simulating bottom-up/top-down processes in sensory perception (Lee and Mumford 2003). In this chapter, we will explore a Bayesian network model of visual processing and use it to simulate the effects of attention on the responses of visual cortical neurons.

While top-down anticipation is clearly at work in the higher cortical processing associated with language comprehension and visual scene analysis, evidence also indicates anticipatory signals in operation at lower levels. For example, some neurons in the retina are sensitive to the direction of motion of moving visual stimuli, and the direction-selective response appears to involve mechanisms that anticipate the location of the stimulus on the basis of its past motion (Berry et al. 1999). This activity can be simulated using neural network models that employ asymmetric inhibition (Barlow and Levic 1965; Ruff et al. 1987). We will implement a simple version of the asymmetric inhibition model of direction selectivity in this chapter.

Whether operating at higher cortical levels or at the subcortical level, processes that involve anticipatory signals seem to use them as part of a pattern of prediction and correction, in which the anticipated features serve as predictions that are corrected by actual sensory input. For example, batters in baseball seem to predict the trajectory of a pitch in the initial instants after it leaves the pitcher's hand, and to correct that prediction using peripheral vision as the ball approaches them (DeLucia and Cochran 1985). In cricket, where the ball takes a bounce between the bowler and the batsman, the batsman predicts where the ball will bounce, and uses the difference between predicted and observed bounce location to help him estimate where and when the ball will reach him (Land and McLeod 2000).

Neurophysiological evidence concerning a similar predictor–corrector mechanism is provided by experiments on a region of the cat brain known as the parabigeminal nucleus (PBN). Neurons in this region are active while a cat tries to visually track a moving spot of light (or target). These neurons continue to produce a response to the moving target even after the light is extinguished, rendering the target invisible (Cui and Malpeli 2003; Ma et al., in review). Obviously, cats (and other animals) cannot visually track completely invisible targets. Rather, the response to the invisible target appears to be the predictive component of a predictor–corrector mechanism, in which the cat estimates the positions of targets using both its expectations concerning where they will move and its visual observations of them. In this chapter, we will simulate the responses of PBN neurons using predictor–corrector models based both on Bayesian networks and neural networks. Before we begin our simulations we will study a familiar process that is, in fact, a predictor–corrector system.

The running average is a simple but elegant example of a predictor-corrector system. (This example is adapted from Rao 1999.) The average of n observations can be computed from the average of the previous $n-1$ observations, and the current observation, using the formula shown in Equation 12.1:

$$v(n) = v(n-1) + \left[o(n) - v(n-1)\right]\left(\frac{1}{n}\right) \qquad \textbf{12.1}$$

where $v(n)$ is the current average, $v(n-1)$ is the previous average, and $o(n)$ is the current observation. The running average is a predictor–corrector system in which the prediction is the previous average $v(n-1)$, and the correction is the difference between the current observation and the prediction $[o(n) - v(n-1)]$. The correction term is weighted by $1/n$. Thus, the running average predicts that the current average will be the same as the previous average, and this prediction is corrected by a correction term that is based on an observation. Note that the weight of the correction term $(1/n)$ decreases as the running average proceeds and the number n of observations increases.

The weight of the correction term $(1/n)$ can be interpreted as a simplified version of a Kalman gain. The Kalman filter (Math Box 12.1) is a predictor–corrector form of adaptive filter that is widely used in engineering. In the classical Kalman filter, the relative contributions of the prediction and correction are weighted by the Kalman gain according to their variances. In the running average the correction weight $(1/n)$ plays a similar role. Early on, when it is based on few observations, the prediction from the running average is inaccurate and varies a lot, and the correction weight is large. As the running average proceeds it becomes more accurate, and the prediction rapidly smoothes out and varies less. The correction weight accordingly decreases.

The use of the Kalman filter as a model of neural systems is increasing in popularity (e.g., Yasushi and Paulin 1989; Rao 1999; Rao and Ballard 1999; Denève et al. 2007). However, the classical Kalman filter is complicated and

MATH BOX 12.1   THE KALMAN FILTER

The development of the Kalman filter (Kalman 1960) was a landmark achievement in the theory of predictor–corrector systems. The following summary is by Rao (1999). The goal is to estimate the state vector $\mathbf{s}(t)$ of some stochastic (i.e., random) linear, dynamical system. At time (t) this state generates an observable output vector $\mathbf{o}(t)$ according to Equation B12.1.1:

$$\mathbf{o}(t) = \mathbf{Gs}(t) + \mathbf{n}(t) \qquad \text{B12.1.1}$$

where $\mathbf{G}$ is the generative matrix and $\mathbf{n}(t)$ is Gaussian noise with mean 0 and covariance matrix $\Sigma = E[\mathbf{nn}^T]$. ($E[\cdot]$ is the expected value where, for example, $E[X]$ is the mean of random variable X.) We assume that the state $\mathbf{s}(t-1)$ will transition to $\mathbf{s}(t)$ according to Equation B12.1.2:

$$\mathbf{s}(t) = \mathbf{Ps}(t-1) + \mathbf{m}(t-1) \qquad \text{B12.1.2}$$

where $\mathbf{P}$ is the prediction matrix and $\mathbf{m}(t)$ is Gaussian noise with mean $\overline{\mathbf{m}}$ and covariance $\Pi = E[(\mathbf{m} - \overline{\mathbf{m}})(\mathbf{m} - \overline{\mathbf{m}})^T]$. At each time step (t) the Kalman filter first *predicts* $\mathbf{s}(t)$ and then uses the observation $\mathbf{o}(t)$ to *correct* its prediction. Call the prediction $\mathbf{s}_p(t)$ and the corrected estimate $\mathbf{s}_e(t)$. The prediction $\mathbf{s}_p$ has covariance $\mathbf{Q}(t) = E[(\mathbf{s}_p - \overline{\mathbf{s}}_p)(\mathbf{s}_p - \overline{\mathbf{s}}_p)^T]$.

The Kalman filter is then implemented recursively as shown in Equations B12.1.3–B12.1.6:

$$\mathbf{s}_p(t) = \mathbf{Ps}_e(t-1) + \overline{\mathbf{m}}(t-1) \qquad \text{B12.1.3}$$

$$\mathbf{Q}(t) = \mathbf{PN}(t-1)\mathbf{P}^T + \Pi(t-1) \qquad \text{B12.1.4}$$

$$\mathbf{N}(t) = \left[\mathbf{G}^T \Sigma(t)^{-1}\mathbf{G} + \mathbf{Q}(t)^{-1}\right]^{-1} \qquad \text{B12.1.5}$$

$$\mathbf{s}_e(t) = \mathbf{s}_p(t) + \mathbf{N}(t)\mathbf{G}^T \Sigma(t)^{-1}\left[\mathbf{o}(t) - \mathbf{Gs}_p(t)\right] \qquad \text{B12.1.6}$$

where the sensory residual $[\mathbf{o}(t) - \mathbf{Gs}_p(t)]$ is the difference between the actual and the predicted observation. The matrix $\mathbf{N}(t)\mathbf{G}^T\Sigma(t)^{-1}$ is known as the Kalman gain matrix, and it determines the weight given to the sensory residual in correcting the prediction $\mathbf{s}_p(t)$. The Kalman gain matrix is updated on each time step along with the state estimate $\mathbf{s}_e(t)$. Note that the Kalman gain is a function of the covariences of the prediction and observation.

will not be considered further in this book. We will consider simpler predictor–corrector mechanisms and will start by implementing the running average. The goal is to compute the running average of a noise vector of $n = 100$ random deviates from a Gaussian distribution. Recall that Gaussian-distributed random deviates (observations) with mean μ and standard deviation σ can be generated according to Equation 12.2:

$$o = \eta(0,1)\sigma + \mu \qquad\qquad \textbf{12.2}$$

where the standard deviation is the square root of the variance σ^2, and $\eta(0,1)$ is a random deviate drawn from a univariate Gaussian distribution with mean 0 and variance 1 (see Chapter 9). The script `runningAverage` (MATLAB® Box 12.1) will implement the running average of a series of Gaussian deviates.

The commands `nObs=100`, `mn=5`, and `var=20` set the number of observations to 100, the mean to 5, and the variance to 20. The vector containing the noise series is generated according to Equation 12.2 using `o=randn(1,nObs)*sd+mn`, where variable `sd=sqrt(var)` is the standard deviation. The average of the noise series is computed using `NoiseMean=mean(o)`. For this particular series it is found to be 5.01. The noise vector is then padded with a 0 at the beginning (now it has 101 elements). The padding 0 corresponds to the value of $v(0)$. Because MATLAB does not allow indices of 0, there will be an offset of 1 between index n in Equation 12.1 and the indices of the vectors in script `runningAverage`. For example, the second element of the noise (observation) vector `o` (the element right after the padding 0) will correspond to $o(1)$ in Equation 12.1. When $n = 1$, the value of the correction weight $(1/n)$ equals 1. By reference to Equation 12.1, the value of $v(1)$ is simply $o(1)$. This makes sense, because the mean of a single value is that value.

In script `runningAverage` the vectors `v` and `kg` are set up to hold, respectively, the running average and the correction weight (Kalman gain) on each update of the running average process. These vectors are each 101 elements long, and the first element corresponds to $n = 0$. The first element of the running average vector is set to 0 (`v(1)=0`), and the first element of the correction weight vector is set to 1 (`kg(1)=1`). A loop from 2 to

---

MATLAB® BOX 12.1   This script implements a running average.

```
% runningAverage.m

mn=5; % set mean of noise series
var=20; % set variance of noise
sd=sqrt(var); % find the noise standard deviation
nObs=100; % set the number of noise values in the series
o=randn(1,nObs)*sd+mn; % generate Gaussian noise series
NoiseMean=mean(o) % find the mean of the noise
o=[0 o]; % pad the noise vector with a zero
v=zeros(1,nObs+1); % define hold vector for running average
kg=zeros(1,nObs+1); % define hold vector for correction gain
v(1)=0; % set initial condition for running average
kg(1)=1; % set initial correction gain value
for n=2:nObs+1; % for each noise value
     kg(n)=1/(n-1); % update correction gain value
     v(n)=v(n-1) + (o(n)-v(n-1))*kg(n); % running average
end % end running average loop
EndRunAvg=v(nObs+1) % grab the last value of running average
```

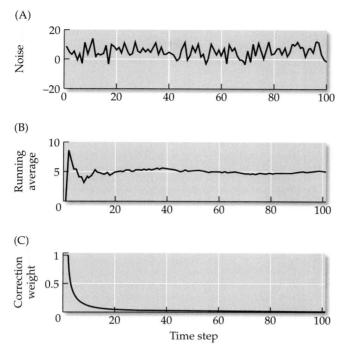

FIGURE 12.1   The running average as a simple example of a predictor–corrector system (A) A series of 100 random deviates (observations) drawn from a Gaussian distribution with mean 5 and variance 20. The actual, overall average of the random deviates in the series is 5.01. (B) The running average of this series varies more at the beginning than at the end. Its final value is also 5.01. (C) The weight of the correction relative to the prediction falls rapidly.

`nObs+1` computes successive values of the running average using command `v(n)=v(n−1)+(o(n)−v(n−1))*kg(n)`. The correction weight `kg` is computed on each iteration using `kg(n)=1/(n−1)` to take account of the offset of 1 between the indices of the vectors and the actual updates to the running average. The final value of the running average, held in variable `EndRunAvg=v(nObs+1)`, equals 5.01 on this run. It is the same value as `NoiseMean`, the average of the noise vector computed before padding it with a 0, because the running average is simply an iterated version of the average.

Plots of the noise vector, the running average vector, and the correction weight vector over successive iterations are shown in Figure 12.1. The correction weight (see Figure 12.1C) decreases rapidly as the running average proceeds. The running average itself (see Figure 12.1B) gradually settles to the mean, after an initial period of wide variation. The running average is initially inaccurate and widely varying because it is based on few observations. As the running average proceeds it becomes more accurate and less variable, because it is based on an ever-increasing number of observations. The correction weight rapidly decreases to reflect the fact that the running average rapidly improves and requires less correction as the running average algorithm proceeds.

Processes similar to the running average may occur in the nervous system. As we discussed in Chapter 11, the least-mean-squares algorithm produces weight updates in the form of a running average. The least-mean-squares algorithm may be similar to a neurobiological learning process that operates on sequences of responses that are stored and repeatedly replayed in the hippocampus. Other forms of prediction, and prediction–correction, probably also occur in the nervous system. We will study some of those in this chapter. Direction selectivity in the visual system can be considered as an example of a predictive mechanism. The next example involves a very simple model of direction selectivity.

12.1 Modeling Visual System Direction Selectivity Using Asymmetric Inhibition

Some neurons in the visual system respond to moving visual stimuli and are selective for the direction in which the stimuli move (Livingstone 1998; Demb 2007). Recent research indicates that visual motion processing begins in the retina and involves mechanisms that occur on the cellular level (Demb 2007). Yet the processing that underlies direction selectivity in the visual system can be illustrated on a conceptual level using classic neural network models that are based on asymmetric inhibition (Barlow and Levic 1965; Ruff et al. 1987). In these models, linear arrays of excitatory and inhibitory units are arranged in such a way that their sequential activation in one direction will allow excitation to pass on to an output unit, but their activation in the opposite direction causes the excitation to be blocked by inhibition. These models capture the ability of the real visual system to anticipate the location to which a visual stimulus may move (Berry et al. 1999), and will serve us as an example of the kinds of predictive mechanisms that are involved in sensory processing. A simplified version of the basic direction-selectivity model, in the form of a four-layered neural network, is schematized in Figure 12.2.

It is easiest to think of the direction-selectivity network (see Figure 12.2) as having two input layers. The excitatory input units are labeled x_j, while

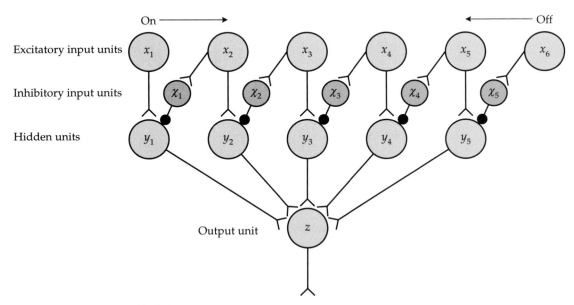

FIGURE 12.2   A network that implements asymmetric inhibition and simulates direction selectivity in the visual system There are two kinds of input units: excitatory (x_j) and inhibitory (χ_i). The hidden units y_i project to the sole output unit z. There is one more excitatory input unit x_j than there are inhibitory input units χ_i or hidden units y_i ($i = 1,...,n-1$ but $j = 1,...,n$). The arrows indicated the directions of motion of the stimulus (simulated light spot) that activate (on) or do not activate (off) the output unit z.

the inhibitory input units (darkly shaded circles in Figure 12.2) are labeled χ_i. The excitatory input units x_j are activated by the visual input (a simulated light spot) as it moves sequentially in either direction. The input units x_j excite the hidden units y_i. Note that j ($j = 1,...,n$) indexes the excitatory input units while i ($i = 1,...,n_y$) indexes both the inhibitory input units and the hidden units. The hidden units represent excitatory interneurons, which excite the (single) output unit z. The excitatory input units x_j also excite the inhibitory input units χ_i, which then inhibit the hidden units y_i. The output unit z is the directionally selective unit, and it will produce a sustained output during sequential activation of the excitatory input units in the on-direction but not in the off-direction. We will assume for simplicity that the visual stimulus moves from one excitatory input unit to the next in one time step (i.e., one network cycle, or one synaptic delay). The timing issue cannot be treated so simply in general (as we will see later in this section), but a fixed input activation sequence allows the basic direction-selectivity mechanism to be illustrated most clearly.

Consider stimulus movement in the on-direction. On the first time step, excitatory input unit x_1 is activated and it excites hidden unit y_1. On the second time step, hidden unit y_1 excites output unit z. Also on the second time step, the stimulus activates input unit x_2, which excites hidden unit y_2, and x_2 also excites χ_1, the inhibitory input unit that inhibits y_1. On the third time step, hidden unit y_2 excites output unit z. Also on the third time step, inhibitory input unit χ_1 inhibits y_1, but this has no effect on output unit z. Because z has already been excited by hidden unit y_1 on the second time step, inhibition of y_1 on the third time step has no effect on the response of output unit z. Excitatory input unit x_3 is also activated on the third time step, and the sequential excitation of z by the hidden units y_i continues unblocked.

Now consider stimulus movement in the off-direction. On the first time step, excitatory input unit x_6 is activated, and it excites the inhibitory input unit χ_5 that inhibits hidden unit y_5. On the second time step, the stimulus activates excitatory input unit x_5, and x_5 attempts to excite hidden unit y_5 but, on this same time step, y_5 is also being inhibited by χ_5, so excitation of hidden unit y_5 by input unit x_5 is blocked. Thus, hidden unit y_5 is unable to excite output unit z. This process of blocking continues throughout the off-direction sequence, and output unit z remains silent. Inhibition by the inhibitory input units in the network is considered asymmetric because it is directed toward hidden units in one direction but not in the other.

Connectivity matrices for the directional-selectivity network with six input units ($n = 6$) are shown in Table 12.1. The inhibitory input units χ_i are numbered according to the hidden unit that each one inhibits. The connectivity matrices are simple in form. The first two can be constructed from concatenations of positive and negative identity matrices, and column vectors of 0s. The third is simply a row vector of 1s. This basic structure is easily extended to larger networks by noting that there is always one more excitatory input unit x_j than there are hidden units y_i or inhibitory input units χ_i ($n_y = n - 1$). Also, the second excitatory input unit connects to the first inhibitory input unit, and so on for the rest, but the first excitatory input unit connects to no inhibitory input unit, and the last excitatory input unit has no corresponding hidden unit to connect to.

Script `directionSelectivity`, listed in MATLAB Box 12.2, will implement the direction-selectivity example. We will consider a network having 30 excitatory input units, so set nEx=30 in `directionSelectivity`. Variable names `xex` and `xin` designate the column vectors of excitatory and inhibitory input states, respectively. The command VX=[zeros(nEx-1,1) eye(nEx-1)] makes the matrix VX that connects the excitatory to the

TABLE 12.1 Connection weight matrices for the direction-selectivity network

(A) Connections to inhibitory input units χ_i from excitatory input units x_j

	x_1	x_2	x_3	x_4	x_5	x_6
χ_1	0	1	0	0	0	0
χ_2	0	0	1	0	0	0
χ_3	0	0	0	1	0	0
χ_4	0	0	0	0	1	0
χ_5	0	0	0	0	0	1

(B) Connections to hidden units y_i from excitatory and inhibitory input units x_j and χ_i

	x_1	x_2	x_3	x_4	x_5	x_6	χ_1	χ_2	χ_3	χ_4	χ_5
y_1	1	0	0	0	0	0	−1	0	0	0	0
y_2	0	1	0	0	0	0	0	−1	0	0	0
y_3	0	0	1	0	0	0	0	0	−1	0	0
y_4	0	0	0	1	0	0	0	0	0	−1	0
y_5	0	0	0	0	1	0	0	0	0	0	−1

(C) Connections to output unit z from hidden units y_i

	y_1	y_2	y_3	y_4	y_5
z	1	1	1	1	1

inhibitory input units. Command `V=[eye(nEx−1) zeros(nEx−1,1) −eye(nEx−1)]` makes the matrix `V` that connects the concatenated input column vector `x=[xex;xin]` to the hidden units in vector variable `y`. The command `U=ones(1,nEx−1)` makes the matrix `U` that connects the hidden units to the single output unit `z`.

A series of input patterns `InPat` that is consistent with a visual stimulus (like a spot of light) that moves from one input unit to the next on each time step is made as a 30-by-30 identity matrix. A series of input patterns that is consistent with a stimulus moving in the opposite direction is made by flipping a 30-by-30 identity matrix left-to-right. This can be done using `InPat=fliplr(eye(nEx))`. (Flipping the identity matrix top-to-bottom would accomplish the same thing.) The responses of the network units are computed in a loop where, on each time step `t`, the excitatory input units are first set to the corresponding input pattern: `xex=InPat(:,t)`. Next the column vector `x=[xex;xin]` is composed and used to compute the vector `q` of the sums of weighted inputs to the hidden units (`q=V*x`), and vector `q` is converted to binary with a threshold at 0 to find `y` (`y=q>0`). Finally, the state of the output unit (`z(t)=U*y`) and the states of the inhibitory input units (`xin=VX*xex`) are updated. Note that the state updates as described all occur on the same time step, and this facilitates comparison of the stimulus with the responses of the units in the network. Nevertheless, the synaptic delays between the various layers of the network are critical to its operation. The delays in the network are taken into account in terms of the order in which the units in the various layers are updated. Critically, inhibitory input units `xin` must be updated after the hidden units `y`, but they can be updated before the output unit `z`.

Figure 12.3A and B show the input to (light spot) and output from (response) the direction-selectivity network for stimulus movement in the off-direction. The output unit shows zero response to the off-direction input. Sequential activation of the excitatory input units in the direction from x_n to x_1, where n is the number of excitatory input units, will cause the inputs to the hidden

MATLAB® BOX 12.2   This script simulates direction selectivity in the visual system.

```
% directionSelectivity.m

dirFlag=0; % set direction flag (1 for on, 0 for off)
nEx=30; % enter the number of excitatory input units

% make the connectivity matrices
VX=[zeros(nEx-1,1) eye(nEx-1)]; % connections to xin from xex
V=[eye(nEx-1) zeros(nEx-1,1) -eye(nEx-1)]; % to y from all x
U=ones(1,nEx-1); % connections to z from y

% make input pattern matrix
if dirFlag==1, % for "on" pattern
    InPat=eye(nEx); % the identity matrix
elseif dirFlag==0, % for "off" pattern
    InPat=fliplr(eye(nEx)); % the flipped identity matrix
end % end input pattern conditional

% find the output
xex=zeros(nEx,1); % define excitatory input vector
xin=zeros(nEx-1,1); % define inhibitory input vector
y=zeros(nEx-1,1); % define y unit vector
z=zeros(nEx,1); % define z unit vector
for t=1:nEx, % for each time step
    xex=InPat(:,t); % set the excitatory input vector
    x=[xex; xin]; % compose the whole input vector
    q=V*x; % find the net input to the y units
    y=q>0; % binarize q to find y with a threshold of zero
    z(t)=U*y; % find the response of the z unit
    xin=VX*xex; % update the inhibitory input vector
end % end output loop
```

units y_i from the excitatory x_j and inhibitory χ_i input units to coincide. This will block excitation of the hidden units. Consequently, the hidden units y_i will fail to excite output unit z. Figure 12.3C and D show the input to, and output from, the network for stimulus movement in the on-direction. The output unit shows a nonzero response (state of 1) to the on-direction input. Sequential activation of the excitatory input units in the direction from x_1 to x_n will cause unblocked excitation of the hidden units. The hidden units, in turn, will excite output unit z, which shows a sustained response to its on-direction stimulus.

This simplified directionally selective network is not technically a predictor–corrector network, but we can think of it loosely as a predictor network because it anticipates particular sequences of input unit activations. For on-direction motion, it anticipates that excitatory input unit $j + 1$ will be activated after excitatory input unit j over the sequence, and output unit z shows a sustained response in that case. For off-direction motion, the network anticipates that excitatory input unit $j + 1$ will be activated *before* excitatory input unit j over the sequence. In this case, it predicts that excitation from excitatory input unit j will coincide with inhibition from inhibitory input unit $i = j$ at hidden unit $i = j$, so that the response of that hidden unit will be nullified. Output unit z shows zero response in this case.

FIGURE 12.3   Simulation of direction selectivity in the visual system (A and C) Each dot marks the location of the light spot on each time step. The light spot moves by one input unit per time step in either direction. There are 30 each of locations, input units, and time steps. (B and D) Each dot marks the response of the single output unit on each time step. For ease of comparison the synaptic delay due to propagation from the input to the output through the network is not exhibited by the output responses. (A) A spot of light moves in steps in the off-direction of the network. (B) The output unit produces no response. (C) A spot of light moves in the on-direction. (D) The output unit produces a response that is sustained for the duration of the stimulus.

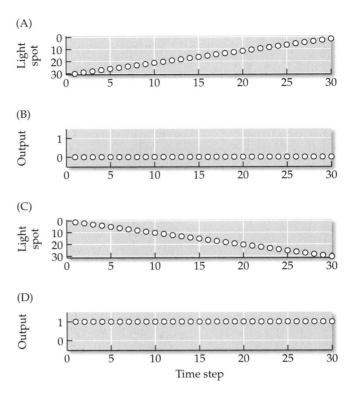

The main advantage of the simplified direction-selectivity model is that it illustrates the basic operation of the asymmetric inhibition mechanism with the minimum of detail. Its main drawback is that its proper operation depends on the "speed" of motion of the visual stimulus. This limitation can be overcome by elaborating the model. Some hints for doing that are provided in Exercise 12.1.

Changes in the speed of the visual stimulus can be simulated by changing the relationship between the time steps and the excitatory input unit activations. To increase the speed of the stimulus it could skip one or more input units as it progresses along the input array on each time step. To decrease the speed the stimulus could skip one or more time steps before activating the next input unit in the sequence. The on-direction response of the simplified model is not sensitive to increases in the speed of the stimulus. The off-direction response can be made insensitive to increases in the speed of the stimulus simply by allowing each inhibitory input unit to inhibit all the hidden units with indices equal to and lower than its own (i.e., each inhibitory input unit would inhibit all the hidden units asymmetrically to its left in Figure 12.2).

Both the on-direction and the off-direction responses can be made insensitive to decreases in the speed of the stimulus by allowing the inhibitory input units and the hidden units to prolong their own responses by exerting positive feedback on themselves. (As in Chapter 2, we will model this positive feedback conveniently using direct, excitatory self-connections, but we point out that it could result from a variety of cellular and/or network mechanisms in the real nervous system.) With this positive feedback, the responses of the inhibitory input units and the hidden units depend both on their inputs from other units and on their own previous states. Along with self-excitation it is helpful to make the hidden units linear with a cutoff of zero, and to convert the output unit activation to binary using a nonzero threshold. (Further details are given in Exercise 12.1.) Careful adjustment of the positive feedback weights and output unit threshold allows the network to respond to on-direction stimuli, and not to respond to off-direction stimuli, over a range of speeds. The responses of the units in an elaborated direction-selectivity network to a stimulus in the on-direction at twice its previous speed are shown in Figure 12.4. Again, the synaptic delay, which is critical to network operation, determines the order in which the states of the units in various layers are updated but is not exhibited in the timing of the responses to facilitate comparison.

The stimulus moves at twice its previous speed by skipping an even-numbered excitatory input unit on each time step (see Figure 12.4A). The output unit produces a sustained response to this faster on-direction input that actually persists for two time steps after the stimulus terminates (see Figure 12.4B). Both the inhibitory input units and the hidden units have prolonged responses due to self-excitation (see Figure 12.4C and D, respectively). The output unit response lag results from the prolonged hidden unit activity, which keeps the (binary) output unit above its threshold even after the stimulus terminates. The prolonged hidden unit activity is truncated by inhibitory input unit activity. However, because the inhibition in the network is asymmetric, the prolonged response of the last hidden unit to be activated in the sequence is not inhibited. Thus, the recurrent (self-excitatory) connections cause the network to generate anticipatory waves of excitation that travel ahead of the stimulus in the on-direction. In the model, this excitatory wave is what enables the network to anticipate the locations of stimuli that move at higher speeds. The network simulates the waves of excitation that have actually been observed in the retina in response to moving visual stimuli (Berry et al. 1999).

In the last section of this chapter we will again exploit a positive feedback mechanism, in a network that anticipates the location of another, simulated moving visual stimulus. This positive feedback will occur from an output unit onto itself, and will be applied in the context of a model of visual tracking by neurons in a region known as the parabigeminal nucleus. In the next section

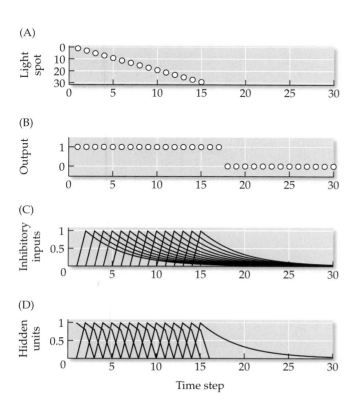

FIGURE 12.4   Simulation of direction selectivity in the visual system at a higher stimulus speed (A) Each dot marks the location of the light spot on each time step. Note that the light spot moves by two input units on every time step, so it moves at twice the speed of the stimulus in Figure 12.3. (B) Each dot marks the response of the single output unit on each time step. The output unit response is sustained for the duration of the stimulus and actually continues for two time steps after the stimulus ceases. (C) Every even-numbered inhibitory input unit is activated as the stimulus skips an even-numbered excitatory input unit on each time step. Each inhibitory input unit asymmetrically inhibits all hidden units with the same or lower index. (D) Every odd-numbered hidden unit is activated by the skipping stimulus. The prolonged responses of the hidden units are truncated by prolonged inhibition from the inhibitory input units, except for the last hidden unit. The activity of the last hidden unit persists even after the stimulus is terminated and slightly prolongs the sustained response of the output unit (shown in B). For ease of comparison the synaptic delay due to propagation from the input to the output through the network is not exhibited by the responses.

we consider yet another model of visual processing, but one that differs from the direction-selectivity model in a fundamental way.

12.2 Modeling Visual Processing as Bottom-Up/ Top-Down Probabilistic Inference

The simplified version of the direction-selectivity (asymmetric inhibition) network is purely feedforward. Even the elaborated version, which allows individual units in certain layers to send a recurrent projection to themselves, is essentially feedforward. In both versions, input units project to hidden units, and hidden units project to the output unit, but the hidden units do not project back to the input units, and the output unit sends no back projections to any layer. This feedforward architecture, adopted for simplicity, is unlike that of the real visual system overall, in which back projections are nearly as common as forward projections (van Essen 1985). The interaction between forward (bottom-up) and backward (top-down) projections has important implications for processing in the visual system (and in neural systems more generally). We will explore some of those implications in this section.

Some of the forward and backward projections in the early visual system are schematized in Figure 12.5 (Grossberg et al. 1997). Neurons in the lateral geniculate nucleus (LGN) of the thalamus project to neurons in visual cortical area V1, which in turn project to neurons in visual cortical area V2, but V2 projects back to V1, and V1 projects back to LGN. A model with this structure, which also includes lateral connections between units at the same level, was used by Grossberg and co-workers to simulate illusory visual perceptions (Grossberg et al. 1997). One example is the Kanizsa square, an illusory square that is perceived to lie above other geometric shapes, parts of which seem to

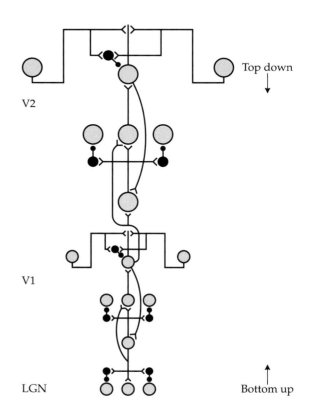

FIGURE 12.5   A model that reproduces some of the connectivity of the visual system The model represents connections within and between the lateral geniculate nucleus (LGN) and visual cortical areas V1 and V2. Note especially the bottom-up and top-down connections between visual areas at different levels of the organizational hierarchy. (After Grossberg et al. 1997.)

(A)   (B)

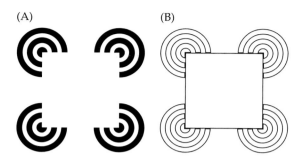

FIGURE 12.6   The Kanizsa-square percept can be simulated by a model of bottom-up/top-down processing in the visual system (A) The edges of a Kanizsa square can be perceived as colinear with edge inducers. (B) The model simulates perception of the Kanizsa square by filling in the line segments between the edge inducers. (After Grossberg et al. 1997.)

be occluded by the square (Kanizsa 1979). The Kanizsa square is perceived despite the fact that the occluding edges are discontinuous (Figure 12.6A). In the model, signals encoding actual edges are sent up from lower to higher levels, while signals encoding expected edges are sent down from higher to lower levels (Grossberg et al. 1997). The result is that missing edge segments are filled in, and lower-level units are activated as though the missing edges were actually present (Figure 12.6B). The model provides an elegant example of bottom-up/top-down processing in the visual system.

Despite their essential difference in architecture, the direction-selectivity (asymmetric-inhibition) model and the illusory-contour model (Grossberg et al. 1997) are similar in that they both work through an interaction between expected, or anticipated, input features and actual input features. Through a predominantly feedforward mechanism, the asymmetric-inhibition model anticipates that an input (light spot) will appear at a particular location. Similarly, the illusory-contour model anticipates that an input (edge) will appear at a particular location, but it combines both feedforward and feedback in its operation. Expectations are based on a complex constellation of input features in the illusory-contour model, while they rely on a single input feature in the direction-selectivity model. Despite their differences, both models incorporate certain units (such as the output unit of the direction-selectivity model) that are active only if expectations are confirmed (and not denied) by actual inputs. We will explore the interaction between expected and actual inputs in more detail in this and later sections. In so doing we will describe neural system function on three different levels: computational, algorithmic, and implementational (Marr 1982). (See also Chapter 9 for a detailed discussion of the levels of description of neural systems function.)

On the computational level, the goal of all the neural processes we explore in this chapter is to perceive more reliably, through an interaction between expectation and sensation. The two models we have discussed so far (the direction-selectivity and illusory-contour models) describe neural function on the implementational level. Although abstract, both of these models indicate how a neural system could accomplish its computational goal in terms of neural mechanism. The model we will consider next concerns neural function on the algorithmic level. Rather than describe a possible mechanism for the neural system, it will describe which quantities are represented by the system and in what way the system combines them so as to achieve its computational goal. This model simulates the effects of attention on visual processing and it involves an interaction between bottom-up and top-down influences. It rep-

(A) V4 neurons

(B) Model

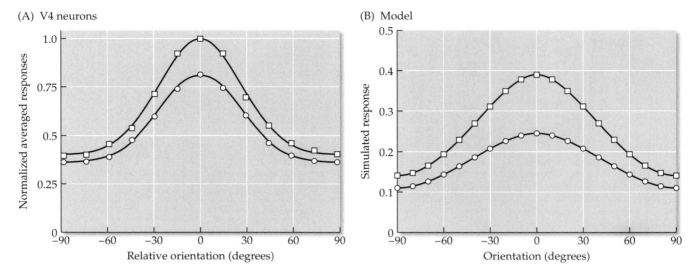

FIGURE 12.7 **Simulating the effects of attention on the responses of neurons in area V4 of monkey visual cortex: population responses** (A) The averaged responses of a sample of V4 neurons that are broadly tuned for orientation (circles) are enhanced when attention is directed to the stimulus location (squares). The differences in orientation selectivity between the neurons were removed before averaging. (B) This response enhancement is reproduced by the image-generation model by increasing the expectation (prior probability) of the stimulus location. (A after McAdams and Maunsell 1999; B after Rao 2005.)

resents the attributes of visual stimulus components (e.g., their orientations and locations) and, in describing how they might combine probabilistically to form images, will suggest a model of visual perception in general. While the model presents a compelling view of bottom-up/top-down processing in the visual system, its main purpose is to recast the somewhat nebulous concept of attention more concretely in terms of probabilistic inference.

Although the term "attention" is difficult to define precisely, factors that increase the attention paid by an animal to the location of a stimulus feature can increase the amplitude of the responses of neurons to that stimulus feature. Some data illustrating the effects of attention on the responses of neurons in visual cortex are illustrated in Figure 12.7. Figure 12.7A shows the averaged responses of broadly tuned orientation-selective neurons in area V4 of monkey visual cortex. (The differences in orientation selectivity between the neurons were removed before averaging.) Orientation-selective neurons are found in many regions of visual cortex. In Chapter 5 we studied orientation-selective neurons in area V1. Visual cortical area V4 receives projections from, and sends projections back to, area V2 (Van Essen 1985). The responses of V4 neurons at all orientations are enhanced when the monkey directs its attention to the location of the stimulus (McAdams and Maunsell 1999). Rao (2005) has simulated this effect (see Figure 12.7B) using a bottom-up/top-down model based on probabilistic inference. The model assumes that the response of a neuron in V4 reflects the probability that its preferred stimulus feature (e.g., a bar of light of a particular orientation) is present in the visual environment. It further assumes that enhancement by attention reflects an increase in this probability, brought about by an increase in the expectation by the monkey for stimuli to appear at the location in which a stimulus with the preferred feature is presented. Our next example will involve a simplified version of this model.

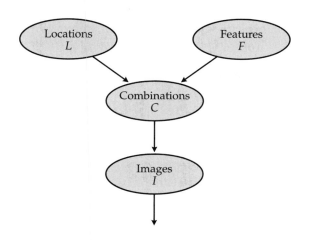

FIGURE 12.8   The image-generation model of processing in the visual system The model, which takes the form of a Bayesian network, is a generative (causal) probabilistic model of the formation of simple images from the locations of features of different orientations. Specifically, features (F) at various locations (L) combine (C) to form images (I). The generative model produces effects (images) from causes (locations and features), and can be used to infer the probabilities of causes from effects. (After Rao 2005.)

The model is schematized in Figure 12.8. This model is a directed graph, not a neural network, and it is intended to describe the function of the visual system on an algorithmic rather than an implementational level. The connections in the directed graph indicate the probabilistic relationships between its nodes, so they are drawn using arrows, rather than the synaptic connection symbols that are often used in neural networks. Each of the four nodes corresponds to a different random variable: location L, feature F, combination C, and image I. The directed graph, indicating the probabilistic relationships between these random variables, can be used to make inferences concerning the probabilities associated with some variables given known values for other variables. In that it can be used for probabilistic (i.e., Bayesian) inference, the directed graph shown in Figure 12.8 is an example of a Bayesian network (Pearl 1988; Jensen 2001).

Despite its abstractness and relative simplicity, this Bayesian network model is meant to represent a large part of the visual system (Rao 2005). Specifically, the image node I represents retinal receptor cells, and neurons in the retina that process visual inputs and send the results, via a relay through the lateral geniculate nucleus, to the visual cortex. The combination node C represents whole populations of neurons in areas V1 and V2 that encode images. The feature node F represents neurons in area V4 that are specialized for specific visual features, such as the orientations of bars of light or of edges. The location node L represents neurons such as those in parietal cortex that encode the locations of stimuli independently of feature values. In terms of the two main streams of visual processing, the feature nodes correspond to the "what" stream while the location nodes correspond to the "where" stream (Mishkin et al. 1983).

The Bayesian network model (see Figure 12.8) is generative, or causal, in the sense that it describes the generation of images from their causes. As such, we can refer to it more specifically as the image-generation model. It is based on the reasonable assumption that images are composed of visual stimuli, such as edges of different orientations, which are situated at specific locations. In the model, features (F) at particular locations (L) combine (C) to form images (I). The random variables I, C, L, and F take specific values i, c, l, and f, respectively. As we saw in Chapter 9, statistical dependencies between random variables permit inferences to be made concerning the probabilities of some variables given the probabilities, or known values, of other variables. Statistical dependencies are two-way relationships. Because inferences can be made in both directions, from causes to effects or from effects to causes, causal models can be used to simulate bottom-up/top-down interactions in the nervous system. With a bit of imagination, causal models could even be used to simulate perception.

Simply stated, perception involves the determination of the characteristics of the physical world from sensory input. More realistically, perception involves computation of the probabilities associated with the characteristics of the physical world, given sensory input that bears a probabilistic relationship with the world. In the simplified case of visual perception that we consider here, the visual system infers, from an image of the environment, the probabilities that specific features have appeared at specific locations. The causal image-generation model depicted in Figure 12.8 can accomplish this simplified rendition of visual perception.

To see how the image-generation model can be used as a model of the visual system, reconsider it first as a probabilistic model of the physical (visible) environment: visual features (edges, orientations) combine to form images. Given the values of some visual features, the model could be used as a computational tool to compute the probabilities of specific images. We can also consider the visual system as a computational tool, but the job it must do is the opposite. The visual system receives an image of the environment and must use that to compute the probabilities of visual features. For example, an image that is transduced by the early visual system (retina and lateral geniculate nucleus) is processed by cortex (V1, V2, V4, and parietal cortex) to determine the probabilities of various visual features. In this way the image-generation model can be used as a model of visual processing. In both cases (physical world or brain), inferences can be made in both the bottom-up and top-down directions. In the visual system, images are used bottom-up to infer visual features, but prior knowledge concerning visual features will influence, top-down, which images the system would expect to see. We will elaborate on these ideas throughout the rest of this section. Specifically, we will use the image-generation model to demonstrate bottom-up/top-down interactions and thereby simulate the attentional modulation of the responses of neurons in area V4 of visual cortex. Before we can do that we must specify the statistical dependencies that define the image-generation model.

The causal relationships in the model are specified in terms of the conditional probabilities between variables that are directly related. Variables that are not caused by other variables have unconditional probabilities assigned to them. Variables L (location) and F (feature) in the image-generation model are causeless. We assume that, disconnected from the graph, variables L and F are independent. This assumption implies that node F represents each stimulus feature independently of its location in the image, and that node L represents each location independently of the feature of the stimulus at that location. The independence of L and F when disconnected from the graph implies that their joint probabilities are equal to the product of their unconditional probabilities: $P(L = l, F = f) = P(L = l)P(F = f)$. Importantly, variables L and F become dependent when they are connected with variable C (combination) in the graph. (Probabilistic linkage of L and F through C will be demonstrated later in this section.) Intermediate variable C is caused by L and F, and variable I (image) is in turn caused by C. Thus, C depends directly on L and F, and I depends directly on C, and these causal relationships are defined in terms of the conditional probabilities assigned for $P(C = c \mid L = l, F = f)$ and $P(I = i \mid C = c)$. We will specify these causal relationships after we assign probabilities to the "causeless" variables.

The assignment of unconditional probabilities to causeless variables is of central importance in the model, because it indicates the expectations associated with those variables. As such, the unconditional probabilities assigned to causeless variables can be considered as the prior probabilities of the model. If we know the value of one or more of the random variables that are caused by other variables, then we can use the conditional probabilities between the variables, and the prior probabilities of the causeless variables, to infer the posterior probabilities of the unknown variables. (See Chapter 9 for a brief introduction to probabilistic inference.) In our simplified version of the image-generation model, we will know the value of the image variable. (I will equal some specific value i.) We will set the prior probabilities of the location and feature variables, and we will use the causal dependencies between all the variables to infer the posterior possibilities of the combination and feature variables. This inference will be used to simulate bottom-up/top-down processing in the visual system. Specifically, changes in the posterior probability of feature F given image I that are due to changes in the prior probability of location L will be used to simulate the effects of attention on the responses of orientation-selective visual neurons in area V4. Thus, attention will be equivalent to expectation, which will be equivalent to prior probability in the image-generation model.

The original version of the model (Rao 2005) included the nine images and combinations in which both locations (left *and* right) could contain either a horizontally orientated feature, a vertically oriented feature, or no feature (null). Constructing the full model with all nine images and combinations is the goal of Exercise 12.2. For the purposes of our example we will consider a simplified version of the model that includes only four images and four combinations. In the simple version, one and only one location (left *or* right) contains either a horizontally or a vertically oriented feature (there are no null stimuli). The images and combinations are shown in Figure 12.9. The illustra-

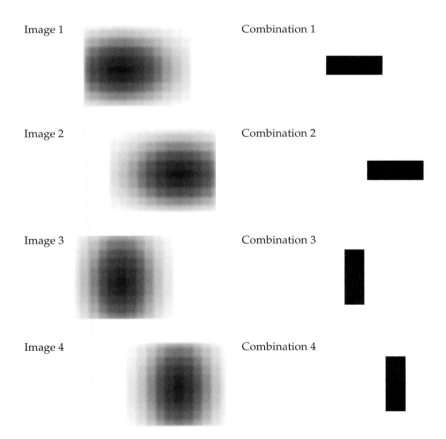

FIGURE 12.9   Pictorial representation of the images and combinations used for the simulation of bottom-up/top-down processing in the visual system Each of the four images (fuzzy blobs) can be characterized by some combination of location (left or right) and feature (orientation: horizontal or vertical).

TABLE 12.2   Prior and conditional probability tables for the image-generation model used in the bottom-up/top-down visual processing simulation

(A) Prior probability $P(L = l)$		(B) Prior probability $P(F = f)$	
$L = 1$	0.5	$F = 1$	0.5
$L = 2$	0.5	$F = 2$	0.5

(C) Conditional probability $P(C = c \mid L = l, F = f)$

	$L = 1, F = 1$	$L = 2, F = 1$	$L = 1, F = 2$	$L = 2, F = 2$
$C = 1$	0.5	0.1	0.1	0.3
$C = 2$	0.1	0.5	0.3	0.1
$C = 3$	0.1	0.3	0.5	0.1
$C = 4$	0.3	0.1	0.1	0.5

(D) Conditional probability $P(I = i \mid C = c)$

	$C = 1$	$C = 2$	$C = 3$	$C = 4$
$I = 1$	0.5	0.1	0.1	0.3
$I = 2$	0.1	0.5	0.3	0.1
$I = 3$	0.1	0.3	0.5	0.1
$I = 4$	0.3	0.1	0.1	0.5

tions of the images as fuzzy, elongated blobs are meant to convey the uncertainty associated with the inference in this example, but the images and other variables are simply referenced by number in the probabilistic calculations.

The conditional and unconditional probabilities that define the image-generation model are listed in Table 12.2. The unconditional probabilities for L and F are shown in Table 12.2A and B, respectively. The prior probabilities for L or F reflect the expectations represented by the model that stimuli will appear at particular locations or have particular orientations. Initially, we will set up the model such that there is no expectation for stimulus location or feature. For the prior distributions to be valid, the prior probabilities of both locations, or of both features, must sum to 1. If we expect neither a particular location nor a particular feature we set $[P(L = 1) = P(L = 2) = 0.5]$ and $[P(F = 1) = P(F = 2) = 0.5]$. These prior distributions for location and feature are listed in Table 12.2A and B, respectively. In the model, expectation could be increased for some particular stimulus orientation as easily as for some particular stimulus location. In the experimental situation the attention of the subject (a monkey) was focused on a specific location in visual space and the effect of that on the orientation-specific responses of area V4 neurons was studied (McAdams and Maunsell 1999; Reynolds et al. 1999). To conform to the experimental situation, attention will be simulated in the model by increasing the prior probability of one location relative to the other.

The conditional probability $P(C = c \mid L = l, F = f)$ in Table 12.2C describes the probability of each combination given both a location and a feature. The first column in Table 12.2C assigns the highest probability to $P(C = 1 \mid L = 1, F = 1)$, since combination 1 (horizontal bar on the left) is most likely for a stimulus at location 1 (left side) with feature 1 (horizontal orientation). The same scheme assigns the highest probabilities to $P(C = 2 \mid L = 2, F = 1)$, $P(C = 3 \mid L = 1, F = 2)$, and $P(C = 4 \mid L = 2, F = 2)$ in the other columns in Table 12.2C. Similarly, the conditional probability $P(I = i \mid C = c)$ in Table

12.2D describes the probability of each image given each combination. The first column in Table 12.2D assigns the highest probability to $P(I = 1 \mid C = 1)$, since image 1 is most likely given combination 1. The same scheme assigns the highest probabilities to $P(I = 2 \mid C = 2)$, $P(I = 3 \mid C = 3)$, and $P(I = 4 \mid C = 4)$ in the other columns in Table 12.2D. Thus, the diagonal elements in Table 12.2C and D are the highest in their respective columns. The off-diagonal elements depart a bit from the scheme by which the diagonal elements were set, but they were chosen in a way that enhances the effect we wish to simulate in this example. The same general result is obtained over a wide range of conditional probability values (see also Exercise 12.2). Each column in Table 12.2C describes the conditional probability distribution for all four combinations given each conjunction of location and feature, so each column of Table 12.2C must sum to 1. Similarly, each column in Table 12.2D describes the conditional probability distribution for all four images given each combination, so each column of Table 12.2D must also sum to 1. Together, the prior and conditional probability distributions listed in Table 12.2 define the image-generation model.

We assume that the causal image-generation model, which we express on the algorithmic level and use the model to make probabilistic inferences, could be implemented by the real visual system. We further assume that the parameters on which the inference is based (i.e., the conditional and prior probability distributions) could be represented by the real visual system and could be learned by an animal through experience with the visual environment. In Chapter 9 we simulated multisensory integration on the algorithmic level as probabilistic (Bayesian) inference, and on the implementational level using sigmoidal neural units. We saw how the parameters of the inference problem could be represented as the weights of the inputs to the units, and how the values of those weights could be learned using plausible algorithms. We will address issues of implementation of causal models later in this section, after we study in detail how probabilistic inference in the image-generation model is carried out on the algorithmic level.

The most general method for probabilistic inference makes use of the joint probability distribution. The joint probability distribution contains the joint probabilities of all possible assignments of specific values to the random variables. By its causal structure, the image-generation model in Figure 12.8 specifies that all joint probabilities are computed according to Equation 12.3:

$$P(I = i, C = c, L = l, F = f) = \qquad\qquad \textbf{12.3}$$
$$P(I = i \mid C = c)P(C = c \mid L = l, F = f)P(L = l)P(F = f)$$

To take a specific example, the joint probability $P(I = 1, C = 1, L = 1, F = 1)$ is equal to the product $P(I = 1 \mid C = 1)P(C = 1 \mid L = 1, F = 1)P(L = 1)P(F = 1)$. Reading these values from the prior and conditional distributions in Table 12.2 we find that $P(I = 1, C = 1, L = 1, F = 1) = (0.5)(0.5)(0.5)(0.5) = 0.0625$. The entire joint probability distribution for the image-generation model is computed by script `BUTDjointDistribution`, listed in MATLAB Box 12.3. This script represents the probabilities in the prior and conditional distributions as defined in Table 12.2. For example, it represents the probability $P(L = 1)$ as `pl1`, which could be read as "the probability that $L = 1$." Similarly, it represents $P(C = 1 \mid L = 1, F = 1)$ as `pc1gl1f1`, which could be read as "the probability that $C = 1$ given $L = 1$ and $F = 1$," and it represents $P(I = 1 \mid C = 1)$ as `pi1gc1`, which could be read as "the probability that $I = 1$ given $C = 1$." We use g in these variable names to distinguish conditional from joint relationships. (In other sections in this chapter, and in other chapters, we omit the g because the relationships are unambiguous.)

MATLAB® BOX 12.3 This script simulates bottom-up/top-down processing in the visual system using the joint distribution.

```
% BUTDjointDistribution.m

% set initial prior distributions for location and feature
pl1=0.5; pl2=1-pl1;    pf1=0.5; pf2=1-pf1;
% set conditional distributions for combo given loc and feat
pc1gl1f1=0.5; pc1gl2f1=0.1; pc1gl1f2=0.1; pc1gl2f2=0.3;
pc2gl1f1=0.1; pc2gl2f1=0.5; pc2gl1f2=0.3; pc2gl2f2=0.1;
pc3gl1f1=0.1; pc3gl2f1=0.3; pc3gl1f2=0.5; pc3gl2f2=0.1;
pc4gl1f1=0.3; pc4gl2f1=0.1; pc4gl1f2=0.1; pc4gl2f2=0.5;
% set conditional distribution for image given combination
pi1gc1=0.5; pi1gc2=0.1; pi1gc3=0.1; pi1gc4=0.3;
pi2gc1=0.1; pi2gc2=0.5; pi2gc3=0.3; pi2gc4=0.1;
pi3gc1=0.1; pi3gc2=0.3; pi3gc3=0.5; pi3gc4=0.1;
pi4gc1=0.3; pi4gc2=0.1; pi4gc3=0.1; pi4gc4=0.5;

% compute the joint distribution (dimension order is I C L F)
joint=zeros(4,4,2,2);
joint(1,1,1,1)=pi1gc1*pc1gl1f1*pl1*pf1;
joint(2,1,1,1)=pi2gc1*pc1gl1f1*pl1*pf1;
joint(3,1,1,1)=pi3gc1*pc1gl1f1*pl1*pf1;
joint(4,1,1,1)=pi4gc1*pc1gl1f1*pl1*pf1;
joint(1,2,1,1)=pi1gc2*pc2gl1f1*pl1*pf1;
joint(2,2,1,1)=pi2gc2*pc2gl1f1*pl1*pf1;
joint(3,2,1,1)=pi3gc2*pc2gl1f1*pl1*pf1;
joint(4,2,1,1)=pi4gc2*pc2gl1f1*pl1*pf1;
joint(1,3,1,1)=pi1gc3*pc3gl1f1*pl1*pf1;
joint(2,3,1,1)=pi2gc3*pc3gl1f1*pl1*pf1;
joint(3,3,1,1)=pi3gc3*pc3gl1f1*pl1*pf1;
joint(4,3,1,1)=pi4gc3*pc3gl1f1*pl1*pf1;
joint(1,4,1,1)=pi1gc4*pc4gl1f1*pl1*pf1;
joint(2,4,1,1)=pi2gc4*pc4gl1f1*pl1*pf1;
joint(3,4,1,1)=pi3gc4*pc4gl1f1*pl1*pf1;
joint(4,4,1,1)=pi4gc4*pc4gl1f1*pl1*pf1;

joint(1,1,2,1)=pi1gc1*pc1gl2f1*pl2*pf1;
joint(2,1,2,1)=pi2gc1*pc1gl2f1*pl2*pf1;
joint(3,1,2,1)=pi3gc1*pc1gl2f1*pl2*pf1;
joint(4,1,2,1)=pi4gc1*pc1gl2f1*pl2*pf1;
joint(1,2,2,1)=pi1gc2*pc2gl2f1*pl2*pf1;
joint(2,2,2,1)=pi2gc2*pc2gl2f1*pl2*pf1;
joint(3,2,2,1)=pi3gc2*pc2gl2f1*pl2*pf1;
joint(4,2,2,1)=pi4gc2*pc2gl2f1*pl2*pf1;
joint(1,3,2,1)=pi1gc3*pc3gl2f1*pl2*pf1;
joint(2,3,2,1)=pi2gc3*pc3gl2f1*pl2*pf1;
joint(3,3,2,1)=pi3gc3*pc3gl2f1*pl2*pf1;
joint(4,3,2,1)=pi4gc3*pc3gl2f1*pl2*pf1;
joint(1,4,2,1)=pi1gc4*pc4gl2f1*pl2*pf1;
joint(2,4,2,1)=pi2gc4*pc4gl2f1*pl2*pf1;
joint(3,4,2,1)=pi3gc4*pc4gl2f1*pl2*pf1;
joint(4,4,2,1)=pi4gc4*pc4gl2f1*pl2*pf1;
```

(Continued on facing page)

MATLAB® BOX 12.3   (continued)

```matlab
joint(1,1,1,2)=pi1gc1*pc1gl1f2*pl1*pf2;
joint(2,1,1,2)=pi2gc1*pc1gl1f2*pl1*pf2;
joint(3,1,1,2)=pi3gc1*pc1gl1f2*pl1*pf2;
joint(4,1,1,2)=pi4gc1*pc1gl1f2*pl1*pf2;
joint(1,2,1,2)=pi1gc2*pc2gl1f2*pl1*pf2;
joint(2,2,1,2)=pi2gc2*pc2gl1f2*pl1*pf2;
joint(3,2,1,2)=pi3gc2*pc2gl1f2*pl1*pf2;
joint(4,2,1,2)=pi4gc2*pc2gl1f2*pl1*pf2;
joint(1,3,1,2)=pi1gc3*pc3gl1f2*pl1*pf2;
joint(2,3,1,2)=pi2gc3*pc3gl1f2*pl1*pf2;
joint(3,3,1,2)=pi3gc3*pc3gl1f2*pl1*pf2;
joint(4,3,1,2)=pi4gc3*pc3gl1f2*pl1*pf2;
joint(1,4,1,2)=pi1gc4*pc4gl1f2*pl1*pf2;
joint(2,4,1,2)=pi2gc4*pc4gl1f2*pl1*pf2;
joint(3,4,1,2)=pi3gc4*pc4gl1f2*pl1*pf2;
joint(4,4,1,2)=pi4gc4*pc4gl1f2*pl1*pf2;

joint(1,1,2,2)=pi1gc1*pc1gl2f2*pl2*pf2;
joint(2,1,2,2)=pi2gc1*pc1gl2f2*pl2*pf2;
joint(3,1,2,2)=pi3gc1*pc1gl2f2*pl2*pf2;
joint(4,1,2,2)=pi4gc1*pc1gl2f2*pl2*pf2;
joint(1,2,2,2)=pi1gc2*pc2gl2f2*pl2*pf2;
joint(2,2,2,2)=pi2gc2*pc2gl2f2*pl2*pf2;
joint(3,2,2,2)=pi3gc2*pc2gl2f2*pl2*pf2;
joint(4,2,2,2)=pi4gc2*pc2gl2f2*pl2*pf2;
joint(1,3,2,2)=pi1gc3*pc3gl2f2*pl2*pf2;
joint(2,3,2,2)=pi2gc3*pc3gl2f2*pl2*pf2;
joint(3,3,2,2)=pi3gc3*pc3gl2f2*pl2*pf2;
joint(4,3,2,2)=pi4gc3*pc3gl2f2*pl2*pf2;
joint(1,4,2,2)=pi1gc4*pc4gl2f2*pl2*pf2;
joint(2,4,2,2)=pi2gc4*pc4gl2f2*pl2*pf2;
joint(3,4,2,2)=pi3gc4*pc4gl2f2*pl2*pf2;
joint(4,4,2,2)=pi4gc4*pc4gl2f2*pl2*pf2;

% compute un-normalized posterior of feature 1 given image 1
pf1gi1JointU=joint(1,1,1,1)+joint(1,2,1,1)+...
    joint(1,3,1,1)+joint(1,4,1,1)+...
    joint(1,1,2,1)+joint(1,2,2,1)+...
    joint(1,3,2,1)+joint(1,4,2,1);

% compute un-normalized posterior of feature 2 given image 1
pf2gi1JointU=joint(1,1,1,2)+joint(1,2,1,2)+...
    joint(1,3,1,2)+joint(1,4,1,2)+...
    joint(1,1,2,2)+joint(1,2,2,2)+...
    joint(1,3,2,2)+joint(1,4,2,2);

% compute normalized posterior of feature 1 given image 1
pf1gi1Joint=pf1gi1JointU/(pf1gi1JointU+pf2gi1JointU);
```

The script `BUTDjointDistribution` defines a (hyper-cuboidal) joint probability distribution matrix using `joint=zeros(4,4,2,2)`, where the dimensions, in order, are I, C, L, and F, and calculates its entries $P(I = i, C = c, L = l, F = f)$ according to Equation 12.3. For example, it computes $P(I = 1, C = 1, L = 1, F = 1)$ using `joint(1,1,1,1)=pi1gc1*pc1gl1f1*pl1*pf1`. The

TABLE 12.3   **Joint probability distribution for the image-generation model used in the bottom-up/top-down visual processing simulation**

F = 1

(A) Joint probability $P(I = i, C = c, L = 1, F = 1)$

	C = 1	C = 2	C = 3	C = 4	
I = 1	0.0625	0.0025	0.0025	0.0225	
I = 2	0.0125	0.0125	0.0075	0.0075	
I = 3	0.0125	0.0075	0.0125	0.0075	L = 1
I = 4	0.0375	0.0025	0.0025	0.0375	

(B) Joint probability $P(I = i, C = c, L = 2, F = 1)$

	C = 1	C = 2	C = 3	C = 4	
I = 1	0.0125	0.0125	0.0075	0.0075	
I = 2	0.0025	0.0625	0.0225	0.0025	
I = 3	0.0025	0.0375	0.0375	0.0025	L = 2
I = 4	0.0075	0.0125	0.0075	0.0125	

F = 2

(C) Joint probability $P(I = i, C = c, L = 1, F = 2)$

	C = 1	C = 2	C = 3	C = 4	
I = 1	0.0125	0.0075	0.0125	0.0075	
I = 2	0.0025	0.0375	0.0375	0.0025	
I = 3	0.0025	0.0225	0.0625	0.0025	L = 1
I = 4	0.0075	0.0075	0.0125	0.0125	

(D) Joint probability $P(I = i, C = c, L = 2, F = 2)$

	C = 1	C = 2	C = 3	C = 4	
I = 1	0.0375	0.0025	0.0025	0.0375	
I = 2	0.0075	0.0125	0.0075	0.0125	
I = 3	0.0075	0.0075	0.0125	0.0125	L = 2
I = 4	0.0225	0.0025	0.0025	0.0625	

entire joint probability distribution for the image-generation model is shown in Table 12.3. Note in Table 12.3A that the value of the joint probability when $I = 1$, $C = 1$, $L = 1$, and $F = 1$ is 0.0625, as we computed it in the numerical example above. Note also that all of the values in the joint distribution must sum to 1 in order for the distribution to be valid.

The joint distribution can be used to infer the posterior probabilities of unknown variables given known values for other variables. This involves normalizing the joint probabilities of the unknown variables so that they sum to 1. For example, suppose we wish to infer the posterior probability that $C = c$, given that $I = 1$, $L = 1$, and $F = 1$. This knowledge narrows the entire joint distribution down to the row corresponding to $P(I = 1, C = c, L = 1, F = 1)$. This is the first row of Table 12.3A. If we normalize those values so that they sum to 1, then each entry corresponds to the posterior probability $P(C = c \mid I = 1, L = 1, F = 1)$. In other words, we can infer the posterior probability of any of the possible values of C given known values for all the other variables by normalizing the joint probabilities for all values of C and the known variables. The normalization is shown in mathematical form in Equation 12.4:

$$P(C = c \mid I = 1, L = 1, F = 1) = \frac{P(I = 1, C = c, L = 1, F = 1)}{\displaystyle\sum_C P(I = 1, C = c, L = 1, F = 1)} \qquad \textbf{12.4}$$

The joint distribution completely specifies the probabilistic relationships among the variables in a probabilistic model but, for large models with many variables, computation of the joint distribution is infeasible. Fortunately, determination of the entire joint distribution is not necessary, since the joint probabilities can be computed as needed directly from the conditional probabilities. By reference to Equation 12.3, Equation 12.4 can be rewritten in terms of conditional probabilities as in Equation 12.5:

$$P(C = c \mid I = 1, L = 1, F = 1) =$$
$$\frac{P(I = 1 \mid C = c)P(C = c \mid L = 1, F = 1)P(L = 1)P(F = 1)}{\displaystyle\sum_C P(I = 1 \mid C = c)P(C = c \mid L = 1, F = 1)P(L = 1)P(F = 1)} \qquad \textbf{12.5}$$

In the denominator of Equation 12.5, the terms $P(L = 1)$ and $P(F = 1)$ do not depend on C and could be taken out of the summation over C, but we will leave all terms inside summations to facilitate comparisons between the equations in this section.

The use of conditional probabilities for inference on directed graphs, such as the image-generation model in Figure 12.8, is made even more efficient through the method of belief propagation (Pearl 1988). By this method each node passes to each other node a message that can be used at the destination node to compute the posterior probability of its variable given known values for other variables. The message passing method is described briefly in Math Box 12.2. We will not use belief propagation for this example. The image-generation model is simple enough that we can compute posterior probabilities directly from the conditional probabilities (using equations such as Equation 12.5).

The posterior probability of any variable given the known value of any other single variable can also be computed directly from the conditional probabilities. For example, the posterior probability that $C = c$ given $I = 1$ can be computed as shown in Equation 12.6:

$$P(C = c \mid I = 1) =$$
$$\frac{\displaystyle\sum_L \sum_F P(I = 1 \mid C = c)P(C = c \mid L = l, F = f)P(L = l)P(F = f)}{\displaystyle\sum_C \sum_L \sum_F P(I = 1 \mid C = c)P(C = c \mid L = l, F = f)P(L = l)P(F = f)} \qquad \textbf{12.6}$$

Similarly, the posterior probability that $F = f$ given $I = 1$ can be computed as in Equation 12.7:

$$P(F = f \mid I = 1) =$$
$$\frac{\displaystyle\sum_C \sum_L P(I = 1 \mid C = c)P(C = c \mid L = l, F = f)P(L = l)P(F = f)}{\displaystyle\sum_C \sum_L \sum_F P(I = 1 \mid C = c)P(C = c \mid L = l, F = f)P(L = l)P(F = f)} \qquad \textbf{12.7}$$

Equation 12.7 is implemented in script `BUTDprobInference`, which is listed in MATLAB Box 12.4. (Equation 12.6, which computes $P(C = c \mid I = 1)$, is implemented similarly.) As a cross-check, the posterior probability $P(F = f \mid I = 1)$

MATH BOX 12.2   BELIEF PROPAGATION

Given a probabilistic causal model, the posterior probabilities of some nodes given values for the others can be computed using an algorithm known as belief propagation (Pearl 1988). An example from Rao (2005) involves the causal, image-generation model in Figure 12.8. Given a specific image, for example $I = 1$, belief propagation prescribes that the following "messages" m be passed from one node to another according to the arrows in the subscripts in Equations B12.2.1–B12.2.4:

$$m_{L \to C} = P(L = l), \quad m_{F \to C} = P(F = f) \tag{B12.2.1}$$

$$m_{C \to L} = \sum_C \sum_F P(C = c \mid L = l, F = f)P(F = f)P(I = 1 \mid C = c) \tag{B12.2.2}$$

$$m_{C \to F} = \sum_C \sum_L P(C = c \mid L = l, F = f)P(L = l)P(I = 1 \mid C = c) \tag{B12.2.3}$$

$$m_{I \to C} = P(I = 1 \mid C = c) \tag{B12.2.4}$$

The messages in Equation B12.2.1 are the prior probabilities of the locations and features before an image becomes available. The posterior probabilities of the unknown variables C (combination), L (location), and F (feature), given the known image $I = 1$ are computed by combining messages at each node, as shown in Equations B12.2.5–B12.2.7:

$$P(C = c \mid I = 1) = \frac{1}{\alpha} m_{I \to C} \sum_L \sum_F P(C = c \mid L = l, F = f) m_{L \to C} m_{F \to C} \tag{B12.2.5}$$

$$P(L = l \mid I = 1) = \frac{1}{\beta} m_{C \to L} P(L = l) \tag{B12.2.6}$$

$$P(F = f \mid I = 1) = \frac{1}{\gamma} m_{C \to F} P(F = f) \tag{B12.2.7}$$

where α, β, and γ are normalization constants that make each of the above posterior probabilities sum to 1 over their unknown variable. This message passing procedure is equivalent to the method we employ in the text to compute the posterior probabilities $P(C = c \mid I = 1)$ and $P(F = f \mid I = 1)$, using Equations 12.6 and 12.7, respectively. To see this, note that substitution of Equations B12.2.1 and B12.2.4 into Equation B12.2.5 produces the numerator of Equation 12.6, and the sum over $C = c$ of all such terms produces the denominator (equal to α). Similarly, substitution of Equation B12.2.3 into Equation B12.2.7 produces the numerator of Equation 12.7, and the sum over $F = f$ of all such terms produces the denominator (equal to γ).

is also computed using the joint distribution in `BUTDjointDistribution`. The posterior probability $P(F = f \mid I = 1)$, computed in the two scripts either by Bayesian inference or from the joint distribution, is held in variables `pf1gi1Bayes` and `pf1gi1Joint`, respectively.

In simulating attentional effects using the image-generation model of visual processing, we are interested in the posterior probabilities associated with the feature node as the prior probabilities associated with the location node are changed. Specifically, we are interested in changes in the posterior probability of feature 1 given image 1 [$P(F = 1 \mid I = 1)$] that result from changes in the prior probability distribution for location [$P(L = 1)$, $P(L = 2)$]. As already mentioned, we assume that, disconnected from the graph, features and locations are independent, meaning that knowing a location L would indicate nothing about a feature F. Connected to the graph, however, variables L and F become dependent through the combination variable C. The dependence of L and F through C has important implications for probabilistic inference using the model.

MATLAB® BOX 12.4   This script simulates bottom-up/top-down processing in the visual system using probabilistic inference.

```
% BUTDprobInference.m

% set initial prior distributions for location and feature
pl1=0.5; pl2=1-pl1;
pf1=0.5; pf2=1-pf1;

% set conditional distributions for combo given loc and feat
pc1gl1f1=0.5; pc1gl2f1=0.1; pc1gl1f2=0.1; pc1gl2f2=0.3;
pc2gl1f1=0.1; pc2gl2f1=0.5; pc2gl1f2=0.3; pc2gl2f2=0.1;
pc3gl1f1=0.1; pc3gl2f1=0.3; pc3gl1f2=0.5; pc3gl2f2=0.1;
pc4gl1f1=0.3; pc4gl2f1=0.1; pc4gl1f2=0.1; pc4gl2f2=0.5;

% set conditional distribution for image given combination
pi1gc1=0.5; pi1gc2=0.1; pi1gc3=0.1; pi1gc4=0.3;
pi2gc1=0.1; pi2gc2=0.5; pi2gc3=0.3; pi2gc4=0.1;
pi3gc1=0.1; pi3gc2=0.3; pi3gc3=0.5; pi3gc4=0.1;
pi4gc1=0.3; pi4gc2=0.1; pi4gc3=0.1; pi4gc4=0.5;

% compute un-normalized posterior of feature 1 given image 1
pf1gi1BayesU=pf1*...
    (pi1gc1*pc1gl1f1*pl1 + pi1gc2*pc2gl1f1*pl1+...
    pi1gc3*pc3gl1f1*pl1 + pi1gc4*pc4gl1f1*pl1+...
    pi1gc1*pc1gl2f1*pl2 + pi1gc2*pc2gl2f1*pl2+...
    pi1gc3*pc3gl2f1*pl2 + pi1gc4*pc4gl2f1*pl2);

% compute un-normalized posterior of feature 2 given image 1
pf2gi1BayesU=pf2*...
    (pi1gc1*pc1gl1f2*pl1 + pi1gc2*pc2gl1f2*pl1+...
    pi1gc3*pc3gl1f2*pl1 + pi1gc4*pc4gl1f2*pl1+...
    pi1gc1*pc1gl2f2*pl2 + pi1gc2*pc2gl2f2*pl2+...
    pi1gc3*pc3gl2f2*pl2 + pi1gc4*pc4gl2f2*pl2);

% compute normalized posterior of feature 1 given image 1
pf1gi1Bayes=pf1gi1BayesU/(pf1gi1BayesU+pf2gi1BayesU);
```

In the image-generation model, inferences concerning *F* are affected by the prior probabilities associated with *L* and vice-versa. For example, combination 1 combines the horizontal orientation (feature 1) with the left location (location 1) and image 1 is its most likely effect (see Figure 12.9). If we observe image 1, then we can infer that the posterior probability of combination 1 has increased, and we can infer, in turn, that the posterior probabilities of both of the causes of combination 1, feature 1 and location 1, have also increased. Increasing the prior probability, or expectation, of location 1 further increases the posterior probability of combination 1, which further increases the posterior probability of feature 1. Thus, features and locations are probabilistically linked through combinations. This linkage allows us to use the image-generation model to simulate the effects of attention on visual processing. By assuming that attention is equivalent to an increase in the expectation that a stimulus will occur at a particular location, we can simulate attention by changing the prior probability distribution for location so that the prior is higher for that location. Because it will change the posterior probability for combination, attention will also change the posterior probability for feature.

FIGURE 12.10 Using probabilistic inference to simulate bottom-up/top-down processing in the visual system This simulation using the image-generation model involves the image I, combination C, location L, and feature F units (see Figures 12.8 and 12.9). (A) The posterior probability $P(C = 1 \mid I = 1)$ of combination 1 given image 1. (B) The posterior probability $P(F = 1 \mid I = 1)$ of feature 1 given image 1. The location expectation determines the prior probability distribution for location. For the first condition (none) there is no expected location $[P(L = 1) = 0.5, P(L = 2) = 0.5]$. For the second condition (left) the expectation is higher at location 1 (on the left) than at location 2 $[P(L = 1) = 0.9, P(L = 2) = 0.1]$. For the third condition (right) the expectation is higher at location 2 (on the right) than at location 1 $[P(L = 1) = 0.1, P(L = 2) = 0.9]$. The prior probability of location affects the posterior probability of combination in the top-down direction. The posterior probability of combination then affects the posterior probability of feature in the bottom-up direction.

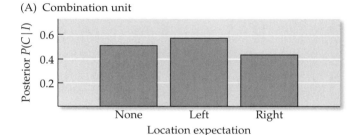

(A) Combination unit

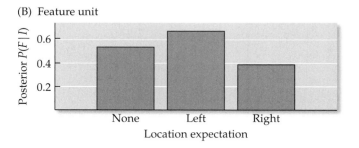

(B) Feature unit

Initially, there is no expectation either for a specific location or a specific feature, so the prior probability distributions for both are uniform: $[P(L = 1) = P(L = 2) = 0.5]$ and $[P(F = 1) = P(F = 2) = 0.5]$ (see Table 12.2A and B). With these uniform prior probabilities, each of the four combinations are equally likely: $P(C = 1) = P(C = 2) = P(C = 3) = P(C = 4) = 0.25$. Now suppose that image 1 appears. The posterior probability of combination 1 given image 1 $[P(C = 1 \mid I = 1)$, see Equation 12.6] increases to 0.50. This posterior probability is shown in Figure 12.10A as the first bar, which corresponds to location expectation "none" (where the prior probability distribution for location is uniform; no expectation for location). The increase in the posterior probability of combination 1 given image 1 $[P(C = 1 \mid I = 1)]$ causes an increase in the posterior probability of feature 1 given image 1 $[P(F = 1 \mid I = 1)$, see Equation 12.7 and `BUTDprobInference`] from its prior of 0.50 to 0.52. This posterior probability is shown in Figure 12.10B as the first bar, which corresponds to location expectation "none" (no expectation for location). Thus, sensory input, in the form of image 1, increases the posterior probability of combination 1, which in turn increases the posterior probability of feature 1. These effects are modulated by changes in the prior probability distribution for location, as we shall see.

Shifting attention toward location 1 can be simulated in the model by setting the prior probability higher for location 1: $[P(L = 1) = 0.9, P(L = 2) = 0.1]$. This change can be made in `BUTDprobInference` by setting `pl1=0.9`. (The script then computes `pl2=1-pl1`.) The effect of this change is to increase $P(C = 1 \mid I = 1)$ and $P(F = 1 \mid I = 1)$ to about 0.56 and 0.66, respectively, as shown for location expectation "left" (location 1) in Figure 12.10A and B. Shifting attention away from location 1 has the opposite effect. This can be simulated by setting the prior probability distribution for location to $[P(L = 1) = 0.1, P(L = 2) = 0.9]$ (and by setting `pl1=0.1` in `BUTDprobInference`). The effect of this change is to decrease $P(C = 1 \mid I = 1)$ and $P(F = 1 \mid I = 1)$ to about 0.43 and 0.37, respectively, as shown for location expectation "right" (location 2) in Figure 12.10A and B. Thus, the enhancement of area V4 neuron responses due to increased attention to the stimulus location, as well as the depression of responses due to increased attention to a different location, can both be simulated by the probabilistic inference, image-generation model of bottom-up/top-down interactions in the visual system.

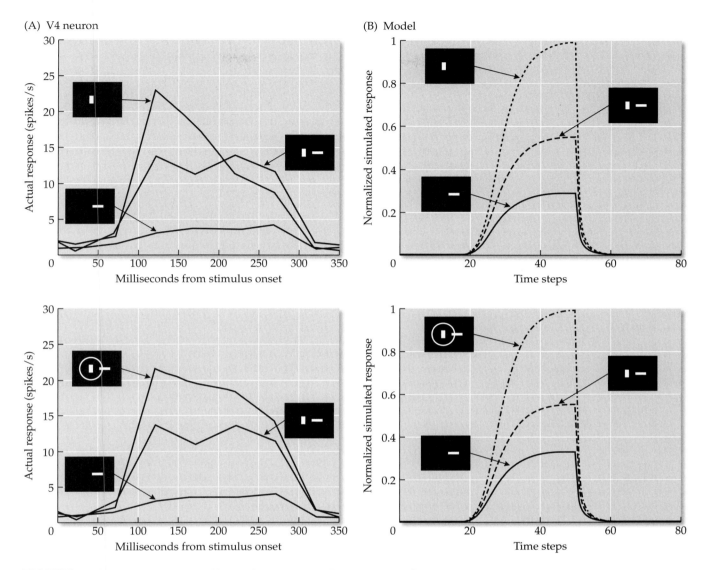

FIGURE 12.11 **Simulating the effects of attention on the responses of neurons in area V4 of monkey visual cortex: individual neuron responses** (A) The response of a V4 neuron with vertical orientation preference is maximal for a vertical bar presented alone, minimal for a horizontal bar presented alone, and of intermediate value for a vertical and a horizontal bar presented together. The response to the combined stimulus is enhanced when attention is directed to the location of the vertical bar. (B) These effects are reproduced by the image-generation model by increasing the expectation (prior probability) of the location in which the vertical bar is presented. (A after Reynolds et al. 1999; B after Rao 2005.)

The same image-generation model can be used to simulate the effects illustrated in Figure 12.11A and B, in which the response of an area V4 neuron, selective for the vertical orientation, to an image of a vertical bar on the left and a horizontal bar on the right is enhanced when attention is directed to the left side (Reynolds et al. 1999; Rao 2005). The "attentional effect" is interpreted in the model as an increase in the posterior probability of the vertical feature, brought about by an increase in the expectation (prior probability) of the location (left side) on which the vertical bar is presented. The simulation involves a larger set of images and combinations than were used in the example we considered, but the basic modeling approach is the same (see also Exercise 12.2).

The probabilistic image-generation model (see Figure 12.8) that we used to simulate attentional effects is representative of a class of Bayesian networks that can be used to simulate bottom-up/top-down processing in the visual system (Lee and Mumford 2003). These hierarchical Bayesian networks, like the image-generation model, are directed graphs, not neural networks. In principle, Bayesian network computations should be implementable using neural elements and neural networks. As we saw in Chapter 9 (specifically in Math Box 9.3), single sigmoidal units can compute the posterior probabilities of binary random variables when the log of the ratio of the two posteriors takes the form of a sum of logs. In graphical models such as the image-generation model, the ratio of the two posterior probabilities of a binary random variable such as feature F would take the less computationally convenient form of a log of sums (see Equation 12.7). A recurrent neural network implementation of the image-generation model that approximates the required log of sums has been proposed (Rao 2005). This model is composed of neural units that represent locations, features, and combinations. The combination units receive image input, and the location, feature, and combination units make recurrent connections with each other. Their stable-state responses equal posterior probabilities, as illustrated in Figure 12.11B. The details of this neural implementation are intricate and will not be considered here.

The probabilistic inference (i.e., Bayesian network or causal model) framework encompasses models based on the Kalman filter (Jensen 2001), but their specifics differ in an important respect. In hierarchical Bayesian models, predictions in the form of prior probabilities flow down, while observations flow up (e.g., Lee and Mumford 2003). In models based on hierarchical Kalman filtering, explicit predictions flow down, while the errors (residuals) between predictions and observations flow up (e.g., Rao 1999; Rao and Ballard 1999). Despite this difference, both the general Bayesian model and the more specific Kalman filter are examples of predictor–corrector models, because predictions are modified by observations in both cases.

An important respect in which the Bayesian and Kalman filter frameworks are similar is in their weighting, according to relative variance, of the prediction and observation (correction) terms. Specifically, in both cases, a higher weight is assigned to whichever of the prediction or the correction has the smaller variance. While the Kalman gain specifies this weighting explicitly, it emerges automatically in the more general Bayesian framework. We will explore this trade-off in our next example.

12.3 A Predictor–Corrector Model of Predictive Tracking by Midbrain Neurons

Some of the clearest behavioral examples of predictor–corrector systems involve target tracking under challenging circumstances. As we discussed at the beginning of the chapter, batters in baseball (and batsmen in cricket) seem to predict the trajectory of a pitch (bowl) in the initial instants after it is thrown, and to correct that prediction by observation (using peripheral vision in baseball, or at the bounce in cricket). The combination of prediction and correction helps players estimate where and when the ball will reach them (DeLucia and Cochran 1985; Land and McLeod 2000). The human ability to track moving targets may have evolved along with hunting. Obviously, many wild predators need to hunt in order to survive, but certain domesticated

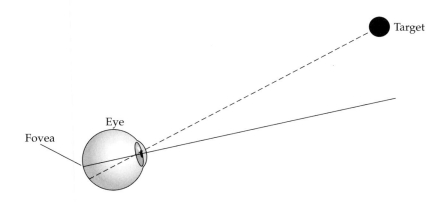

FIGURE 12.12   Schematic illustrating retinal position error Retinal position error is the difference (in degrees) between the retinal position of the fovea and the image of the target on the retina.

animals, who like civilized humans do not need to hunt, still seem to relish the thrill of the chase.

A cat must visually track a mouse in order to catch it. The responses of neurons in the parabigeminal nucleus, located in the cat midbrain, seem to encode the predicted location of a moving visual target during brief periods in which the target becomes invisible. We will use a predictor–corrector approach to simulate that behavior. In the next section (Section 12.4) we will explore how a target-tracking predictor–corrector mechanism might be implemented by neurons. There we will use a very simple neural model that exploits a recurrent connection to anticipate moving target location. In this section we will consider an algorithmic description of a predictor–corrector system that is based on probabilistic inference. In this scenario, the system makes a prediction about the current position of a moving target using its past estimate of target position, and it also observes the current position of the target, but both its prediction and its observation are uncertain. To reduce this uncertainty, the system combines its prediction with its observation (correction) using Bayesian inference to estimate current target position. Both models can be used to derive experimentally testable predictions, and both provide insight into how prediction and correction might actually interact in the brain to improve perception.

In order for a cat to visually track a mouse, it must move its eyes so that its fovea (the high-acuity part of its retina) is in line with (looks at) the target (Figure 12.12). Visual tracking in cats is not smooth, but consists of a series of discrete gaze shifts, or saccades (Figure 12.13A). The brain structure in mammals responsible for producing saccadic eye-movement commands is the superior colliculus (SC; see Chapter 3 for background on the SC). Also located in the midbrain, the SC is a layered structure that can be subdivided into superficial (SSC) and deep (DSC) layers. The SSC is a purely sensory structure, while the DSC is sensory-motor (Wurtz and Goldberg 1989).

Both the SSC and the DSC are organized retinotopically, but for simplicity we can think of them as representing two-dimensional maps of space. A visual stimulus in a certain region of space will activate neurons in the corresponding region of the SSC (and the DSC). Likewise, a burst of activity in a circumscribed region of the DSC constitutes a saccade command that will move the eyes so that the fovea is in line with the corresponding region of space (Wurtz and Goldberg 1989). The activity of SC neurons is usually studied using stationary targets. Such targets appear in a certain region of space and stay there while the cat makes a saccade toward them. More recent work is focused on moving targets, which cats try to acquire using a series of gaze shifts known as catch-up saccades (Cui and Malpeli 2003). A catch-up saccade is made to reacquire a target after it has moved a certain distance away from the fovea

FIGURE 12.13 The activity of a neuron in the parabigeminal nucleus (PBN) of a cat as it tracks a visible target In this case the target is a light spot moving horizontally at an angular velocity of 3 degrees/s. (A) The eye makes a series of saccades that intermittently "catch up" with the target. The solid and dashed lines, respectively, show eye and target angular positions in degrees. (B) The retinal position error (see Figure 12.12) is small right after a saccade but increases between saccades as the target continues to move while the eye remains stationary. (C) The activity (instantaneous firing rate in action potentials, or spikes, per second) of the PBN neuron is closely correlated with retinal position error. (After Cui and Malpeli 2003.)

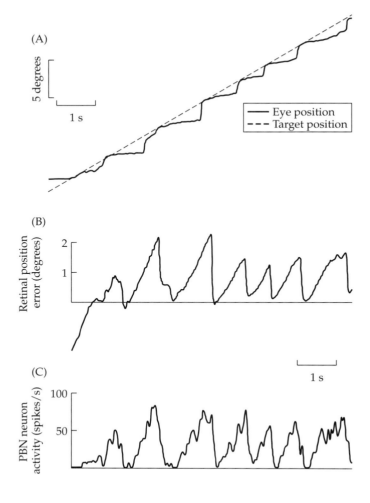

(see Figure 12.13A). The target is briefly centered on the fovea during the subsequent fixation (eye-stationary) period, and then another catch-up saccade is made to reacquire the target after it has again moved away from the fovea.

The critical signal for saccadic tracking is the difference between the retinal position of the fovea and of the image on the retina of the target. The difference between foveal position and target image position is called retinal position error (Figure 12.13B), but we can also think of it simply as target position relative to some fixed reference (such as the fovea; see also Figure 12.12). To illustrate this, we can consider the SC, which is actually a paired structure that encodes space in two dimensions, as a single, one-dimensional map of space. This simple SC (SSC or DSC) can be represented as a linear array of units that encodes target position according to the location of the unit in the array that is active. This one-dimensional model is illustrated for the SSC in Table 12.4, where the fovea is represented by the location at the center. We deliberately use a table (see Table 12.4), rather than a figure, to illustrate our one-dimensional model of the SSC, because this tabular format is compatible with tables we will use subsequently for numerical examples of probabilistic inference in scaled-down versions of the target-tracking predictor–corrector model.

In the one-dimensional model of space (see Table 12.4A), the target is displaced two spaces from the center in the positive direction. Its position is encoded correctly by the activity of the SSC unit located two units in the positive direction from the foveal representation within the SSC (see Table 12.4B). If the SSC unerringly encoded target position, then use of a predictor–corrector mechanism would be unnecessary, but this is probably not the case. More real-

TABLE 12.4   **Representing one dimension of visual and retinal space, the position of a target in space, and the location of an active unit in a one-dimensional model of the superficial superior colliculus (SSC)**

(A) Space, showing target position relative to the center

				Center		Target	
Visual space	−3	−2	−1	0	+1	+2	+3
Indices of positions	1	2	3	4	5	6	7

(B) SSC observation, showing location of active unit relative to fovea

				Fovea		Active unit	
Retinal space	−3	−2	−1	0	+1	+2	+3
Indices of SSC units	1	2	3	4	5	6	7

Each column corresponds (A) to a position in visual space or (B) to a location on the retinotopic SSC map. Each column is located (A) relative to the center of space, or (B) to the region corresponding to the fovea in the SSC (first row in each table). Each position (A) or unit (B) can be identified using an integer index (second row in each table).

istically, the SSC encodes target position with some uncertainty. For example, the activity of the SSC unit corresponding to target position +2 could signify that the target is at position +2 in space with some probability less than 1, but that it is also at positions +1 and +3 with some probability greater than 0.

To reduce this uncertainty, the brain might employ a predictor–corrector mechanism for target tracking. Such a system could make use of its previous estimates of target position to form a prediction. For example, the system could use a series of past target-position estimates to form an estimate of target velocity, or of target displacement per unit time. It could then predict that target position on the next time step should be the sum of its current estimate of target position and its estimate of target displacement per unit time. This prediction would also be uncertain, but the uncertainties of the prediction and the observation (from the SSC) would be reduced by combining them probabilistically.

This model assumes that the target-tracking system makes predictions of target position from past estimates, and that it receives corrections in the form of inputs from the SSC concerning observations of target position. The target-tracking system might also have access to the saccadic commands generated by the DSC. If the DSC produces a burst of activity in some local region, then the system would have a measure of the size of the saccadic command, and it could subtract the size of that command from its current estimate of target position to predict target position after the saccade. Thus, target-position prediction in this system would have two modes. In the absence of a saccadic command from the DSC, the system would compute its target-position prediction on the basis of its previous velocity and position estimates. In the presence of a saccadic command from the DSC, the system would compute its prediction on the basis of its previous target position estimate and the DSC saccadic command. While this scheme seems to make sense intuitively, it is difficult to see how uncertainty would be represented in it. Rather than try to calculate saccade metrics and estimate target velocities explicitly, we will construct the target-tracking predictor–corrector model in terms of probabilistic relationships among random variables, as in the visual processing model of the previous section (see Section 12.2).

We will base the design of the target-tracking predictor–corrector system on that of the decision-theoretic agent, which involves probabilistic infer-

MATH BOX 12.3   DECISION-THEORETIC AGENT DESIGN

The decision-theoretic agent uses a predictor-corrector mechanism in choosing the optimal action on each time step. Decision-theoretic agent design provides a generalized framework in which prediction and correction are combined with action selection, and in which the prediction is based both on the previous estimate and on the possible outcomes of the selected action (Russell and Norvig 1995). On each time step (t), the decision agent takes an observation from the environment in random variable $O(t)$, and returns a decision on the action to be taken $A(t)$. The agent maintains the distribution $P(S(t)|O(t))$ of the posterior probabilities of the states $S(t)$ given the observation $O(t)$, which it updates on each time step. The operation of the decision-theoretic agent can be described by Equations B12.3.1–B12.3.3, which are implemented in a recurring sequence:

$$P\big(S(t)\big) = \sum_{S(t-1)} P\big(S(t)\,|\,S(t-1),\,A(t-1)\big)P\big(S(t-1)\,|\,O(t-1)\big) \qquad \text{B12.3.1}$$

$$P\big(S(t)\,|\,O(t)\big) = \frac{P\big(O(t)\,|\,S(t)\big)}{P\big(O(t)\big)}P\big(S(t)\big) \qquad \text{B12.3.2}$$

$$A(t) = \arg\max_{A(t)} \sum_{S(t)}\left[P\big(S(t)\,|\,O(t)\big) \sum_{S(t+1)} P\big(S(t+1)\,|\,S(t),\,A(t)\big)U\big(S(t+1)\big)\right] \qquad \text{B12.3.3}$$

The state transitions are Markovian, meaning that the next state depends only on the previous state. Note that Equations B12.3.1 and B12.3.2 are written in terms of the specific state $S(t) = s(t)$ given observation $O(t) = o(t)$, but they are used to update the prior $P(S(t) = s(t))$ and posterior $P(S(t) = s(t)\,|\,O(t) = o(t))$ probabilities for all possible states s on each time step.

By Equation B12.3.1, each prediction $P(S(t))$ is the sum of the probability of each state given the previous states and action $P(S(t)\,|\,S(t-1),\,A(t-1))$, weighted by the previous state estimates $P(S(t-1)\,|\,O(t-1))$. By Equation B12.3.2, the current state estimates are the posterior probabilities $P(S(t)\,|\,O(t))$ of the states $S(t)$ given the observation $O(t)$, where the updated prior probabilities $P(S(t))$ are the predictions computed in Equation B12.3.1. By Equation B12.3.3, the chosen next action is the one that maximizes the expected value, where the value of each state at time $(t + 1)$ is given by $U(S(t + 1))$ (for details see Russell and Norvig 1995).

ence in time based on predictions, observations, and actions. (See Russel and and Norvig 1995 for details.) The operation of the decision-theoretic agent is briefly summarized in Math Box 12.3. Decision-theoretic agent design generally assumes Markov state transitions, so that the next state depends only on the previous state. For simplicity, we will adopt the Markov assumption in the design of the target-tracking predictor–corrector model. The decision-theoretic agent finds the action on each time step that has the highest expected value. (See Chapter 11 for a detailed discussion of expected values and how they can be learned in a Markov environment.) For simplicity, we will not decide among various actions on the basis of expected values but will have only one action, which will be a catch-up saccade, generated whenever target position relative to the fovea exceeds a threshold. This action will deterministically bring the fovea back in line with target position.

The target-tracking predictor–corrector model is schematized in Figure 12.14. The nodes in the model correspond to random variables. Specifically, random variable T represents target position, while random variable V represents the location on the SSC of the unit that is activated by the visible target. These random variables are functions of time. So as not to confuse them with other variable names, we will denote specific values of T as t_S, and specific values of V as v_S. This will enable us to continue to use t to denote discrete time. To further distinguish a specific target value t_S from discrete time, in this chapter we will always enclose discrete time in parentheses as in (t) or ($t - 1$). By using the shorthand $P(T) \equiv P(T = t_S)$, which we

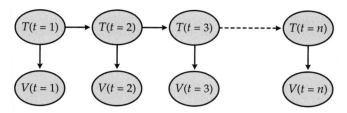

FIGURE 12.14   Schematic of the target-tracking predictor–corrector model
This causal model takes the form of a dynamic Bayesian network. Random variables
T and V stand for target position and visual input, respectively, and (t) represents
discrete time in steps from 1 to n. The position of the target on any time step can be
probabilistically inferred from the position of the target on the previous time step
and the visual input on the current time step.

introduced in Chapter 8, we will rarely need to use the variable t_S for specific target
values. In contrast, we will frequently use terms of the form $V(t)$, which denotes the
value of the visual input V (from the SSC) on time step (t), and $T(t)$, which denotes
the position of target T on time step (t).

Like the image-generation model of visual processing (see Section 12.2),
the target-tracking predictor–corrector model is causal. It takes the form of
a directed graph, with arrows that signify causal dependencies between its
nodes. The nodes represent the target T and visual input V random variables.
Unlike the image-generation model, the target-tracking model is time-depen-
dent. Thus, target position on the previous time step $T(t-1)$ "causes" target
position on the current time step $T(t)$. Also, target position on any time step
$T(t)$ causes a visual sensory input $V(t)$ on that time step. Given this causal
structure, predictions based on target position on the previous time step can
be corrected by observations on the current time step, in order to infer the
probability of target position on the current time step.

There is an important respect in which the target-tracking predictor–corrector model will differ from the image-generation model of visual processing
(see Section 12.2). With its prior and conditional probabilities specified, we
used the image-generation model to infer the probability that one random
variable took one of its possible values (e.g., that the feature variable F took
value 1), given the known value of another random variable (e.g., the image
variable I takes value 1). We will go to the other extreme in our use of the
target-tracking model to infer, on every time step, the probability that the
target is at each one of its possible positions ($T = t_S$ where $t_S = 1,..., n_P$ and
n_P is the number of possible target positions). To make that inference we will
use the current observation, but will also use the posterior probability that the
target was at each of its possible positions on the previous time step (previous estimate), and the prior probability that the target is at each of its possible
positions on the current time step (prediction). Thus, the target-tracking model
will update the entire target-position probability distribution on every time
step. In that it will maintain a representation of an entire probability distribution, the target-tracking predictor–corrector model is similar to some of the
population encoding schemes we discussed at the end of Chapter 9.

Equations 12.8 and 12.9 describe the predictor–corrector mechanism.

$$P\big(T(t)\big) = \sum_{T(t-1)} P\big(T(t)\,|\,T(t-1),\,A(t-1)\big)P\big(T(t-1)\,|\,V(t-1)\big) \qquad \textbf{12.8}$$

$$P\big(T(t)\,|\,V(t)\big) = \frac{P\big(V(t)\,|\,T(t)\big)}{P\big(V(t)\big)}\,P\big(T(t)\big) \qquad \textbf{12.9}$$

The evidence (unconditional probability) $P(V(t))$ in Equation 12.9 can be computed according to the principle of total probability as in Equation 12.10:

$$P\big(V(t)\big) = \sum_{T(t)} P\big(V(t) \,|\, T(t)\big) P\big(T(t)\big) \qquad \textbf{12.10}$$

Together, Equations 12.8, 12.9, and 12.10 describe the target-tracking predictor-corrector model.

The heart of the target-tracking predictor–corrector system is Equation 12.9, which is Bayes' rule (see Chapter 9). At any time (t), Equation 12.9 specifies that the posterior probability $P(T(t) \,|\, V(t))$ of the target given the visual input is the ratio $P(V(t) \,|\, T(t)) \,/\, P(V(t))$ between the likelihood and the evidence of the visual input, multiplied by the prior probability $P(T(t))$ of the target. Note that the term $P(T(t) \,|\, V(t))$ is shorthand for the term $P(T(t) = t_S \,|\, V(t) = v_S)$ where, again, v_S stands for a specific visual input and t_S stands for a specific target position, while (t) stands for a discrete time step. On every time step the target-tracking model computes the posterior probability of the target at each possible position. (That is, it computes the entire target posterior probability distribution.) This could be done by applying Equation 12.9 separately to find $P(T(t) = 1 \,|\, V(t) = v_S)$, $P(T(t) = 2 \,|\, V(t) = v_S)$, ..., $P(T(t) = n_P \,|\, V(t) = v_S)$, where n_P is the number of possible target positions. Alternatively, the process could be vectorized. We will use a vectorized approach to find the distribution of the target posterior $P(T(t) \,|\, V(t))$ (see later in this section). The target posterior probability distribution is then used by the model to make its estimate of target position. Specifically, the target-position estimate of the target-tracking model at any time (t) is taken as the target position with the highest posterior probability.

The element of time in the target-tracking model is incorporated by Equation 12.8, which specifies that the prior probability distribution $P(T(t))$ on the current time step is a function of two probability distributions: $P(T(t - 1) \,|\, V(t - 1))$ and $P(T(t) \,|\, T(t - 1), A(t - 1))$. The distribution $P(T(t - 1) \,|\, V(t - 1))$ is the posterior probability on the previous time step. It is the distribution from which the system drew its target position estimate on the previous time step. The distribution $P(T(t) \,|\, T(t - 1), A(t - 1))$ is the conditional probability of target position on the current time step $T(t)$ given the target position $T(t - 1)$ and the action $A(t - 1)$ on the previous time step. Action $A(t - 1) = 1$ corresponds to the catch-up saccade commanded by the DSC that brings target position relative to the fovea deterministically back to 0. Specifically, $P(T(t) \,|\, T(t - 1), A(t - 1) = 1)$ equals 1 for $T(t) = t_F$, where t_F is position 0 relative to the fovea, and equals 0 for all other target positions. In between catch-up saccades, when $A(t - 1) = 0$, the conditional probability $P(T(t) \,|\, T(t - 1), A(t - 1) = 0)$ can be thought of as a probabilistic model of the movement of the target relative to the fovea [$T(t)$ given $T(t - 1)$]. This conditional probability embodies the Markov assumption that current target position depends only on previous target position. In principle, a conditional probability $P(T(t) \,|\, T(t - 1), T(t - 2),..., T(t - n), A(t - 1) = 0)$ could be specified instead that would take target positions at n previous time points into account, but since the end result in any case is the determination of the prior probability $P(T(t))$, the Markov assumption entails no loss of generality.

The target-tracking predictor–corrector model operates by successively applying Equations 12.8 and 12.9 (the denominator of Equation 12.9 is computed by Equation 12.10). On every time step the model computes the prior probability $P(T(t))$ of the target at each possible position (see Equation 12.8). The predicted target position is whichever target position has the highest prior probability. Also on every time step, the model computes the posterior probability $P(T(t) \,|\, V(t))$ of the target at each possible position (see Equation 12.9).

TABLE 12.5   The likelihood and conditional probability tables (reduced size versions) for the target-tracking predictor–corrector model of parabigeminal nucleus (PBN) neurons

(A) Likelihood $P(V(t) \mid T(t))$

	$T(t) = 1$	$T(t) = 2$	$T(t) = 3$	$T(t) = 4$	$T(t) = 5$	$T(t) = 6$	$T(t) = 7$
$V(t) = 1$	0.8	0.1	0	0	0	0	0.1
$V(t) = 2$	0.1	0.8	0.1	0	0	0	0
$V(t) = 3$	0	0.1	0.8	0.1	0	0	0
$V(t) = 4$	0	0	0.1	0.8	0.1	0	0
$V(t) = 5$	0	0	0	0.1	0.8	0.1	0
$V(t) = 6$	0	0	0	0	0.1	0.8	0.1
$V(t) = 7$	0.1	0	0	0	0	0.1	0.8

(B) Conditional probability $P(T(t) \mid T(t-1), A(t-1) = 0)$

	$T(t-1) = 1$	$T(t-1) = 2$	$T(t-1) = 3$	$T(t-1) = 4$	$T(t-1) = 5$	$T(t-1) = 6$	$T(t-1) = 7$
$T(t) = 1$	0.2	0.1	0	0	0.1	0.2	0.4
$T(t) = 2$	0.4	0.2	0.1	0	0	0.1	0.2
$T(t) = 3$	0.2	0.4	0.2	0.1	0	0	0.1
$T(t) = 4$	0.1	0.2	0.4	0.2	0.1	0	0
$T(t) = 5$	0	0.1	0.2	0.4	0.2	0.1	0
$T(t) = 6$	0	0	0.1	0.2	0.4	0.2	0.1
$T(t) = 7$	0.1	0	0	0.1	0.2	0.4	0.2

(C) Conditional probability $P(T(t) \mid T(t-1), A(t-1) = 1)$

	$T(t-1) = 1$	$T(t-1) = 2$	$T(t-1) = 3$	$T(t-1) = 4$	$T(t-1) = 5$	$T(t-1) = 6$	$T(t-1) = 7$
$T(t) = 1$	0	0	0	0	0	0	0
$T(t) = 2$	0	0	0	0	0	0	0
$T(t) = 3$	0	0	0	0	0	0	0
$T(t) = 4$	1	1	1	1	1	1	1
$T(t) = 5$	0	0	0	0	0	0	0
$T(t) = 6$	0	0	0	0	0	0	0
$T(t) = 7$	0	0	0	0	0	0	0

The estimated target position is whichever target position has the highest posterior probability. The posterior probability is computed using Bayes' rule (see Equation 12.9). As such, it represents the prior probability $P(T(t))$ after it has been modified by the ratio of the likelihood $P(V(t) \mid T(t))$ to the evidence $P(V(t))$ (see Chapter 9 for background on Bayes' rule). Thus, using the target-tracking predictor–corrector model, the prior $P(T(t))$ constitutes the prediction that is corrected by visual input $P(V(t) \mid T(t)) / P(V(t))$ to produce the estimate $P(T(t) \mid V(t))$, which is the posterior probability computed using Bayes' rule (see Equation 12.9).

The operation of the target-tracking predictor–corrector system is illustrated using a numerical example in Tables 12.5 and 12.6. The "space" in this example consists of only seven positions (as in Table 12.4). Because the target can appear at only one position at a time, random variable T has only seven states. For simplicity, we will restrict the SSC to only one active unit at a time, so that random variable V also will have only seven states. (For the purpose of reducing the number of possible states, we made a similar simplification to a model of the SC in Chapter 8.) Note that the states of random variable T

TABLE 12.6   Prediction and correction in a (reduced size) model of the responses of neurons in the parabigeminal nucleus (PBN)

(A) Space, showing target positions relative to the fovea

−3	−2	−1	0	+1	+2	+3

(B) Previous posterior probability distribution (also the previous estimate)

0	0	0	1	0	0	0

(C) Current prior probability distribution

0	0	0.10	0.20	0.40	0.20	0.10

(D) Current predicted target position

0	0	0	0	1	0	0

(E) Current SSC observation, showing location of active unit

0	0	0	0	0	1	0

(F) Current likelihood distribution, based on SSC observation

0	0	0	0	0.10	0.80	0.10

(G) Current posterior probability distribution

0	0	0	0	0.19	0.76	0.05

(H) Current estimated target position

0	0	0	0	0	1	0

correspond to specific target positions. Similarly, the states of random variable V correspond to the locations of the active unit in the simulated SSC, and so also correspond to observations of the target at specific positions. We will make the conversion between states and positions frequently in this section, both in numerical examples and in MATLAB programs.

We will use the reduced space and model configurations depicted in Tables 12.4–12.6 to demonstrate how the target-tracking predictor–corrector model estimates target position. Specifically, we will use one observation $V = v_S$ and the prior probabilities for all target positions to compute the posterior probabilities for all target positions, and choose as our estimate whichever target position has the highest posterior probability. The likelihood $P(V(t) \mid T(t))$ and the conditional probability $P(T(t) \mid T(t-1), A(t-1))$ matrices for this example are shown in Table 12.5A–C. The likelihood matrix (see Table 12.5A) consists of shifted versions of the profile [0 0 0.1 0.8 0.1 0 0]. To see how the likelihood matrix is constructed, consider the column for which the target at time (t) is in state 4 ($T(t) = 4$). This corresponds to the central target position at 0 (see Table 12.4). The highest likelihood in this column (0.8) is for $V(t) = 4$, which corresponds to an input from the SSC that is also in state 4. However, there are nonzero probabilities that the visual (SSC) input is in nearby states. Specifically, when $T(t)=4$ the likelihood is 0.1 for each of $V(t) = 3$ and $V(t) = 5$. (Circular boundary conditions on the distributions are imposed for simplicity.) Note that each row of the likelihood distribution matrix specifies the probability of *one* visual input state given *each* target position state. Thus, one row of the likelihood distribution matrix can be used to update the posterior probabilities of all target positions (see Equations 12.9 and 12.10). Note also that the likelihood distribution matrix is symmetric, so its corresponding rows and columns are the same.

The conditional probability distribution matrix (target motion model) is split into two sections, one for $A(t-1) = 0$ (between saccades, see Table 12.5B) and another for $A(t-1) = 1$ (just after a saccade, see Table 12.5C). The conditional distribution matrix $P(T(t) \mid T(t-1), A(t-1) = 0)$, which probabilistically describes target motion between catch-up saccades, consists of shifted versions of the profile [0 0.1 0.2 0.4 0.2 0.1 0]. Note that this profile has a larger variance than the likelihood profile. Thus, the probabilistic model of target motion, from which the prediction is derived (see Equation 12.8), has a larger variance than the likelihood, from which the correction is derived (see Equations 12.9 and 12.10). This will have important implications for the behavior of the overall target-tracking predictor–corrector model.

The conditional probability matrix with $A(t-1) = 0$ (between saccades) is constructed in such a way that when, for example, the target at time $(t-1)$ was in state four ($T(t-1) = 4$), the probability at time (t) is highest (0.4) for the target in state *five* ($T(t) = 5$), but there are nonzero probabilities for $T(t)$ to be in other states as well (see the column corresponding to $T(t-1) = 4$ in Table 12.5B). The target states of $T(t-1) = 4$ and $T(t) = 5$ correspond to target positions relative to the fovea of 0 and +1, respectively. Thus, the conditional probability distribution matrix is constructed such that, between catch-up saccades ($A(t-1) = 0$), the target tends to move in the positive direction on each time step. After a catch-up saccade, when $A(t-1) = 1$, the probability at time (t) is 1 for the target in state 4 and 0 elsewhere (see Table 12.5C). This corresponds to the central target position of 0 (see Table 12.4). Thus, the conditional probability matrix just after a catch-up saccade $P(T(t) \mid T(t-1), A(t-1) = 1)$, is constructed such that the target is returned deterministically to position 0 relative to the fovea, regardless of the target position on the previous time step.

A numerical example involving vectorized versions of Equations 12.9 and 12.10, and some of the values in Tables 12.5 and 12.6, will illustrate the operation and the central features of the target-tracking predictor–corrector model. Specifically, the numerical example will illustrate how the model uses its observation to correct its prediction, and will also show how the relative variances of the observation and prediction determine the strength of their influence on the resulting estimate. Since Equations 12.9 and 12.10 both involve probabilities that all occur on the same time step (t) we can drop (t) from our notation for clarity. Let vector $P(\textbf{T})$ be the prior target probability distribution: $P(\textbf{T}) = [P(T = 1)\ P(T = 2) \ldots P(T = 7)]^T$, and assign to it specific probabilities as follows: $P(\textbf{T}) = [0\ 0\ 0.1\ 0.2\ 0.4\ 0.2\ 0.1]^T$. This is column 4 of the conditional probability distribution matrix $P(T(t) \mid T(t-1), A(t-1) = 0)$ in Table 12.5B. The target state with the highest prior probability is state 5 [$P(T = 5)$, the fifth element of $P(\textbf{T})$], and this corresponds to the prediction that the target is located at position +1 (see Table 12.6C and D; see also Table 12.6A for positions in space).

Now assume that a visual observation is made of a target at position +2 (as shown in Table 12.4). This observation would result in activation of SSC unit 6 ($V = 6$) (see Table 12.6E). Let vector $P(\textbf{V}_T)$ be the distribution of the likelihoods of this observation given each possible target state: $P(\textbf{V}_T) = [P(V = 6 \mid T = 1)\ P(V = 6 \mid T = 2) \ldots P(V = 6 \mid T = 7)]^T$, and assign probabilities as follows: $P(\textbf{V}_T) = [0\ 0\ 0\ 0\ 0.1\ 0.8\ 0.1]^T$. Note that this is the sixth row (transposed) of the likelihood distribution matrix (see Table 12.5A). According to Equation 12.10, the unconditional probability $P(V = 6)$ (or the evidence, which is a scalar) of observing this visual input $V = 6$ can be computed as the dot product $P(V) = P(\textbf{V}_T)^T P(\textbf{T})$. According to Equation 12.9, the target posterior distribution $P(\textbf{T}_V) = [P(T = 1 \mid$

$V = 6$) $P(T = 2 \mid V = 6)$ ... $P(T = 7 \mid V = 6)]^{\mathrm{T}}$ can then be computed as follows: $P(\boldsymbol{T}_{\mathrm{V}}) = [P(\boldsymbol{V}_{\mathrm{T}})/P(V)] \circ P(\boldsymbol{T})$, where $\circ$ corresponds to element-by-element multiplication. Note that the likelihood vector divided by the evidence $[P(\boldsymbol{V}_{\mathrm{T}})/P(V)]$ is the correction of the target-tracking predictor–corrector model. The posterior target probability distribution that results from this computation is $P(\boldsymbol{T}_{\mathrm{V}})^{\mathrm{T}} = [0\ 0\ 0\ 0\ 0.19\ 0.76\ 0.05]$ (as shown in Table 12.6G). The target state with the highest posterior probability is state 6 $[P(T = 6 \mid V = 6)$, the sixth element of $P(\boldsymbol{T}_{\mathrm{V}})]$, so this simple version of the model would estimate that the target is located at position +2, which corresponds to state 6 (see Table 12.6H and A). This example illustrates how the target-tracking model corrects its prediction in forming its estimate. Scrutiny of the prior and likelihood distribution vectors illustrates how these two components are weighted in determining the estimate.

Recall that the prior probability distribution vector is $P(\boldsymbol{T}) = [0\ 0\ 0.1\ 0.2\ 0.4\ 0.2\ 0.1]^{\mathrm{T}}$ (see Table 12.6C) while the likelihood distribution vector is $P(\boldsymbol{V}_{\mathrm{T}}) = [0\ 0\ 0\ 0\ 0.1\ 0.8\ 0.1]^{\mathrm{T}}$ (see Table 12.6F). Comparison of these two distribution vectors reveals that the prior vector has a larger variance than the likelihood vector. The prior vector corresponds to the prediction that the target is at position +1 (see Table 12.6D and A), while the likelihood vector corresponds to the observation (and correction) that the target is at position +2 (see Table 12.6E and A). The resulting estimate that the target is at position +2 (see Table 12.6H and A) indicates that the model weighted the correction more heavily than the prediction. Thus, the *weighting* of the correction relative to the prediction is related to the *variance* of the prediction relative to the correction. Specifically, the model effectively assigns a heavier weight to the distribution with the smaller variance. The weighing by relative variance of prediction to correction is a general feature of dynamic Bayesian predictor–corrector models, and in this important regard they are analogous to the Kalman filter. (See the beginning of this chapter for a brief discussion of the Kalman filter.)

To emphasize the importance of weighting by relative variance of prediction to correction in the target-tracking model, we can reverse the variance ordering by keeping the prior probability distribution the same but setting the likelihood to have maximal variance by making its distribution vector uniform: $P(\boldsymbol{V}_{\mathrm{T}}) = [0.14\ 0.14\ 0.14\ 0.14\ 0.14\ 0.14\ 0.14]^{\mathrm{T}}$. (Note that the probability values have been rounded to the nearest hundredth but they nearly sum to 1.) Repeating the above procedure for implementing Equations 12.9 and 12.10 will produce a posterior probability distribution vector that is exactly the same as the prior distribution vector: $P(\boldsymbol{T}_{\mathrm{V}})^{\mathrm{T}} = [0\ 0\ 0.1\ 0.2\ 0.4\ 0.2\ 0.1]^{\mathrm{T}}$ (see Table 12.6C). The maximal posterior probability value of 0.4 occurs at element 5, which corresponds to target position +1 (not shown). The target position estimate using the likelihood with increased (maximal) variance is the same as the prediction, +1 (see Table 12.6D and A). Obviously, the estimate now weights the prediction more heavily than the correction (and the observation).

This illustrates how the target-tracking predictor–corrector model, which is based on Bayes' rule, takes the relative variance of the prediction (prior) and correction (likelihood) into account. When the variance of the prediction is larger, the estimate favors the correction, but when the variance of the correction is larger, the estimate favors the prediction. For the extreme case we just considered, in which the likelihood is uniform and so has maximal variance, $P(V(t) \mid T(t)) = P(V(t))$ and the correction ratio $P(V(t) \mid T(t)) / P(V(t))$ is equal to 1 at all target positions. According to Bayes' rule, the posterior $P(T(t) \mid V(t))$ is equal to the prior $P(T(t))$ in that case.

In the context of a model of target-tracking by animals, a uniform likelihood would be interpreted as SSC activity that is independent of the target. A situation analogous to that of the uniform likelihood could arise in the brain if the lights were turned off during tracking. Then the SSC could not be activated by the target, and we would assume that any activity it might have would be independent of the target. A system that relied exclusively on observation for its target-position estimate might output either its last estimate, or nothing at all, if the lights were turned off during tracking. In contrast, a predictor–corrector system without an observation could not generate a correction, but it could fall back on its prediction to estimate target position. According to the assumptions of the model, if a predictor–corrector system for target tracking exists in the brain, then it should continue to produce target position estimates even if visual (or other sensory) observation of the target is discontinued.

As mentioned earlier in this section, a midbrain region associated with the SC in cats has been discovered that does indeed seem to use a predictor–corrector mechanism to estimate target position during tracking (Cui and Malpeli 2003). That region, the parabigeminal nucleus (PBN), receives input predominantly from the SC (from SSC and possibly also from DSC; Graham 1977). The firing rates of single PBN neurons are proportional to retinal position error, or the displacement from the fovea of the retinal image of a visual target, during tracking (see Figure 12.13). Most interestingly, the firing rates of PBN neurons continue to increase as retinal position error increases during brief periods when the moving target is not visible, although at a reduced rate. The averaged firing rates of a sample of PBN neurons during tracking of visible, or of temporarily invisible, moving targets are shown in Figure 12.15.

The firing rates of single PBN neurons are not linearly related to retinal position error over the entire range of target positions in visual space. Instead, the responses of PBN neurons either fall off or plateau (saturate) as the target moves and retinal position error exceeds a certain value (Cui and Malpeli 2003). Thus, their responses may be proportional not to target position itself, but to the probability that target position falls within a range, or exceeds a certain position that is specific for each PBN neuron (i.e., its characteristic or preferred position). The goal of the next example is to use the target-tracking predictor–corrector model to simulate the PBN by using it to compute the probability that a target is at or past a specific point relative to the fovea.

Two scripts are used to simulate the responses of PBN neurons using the target-tracking predictor–corrector model. Script `predictCorrectSetUp`, which is listed in MATLAB Box 12.5, sets up the simulated space. This script also constructs the conditional probability matrix, which instantiates the inter-

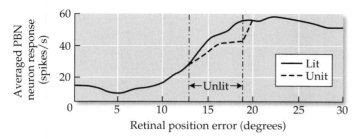

FIGURE 12.15 The averaged responses of neurons in the parabigeminal nucleus (PBN) of cats while they visually track moving targets The targets (light spots) stay lit for their whole trajectory, or are unlit during part of their trajectory. The averaged instantaneous firing rate (in spikes per second) of PBN neurons in either condition is plotted as a function of retinal position error, which is the difference in degrees between the fovea and the target image on the retina (see Figure 12.12). The averaged PBN neuron response continues to increase for unlit targets (dashed line), but at a lower rate than for lit targets (solid line). (After Ma et al., in review.)

ⓂATLAB® BOX 12.5 This script sets up the target-tracking predictor–corrector model.

```
% predictCorrectSetUp.m

range=80; % set range of space units (space is -range:0:range)
CellPrefT=10; % enter PBN cell preferred T position (in space units)
lightOff=12; % enter lights off position (in space units)
lightOn=21; % enter lights on position (in space units)
nTpos=31; % set number of positions (spaces) target will assume
pTvar=25; % set variance of prediction (target motion model)
pVTvar=9; % set variance of observation (visual likelihood)
TposVec=0:nTpos-1; % set target position vector (in space units)
space=(-range:range)'; % make the space
nSpace=length(space); % find the number of spaces
shift=(nSpace+1)/2; % compute the shift parameter

pTgauss=exp((space.^2/pTvar)*(-0.5)); % pTgauss as discrete Gaussian
pTgauss=pTgauss/sum(pTgauss); % normalize the discrete Gaussian
pTgauss=circshift(pTgauss,shift+1); % shift Gaussian (note +1)
pTTpre=zeros(nSpace); % zero conditional target probability matrix
for s=1:nSpace, % for each location in space
    pTTpre(:,s)=pTgauss; % set each column of target prob matrix
    pTgauss=[pTgauss(nSpace);pTgauss(1:nSpace-1)]; % rotate
end % end loop that makes conditional target probability matrix
pVTgauss=exp((space.^2/pVTvar)*(-0.5)); % set pVTon as Gaussian
pVTgauss=pVTgauss/sum(pVTgauss); % normalize the discrete Gaussian
pVTgauss=circshift(pVTgauss,shift); % shift Gaussian (note no +1)
pVTon=zeros(nSpace); % zero the visual input likelihood matrix
for s=1:nSpace, % for each location in space
    pVTon(:,s)=pVTgauss; % set each column of likelihood matrix
    pVTgauss=[pVTgauss(nSpace);pVTgauss(1:nSpace-1)]; % rotate
end % end loop that makes likelihood matrix
pVToff=ones(nSpace,1)*1/nSpace; % set pVToff as uniform distribution
```

nal, probabilistic model of target motion, and the likelihood distribution matrices both for visible and invisible targets. Script pbnPredictCorrect, listed in MATLAB Box 12.6, uses the model to simulate tracking, and to simulate the responses of PBN neurons. The operation of these programs can be best explained by first redoing, using MATLAB commands, the numerical example we studied above, because the numerical example is a scaled-down version of the target-tracking model as implemented in the MATLAB scripts.

Begin by setting the profile pro=[0.2 0.4 0.2 0.1 0 0 0.1]'. Then the conditional probability distribution matrix (internal model of target motion between saccades), can be defined as pTTpre=zeros(7), and can be constructed using the loop: for s=1:7, pTTpre(:,s)=pro; pro=[pro(7);pro(1:6)]; end. The resulting matrix [target-motion model between saccades, $P(T(t) \mid T(t-1), A(t-1) = 0)$] is shown in Table 12.5B. Using the profile pro=[0.8 0.1 0 0 0 0 0.1]', a similar method could be used to construct the likelihood distribution matrix $P(V(t) \mid T(t))$ shown in Table 12.5A. Scaled up versions of these commands are implemented by script predictCorrectSetUp.

MATLAB® BOX 12.6   This script implements a predictor–corrector simulation of the responses of neurons in the parabigeminal nucleus.

```
% pbnPredictCorrect.m
% this script runs predictCorrectSetUp first

predictCorrectSetUp % run predictCorrecSetUP
CellPrefT=CellPrefT+shift; % shift PBN cell preferred T position

% find target posteriors for a lighted target that stays on
TposHld=zeros(1,nTpos); % zero target position hold vector
TestHldOn=zeros(1,nTpos); % zero target estimate hold vector
pbnCellOn=zeros(1,nTpos); % zero PBN cell response hold vector
Tpos=0; % start the target at zero position
Test=0; % zero the target position estimate
pTV=ones(nSpace,1)/nSpace; % set posterior to uniform initially
for t=1:nTpos, % for each time step
    pT=pTTpre*pTV; % find new prior (prediction)
    pVT=pVTon(:,Tpos+shift); % get likelihood at current target
    pV=pVT'*pT;  % compute unconditional probability (evidence)
    pTV=pVT/pV.*pT;  % compute target posterior probability
    [maxpTV,Test]=max(pTV); % take new estimate as max posterior
    Test=Test-shift;  % take account of shift about zero
    pTVcellShift=circshift(pTV,-CellPrefT); % shift posterior
    pbnCellOn(t)=sum(pTVcellShift(1:round(nSpace/2-1))); % pbn
    TposHld(t)=Tpos;  % save target position
    TestHldOn(t)=Test;  % save estimate for lights on
    Tpos=Tpos + 1;  % advance target one space unit per time step
end % end target on loop

% find target posteriors for a lighted target that goes off
TestHldOff=zeros(1,nTpos); % zero target estimate hold vector
pbnCellOff=zeros(1,nTpos); % zero PBN cell response hold vector
pTVseriesOff=zeros(nSpace,nTpos); % zero prediction series matrix
Tpos=0; % start the target at zero position
Test=0; % zero the target position estimate
pTV=ones(nSpace,1)/nSpace; % set posterior to uniform initially
for t=1:nTpos, % for each time step
    pT=pTTpre*pTV; % find new prior (prediction)
    if t>=lightOff & t<=lightOn,  % lights out interval
       pVT=pVToff; % set to "off" likelihood
    else pVT=pVTon(:,Tpos+shift); end % set to "on" likelihood
    pV=pVT'*pT;  % compute unconditional probability (evidence)
    pTV=pVT/pV.*pT;  % compute target posterior probability
    pTVseriesOff(:,t)=pTV; % save prediction in series matrix
    [maxpTV,Test]=max(pTV); % take new estimate as max posterior
    Test=Test-shift;  % take account of shift about zero
    pTVcellShift=circshift(pTV,-CellPrefT); % shift posterior
    pbnCellOff(t)=sum(pTVcellShift(1:round(nSpace/2-1))); % pbn
    TestHldOff(t)=Test;  % save estimate for lights off
    Tpos=Tpos+1;  % advance target one space unit per time step
end % end target off loop
```

Assume that on the previous time step the target was estimated to be at position 0, and that no catch-up saccade was made. Set the posterior distribution vector for the previous time step as pTV=[0 0 0 1 0 0 0]', where the number 1 at target state 4 corresponds to the estimate of the target at position 0. Thus, for simplicity in this example, the posterior probability distribution and estimate vectors are the same (as also shown in Table 12.6B), but this would not be the case in general. The prior probability that the target is located at each of the possible target positions (the prior probability distribution) for the current time step can be computed using pT=pTTpre*pTV (see Equation 12.8). The result, expressed as a row, is the prior probability distribution pT=[0 0 0.1 0.2 0.4 0.2 0.1] (see Table 12.6C). The maximal prior probability occurs for target state 5, which corresponds to a prediction of the target at position +1, as in the numerical example (see Table 12.6D and A). Note that the command pT=pTTpre*pTV produces the current prior as the product of the conditional (target-motion) probability matrix and the previous posterior, and that the maximal previous posterior (estimate) and maximal current prior (prediction) correspond to target positions 0 and +1, respectively. This demonstrates that the conditional probability matrix (the internal model of target motion) essentially predicts that the target will move by one position in the positive direction on each time step.

As in the numerical example, assume that the visual observation of a target activates the SSC unit corresponding to position +2 and state $V = 6$ (see Table 12.6E and A), and set the likelihood distribution vector as pVT=[0 0 0 0 0.1 0.8 0.1]'. This is the same likelihood vector we used in the numerical example (see Table 12.6F), and it could have been read from the row corresponding to $V = 6$ of the likelihood distribution matrix (see Table 12.5A; since this matrix is symmetric it could have been read equivalently from the column corresponding to $T = 6$). Now the evidence for this particular state of SSC activity (see Equation 12.10) can be computed as the dot product between the likelihood and prior distribution vectors using pV=pVT'*pT. The posterior probability vector can be computed (see Equation 12.9) using the command pTV=pVT/pV.*pT. (Note that .* signifies element-by-element multiplication in MATLAB.) The resulting target posterior probability vector, expressed as a row, is pTV=[0 0 0 0 0.19 0.76 0.05] (see Table 12.6G). This vector contains the posterior probabilities of the target at each of the possible target positions, and can be used to estimate target position. As in the numerical example, target state 6 has the highest posterior probability, and this maximal value corresponds to the estimated target position of +2 (see Table 12.6H and A). The script pbnPredictCorrect implements scaled up versions of these commands to simulate target tracking.

In addition to defining and running the inferential components of the target-tracking predictor–corrector model, the scripts predictCorrectSetUp and pbnPredictCorrect also set up a simulated space (which corresponds to a simulated retina), and locate the actual and estimated positions of the target in this space (or relative to the fovea, in which case target position is equivalent to retinal position error). The script predictCorrectSetUp sets up a one-dimensional environment, held in vector space, which consists of an array of 161 spaces: 80 to the left and 80 to the right of the 0 space. It finds the value shift that relates the indices of space, from 1 to 161, to target positions from −80 to +80. It also defines vectors for prior (prediction) and posterior (estimate) probabilities, and sets up arrays for likelihood and conditional distribution matrices, which are scaled-up versions of the example distribution matrices described above and shown in Table 12.5. The program uses these probabilities to simulate estimation by the PBN of the position of a moving target (a spot of light) that is lit (visible) along its entire trajectory, or that is unlit (invisible) for part of its trajectory.

Script `predictCorrectSetUp` makes the discrete Gaussian profile `pTgauss` and uses it to construct the conditional probability matrix $P(T(t) | T(t-1), A(t-1) = 0)$ for target movement between saccades, which is held in array `pTTpre`. It makes the discrete Gaussian profile `pVTgauss` and uses it to construct the target-visible likelihood distribution matrix for $P(V(t) | T(t))$, which is held in array `pVTon`. Profiles `pTgauss` and `pVTgauss` have variances `pTvar` and `pVTvar`, respectively. The script also makes a uniform profile for the target-invisible likelihood distribution vector `pVToff`. Script `predictCorrectSetUp` also sets other parameters such as the preferred target position of the simulated PBN neuron (cell) in variable `CellPrefT`, and the target positions at which the target light will go off and come back on again: `lightOff` and `lightOn`.

Script `pbnPredictCorrect` simulates target tracking by starting the target at position 0 (in space, or relative to the fovea), and on each time step it advances the actual target position variable `Tpos` by one space unit. On each time step, the script updates the prior $P(T(t))$, the likelihood $P(V(t) | T(t))$, and the posterior $P(T(t) | V(t))$ distributions, which are held in column vectors `pT`, `pVT`, and `pTV`, respectively. It updates the prior distribution $P(T(t))$ by multiplying the conditional probability matrix $P(T(t) | T(t-1), A(t-1) = 0)$ by the previous posterior distribution $P(T(t-1) | V(t-1))$ using `pT=pTTpre*pTV`. It updates the likelihood distribution $P(V(t) | T(t))$ differently depending on whether the target is lit or unlit. For a lit target, it chooses the column of the likelihood matrix corresponding to the current target position using the command `pVT=pVTon(:,Tpos+shift)`, where the shift between indices and space units is taken into account. For an unlit target it sets the likelihood equal to a uniform distribution using `pVT=pVToff`. It computes the evidence $P(V(t))$ using `pV=pVT'*pT`, and the current posterior distribution $P(T(t) | V(t))$ using `pTV=pVT/pV.*pT`, as described in detail above. This completes one cycle of updates.

The target posterior is initially set to a uniform distribution, and so the initial prior distribution is also uniform, which corresponds to the prediction that a potential target could appear anywhere. Target tracking begins with a visual observation of a target, after which the Gaussian lights-on likelihood causes the updated target posterior distribution also to be Gaussian. The estimated target position, held in variable `Test`, is taken as the position corresponding to the current target state with the highest posterior probability.

The simulated PBN neuron response is computed from the current posterior target-position distribution. Specifically, as Equation 12.11 shows, it is taken as the sum of the posterior probabilities that the target is at or beyond the preferred target position t_P of the PBN neuron:

$$P(T \geq t_P | V) = P(T = t_P | V) + P(T = t_P + 1 | V) + P(T = t_P + 2 | V) + \cdots \quad \textbf{12.11}$$

where the discrete time step variable (t) is again omitted for clarity. In script `pbnPredictCorrect`, this sum (see Equation 12.11) is computed only over one-half of the elements of the posterior probability vector, starting from the element corresponding to the preferred target position of the PBN unit. Because, for simplicity, we made the space circular, this procedure avoids summing probability values corresponding to the opposite side of the space, but it only approximates the probability $P(T \geq t_p | V)$.

Script `pbnPredictCorrect` is written in two blocks. The first block simulates tracking of a target that stays lit over its entire trajectory, while the second block simulates tracking of a target that is unlit for a portion of its trajectory. The first block saves the actual and estimated target positions and simulated

PBN neuron responses for the lit target in vectors `TposHld`, `TestHldOn`, and `pbnCellOn`, respectively. These vectors can be plotted against the target positions in `TposVec`, which is set in `predictCorrectSetUp`. The second block saves the analogous values over the whole trajectory for the target that is unlit during the portion of its trajectory between `lightOff` and `lightOn`. In addition, the second block saves the entire posterior probability distribution on each time step in array `pTVseriesOff`.

With this extensive preparation we can now describe some simulations using the target-tracking predictor–corrector model. The preferred target position of the simulated PBN cell is set to 10, and the variances of the target-motion and the lights-on likelihood distributions are set to 25 and 9, respectively, using `CellPrefT=10`, `pTvar=25`, and `pVTvar=9`. Scripts `predictCorrectSetUp` and `pbnPredictCorrect` are run and the results are shown in Figure 12.16. Because the target advances by one space unit on each time step, and because the conditional probability $P(T(t) \mid T(t-1), A(t-1) = 0)$ (internal model of target motion) assigns the highest probability to the target at (t) that is one space unit ahead of the target at ($t-1$) (see also Table 12.5B), the script produces accurate estimates of target position regardless of whether the target stays lit over its whole trajectory or is unlit during a portion of its trajectory (see Figure 12.16A). Thus, actual target position `Tpos`, and the position corresponding to the maximal target posterior probability `Test`, are the same whether the target stays lit or is temporarily unlit. However, the values of the target posterior probability, and so also of the simulated PBN neuron response, are lower during the lights-off interval (see Figure 12.16B).

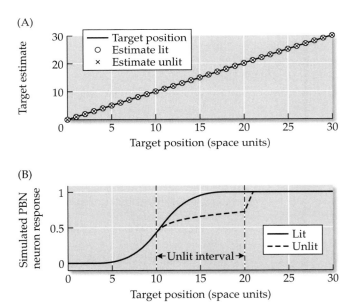

FIGURE 12.16 Using the target-tracking predictor–corrector model to simulate the responses of neurons in the cat parabigeminal nucleus (PBN) The model simulates the activity produced by the average PBN neuron (see Figure 12.15) while the cat visually tracks a moving target (light spot). (A) The model accurately estimates target position whether or not the target (solid line) stays lit for its whole trajectory (circles), or is unlit (crosses) during part of its trajectory. (B) The simulated PBN neuron response is the probability that the target is at or beyond the neuron's preferred target position, which is at position 10 in this simulation. The simulated PBN neuron response is lower when the target is unlit, over the range of unlit target positions in this simulation.

This occurs because the variance that defines the unlit target likelihood (which is maximal) is larger than that of the lit target likelihood (`pVTvar`).

During the unlit interval, the likelihood $P(V(t) \mid T(t))$ is set to a uniform distribution, so it has maximal variance. Because the ratio $P(V(t) \mid T(t)) / P(V(t))$ is equal to 1 at all target positions when the likelihood is uniform, the posterior $P(T(t) \mid V(t))$ is equal to the prior $P(T(t))$ during the unlit interval (see Equation 12.9). As the unlit interval endures, the prior, which is a function of the previous posterior $P(T(t-1) \mid V(t-1))$ and the target-motion conditional probability $P(T(t) \mid T(t-1), A(t-1) = 0)$, has a variance that increases, and amplitude that decreases, on each time step. Because the prior and posterior distributions are equal during the unlit interval, the posterior distribution also has a continuously increasing variance, and continuously decreasing amplitude, during this interval, as shown in Figure 12.17. Thus, without a correction, the uncertainties associated with the prediction [prior $P(T(t))$] and the probabilistic model of target motion [conditional probability $P(T(t) \mid T(t-1), A(t-1) = 0)$] are compounded, and the variances of the prior and posterior distributions would ultimately become maximal, matching that of the unlit target likelihood (which has a uniform distribution).

As the variance of the posterior distribution increases with that of the prior, the posterior probability values at and near the estimated target position decrease. It is this increase in the variance of the posterior, and concomitant decrease in its amplitude, that causes the simulated PBN neuron response to be smaller for the unlit target over the range of target positions shown in Figure 12.16B. That the PBN neuron response should be smaller for unlit than for lit targets is consistent with intuition but, in the model, the reduction in the unlit response pertains only over the midrange of retinal position errors. The

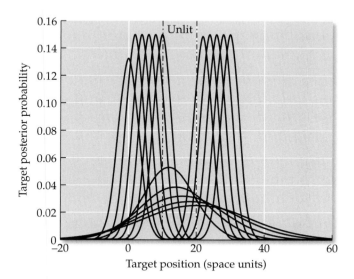

FIGURE 12.17   The target posterior probability distribution from the target-tracking predictor–corrector model for a lit target (simulated light spot) that is temporarily unlit Each curve shows the entire target posterior probability distribution on a different time step. The estimated target position is the target position with the highest posterior probability on any time step. (For clarity, only curves for every second time step are shown.) During the unlit interval the distribution abruptly and then more gradually increases in variance, and decreases in amplitude, with each time step. However, the estimate is still accurate in that the peak of the target posterior probability distribution matches actual target position on every time step, whether the target is lit or unlit, as shown in Figure 12.16A.

midrange corresponds roughly to target positions within and closely border-ing the preferred target position range of a PBN neuron. The counterintuitive behavior of model PBN neurons outside the midrange leads to a modeling prediction that we will consider at the end of this section.

Reduction in the amplitude of the target posterior probability distribution for unlit targets (see Figure 12.17), which can reduce the simulated PBN neu-ron response, does not preclude accurate estimation of the positions of unlit targets (see Figure 12.16). The conditional probability $P(T(t) \mid T(t-1), A(t-1) = 0)$, which is the internal model of target motion, is constructed so that the pre-dicted target is one space unit ahead of the current estimate. Because the target itself advances by one space unit on each time step, the estimate is accurate despite the fact that the variance of the target posterior distribution increases, and so its probability value at the estimated target position decreases, with each time step during the unlit interval. Target position estimates are accurate in both cases because the peak of the target-position posterior probability distribution occurs at the same target position whether the target is lit or tem-porarily unlit, even though the value at the peak is smaller when the target is unlit. The feature by which the overall target-tracking model accurately estimates target position even when the target is unlit is consistent with the experimental observation that cats make saccades as accurately to unlit as to lit targets (Ma et al., in review).

The target-tracking predictor–corrector model successfully simulated the finding that PBN neuron responses are smaller for unlit than for lit targets over the midrange of retinal position errors (see Figures 12.15 and 12.16B). Interestingly, the model predicted that PBN neuron responses should be *larger* for unlit than for lit targets at retinal position errors outside the midrange. This prediction follows from the assumption that PBN neuron responses are

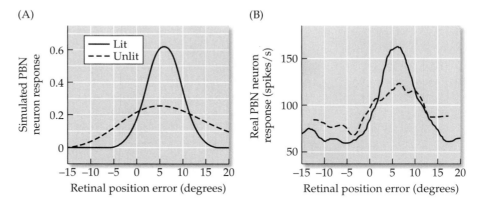

FIGURE 12.18 Confirming a prediction of the target-tracking predictor–corrector model The prediction concerns the responses of cat parabigeminal nucleus (PBN) neurons to moving targets (light spots). The model assumes that the variance of the correction (observation of the target) is larger (i.e., maximal) when the target is unlit. (A) Given this assumption, the model explains why the PBN neu-ron response to the unlit target would be smaller than the response to the lit target for midrange retinal position errors. Counterintuitively, the model predicts that the unlit response should be larger for retinal position errors outside the midrange. This prediction was subsequently confirmed. (B) The plot shows the response from a representative, actual PBN neuron. For the simulated results (in A) the target is either lit (solid curve) or unlit (dashed curve) over the whole range displayed (the target starts out lit at negative retinal position errors outside the range of the plot in both the lit and unlit cases). The real data (in B) is a composite of responses to lit and unlit targets at various retinal position errors spanning the range of the plot. (After Ma et al., in review.)

proportional to target-position posterior probabilities (and to sums thereof; see Equation 12.11). Recall that, for unlit targets, the variance of the target-position posterior probability increases on each time step. This decreases the target posterior at the peak of its distribution (i.e., at the estimated target position), but it necessarily *increases* the target posterior on the shoulders of its distribution. (In other words, the target posterior is flatter for unlit targets.) In consequence, although the PBN neuron response is smaller for retinal position errors over the midrange, the model predicted that the PBN response should be larger for retinal position errors outside the midrange (Figure 12.18A). This prediction was subsequently confirmed experimentally (Figure12.18B; see also Ma et al., in review).

The real PBN neuron response shown in Figure 12.18B falls off at larger retinal position errors, in contrast to the averaged PBN neuron response shown in Figure 12.15 that reaches a plateau (from which it also falls off slightly). Thus, the PBN neuron response shown in Figure 12.18B is more sharply tuned for retinal position error than the averaged response shown in Figure 12.15. This more sharply tuned response was simulated by computing the model PBN neuron response as a sum over a small range of target posterior probabilities, rather than as the sum of all target posteriors at and beyond a preferred target position as in Equaiton 12.11. Because it is more sharply tuned than average, the PBN neuron response shown in Figure 12.18B nicely illustrates the finding that, compared with the lit target response, the unlit target response is smaller for midrange retinal position errors but larger for retinal position errors outside the midrange. This finding confirms the model prediction (see Figure 12.18A). The PBN neuron response shown in Figure 12.18B also has a different preferred target location than the averaged response shown in Figure 12.15. Because real PBN neurons differ in their preferred target locations and in the sharpness of their tuning (Cui and Malpeli 2003; Ma et al., in review), it is possible that the population of PBN neurons together encode the entire target-position posterior probability distribution. We discussed possible forms of probability distribution encoding in Chapter 9.

12.4 Training a Sigmoidal Unit to Simulate Trajectory Prediction by Neurons

The target-tracking predictor–corrector model is essentially a dynamic Bayesian network (Russell and Norvig 1995; Jensen 2001). As such, it offers a description of PBN function on the algorithmic level. To the extent that the predictor–corrector model is able to simulate the responses of real PBN neurons, we can use it to formulate valid hypotheses concerning the computation that PBN neurons may be performing. However, the predictor–corrector model indicates nothing about the implementation of that computation by PBN neurons. As we saw in Chapter 9, neural units can learn to compute probabilities. It is possible that predictive brain functions are implemented by neurons that learn to represent likelihood and conditional probabilities, and compute prior and posterior probabilities, which are analogous to those used in the target-tracking predictor–corrector model. It is also possible that the implementation of predictive brain functions such as tracking involves network dynamics. The goal of the final example is to train a simple, recurrent neural network model of the PBN to take input from both the SSC and DSC and use that to estimate the posterior probability that the target being tracked is at or beyond a preferred target position. This type of response, computed as a summed posterior probability (see Equation 12.11) corresponds to the average response observed for PBN neurons (see Figure 12.15).

FIGURE 12.19 **Model of a single neuron in the parabigeminal nucleus (PBN)** The model PBN neuron receives input from itself, from a bias unit, and from the superficial and deep layers of the superior colliculus (SSC and DSC, respectively). The SSC is represented as an array of 161 input units (of which only five are shown), while the DSC and bias are single input units.

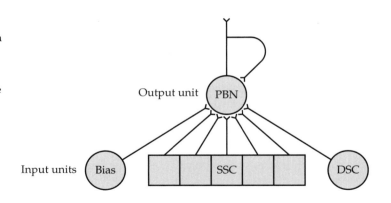

The model is schematized in Figure 12.19. It has two layers. The output layer consists of a single, sigmoidal unit that represents a PBN neuron. The input layer consists of a bias unit, a series of units representing the input to the PBN from the SSC, and a single unit representing the input to the PBN from the DSC. In the diagram the SSC is shown as a series of five units, but in the actual model the SSC is composed of 161 units to match the space (and retinal) dimension of the target-tracking predictor–corrector model. The output unit also receives a recurrent connection from itself.

Because the single recurrent connection occurs at the output, the neural network model of the PBN can be trained using the delta rule (see Chapter 6). If the model had recurrent connections from the output unit back to the input units (or to hidden units), then a more complicated algorithm, such as recurrent back-propagation as described in Chapter 10, would be needed to train it. With the delta rule, the state of the output unit on time step $(t-1)$ is treated as an input to the output unit on time step (t), and the recurrent weight is trained in the same way as the input weights from the SSC, DSC, and bias units (see Figure 12.19). This method of training the recurrent weight is similar to the delta-rule-through-time procedure we discussed in Chapter 10.

For the purposes of computing the output unit response and for training the network connection weights, it is convenient to assemble all the inputs to the output unit y at time $(t-1)$ into the entire network state vector $\mathbf{z}(t-1)$ $= [\mathbf{x}(t-1)^\mathrm{T}\ y(t-1)]^\mathrm{T}$, which is composed of the bias, SSC, and DSC inputs in column vector $\mathbf{x}(t-1)$, and the previous response of the output unit $y(t-1)$. The connectivity matrix $\mathbf{M}$ is then just a row vector composed of the weights to the output unit from the bias, SSC, and DSC input units and from the output unit to itself. The delta-rule update to the connectivity matrix (row vector) $\mathbf{M}$ is described by Equation 12.12:

$$\Delta\mathbf{M}(t) = a\left[d(t) - y(t)\right]f'\!\left(q(t)\right)\mathbf{z}(t-1) = a\,e(t)\,f'\!\left(q(t)\right)\mathbf{z}(t-1) \qquad \textbf{12.12}$$

where $d(t)$ is the desired output, $e(t)$ is the error, or difference between the desired and actual outputs, and a is the learning rate. The quantity $q(t)$ is the weighted input sum, and $f(q(t))$ is the squashing function applied to the weighted input sum as shown in Equations 12.13 and 12.14:

$$q(t) = \mathbf{M}\mathbf{z}(t-1) \qquad \textbf{12.13}$$

$$y(t) = f\!\left(q(t)\right) = \frac{1}{1+\exp\!\left(-q(t)\right)} \qquad \textbf{12.14}$$

The term $f'(q(t))$ in Equation 12.12 is the derivative of the squashing function (see Math Box 6.3 in Chapter 6).

The neural model will be trained during simulated visual tracking of a moving target (light spot). A catch-up saccade will be made whenever actual target position exceeds a threshold. The DSC unit will take value 1 whenever a saccade is made, but will take value 0 otherwise. After each catch-up saccade ($A(t − 1) = 1$), the target will be reset at position 0. It will then move probabilistically according to the conditional probability $P(T(t) \mid T(t − 1), A(t − 1) = 0)$ that was used in the target-tracking predictor–corrector model. The desired output will take value 1 whenever the actual target position equals or exceeds the preferred target position of the simulated PBN neuron, and will take value 0 otherwise. The input from the SSC will be a vector of 0s, with a 1 at the location of the SSC input unit that is activated by the target. The location of the active unit will be determined probabilistically from actual target position using the likelihood $P(V(t) \mid T(t))$ as used in the predictor–corrector model. The bias unit will maintain a constant state of 1.

The script `pbnDeltaRule`, listed in MATLAB Box 12.7, will implement training of the PBN neural network model (see Figure 12.19) using the delta rule. Like script `pbnPredictCorrect`, many (but not all) of the parameters for `pbnDeltaRule` are set using `predictCorrectSetUp` (see MATLAB Box 12.5). Script `pbnDeltaRule` also creates a one-dimensional array to represent the SSC. For simplicity, there is a one-to-one correspondence between possible target positions and SSC units.

The variances of the prediction and the observation, and the preferred PBN unit target position, are set in `predictCorrectSetUp` as for the target-tracking predictor–corrector model: `pTvar=25`, `pVTvar=9`, and `CellPrefT=10`. The command `SACstart=40` in `pbnDeltaRule` sets the threshold for a saccade at position +40 in the simulated space. The command `lightInt=200` sets the intervals (in time steps) over which the light spot is lit or unlit. (Training on an unlit target improves estimation of the summed, unlit target probability by the unit.) The conditional probability $P(T(t) \mid T(t − 1), A(t − 1) = 0)$ is held in matrix `pTTpre` and, unless a saccade is made, `pTTpre` is used to set the prior probability of the target `pT`. The prior vector `pT` is then used to determine actual target position `Tpos` by first computing the cumulative prior using `cpT=cumsum([0 pT'])`, and then finding the slot in `cpT` into which falls a uniformly distributed random deviate. (This method involving the cumulative prior is described in more detail in Chapter 9.) A similar method involving the likelihood $P(V(t) \mid T(t))$, held in vector `pVT`, is used to find the active SSC unit given current target position `Tpos`.

The network is trained on each time step for `nIts=20000` time steps (same as training cycles or iterations) using the delta rule, which is described in detail in Chapter 6. Briefly, Equations 12.13 and 12.14 are implemented using `q=M*z` followed by `y=1./(1+exp(-q))`, where q is the weighted input sum, M is the weight matrix, z is the network state (column) vector (whose elements are the previous states of all the input units and the single output unit), and y is the state of the output unit. Equation 12.12 is implemented using `e=d-y`, `dSquash=y*(1-y)`, and `deltaM=a*e*dSquash*z'`, where a is the learning rate (`a=0.1`), e is the error, d is the desired output, dSquash is the derivative of the squashing function, and `deltaM` is the weight-change matrix (row vector). The weight update concludes with `M=M+deltaM`. Following training the network is tested using a lit target that moves deterministically over a range from 0 to 30, one space unit per time step, and activates the SSC deterministically, so that the active SSC unit advances by one place on each time step. A similar method (not listed in MATLAB Box 12.7) tests the network using a target that is unlit over an interval, during which no SSC unit is activated.

A sample of the erratic simulated target motion, generated according to the conditional probability $P(T(t) \mid T(t − 1), A(t− 1) = 0)$, is shown in

MATLAB® BOX 12.7 **This script uses the delta rule to train a single sigmoidal unit with feedback to simulate the responses of neurons in the parabigeminal nucleus.**

```
% pbnDeltaRule.m
% this script runs predictCorrectSetUp first

predictCorrectSetUp % run predictCorrectSetUp
nUnit=1; % set number of units (one output unit in this case)
nIn=nSpace+2; % number of inputs (all SSC, one DSC, one bias)
a=0.1; % set learning rate
b=1; % set bias input to unit
nIts=20000; % set number of training iterations
SACstart=40; % set saccade start position
lightInt=200; % set light flip interval for training

% train while simulating close-order tracking
M=0.2*(rand(nUnit,nIn+nUnit)-0.5); % random initial weight matrix
TposHld=zeros(1,nIts); % zero target position hold vector
SSChld=zeros(1,nIts); % zero SSC response hold vector
xSSC=zeros(nSpace,1); % zero the input from SSC
Tpos=0; SSC=0; DSC=0; y=0; d=0; % zero initial values
z=[b;xSSC;DSC;y]; % set initial state vector
lightFlip=1; % set light flag to begin training on lit target
for t=1:nIts, % for each training cycle
    TposHld(t)=Tpos; % save current target position
    SSChld(t)=SSC; % save current SSC input value
    q=M*z; % find weighted input to output unit
    y=1./(1+exp(-q)); % squash responses of output unit
    e=d-y; % compute error
    dSquash=y*(1-y); % derivative of squash
    deltaM=a*e*dSquash*z'; % find delta M
    M=M+deltaM; % update the connectivity matrix
    if rem(t,lightInt)==0, lightFlip=1-lightFlip; end % lit/unlit
    if Tpos>=SACstart, % if a resetting saccade is to be made,
        Tpos=0; SSC=0; DSC=1; % reset target and SC
        xSSC=zeros(nSpace,1); % reset SSC input vector to zero
    else   % otherwise advance target according to P(T(t)|T(t-1))
        pT=pTTpre(:,Tpos+shift); % find shifted prior
        cpT=cumsum([0 pT']); % compute the cumulative prior
        indxVec=find(cpT<=rand); % generate random deviate
        Tpos=indxVec(length(indxVec)); % find actual target position
        if Tpos<nSpace/3, Tpos=nSpace; end % keep target in bounds
        Tpos=Tpos-shift; % take account of shift about zero
        SSC=0; xSSC=zeros(nSpace,1); DSC=0; % zero SSC and DSC
        if lightFlip==1, % if the target is lit
            pVT=pVTon(:,Tpos+shift); % find shifted likelihood
            cpVT=cumsum([0 pVT']); % compute cumulative likelihood
            indxVec=find(cpVT<=rand); % generate random deviate
            SSCindx=indxVec(length(indxVec)); % actual active SSC unit
            if SSCindx<nSpace/3, SSCindx=nSpace; end % bounded
            SSC=SSCindx-shift; % take account of shift
            xSSC(SSCindx)=1; % set SSC input vector
        end % end target lit conditional
    end % end tracking loop
```

(Continued on facing page)

MATLAB® BOX 12.7   (continued)

```
        z=[b;xSSC;DSC;y]; % reset state vector
        if Tpos>=CellPrefT, d=1; % set desired output to one
        else d=0; end % or set desired output to zero
end % end training loop

% following training, find pbn network responses for a lit target
xSSC=zeros(nSpace,1); DSC=0; y=0; % zero initial values
pbnCellOn=zeros(nTpos,nUnit); % zero response hold vector
for t=1:nTpos, % step through target positions in testing range
        Tpos=TposVec(t); % set next target position
        SSC=Tpos; % for testing SSC value equals target position
        SSCindx=SSC+shift; % take shift into account
        xSSC=zeros(nSpace,1); % zero SSC vector
        xSSC(SSCindx)=1; % set element of SSC input vector
        z=[b;xSSC;DSC;y]; % reset state vector
        q=M*z; y=1./(1+exp(-q)); % compute output and squash it
        pbnCellOn(t,:)=y; % store y output
end % end lit target testing loop
```

Figure 12.20 (solid line). The observation of this target (open circles in Figure 12.20), encoded as the corresponding location of the active unit in the SSC, is noisy because it is determined by the likelihood distribution $P(V(t) \mid T(t))$. The desired output (not shown) is 1 whenever the actual target is at or above the line showing the preferred PBN unit target position (dashed line in Figure 12.20), and 0 otherwise. The simulated PBN neuron must learn to use this noisy input from the SSC, its copy of occasional saccade commands from the DSC, and its own previous activity to estimate the probability that the target is at or past its preferred target position.

Following 20,000 training cycles, the responses of the PBN unit to the target, continuously lit or temporarily unlit, as it moves from position 0 to position 30

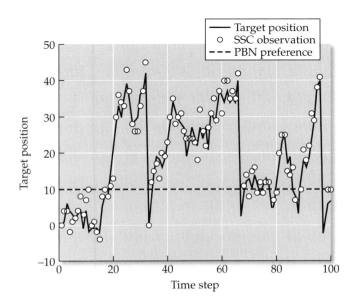

FIGURE 12.20 Learning to track an erratic target using noisy observations Target position and observation data such as these were used to train a sigmoidal unit with a recurrent self-connection to simulate the responses of neurons in the parabigeminal nucleus (PBN). The target (solid line) tends to move in the positive direction, but this movement is erratic. The observations of the target (circles), which would arrive at the PBN via the superficial superior colliculus (SSC), are noisy. The preferred target position (of 10) of the PBN unit is indicated by a dashed line. The desired output (not shown) is respectively 1 or 0 for targets at positions above or below the preferred target position of the PBN unit.

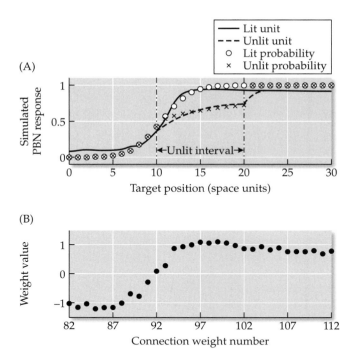

FIGURE 12.21 Simulating the target prediction capability of a PBN neuron using a sigmoidal unit with a recurrent self-connection The unit was trained with the delta rule to use noisy observations to determine whether an erratically moving target was at or past the preferred target position of the unit. (A) The response of the unit to a target (simulated light spot) that remains lit (solid line), or that is unlit during an interval (dashed line), well approximates the lit (circles) and unlit (crosses) PBN neuron responses as simulated using the predictor–corrector model (which are also shown in Figure 12.16B). (B) Connection weights 82 through 112 are the weights of the SSC inputs corresponding to target positions from 0 to 30. The weights from the SSC units (B) largely determine the sigmoidal shape of the response to the lit target (A, solid line). The bias and recurrent weights determine the activity of the unit when the target is unlit. The bias, DSC, and recurrent weights take values of about −1.5, −3, and +3, respectively. (The other SSC weights, and the bias, DSC, and recurrent weights, are not shown.)

are shown in Figure 12.21A (solid and dashed lines). They agree well with the posterior probability that the target is at or beyond the preferred target position of the PBN neuron, whether the target is lit or unlit (circles and crosses in Figure 12.21A). These posterior probabilities were computed as sums according to Equation 12.11 using the target-tracking predictor–corrector model, and depict the same, simulated PBN neuron responses shown in Figure 12.16B. Due to the high degree of randomness inherent in training this network, the simulated behavior you observe from trial to trial will vary and will not always match the simulated responses shown in Figure 12.21, but those modeling results are representative.

The weights to the PBN unit from SSC units 82 to 112, which correspond to target positions 0 to 30, are shown in Figure 12.21B (dots). The SSC input largely determines the response of the PBN unit to the lit target. The slight falling off of SSC weight values for weights higher than 97 is reflected in the PBN unit response as target position increases past about 15 space units. This falling off in the simulated response matches that observed in the averaged responses of real PBN neurons (see Figure 12.15). In the model, the SSC connection weights corresponding to more distant target positions receive less training, because those target positions are visited less often during simulated tracking. Falling off in the responses of real PBN neurons for more distant target positions may likewise reflect the relatively greater frequency of visual inputs from nearby targets during tracking by catch-up saccades.

The response of the PBN unit during the unlit interval is driven by the weight of its recurrent connection (see Exercise 12.4). During the unlit interval, the PBN unit response rises to a stable-state that is determined by its bias and recurrent inputs, and by its response just before the target becomes unlit. Both the rate of rise and the stable-state level are such that the PBN unit response well approximates the posterior probability that the target is at or beyond its preferred target position during the unlit interval. In that the response during the unlit interval rises to a stable-state, the solution that the network finds in the target-tracking case is reminiscent of the one found by the recurrent neural network in the simulation of short-term memory in Chapter 10. However, in the target-tracking case, the rate of rise is as important a characteristic of the response as the stable-state level that is ultimately attained.

The neural network in Figure 12.19 is undoubtedly a gross oversimplification of the actual connectivity within the PBN, and between the PBN and SC. However, the simulation captures the essential features of the responses of PBN neurons. It is possible that the predictive capability of the PBN, manifested as a continually rising response to an invisible target, is due to recurrent connections within the PBN. If the recurrent connections within PBN utilize synaptic transmitters different from the input connections to PBN from SC, then it might be possible pharmacologically to block the recurrent connections but not the input connections. This would allow experimental verification of the modeling hypothesis that the response of PBN neurons to temporarily invisible moving targets is due to recurrent connections within the PBN.

Predictor-corrector mechanisms are likely to occur throughout the brain. Dynamic Bayesain network models such as the target-tracking predictor–corrector model (see Section 12.3), and recurrent neural network implementations of them (this section), might be applicable to brain regions besides the PBN. A possible candidate for simulation using a predictor–corrector approach is the medial superior temporal area (MST) of cortex, which is involved in smooth pursuit eye-movement tracking. Like neurons in PBN, neurons in MST continue to respond even when the visible target being pursued becomes invisible (Newsome et al. 1988).

Exercises

12.1 Script `directionSelectivity` (see MATLAB Box 12.2) implements a simplified version of the asymmetric inhibition model of direction selectivity in the visual system. The main limitation of the simplified model is that it can fail to operate properly for stimulus speeds other than those that activate the excitatory input units in order in a strict sequence. Modify script `directionSelectivity` so that it will operate properly for stimuli over a range of different speeds. The simplified version already operates properly for stimuli at higher speeds that move in the on-direction. To make the model operate properly for stimuli at higher speeds that move in the off-direction, allow each inhibitory input unit asymmetrically to inhibit not only the single hidden unit to its left, but to inhibit all of the hidden units to its left. This can be done using the command

`V=[eye(nEx-1) zeros(nEx-1,1) -triu(ones(nEx-1))]`
where `nEx=30` is the number of excitatory input units in the network. (Note that `V` is the weight matrix for the connections to the hidden units, with states in vector `y`, from the combined input vector `x=[xex;xin]`). To make the network operate properly for stimuli at lower speeds that move in either direction, allow each inhibitory input unit and hidden unit to send an excitatory, feedback connection to itself. This can be done by setting recurrent weight matrices `WY=eye(nEx-1)*selfY` and `WXIN=eye(nEx-1)*selfXin`, where `selfY` and `selfXin` are the values of the self-excitation weights of each hidden unit or inhibitory input unit, respectively. Now the states of the hidden units are updated using `qy=WY*yP+V*x` and `y=max(qy,0)`, after which the states of the inhibitory inputs are updated using `xin=WXIN*xinP+VX*xex`, where `yP` and `xinP` are vectors of the hidden unit and inhibitory input unit states from the previous time step. The output unit is updated on time step `t` using `qz=U*y` and `z(t)=qz>zThr` where `zThr` is the threshold for converting the output of unit `z` to binary. Note that connectivity matrices `VX` and `U` are the same as in the simplified model. As for the simplified model, all units are updated on the same time step, to facilitate comparison, while the synaptic delays are implemented in terms of the order in which the units in the different layers are updated. Start off with self-excitation values of `selfY=0.8` and `selfXin=0.8`, and an output threshold of `zThr=0.6`. The elaborated network with these parameter settings should operate properly (i.e., produce a sustained output for on-direction, but produce zero output for off-direction, moving stimuli) even if the stimuli move at twice or half their previous speed. At twice-speed the stimulus skips an excitatory input unit on each time step, while at half-speed the stimulus takes two time steps to activate the next excitatory input unit in the sequence. Can the elaborated network operate properly in both directions at these different stimulus speeds? Can you reproduce the anticipation results? (See the hidden unit responses in Figure 12.4D.) Does the network continue to operate properly at even faster or slower stimulus speeds? Can you achieve correct operation with different parameter settings?

12.2 In the simulation of bottom-up/top-down processing using probabilistic inference (`BUTDprobInference`, listed in MATLAB Box 12.4), we considered a simplified version of the Rao (2005) image-generation model that had only four images in which only one blob, oriented either horizontally *or* vertically, could appear only on the left *or* right. These images represented only four combinations (see Figure 12.9). Expand this simulation to include the nine images and combinations in which both locations (left *and* right) can contain either a horizontally orientated blob, a vertically oriented blob, or no blob (null). The conditional probability table for image given combination $P(I = i \mid C = c)$ will be 9-by-9, and the conditional probability table for combination given location and feature $P(C = c \mid L = l, F = f)$ will be 9-by-4. Parameterize these conditional probability distributions as appropriate. Try representing them as rectangular matrices, and carry out the required computations using dot products of rows and columns extracted from them. Use the model to simulate the attention results shown in Figure 12.11 in which the response, or posterior probability $P(F = f \mid I = i)$, of the vertical feature detector to an image of a vertical blob at one location and a horizontal blob at the other is increased when the prior probability $P(L = l)$ of the location of the vertical blob is increased.

12.3   In the predictor–corrector simulation of the responses of neurons in the parabigeminal nucleus (PBN), the simulated PBN neuron response was lower when the target was unlit than when it was lit. This in part reflects the fact that the variance of the observation is maximal when the target is unlit, but it is also a function of the specific part of the trajectory during which the target is unlit. Rerun the predictor–corrector simulation (pbnPredictCorrect, listed in MATLAB Box 12.6) after first changing the range of target positions over which the target is unlit. (Variables lightOff and lightOn, respectively, start and end the unlit part of the trajectory, and they are set in predictCorrectSetUp, listed in MATLAB Box 12.5.) Are there parts of the trajectory (target position ranges) for which the PBN response is *higher* when the target is unlit than when it is lit? Does this make sense? (Keep in mind that the simulated PBN neuron computes the posterior probability that the target is at or beyond its preferred target position, and that the variances of the observation, and so also of the target prior and posterior distributions, are larger when the target is unlit.)

12.4   In training a single sigmoidal unit with feedback to simulate the responses of neurons in the parabigeminal nucleus (PBN), we found that the delta rule adjusted the values of the bias and feedback weights, as well as the weights from input units representing the deep and superficial superior colliculi, to the PBN unit (see Figure 12.21B). Train the PBN network model using pbnDeltaRule (listed in MATLAB Box 12.7, which will first run predictCorrectSetUp, listed in MATLAB Box 12.5), and explore the effects of altering connection weights on the performance of the trained network. The commands M(1)=0 and M(164)=0 will, respectively, zero the weights of the connections from the bias unit to the PBN unit and from the PBN unit to itself. What happens to the responses of the trained unit if the bias and/or feedback weights are set to 0? Do the bias and feedback connections affect the lit as well as the unlit responses of the unit? These experiments reveal the mechanism developed by the model PBN unit in learning to estimate the probabilities of the positions of lit and unlit, moving targets.

References

Barlow HB, Levick WR (1965) The mechanism of directionally selective units in the rabbit's retina. *Journal of Physiology London* 178: 477–504.

Berry MJ II, Brivanlou IH, Jordan TA, Meister M (1999) Anticipation of moving stimuli by the retina. *Nature* 398: 334–338.

Cui H, Malpeli JG (2003) Activity in the parabigeminal nucleus during eye movements directed at moving and stationary targets. *Journal of Neurophysiology* 89: 3128–3142.

DeLucia PR, Cochhran EL (1985) Perceptual information for batting can be extracted throughout a ball's trajectory. *Perceptual and Motor Skills* 61: 143–150.

Demb JB (2007) Cellular mechanisms for direction selectivity in the retina. *Neuron* 55: 179–186

Denève S, Duhamel J-R, Pouget A (2007) Optimal sensorimotor integration in recurrent cortical networks: A neural implementation of Kalman filters. *Journal of Neuroscience* 27: 5744–5756.

Gilbert CD, Sigman M (2007) Brain states: Top down influences in sensory processing. *Neuron* 54: 677–696.

Graham J (1977) An autoradiographic study of the efferent connections of the superior colliculus in the cat. *Journal of Comparative Neurology* 173: 629–654.

Grossberg S, Mingolla E, Ross WD (1997) Visual brain and visual perception: How does the cortex do perceptual grouping? *Trends in Neuroscience* 20: 106–111.

Jensen FV (2001) *Bayesian Networks and Decision Graphs*. Springer, New York.

Kalman RE (1960) A new approach to linear filtering and prediction theory. *Transactions of the ASME Journal of Basic Engineering* 82: 35–45.

Kanizsa G (1979) *Organization in Vision*. Praeger, New York.

Land MF, McLeod P (2000) From eye movements to actions: How batsman hit the ball. *Nature Neuroscience* 3: 1340–1345.

Lee TS, Mumford D (2003) Hierarchical Bayesian inference in the visual cortex. *Journal of the Optical Society of America* 20: 1434–1448.

Livingstone MS (1998) Mechanisms of direction selectivity in macaque V1. *Neuron* 20: 509–526.

Ma R, Cui H, Lee S-H, Anastasio TJ, Malpeli JG (in review) Predictive encoding of moving target trajectory by neurons in the midbrain.

Marr D (1982) *Vision*. WH Freeman and Company, San Francisco, CA.

McAdams CJ, Maunsell JHR (1999) Effects of attention on orientation-tuning functions of single neurons in macaque cortical area V4. *Journal of Neuroscience* 19: 431–441.

Mishkin M, Ungerleider LG, Macko DA (1983) Object vision and spatial vision: Two cortical pathways. *Trends in Neuroscience* 6: 414–417.

Motter BC (1993) Focal attention produces spatially selective processing in visual cortical areas V1, V2, and V4 in the presence of competing stimuli. *Journal of Neurophysiology* 70: 909–919.

Newsome WT, Wurtz RH, Komatsu H (1988) Relation of cortical areas MT and MST to pursuit eye movements. II. Differentiation of retinal from extraretinal inputs. *Journal of Neurophysiology* 60: 604–620.

Pearl P (1988) *Probabilistic Reasoning in Intelligent Systems: Networks of Plausible Inference*. Morgan Kaufmann, San Mateo, CA.

Rao RPN (1999) An optimal estimation approach to visual perception and learning. *Vision Research* 39: 1963–1989.

Rao RPN (2005) Bayesian inference and attentional modulation in the visual cortex. *NeuroReport* 16: 1843–1848.

Rao RPN, Ballard DH (1999) Predictive coding in the visual cortex: A functional interpretation of some extra-classical receptive field effects. *Nature Neuroscience* 2: 79–87.

Reynolds JH, Chelazzi L, Desimone R (1999) Competitive mechanisms subserve attention in macaque areas V2 and V4. *Journal of Neuroscience* 19: 1736–1753.

Ruff PI, Rauschecker JP, Palm G (1987) A model of direction-selective "simple" cells in the visual cortex based on inhibition asymmetry. *Biological Cybernetics* 57: 147–157.

Russell S, Norvig P (1995) *Artificial Intelligence: A Modern Approach*. Prentice-Hall, Upper Saddle River, New Jersey, pp 498–522.

Van Berkum JJA, Brown, CM, Zwitserlood P, Kooijman V, Hagoort P (2005) Anticipating upcoming words in discourse: Evidence from ERPs and reading times. *Journal of Experimental Psychology* 31: 443–467.

Van Essen DC (1985) Functional organization of primate visual cortex. In: Peters A, Jones EG (eds) *Cerebral Cortex: Volume 3*. Plenum Press, New York, pp 259–329.

Wurtz RL, Goldberg ME (1989) *The Neurobiology of Saccadic Eye Movements*. Elsevier, Amsterdam.

Yasushi M, Paulin M (1989) A Kalman filter theory of the cerebellum. In: Arbib MA, Amari S-I (eds) *Dynamic Interactions in Neural Networks: Models and Data*, Springer-Verlag, New York, pp 239–259.

13

Simulated Evolution and the Genetic Algorithm

*The genetic algorithm simulates the process
of biological evolution and can be used to
optimize the structure, connectivity, and
adaptability of neural systems models*

The ultimate goal of neural systems modeling is to understand why
the brain is as it is. There are two reasons for the "is-ness" of
any neural system. The first reason is its function. Neural system
function has been our primary concern in this book, but function
does not alone determine the nature of a neural system. The
second reason is its history. Every neural system has acquired
its particular *modus operandi* through some combination of
evolution, development, and learning. The nature of any neural
system has as much to do with its history as with its function.

To illustrate this dual influence on the nature of a non-neural
system, consider the electric power system. Efficiency dictates
that electric power be generated and transmitted in the form of
alternating rather than direct current, but the best alternation
frequency depends on other factors, including the requirements
of the motors and other equipment that use the power. In North
America today the standard frequency for alternating-current
electric power is 60 cycles per second, but in the past, frequencies

as low as 25 cycles per second were in use. Adoption of the standard has required the development of specialized equipment and the deployment of expensive material conversions that are still ongoing (Blalock 2003). Thus, the reason why the electric current out of a North American wall outlet alternates at 60 cycles per second has as much to do with the history of electric power usage as with the function of electric generators. And as every traveler knows, different countries with different histories can have different standard frequencies for alternating current.

Alternation, or oscillation, in neural systems also depends as much on history as on function, particularly with regard to the mechanism by which the oscillation is produced. In Chapter 2 we constructed a neural model of an oscillator. Specifically, we simulated the flight-control central pattern generator (CPG) of the locust, which was originally modeled by Donald Wilson (Wilson 1961). Part of the *modus operandi* of the Wilson model involves the "fatigue" of individual units by which they "get tired" after a while and simply switch off their own activity. Wilson considered fatigue to be a cellular property, but we simulated it instead using interactions among units in a recurrent network. In taking this alternative approach we were able to achieve the same function using a completely different mechanism. Diversity of mechanism characterizes biological oscillators in general.

Central pattern generators occur in practically all vertebrate and invertebrate animals and mediate periodic behaviors ranging from locomotion to stomach churning. Other biological oscillators underlie basic physiological processes that include periodic heart and smooth muscle contractions and release of hormones. Oscillation can be a cellular or a network property. In single cells, chemical interactions occurring in the cytoplasm can produce oscillations in chemical concentrations, and interactions involving ion channels can produce membrane potential oscillations (Berridge and Rapp 1979). Single-neuron oscillators fire periodic bursts of action potentials. Oscillations in central pattern generator networks can result from dynamic interactions between non-bursting neurons only (as in our model of the locust-flight central pattern generator in Chapter 2), or between non-bursting and bursting neurons, and the network configurations of known central pattern generators vary widely (Friesen and Stent 1978; Selverston and Moulins 1985). These facts indicate that central pattern generation can be accomplished through a potentially huge variety of mechanisms. They further suggest that the mechanism that actually mediates the function of any particular central pattern generator depends to a large extent on the evolutionary history of the organism in which it operates.

We will not attempt to simulate the parallel evolution of central pattern generators in this chapter. (But simulated evolution of a nonlinear version of the Wilson central pattern generator is the subject of Exercise 13.4.) Our goal in this chapter is to simulate some of the ways in which genetic evolution can influence the structure, connectivity, and adaptability of neural systems. This influence is profound but limited. There are hundreds of trillions of synapses in the human brain, but only about 30,000 genes in the human genome. It is clear that in humans, as in other animals, the genome does not specify the weight of every synapse. However, proteins encoded by genes direct the formation of neuronal connections and mediate the plasticity of synapses. Our goal in this chapter is to explore ways in which the genome could set the parameters for the developmental and adaptive processes that ultimately make the brain what it is. Our studies in this chapter will all involve simulated evolution using the genetic algorithm.

The genetic algorithm, developed by John Holland (1975), is a computational optimization procedure that was designed on the basis of biological

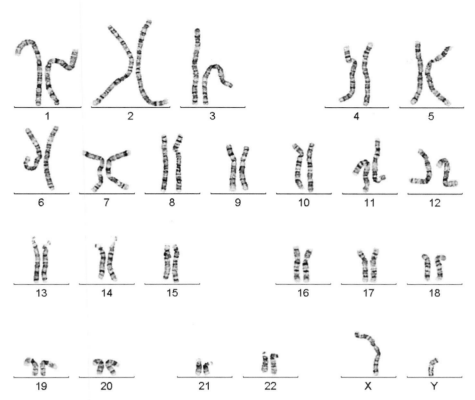

FIGURE 13.1   A normal, human male karyotype The karyotype characterizes the set of chromosomes of a eukaryotic organism. The normal human male has 22 pairs of chromosomes plus one X and one Y chromosome. (Courtesy of the J. Craig Venter Institute.)

evolution. Biological evolution occurs through the variation of the genetic code among individuals in a population, selection from that population, and mutation and recombination of the genetic codes of the fittest individuals. The results of biological evolution are sets of individuals who are well adapted to the task of survival in a particular environment. The genetic algorithm essentially imitates this survival-of-the-fittest strategy for the purpose of optimizing the performance of computational systems (including neural networks) whose parameters it can specify and represent in a form amenable to simulated genetic evolution. This involves the representation of system parameters in terms of genes and chromosomes.

Structurally, genes are situated on chromosomes. Biological organisms can have many chromosomes. As an example, Figure 13.1 shows a normal human male karyotype (i.e., the characteristic chromosome complement of the normal human male). Each chromosome can hold many genes. In biological organisms, genes encode proteins. Whereas genes are composed of the four nucleic acid molecules—adenine, thymine, guanine, and cytosine—proteins are composed of the 21 amino acid molecules. Sequences of three nucleic acids encode each of the different amino acids. Through the processes of gene transcription and translation, the genetic code is read out and used as the blueprint for the construction of proteins (Watson et al. 2008).

Proteins are macromolecules that have various functions in cells, from catalyzing biochemical reactions to supporting cell structure. Proteins play essential roles in the brain. These include the formation both of the ionic channels that underlie nerve cell excitability and the receptors that mediate synaptic transmission. Proteins also serve as chemical signals that guide the growth of axons and direct the formation of connections between neurons. These chemical signals were first discovered by Roger Sperry (1963). Sperry studied the development of connections to the optic tectum from the retina in frogs. (The optic tectum is the amphibian analog of the superior colliculus in mammals; see Chapters 3, 5, and 9 for references on the superior colliculus.) These connections, which travel over the optic nerve, are orderly in that the retinal map is preserved in the tectum. Sperry observed that the optic nerve axons would regrow after they had been surgically disconnected, and would re-innervate the tectum with the correct topography. Sperry wondered whether neural activity or molecular markers guided this re-establishment of connectivity. The experiment he designed to test this involved disconnecting the optic nerve from the tectum and then rotating the eye of the frog upside down (while the frog was deeply anesthetized, of course).

Sperry reasoned that if neural activity guided regrowth, then the optic nerve axons should re-innervate a completely different set of tectal neurons in such a way that the behavioral responses of the frog would be appropriate for the new orientation of its eye. Alternatively, if molecular markers guided regrowth, then the optic nerve axons should twist around and reconnect to the same tectal neurons as before. After the period of regrowth, Sperry found that the behavioral responses of the frog were essentially upside down. For example, if a fly appeared in the upper part of the visual field the frog would snap toward the lower part of the visual field. The results suggested that the optic nerve axons were guided by molecular markers on the surface of the tectum that caused them to reconnect to the same tectal neurons they had been disconnected from, regardless of the consequences for behavior this entailed. That and similar results led Sperry to formulate his chemoaffinity hypothesis (Sperry 1963), according to which the connectivity of the nervous system is established by means of molecular markers that guide the direction of axon growth, and determine the patterns of connectivity between different regions of the brain and among neurons within each region.

It is recognized now that the development of connections within the nervous system involves a combination of activity-dependent and molecular mechanisms (Jacobson 1991). We studied models of activity-dependent mechanisms in the context of self-organizing maps in Chapter 5. Indeed, the development of certain structural and functional properties of the nervous system critically depends on neural activity. Examples we studied in Chapter 5 include the orientation pinwheel structures and orientation selectivity functions of neurons in the visual system. However, those activity-dependent mechanisms do not start from a completely random configuration but from a highly structured configuration that is established by molecular mechanisms.

The guidance of axon growth and connectivity is schematized in Figure 13.2. While axons can be guided by structural features, such as the boundaries between tissues (e.g., between brain tissue and blood vessels), most axon guidance involves protein markers. These markers can either diffuse into the extra-cellular space and form concentration gradients that guide axon growth, or they can be attached to the surfaces of other neurons and direct the formation of specific connections (Jacobson 1991; Huber et al. 2003; Inatani 2005). By encoding these marker proteins, genes specify the developmental mechanisms and connectivity patterns that determine much of the structure of the nervous system.

The influence of the genome is not limited to axonal path-finding. Research involving direct manipulation of the genome has revealed that a broad range of genes are involved both in neural development and adaptive plasticity. Experiments using genetic knock-out animals (mice mostly) show that mutations in genes for proteins such as brain-derived neurotrophic factor, neural-cell adhesion molecule, certain glutamate receptor subunits, and protein kinases including calcium/calmodulin-dependent protein kinase, can cause profound deficits both in brain development and plasticity (Chen and

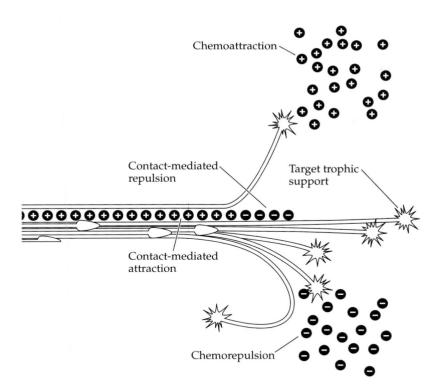

FIGURE 13.2   Growing axons are guided by molecular cues These cues induce attraction or repulsion and include proteins that are attached to cell surfaces or secreted into the extra-cellular milieu. (After Huber et al. 2003.)

Tonegawa 1997). By encoding the proteins involved in neural plasticity, genes specify the learning mechanisms that determine much of the function of the nervous system. Thus, the genome provides the basis for the developmental and adaptive processes that determine both the structure and the function of the nervous systems.

The genome itself is shaped by evolution through the processes of variation and selection. Genetic variation occurs mainly in two ways, mutation and recombination, both of which affect the sequences of nucleic acids in genes and so change the code (Watson et al. 2008). Mutation involves random changes in the code on a single gene, while recombination involves the swapping of bits of code between homologous regions of two chromosomes. The crossover point (site) for recombination can occur between genes or within genes. Thus, recombination changes the set of genes on a chromosome, but can also change the code within a single gene if part of that gene gets swapped for its counterpart on another chromosome. We will explore the effects both of mutation and recombination in this chapter.

There are a great variety of techniques for simulating evolution that imitate these genetic operators, and others, in different combinations and according to different algorithms (Goldberg 1989). In this chapter we will implement a simple and straightforward version of the genetic algorithm in which both recombination and mutation occur on each cycle of variation and selection. The goal of the algorithm is to find genes that are highly fit in some well-defined sense. The method we will use is illustrated in Table 13.1, which whimsically depicts the evolution of a common food item, the salad.

The population in this case consists of five individuals. Just as an individual biological organism can be considered both as a set of genes (its genotype), and as a body that is encoded by those genes (its phenotype), so each individual in this population is both a "salad" and the set of genes that encodes that salad. More specifically, each individual is represented by a chromosome that contains five genes, and each gene encodes an ingredient of a salad. In

TABLE 13.1   One step in the evolution of the salad (each row is a chromosome)

(A) An intermediate stage in the evolution of the salad

1	Vinegar	Banana	Olive oil	Oatmeal	Jelly beans
2	Cucumber	Corn chips	Vinegar	Blueberries	Salami
3	Corn chips	Catsup	Milk	Lettuce	Olive oil
4	Tomato	Olive oil	Tomato	Olive oil	Tomato
5	Lettuce	Tuna fish	Vinegar	Pepper	Cucumber

(B) Salads four and five are chosen for reproduction with crossover

Most fit (5)	Lettuce	Tuna fish	Vinegar	Pepper	Cucumber
			xxx		
Next fit (4)	Tomato	Olive oil	Tomato	Olive oil	Tomato

Crossover point (xxx) between bits three and four

Son	Lettuce	Tuna fish	Vinegar	Olive oil	Tomato
Daughter	Tomato	Olive oil	Tomato	Pepper	Cucumber

(C) Offspring replace salads one and three. The next generation is tastier!

1 (Now son)	Lettuce	Tuna fish	Vinegar	Olive oil	Tomato
2	Cucumber	Corn chips	Vinegar	Blueberries	Salami
3 (Now dtr)	Tomato	Olive oil	Tomato	Pepper	Cucumber
4	Tomato	Olive oil	Tomato	Olive oil	Tomato
5	Lettuce	Tuna fish	Vinegar	Pepper	Cucumber

this whimsical example, the code is not a sequence of nucleic acids—it is an English word that describes an ingredient.

Table 13.1A shows the population at an arbitrarily chosen generation. As evolution proceeds, through variation and selection, the overall fitness of the population should improve. The fitness of each salad is its tastiness, and the tastier the salad the more likely it is to survive and reproduce under the selective pressure of the competitive "gastronomic environment." Variability of the salads in the population, which may change their fitness, occurs through mutation and recombination. Mutation is simply a random change in a gene of a single individual. For example, mutation of the "milk" gene to "cheese" might slightly improve the fitness (tastiness) of salad 3.

Recombination is more complicated. The first step is to select two chromosomes with high fitness to be recombined. As we will see later, chromosomes should be selected probabilistically (not deterministically) according to fitness, but for this example we will simply choose the two most fit chromosomes for mating (i.e., recombination). In order to rank the chromosomes we must turn their genes (genotypes) into salads (phenotypes) and taste them.

While there is no accounting for taste, most readers would probably rank salad 5 as the most fit, and salad 1 as the least fit. For sake of illustration, let us agree that the ranking of the salads from most to least fit is: 5, 4, 2, 3, and 1. As shown in Table 13.1B, we select the two most fit chromosomes, 5 and 4, for mating. Recombination begins by copying the parent chromosomes (the parents themselves will survive into the next generation). Recombination continues by randomly selecting a crossover point and swapping the copied chromosomes at that point. In this case the crossover point occurs between the third and fourth genes, so the copies of chromosomes 4 and 5 are both broken at that point, and each copy swaps a homologous segment with the other. Thus, one offspring (the "son") consists of the first segment of chromosome 5 and the second segment of chromosome 4, and the other offspring (the "daughter") consists of the first segment of chromosome 4 and the second segment of chromosome 5. These offspring chromosomes will replace two less fit chromosomes. The replacement chromosomes should also be chosen probabilistically, but for this example we will choose the two least fit chromosomes, 1 and 3. In Table 13.1C, the son and daughter of chromosomes 4 and 5 have replaced chromosomes 1 and 3. Again, while there is no accounting for taste, most readers would agree that the current generation of salads is tastier than the previous generation.

This whimsical "gastronomic evolution" example illustrates the basic plan that we will use in implementing the genetic algorithm. The "birth" of new offspring through recombination will mark the beginning of a new generation. Selection will be probabilistic, but offspring will be produced from fit individuals, who will remain in the population, and offspring will replace unfit individuals. After the new population is established, all of the chromosomes will be subject to random mutation, but at a very low rate. This procedure incorporates the main features of simulated evolution and is simple to implement.

Technically, the genetic algorithm in this example of gastronomic evolution is solving a subset selection problem in that it is selecting a subset of ingredients from a vast cornucopia. Note, specifically, that the crossover points never occur within a gene encoding an ingredient, only between genes (ingredients). The genetic algorithm is more typically used for parameter optimization problems in which each gene encodes a different parameter as a bit string. Changes in the values of the parameters, which are necessary for their optimization, occur when crossover occurs within the genes. Changes in the values of the encoded parameters can also occur through mutation. We will use both of these mechanisms of simulated genetic variation to optimize various parameters of neural networks, including numbers of units, learning rules, and connection weights.

13.1 Simulating Genes and Genetic Operators

Genes can be simulated as bit (binary) strings (of 0s and 1s). In artificial evolution, the genes encode not proteins but the elements or parameters of computational systems. In this chapter the computational systems will be neural networks. Our chromosomes will be simple, consisting of one or a few genes. Simulated evolution will occur over a changing chromosome population (set of chromosomes), in which the genotype of each chromosome specifies a neural network phenotype. Simulated evolution of this population will be implemented according to the procedure described in the previous section.

The chromosomes vary within the population. This is due, in the first instance, to randomization of each initial chromosome. Variation is continually re-introduced into the population by random mutation and recombination. For binary chromosomes, mutation involves selecting bits at random and flipping them from 0 to 1 or vice-versa. Mutation occurs at a low rate, but every chromosome can potentially undergo mutation on each generation in our version of the genetic algorithm.

In our examples the chromosomes will encode one or more of the parameters that describe neural network structure, function, or adaptability (e.g., numbers of units, connection weight values, or learning rules). After the genes are decoded, the neural networks encoded by each chromosome can be constructed and their fitness can be evaluated. Fitness will obviously vary because the chromosomes vary. The chromosomes can be ordered on the basis of the fitness of the networks they encode. Genetic recombination is simulated by selecting a pair of parent chromosomes from the population, with a probability that is proportional to their fitness, and copying them. A crossover point is chosen at random, the chromosomes of each copy are broken at the crossover point, and a pair of offspring is produced by swapping and then rejoining the symbol (binary) strings of the copies. The offspring chromosomes will replace two other chromosomes from the population. The chromosomes to be replaced are selected with a probability that is inversely proportional to their fitness. Fitness can be retested after mating (and mutation), and the recombination process can be repeated, as the genetic algorithm moves the population through the generations.

Because the chromosomes in the initial population are random, and mutation and crossover points are chosen at random, and mating and replaceable chromosomes are selected partly at random, it might seem as though the genetic algorithm is simply performing a random search. In fact, analysis shows that the genetic algorithm will cause good genes to spread throughout the population genome at a geometric rate, thus improving the overall fitness of the population (Math Box 13.1). The fittest member (chromosome) of the population can be considered as the solution of the genetic optimization procedure in any given generation.

The use of the genetic algorithm in the design of neural networks is quite a reasonable approach (Yao 1999). As described in the previous section, genes are in large part responsible for the anatomical and physiological characteristics of the nervous system, but genes cannot directly specify every connection and synaptic weight. Because the number of synapses in the brain far exceeds the number of genes in the genome, it seems clear that genes can specify only certain of the parameters that are involved in governing the formation and operation of the nervous system. Developmental and adaptive processes, similar to the neural network algorithms we have considered in previous chapters, would also be needed to completely specify the structure and function of the brain. In this chapter we will use the genetic algorithm to specify some of the parameters needed for the construction and adaptation of neural network models, but to illustrate the algorithm we will first use it to find the minimum of a function of one variable.

13.2 Exploring a Simple Example of Simulated Genetic Evolution

The goal of the genetic algorithm is to maximize the fitness of some computationally realizable entity. A straightforward way to demonstrate the algorithm is to use it to maximize a function (Goldberg 1989). However, the performance of neural networks is most commonly evaluated in terms of error. The fitness of the neural network models we will evolve in this chapter will be inversely proportional to a measure such as the error on a learning task, or to the number of cycles required for learning to occur. Rather than convert the error measure to fitness and then maximize that fitness, it will be more efficient for us simply to use the genetic algorithm to minimize the error directly. To illustrate this we will use the genetic algorithm to minimize the quadratic function shown in Equation 13.1:

$$f(x) = x^2 - 30x + 230 \qquad \textbf{13.1}$$

MATH BOX 13.1   THE SCHEMA THEOREM FOR THE GENETIC ALGORITHM

While there are several elements of randomness associated with the genetic algorithm (random initial genes, probabilistic selection of chromosomes for reproduction, random selection of crossover points, and random mutation), the genetic algorithm is definitely not just a random search. Due to the operational characteristics of the genetic algorithm, simulated genes that are more fit than average spread geometrically throughout the population. The following analysis is from Goldberg (1989). It is based on the idea of genetic schemata. We encountered schemata of a different sort in Chapter 7, where they represented functional groups of neurons. In the context of the genetic algorithm, a schema H is a particular pattern of bits along a string representing a chromosome. At any generation g there are $m(H, g)$ instances of schema H in the population of chromosomes (strings) $\mathbf{A}(g)$. The goal of the analysis is to determine the number of instances of schema H in the next generation, which is denoted by $m(H, g + 1)$.

The analysis is based on a version of the genetic algorithm in which the entire population of n chromosomes at generation $g + 1$ is selected from the population at generation g. Chromosomes in generation $g + 1$ then mutate and/or recombine (crossover) at random. Selection occurs according to fitness and with replacement (i.e., the same chromosome can be selected multiple times). Specifically, a string A_i is selected according to the probability $p_i = f_i / \Sigma f_j$, where f_i is the fitness of A_i and Σf_j is the summed fitness of all the strings. After selecting a population of n strings from $\mathbf{A}$ (with replacement), the expected number of strings containing schema H in the next generation is $m(H, g + 1) = n \times m(H, g) \times f(H) / \Sigma f_j$ where $f(H)$ is the average fitness of strings containing schema H. Because the average fitness of the population can be expressed as $f(\mathbf{A}) = \Sigma f_j / n$, the expected number of strings containing schema H in the next generation can be described as in Equation B13.1.1:

$$m(H, g + 1) = m(H, g)\frac{f(H)}{f(\mathbf{A})}$$ B13.1.1

In words, Equation B13.1.1 says that, due to selection, schemata with fitness greater than average will receive an increasing number of copies in the next generation, while schemata with fitness less that average will receive a decreasing number. Now suppose that the fitness of a schema H remains, over generations, a constant $c \times f(\mathbf{A})$ above the average fitness, so that $f(H) = f(\mathbf{A}) + cf(\mathbf{A})$. Then Equation B13.1.1 can be rewritten as Equation B13.1.2:

$$m(H, g + 1) = m(H, g)\frac{\left[f(\mathbf{A}) + cf(\mathbf{A})\right]}{f(\mathbf{A})} = m(H, g)(1 + c)$$ B13.1.2

Starting at $g = 0$ and advancing through the generations, we get the geometric progression shown in Equation B13.1.3, which is of the same general form as the progression we first encountered in Math Box 1.1 (see Chapter 1):

$$m(H, g) = m(H, 0)(1 + c)^g$$ B13.1.3

Thus, schemata with above ($c > 0$) or below ($0 > c > -1$) average fitness will, respectively, increase or decrease geometrically in the population. Extending the analysis to account also for crossover and random mutation (see Goldberg 1989 for details) it can be shown that the relationship in Equation B13.1.4 holds true:

$$m(H, g + 1) \geq m(H, g)\frac{f(H)}{f(\mathbf{A})}\left[1 - p_C\frac{\delta(H)}{l-1} - o(H)p_M\right]$$ B13.1.4

where p_C is the probability of crossover, p_M is the probability of mutation, l is the length of the string, and $\delta(H)$ and $o(H)$ are the length and order of the schema, respectively. The length of a schema is the distance between its first and last critical bits, while the order is the number of critical bits in the schema. For example, for the schema [1 0 * * 1], where the uncritical bits * can be either 0 or 1, the length $\delta(H) = 4$ while the order $o(H) = 3$. Equation B13.1.4 is the "schema theorem." The term in brackets is the probability that a schema H will survive crossover and mutation. Long, high-order schemata are susceptible to destruction by these genetic operators while short, low-order schemata are more resistant. The schema theorem basically states that the number of short, low-order schemata with above average fitness will increase geometrically in subsequent generations.

FIGURE 13.3   A concave-up function used to illustrate the principles of genetic search The quadratic function is $f(x) = x^2 - 30x + 230$, where x is the argument of the function and $f(x)$ is its value. The minimum can be found using the genetic algorithm.

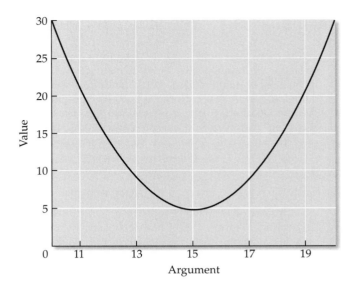

A graph of this concave-up function is shown in Figure 13.3. Of course, we do not need the genetic algorithm to minimize Equation 13.1. The minimum value of the quadratic function $f(x)$, and the argument x that gives the minimum value, can be determined easily using calculus, as shown in Math Box 13.2. The object of the first example is to use the genetic algorithm on a simple problem for which we already know the answer. The script `gaMinimum`, listed in MATLAB® Box 13.1, will use the genetic algorithm to find the minimum of a function.

We begin by generating an initial population of binary chromosomes in which every bit in every gene (bit string) is determined randomly. Each chromosome needs to represent only one item, which is the decimal argument of the function in Equation 13.1, so each chromosome will have only one gene. For this problem it is convenient to use integer arguments that range from 0 to 31. This range can be represented with binary numbers that are five digits long (five-element bit strings). Also for convenience, we can set the population size at five chromosomes, so our population can be represented as a 5-by-5 square matrix of binary values. For the initial population we simply generate a 5-by-5 matrix in which each element will be a 1 with probability 0.5. This can be done using the command `POP=rand(popSize)>0.5`, where `popSize=5` is the popula-

MATH BOX 13.2   FINDING THE MINIMA (MAXIMA) OF FUNCTIONS

Finding the minima (or maxima) of a differentiable function is one of the simplest applications of calculus. The first derivative $f'(x)$ is the instantaneous rate of change of a function. Because the rate of change is zero at the minima (or maxima), the arguments x that produce the minimal (or maximal) values of the function $f(x)$ are the solutions of $f'(x) = 0$. For example, consider the quadratic function in Equation 13.1 that we minimize in Section 13.2 using the genetic algorithm: $f(x) = x^2 - 30x + 230$. This function has a single minimum (see Figure 13.3). Its first derivative with respect to x is $f'(x) = 2x - 30$. To find the

argument x for which the first derivative $f'(x)$ is zero we solve $0 = 2x - 30$ to get $x = 15$. Using this as the argument of our original function, we find that its minimum value is $f(x) = 15^2 - 30(15) + 230 = 5$.

Other functions can have multiple minima (or maxima). Consider $f(x) = \sin(x)$, the sine wave. It has a maximum that alternates with a minimum every $\pi/2$ radians (90 degrees). Its first derivative is $f'(x) = \cos(x)$, and $\cos(x) = 0$ at every argument x that is a multiple of $\pi/2$ radians (90 degrees), coinciding with the maxima and minima of $\sin(x)$.

MATLAB® BOX 13.1 The script uses the genetic algorithm with binary genes to find the minimum of a function.

```
% gaMinimum.m

popSize=5; % set the population size
pow=fliplr(0:popSize-1); % set powers for decoding
pw2=2.^pow'; % find powers of two for decoding genes
POP=rand(popSize)>0.5; % randomize initial population
chromL=5; % set length of each chromosome
numGen=20; % set the number of generations
muRate=0; % set the mutation rate
meanVal=zeros(1,numGen); % define value hold vector

for gen=1:numGen; % for each generation
    dec=(POP*pw2)'; % convert the binary chromosomes to decimal numbers
    val=dec.^2-30*dec+230; % find value of function for each chromosome
    meanVal(gen)=mean(val); % find and store mean value for generation
    if numGen==gen, break; end % do not change last generation
    normVal=val./sum(val); % normalize the values for each chromosome
    ranVec=rand(1,popSize); % generate a vector of random numbers
    normRan=ranVec./sum(ranVec); % normalize the random vector
    pertVal=normVal+normRan; % randomly perturb values for chromosomes
    [theVals,index]=sort(pertVal); % sort chroms by perturbed value
    dad=POP(index(1),:); % dad has smallest perturbed value
    mom=POP(index(2),:); % mom has next smallest value
    coSite=ceil(rand*chromL); % choose a random crossover site
    son=[dad(1:coSite) mom(coSite+1:chromL)]; % generate son
    dtr=[mom(1:coSite) dad(coSite+1:chromL)]; % generate daughter
    POP(index(popSize),:)=son; % replace least fit by son
    POP(index(popSize-1),:)=dtr; % replace next least fit by dtr
    MUMX=rand(popSize)<muRate; % generate random mutation matrix
    POP=abs(POP-MUMX); % mutate the chromosomes
end % end loop over generations
```

tion size. Thus, each row of POP is a chromosome containing one gene, and each gene is a binary number (bit string) that encodes an integer argument for the function in Equation 13.1.

Decoding each binary, single-gene chromosome involves finding its decimal equivalent. A 5-digit binary number, expressed as a row vector, can be converted to its decimal equivalent by multiplying it by a column vector in which the elements are the number 2 raised to powers from 4 to 0 in descending order. For example, the decimal equivalent of the binary number [1 0 1 0 1] is the dot product of this row vector with the column vector $[16\ 8\ 4\ 2\ 1]^T$, which is $[1\ 0\ 1\ 0\ 1]\ [16\ 8\ 4\ 2\ 1]^T = 16 + 4 + 1 = 21$. In script gaMinimum the powers of 2 are set using pow=fliplr(0:popSize-1), and the column vector of 2 raised to those powers is pw2=2.^pow'. The entire population of chromosomes can be converted from binary to decimal using dec=(POP*pw2)'. (We convert the result from a column to a row to facilitate its display.) The row dec is the vector of decimal equivalents for the binary population.

Having decoded the genotype, we must determine the phenotype. In this simple case the phenotype is just the value of the quadratic function in Equation 13.1 for each of the decimal arguments encoded by the single-gene chromosomes. The vector of values (phenotypes) is computed using val=dec.^2-30*dec+230. Knowing the phenotypes, we can rank the chromosomes according to fitness. We are searching for the chromosome that produces the minimum value of the function, so the most fit chromosome produces the smallest value. Because our goal is to minimize the function, by arranging the values from smallest to largest we order the chromosomes from most fit to least fit. However, as mentioned above and demonstrated below, we want to select chromosomes probabilistically, not deterministically, according to fitness.

We want to order the chromosomes in such a way that the two most fit will most likely (but not definitely) be selected for mating, while the two least fit will most likely (but not definitely) be selected for replacement by the offspring. Therefore, we need to use fitness to determine the probabilities with which we will select chromosomes for mating or replacement. We described an accurate way to choose items based on probability in Chapter 9, and that method could be used for this purpose as well. A quicker method, which also allows some useful manipulation of the indeterminacy of the selection, is used in script `gaMimimum`. It involves ordering the phenotype values after they have been randomly perturbed. It begins by normalizing the values so that they sum to 1 using `normVal=val./sum(val)`, generating a uniformly random (range 0 to 1) vector of the same size and normalizing it using `ranVec=rand(1,popSize)` and `normRan=ranVec./sum(ranVec)`, and then perturbing the normalized values using `pertVal=normVal+normRan`. Now if we sort the perturbed values, they will be ordered most likely (but not definitely) from most fit to least fit. The command `[theVals,index]=sort(pertVal)` will place the sorted values in vector `theVals`, and will place the indices of the sorted, perturbed values in vector `index`. The elements of `index` are the indices of the chromosomes ordered most likely (but not definitely) from most fit to least fit. Selection using `index` is straightforward.

After selecting the parents probabilistically according to fitness, we mate them. To review (see Section 13.1), this process begins by making copies of the parents (who survive). It proceeds by randomly choosing a crossover point and recombining the copies so that the chromosome of one offspring is the first part of one parent chromosome and the second part of the other parent chromosome, with the parts being divided at the crossover point. The chromosome of the other offspring combines the parts that are left over. For example, if dad = [1 1 1 1 1] and mom = [0 0 0 0 0], and the crossover point is randomly selected to fall between bits two and three, then son = [1 1 0 0 0] and dtr = [0 0 1 1 1] (dtr is a convenient three-letter abbreviation for daughter).

In script `gaMinimum` we use the ordering in vector `index` to select chromosomes probabilistically according to fitness. The parents, `dad` and `mom`, are most likely the most fit, so we select `dad=POP(index(1),:)` and `mom=POP(index(2),:)`. We choose a random crossover site using `coSite=ceil(rand*chromL)`, where `chromL` is the length of each chromosome in the population. Then `son` is generated using the command `son=[dad(1:coSite)  mom(coSite+1:chromL)]`. Daughter `dtr` is generated using an analogous command: `dtr=[mom(1:coSite) dad(coSite+1:chromL)]`. Note that the parent chromosomes have, in effect, been copied, but they themselves are not affected by the recombination process. The chromosomes to be replaced are most likely the least fit. The script replaces the least fit and next-to-least fit chromosomes using `POP(index(popSize),:)=son` and `POP(index(popSize-1),:)=dtr`.

This process can be repeated with other parents, but one mating and one offspring pair per generation seems sufficient for a population of only five individuals. After recombination the population is subjected to random mutation at a low rate. Specifically, each binary element (bit) in each gene in the population of chromosomes has a small probability of being flipped from 0 to

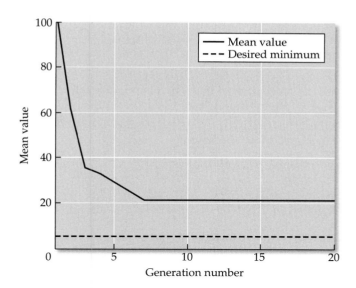

FIGURE 13.4   Using the genetic algorithm with zero mutation probability to find the minimum of a function The mean value of the function over the population of chromosomes decreases rapidly during genetic search. With mutation probability zero, the mean value stabilizes at a certain level and can decrease no further.

1 or vice versa. Script `gaMinimum` implements random mutation by first issuing the command `MUMX=rand(popSize)<muRate`, which makes a mutation matrix `MUMX` of the same dimensions as `POP` and in which each element is 0 but has the low probability `muRate` of being a 1. The script then uses mutation matrix `MUMX` to flip bits in `POP` with the command `POP=abs(POP−MUMX)`. Mutation rates (probabilities) of 0.01 or 0.02 are typical.

Random mutation is a critically important component of the genetic algorithm and is, in some sense, even more important than recombination. To demonstrate the usefulness of random mutation we will set the mutation rate to 0 (`muRate=0`) for our first simulation. Set the algorithm to run through 20 generations (`numGen=20`). After each generation, the script `gaMinimum` stores the mean value for the population in array `meanVal`. This mean value over 20 generations, with recombination but without random mutation, is shown in Figure 13.4. The mean value of the function decreases as the generations progress. Thus, the genetic algorithm is indeed improving population fitness. However, the algorithm reaches a floor, after about seven generations, below which it is not able to further reduce the mean value.

The population of chromosomes after 20 generations of simulated evolution, with recombination but without random mutation, is shown in Table 13.2A. The population is homogeneous, and this homogeneity explains why the population mean value reaches a non-optimal floor through which it cannot fall. The reason is that once the population reaches a configuration in which all of the chromosomes are identical, recombination can do nothing but swap identical segments (bit strings). In a homogeneous population, no amount of recombination can produce variability.

Since all of the chromosomes are identical, they must all be considered the fittest. Recall that each chromosome in this example contains a single gene, and each gene encodes an argument for the function in Equation 13.1 that we want to minimize. Every gene in this homogeneous population encodes an argument of 19, which gives a value for the function of 21. This value is far from the minimum (see Figure 13.3 and Math Box 13.2). Even though the chromosomes could recombine, without random mutation the population got stuck in a homogeneous and non-optimal configuration. This situation is avoided with random mutation.

We rerun the simulation for `numGen=20` generations, but this time we set the mutation rate to the low but nonzero value of `muRate=0.01`. The

TABLE 13.2 Finding the minimum of a function using the genetic algorithm

Population of chromosomes, each expressed as a row vector and containing one binary gene					Decimal argument decoded from genes	Value of the function for decimal argument
(A) With recombination but without mutation						
1	0	0	1	1	19	21
1	0	0	1	1	19	21
1	0	0	1	1	19	21
1	0	0	1	1	19	21
1	0	0	1	1	19	21
(B) With recombination and with mutation						
0	1	1	1	1	15	5
0	1	1	1	1	15	5
0	1	0	1	0	10	30
0	1	1	1	1	15	5
0	1	1	1	1	15	5

The population consists of five chromosomes, each expressed as a row vector. Each chromosome in this simple example contains one, 5-bit binary gene. With recombination but without mutation, the population of chromosomes becomes homogeneous and generally does not reach the minimum. With recombination and with mutation, the population stays diverse, and some chromosomes in the population do reach the minimum.

population mean value over 20 generations, with recombination and with random mutation, is shown in Figure 13.5. Again the mean value of the function decreases as the generations progress and, as in the previous simulation, the genetic algorithm improves population fitness. Unlike the previous simulation without mutation, this simulation with random mutation does reach the minimum, but sporadically. The mean value falls and rises again, due to the variability re-introduced by random mutation, but it can often attain the minimum of the function.

The population of chromosomes after 20 generations of simulated evolution, with recombination and with random mutation, is shown in Table 13.2B. The population is heterogeneous. One of the chromosomes encodes the argument of 10, which produces the non-minimal value of 30. Four of the chromosomes encode the argument of 15, which produces the value of 5, which is the minimum value of the function (see Figure 13.3 and Math Box 13.2). These chromosomes are the fittest, and would be considered the solution of the genetic algorithm to the minimization problem. The performance of the genetic algorithm is clearly better with random mutation than without it.

Random mutation improves the performance of the genetic algorithm because it ensures that the population remains diverse. This is critical, because genetic diversity is the source of the alternative schemata (bit sequences) that the genetic algorithm selects and recombines as it searches for a solution to the optimization problem. Random selection, both of the parents of the offspring and of the individuals to be replaced by the offspring, ensures that less fit schemata remain in the population. This provides another important source of diversity but, as we have seen, only random mutation will ultimately prevent the population from becoming homogeneous and getting stuck in a non-optimal solution. This example illustrates the principle, often invoked in

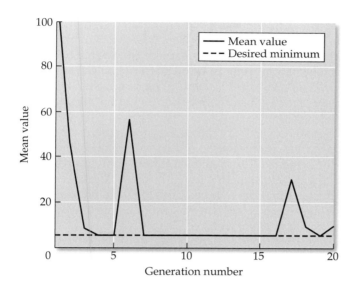

FIGURE 13.5   Using the genetic algorithm with nonzero mutation probability to find the minimum of a function The mean value of the function over the population of chromosomes decreases rapidly during genetic search. With a small but nonzero mutation probability (0.01 in this case), the mean never stabilizes but it can reach the minimal value.

non-scientific settings, that diversity does indeed improve the adaptability of evolving systems.

These mechanisms for re-introducing variation and diversity into the population improve performance at the cost of erratic behavior. Due to these sources of randomness, different runs of the genetic algorithm will vary greatly from one to another. In using the genetic algorithm to find solutions to real problems, it is useful to run the same problem in parallel over many separate populations and use the solutions found by the most successful populations (for an example in a neural systems modeling context see Anastasio and Gad 2007). For the purposes of this chapter, it is important to do several runs of each example in order to establish a general feeling for its behavior. The results reported are representative of the results expected for each example, but are unlikely to exactly match your results on any particular run.

13.3 Evolving the Sizes of Neural Networks to Improve Learning

A particularly nice example of using the genetic algorithm to evolve the parameters that specify neural networks involves multilayered pattern associators trained using back-propagation. Recall from Chapter 6 that back-propagation is a supervised learning algorithm that can train multilayered, feedforward networks of nonlinear units to accomplish a huge range of input–output transformations. In using such networks to model the brain, we often assume that a learning process, such as back-propagation, guides connection weight modification, but that evolution determines network architecture. Schaffer and coworkers (1990) used the genetic algorithm to optimize the architectures of neural networks trained using back-propagation to generalize from a set of patterns. These networks had four layers, including two layers of hidden units. They represented these networks using binary chromosomes containing genes that encoded the numbers of units in the first and second hidden unit layers.

The networks optimized by the genetic algorithm had four input units. The first two inputs were noise units that were uncorrelated with the desired output, while the second two inputs encoded the numbers from 0 to 3 in binary. The two output units encoded the numbers from 0 to 3 in Gray code, which is a type of binary code in which only one bit is changed in going from any value to a higher or lower value. Thus, the numbers from 0 to 3 in binary are [00], [01], [10], and [11], while the same numbers in Gray code are [00], [01], [11], and [10]. The transformation from an input pattern consisting of two noise elements and two binary elements to an output pattern consisting of two Gray-coded elements was termed "the minimum interesting coding problem" (Schaffer et al. 1990).

The transformation from binary to Gray code is easy for a pattern associator trained with back-propagation, and Schaffer and co-workers (1990) chose it largely for reasons of convenience. The challenge for the evolving networks in this case was to learn the transformation despite the noise. The noise inputs require a network to generalize in order to accomplish the transformation, and it was in evolving the ability to generalize that the genetic algorithm produced an unexpected but potentially relevant result.

Schaffer and coworkers (1990) used recombination and random mutation as the mechanisms of genetic variation in a population of 30 chromosomes. The fitness measure was inversely proportional to the error of each network on the required pattern association task. After many generations of simulated evolution using the genetic algorithm, they compared the performance of the fittest network with that of the full network, which had 16 hidden units in each of the two layers. The full network was not determined by genetic search but was expected, *a priori*, to yield the best performance. The comparison showed that the fittest network found by genetic search greatly outperformed the full network. (That is, the genetically determined network had much lower error than the full network.) The architecture of the network found through genetic search, shown in Figure 13.6, was surprising, especially considering that the full network was believed beforehand to be the optimal network.

The fittest network found by the genetic algorithm had four hidden units in its second hidden layer, but only one unit in its first hidden layer. The network

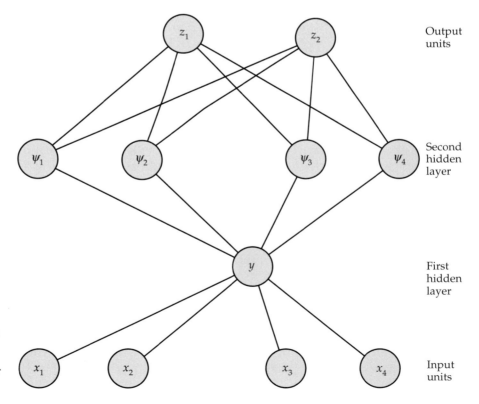

FIGURE 13.6 Using the genetic algorithm to optimize the number of hidden units in multilayered networks In this example, four-layered feedforward networks (having two hidden layers) of sigmoidal units were trained on the minimal interesting coding problem. The optimal network has only one hidden unit in its first hidden layer. The units in each layer are: input layer, x_1 through x_4; first hidden layer, y only; second hidden layer, ψ_1 through ψ_4; and output layer, z_1 and z_2. (After Schaffer et al. 1990.)

with this architecture performed well on the generalization task because the single unit in the first hidden layer forced the network, trained using back-propagation, to generalize. The architecture of this network could be characterized as a convergence from the four input units down to the single unit in the first hidden layer, followed by a divergence from the single unit in the first hidden layer up to the four units in the second hidden layer. This bottleneck structure is actually observed in certain parts of the brain.

One well known instance of a bottleneck in a real neural system occurs along the visual pathway, as schematized in Figure 13.7. The visual pathway in mammals starts with the photoreceptors in the retina, which project over bipolar cells (see also Chapter 3) to the retinal ganglion cells whose axons form the optic nerve. The optic nerve projects to the lateral geniculate nuclei of the thalamus. Lateral geniculate neurons, in turn, project to the visual cortex. Along the visual pathway there is a convergence from about 100 million photoreceptors down to about 1 million ganglion cells, which is followed by a divergence from the ganglion cells up to about 1 billion visual cortical neurons (Dowling 1992). While exploring the functional consequences of convergence and divergence in the visual pathway is still an area of active research, it is temping to speculate, by analogy with the results of artificial evolution by Schaffer and co-workers (1990), that the visual pathway bottleneck contributes to visual perception by introducing a step of generalization.

(A)

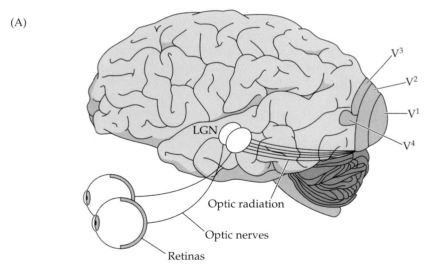

(B)

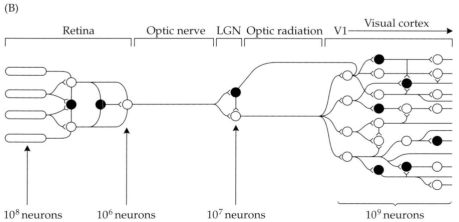

FIGURE 13.7   Convergence and divergence in the visual pathway
(A) The optic nerves carry signals from the retinas of the two eyes to the lateral geniculate nuclei (LGN). The optic radiation carries signals from the LGN to the visual cortical areas (mostly V1). Signals spread from V1 to the other visual cortical areas (V2, V3, V4, etc.). (B) In the retina there is a convergence from about 100 million photoreceptors down to about 1 million optic nerve fibers. From the optic nerve through the LGN there is a divergence up to about 1 billion visual cortical neurons. (After Dowling 1992.)

While generalization is an ability that underlies many important input–output transformations, it is certainly not the sole determinant of the optimal number of hidden units in all cases. We saw, for example, in Chapter 9 that an abundance of hidden units can improve the ability of three-layered neural networks to estimate probabilities. We also saw in Chapters 6 and 7 that an abundance of hidden units can speed learning in three-layered networks trained either with back-propagation or perturbative reinforcement learning. The goal of the next example is to use the genetic algorithm to optimize the speed of learning in three-layered networks trained by back-propagation on the labeled-line patterns. The genetic algorithm is set up so that it can adaptively vary the numbers of hidden units in the networks. Of course, the genetic algorithm could also optimize other parameters of these adaptive networks, like the learning rate, but we will limit the optimization to number of hidden units to keep it simple.

Script `gaHidden`, listed in MATLAB Box 13.2, will use the genetic algorithm to optimize the speed of learning in three-layered feedforward networks trained using back-propagation by adapting the number of hidden units. Our goal is to minimize a measure, in this case number of training iterations, by adapting one item, the number of hidden units. Thus, the same genetic algorithm procedures we used to find the argument that minimizes a function can be used to find the number of hidden units that minimizes the number of training iterations in this example. Comparison between scripts `gaHidden` and `gaMiminum` will reveal a strong structural similarity.

As in the function minimization example, we will optimize only one parameter for the speed-of-learning example, so each chromosome will have only one gene. We can encode numbers of hidden units from 0 to 31 using 5-bit, binary genes, as before. Since we are again encoding only one item, a population of five chromosomes should work well. Thus, for the initial population we can again simply generate a 5-by-5 matrix in which each element will be a 1 with probability 0.5. Procedures for chromosome decoding, selection, recombination, and random mutation for the speed-of-learning example can be implemented as in the function minimization example.

To run simulated evolution of networks trained using back-propagation we need to specify the training patterns and the learning parameters. We also need to implement back-propagation training to establish the fitness of each network. To do this training, script `gaHidden` actually calls another script called `backPropTrainFORga`, listed in MATLAB Box 13.3. To make this example more manageable, parameter setting is shared between the two scripts. The labeled-line input and desired output patterns are set in `gaHidden` using `InPat=[0 0; 1 0; 0 1]` and `DesOut=[0;1;1]`. This script uses the training patterns themselves to determine the numbers of input and output units (`nIn` and `nOut`). It sets the maximal number of allowed training iterations using `maxIts=7000`, and also sets the parameters for the genetic algorithm, as in `gaMinimum`. The mutation rate should be set to `muRate=0.01`. The companion script `backPropTrainFORga` sets the back-propagation training parameters including the learning rate `a=0.1`, bias `b=1`, and tolerance `tol=0.1`. Script `backPropTrainFORga` also sets the initially random input–hidden and hidden–output weight matrices `V` and `U`. This script is the same as `backPropTrain` from Chapter 6, except that certain parameters, notably the numbers of units, are set outside it.

For each generation script `gaHidden` decodes the chromosome population using `nHidVec=POP*pw2`. Each element of vector `nHidVec` is the number of hidden units `nHid` encoded by each single-gene chromosome, indexed

MATLAB® BOX 13.2   This script uses the genetic algorithm to optimize the speed of learning by evolving the number of hidden units in three-layered, feedforward networks trained using back-propagation.

```matlab
% gaHidden.m
% this script calls script backPropTrainFORga.m

InPat = [0 0;1 0;0 1]; % labeled line input patterns
DesOut = [0;1;1]; % labeled line desired output patterns
[nPat,nIn]=size(InPat); % pattern number and input number
[nPat,nOut]=size(DesOut); % pattern number and output number
maxIts=7000; % set maximum number of allowed iterations
popSize=5; % set the population size
pow=fliplr(0:popSize-1); % set powers for decoding
pw2=2.^pow'; % find powers of two for decoding genes
POP=rand(popSize)>0.5; % randomize initial population
chromL=5; % set length of each chromosome
numGen=20; % set the number of generations
muRate=0.01; % set the mutation rate
nHidVec=zeros(1,popSize); % define hidden number hold vector
nitVec=zeros(1,popSize); % define iteration number hold vector
meanHid=zeros(1,numGen); % define mean hidden units hold vector
meanNit=zeros(1,numGen); % define mean iterations hold vector

for gen=1:numGen % for each generation
    nHidPre=nHidVec; % save previous hidden number vector
    nHidVec=POP*pw2; % decode the new population of chromosomes
    for chrom=1:popSize % for each chromosome in the population
        if nHidVec(chrom)==0 % if chromosome encodes 0 hidden units
            nitVec(chrom)=maxIts; % set number of iterations to max
        elseif nHidVec(chrom)~=nHidPre(chrom) % if chrom changed
            nHid=nHidVec(chrom); % set hidden unit number to chrom
            backPropTrainFORga % train using back-propagation
            nitVec(chrom)=c; % save required number of iterations
        end % end evaluation conditional
    end % end loop over chromosomes in population
    meanHid(gen)=mean(nHidVec); % save mean number hidden units
    meanNit(gen)=mean(nitVec); % save mean number iterations
    if numGen==gen, break; end % do not change last generation
    normNit=nitVec./sum(nitVec); % normalize iteration numbers
    ranVec=rand(1,popSize); % generate a vector of random numbers
    normRan=ranVec./sum(ranVec); % normalize the random vector
    pertNit=normNit+normRan/3; % randomly perturb nits
    [theNits,index]=sort(pertNit); % sort chroms by perturbed nits
    dad=POP(index(1),:); % dad has smallest number of iterations
    mom=POP(index(2),:); % mom has next smallest number
    coSite=ceil(rand*chromL); % choose a random crossover site
    son=[dad(1:coSite) mom(coSite+1:chromL)]; % generate son
    dtr=[mom(1:coSite) dad(coSite+1:chromL)]; % generate daughter
    POP(index(popSize),:)=son; % replace least fit by son
    POP(index(popSize-1),:)=dtr; % replace next least fit by dtr
    MUMX=rand(popSize)<muRate; % generate random mutation matrix
    POP=abs(POP-MUMX); % mutate the chromosomes
end % end loop over generations
```

MATLAB® BOX 13.3 **This script trains a three-layered network of sigmoidal units to associate patterns using back-propagation.**

```
% backPropTrainFORga.m
% this script is called from gaHidden.m,
% which sets some of its parameters

a=0.1; % set learning rate
b=1; % set bias
tol=0.1; % set tolerance
V=rand(nHid,nIn+1)*2-1; % set initial input-hidden connectivity matrix
U=rand(nOut,nHid+1)*2-1; % set initial hidden-output matrix
deltaV=zeros(nHid,nIn+1); % define change weight for in-hid matrix
deltaU=zeros(nOut,nHid+1); % define change weight for hid-out matrix
maxErr=10; % set the maximum error to an initially high value

for c=1:maxIts, % for each learning iteration
    pindx=ceil(rand*nPat); % choose an input pattern at random
    x=[InPat(pindx,:) b]'; % append the bias to the input vector
    y=1 ./(1+(exp(-V*x))); % compute the hidden unit response
    y=[y' b]'; % append the bias to the hidden unit vector
    z=1 ./(1+(exp(-U*y))); % compute the output unit response
    e=DesOut(pindx,:)-(z'); % find the error vector
    if max(abs(e))>tol, % train if any error exceeds tolerance
        x=x';y=y';z=z'; % convert column to row vectors
        zg=(z.*(1-z)).*e; % compute the output gradient
        yg=(y.*(1-y)).*(zg*U); % compute the hidden gradient
        deltaU=a*zg'*y; % compute the change in hidden-output weights
        deltaV=a*yg(1:nHid)'*x; % change in input-hidden weights
        U=U+deltaU; V=V+deltaV; % update the hid-out and in-hid weights
    end % end the training conditional
    if rem(c,(5*nPat))==0, % every so often check network performance
        Inb=[InPat b*ones(nPat,1)]; % append bias to all input patterns
        Hid=(1./(1+exp(-V*Inb')))'; % find hid response to all patterns
        Hidb=[Hid b*ones(nPat,1)]; % append bias to all hidden vectors
        Out=(1./(1+exp(-U*Hidb')))'; % out response to all patterns
        maxErr=max(abs(abs(DesOut-Out))); % max error over all patterns
    end % end check conditional
    if maxErr<tol, break, end, % break if all errors within tolerance
end % end training loop
```

by variable `chrom`. To evaluate the fitness of a chromosome the script sets parameter `nHid` to the number of hidden units encoded by that chromosome. It then calls `backPropTrainFORga`, which assembles the network by constructing the initially random input–hidden and hidden–output weight matrices according to the number of hidden units `nHid`, and trains the network using back-propagation. The measure used to determine the fitness of each chromosome is the number of iterations `c` (training cycles) required by back-propagation to train the network encoded by it to reach tolerance. These iterations are stored in vector `nitVec` using command `nitVec(chrom)=c`. Vector `nitVec` is used to order the fitness of the chromosomes, as was vector `val` in the function minimization example, after first normalizing `nitVec` using `normNit=nitVec./sum(nitVec)`. One small difference between the two scripts is that the degree of indeterminacy in choosing chromosomes for mating or replacement in the speed-of-learning example is reduced in comparison

(A)

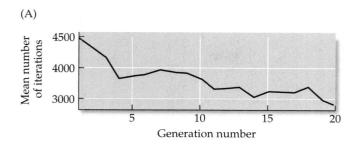

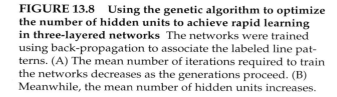

FIGURE 13.8   Using the genetic algorithm to optimize the number of hidden units to achieve rapid learning in three-layered networks The networks were trained using back-propagation to associate the labeled line patterns. (A) The mean number of iterations required to train the networks decreases as the generations proceed. (B) Meanwhile, the mean number of hidden units increases.

(B)

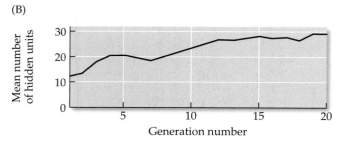

with the function minimization example by generating the perturbed ordering vector using `pertNit=normNit+normRan/3` in script `gaHidden`.

If by chance a chromosome `chrom` encodes zero hidden units, then script `gaHidden` simply sets the required number of iterations to the maximum allowed: `nitVec(chrom)=maxIts`. Since back-propagation training is time consuming, the script re-evaluates the fitness of a chromosome only if it has been modified from its configuration in the previous generation. For each generation the script stores the mean number of hidden units and the mean number of iterations required to reach tolerance in arrays `meanHid` and `meanNit`, respectively. These mean values over the course of `numGen=20` generations of simulated evolution are shown for a representative run in Figure 13.8.

The population mean number of training cycles decreases as the population progresses through 20 generations (see Figure 13.8A). The population has gotten faster at learning the labeled-line transformation as a result of simulated evolution. The improved performance must be accompanied by a change in the numbers of hidden units in the networks, because that is the only parameter that can be manipulated by the genetic algorithm in this example. The population mean number of hidden units increases as the population progresses through the same 20 generations (see Figure 13.8B). It appears that the networks are evolving to have larger numbers of hidden units, and this allows them to learn the labeled-line transformation in fewer training iterations. This relationship is borne out by a scatter plot of the population mean number of hidden units versus mean number of training iterations, which is shown in Figure 13.9.

This evolution simulation nicely illustrates that networks with more hidden units learn faster. In general, increasing the number of hidden units increases the number of degrees of freedom that the algorithm has available to learn any given input–output transformation. The more hidden units there are in the network, the more likely it is that the initial weight randomization will produce hidden units with responses close to those needed to solve the problem. Training speed is not the only consideration bearing on the size of hidden layers in neural networks. In real and artificial neural networks, we might imagine that the optimal number of hidden units depends on many competing factors. These include speed of learning (many hidden units), the ability

FIGURE 13.9   Relationship between mean number of iterations and mean number of hidden units during optimization of learning speed in three-layered networks The feedforward networks were trained using back-propagation to associate the labeled line patterns. The genetic algorithm optimized the number of hidden units to achieve rapid learning. The mean numbers of training iterations and of hidden units were calculated for every generation. Over all generations, the mean number of iterations required to train the network is inversely correlated with the mean number of hidden units.

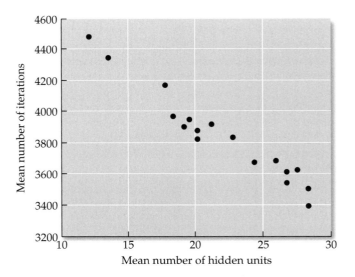

to generalize (few hidden units), and the need to represent the information content of the inputs (many hidden units; see also Chapter 8).

13.4 Evolving Optimal Learning Rules for Auto-Associative Memories

In the previous example we used the genetic algorithm to optimize the structure of a neural network. The genome could also specify the learning rule used to train a neural network. We can explore this possibility using the Hopfield network, which we studied in detail in Chapter 4. Recall that the Hopfield network is composed of a single layer of neural units (here binary) that feedback on each other but not on themselves. The combination of nonlinearity and feedback endows the network with attractor dynamics and multiple fixed points (stable states). Memory recall by the Hopfield network consists in relaxation to a stable state, where the pattern characterizing the stable state (some pattern of 1s and 0s over the units) constitutes the memory. Memory is stored in terms of the weights of the recurrent connections between the units in the Hopfield network, which determine the stable-state patterns. The Hopfield network is useful as a memory model because the weights can be learned using plausible (Hebbian) learning rules (see Chapter 4 for details). These rules allow the network to learn to associate the elements of a pattern with themselves. The rule by which a Hopfield network learns to auto-associate patterns is critical to its function.

As we recall from Chapter 4, the optimal learning rule for a Hopfield network depends on the density of the patterns that the network needs to store. Specifically, the optimal weights in a Hopfield network are computed as shown in Equation 13.2:

$$w_{ij} = \sum_l (y_i^l - p_d)(y_j^l - p_d)$$

13.2

In Equation 13.2, w_{ij} is the weight to post-synaptic unit y_i from pre-synaptic unit y_j, l is the index of the binary patterns to be stored, and p_d is the probability that any pattern element will take value 1. We can refer to p_d as the "pattern density" probability, because the closer it is to 1 the more dense will be the patterns. Equation 13.2 indicates how the optimal learning rule could be specified by an estimate of the pattern density probability p_d. This parameter could be estimated by direct examination of the patterns. We assume, however, that a neurobiologically plausible learning rule operates only on information local to individual synapses (as for the Hopfield rule and other Hebbian rules, see Chapter 4), and that the mechanism for modifying individual synapses does not have access to the full set of patterns. Another approach to the problem is to realize that the estimate of p_d would affect the ability of a trained network to store and accurately recall a given set of patterns. By interpreting the recall ability of a network as its fitness, the genetic algorithm could be used to adaptively generate fitter networks trained with increasingly better estimates of the parameter p_d. The purpose of the example in this section is to use the genetic algorithm to optimize the learning rule in Hopfield networks. Script `gaOpfield`, listed in MATLAB Box 13.4, will implement the genetic search in this context.

As in the previous examples, we seek to adapt only one item, so only one gene per chromosome is needed, and a population of five, single-gene chromosomes will be sufficient. Again, the initial chromosome population can be constructed as a 5-by-5 matrix in which each element will be a 1 with probability 0.5. Each chromosome will encode an estimate of p_d, a good range for which would be from 0.01 to 0.50. In script `gaOpfield`, the population in matrix POP is decoded using `probEvec=0.01+(0.49/31)*POP*pw2`, where `probEvec` holds the pattern density probability estimate `probE` encoded by each single-gene chromosome.

The script sets up Hopfield networks having `nUnits=20` units, with states held in vector y, and it will train them on `nPats=3` patterns, which match their capacity (see Chapter 4). The script holds the actual pattern density probability to be estimated in parameter `probA`, and uses that value to generate the random patterns P to be stored by the Hopfield networks using `P=rand(nPats,nUnits)<probA`. Thus, P is an array of 3 binary patterns of 20 elements each, in which every element has probability `probA` of being a 1. Note that the script has two versions of the pattern density probability p_d: `probA`, which is the actual value of p_d used to generate the patterns, and `probE`, which is the value of p_d as estimated by the genetic algorithm. In evolving fitter Hopfield networks, the genetic algorithm essentially will try to find the pattern density probability p_d by bringing `probE` closer to `probA`.

The fitness of each single-gene chromosome is evaluated by using its probability estimate `probE` to construct a Hopfield connectivity matrix, testing the resulting Hopfield network on each of the three patterns, and computing the difference between the desired and the recalled patterns. In script `gaOpfield`, a connectivity matrix OP is constructed in one step of matrix multiplication (see Chapter 4) using `OP=(P'-probE)*(P-probE)`, where P is the pattern matrix. This command implements Equation 13.2. The diagonal of connectivity matrix OP is set to 0 using `MSK=(ones(nUnits)-eye(nUnits))` followed by `OP=OP.*MSK`. The script initializes the state of the Hopfield network with each desired pattern at half strength using `y=(P(pat,:)*0.5)'`, where `pat` indexes the patterns. The network state vector y is then repeatedly updated asynchronously by choosing one unit at random on each update. This was done in Chapter 4 using script `AsynchUP` (see MATLAB Box 4.3), which computes asynchronous updates but also saves the state every ten updates. Because we only need the stable-state response for this example we will implement asynchronous updates of the Hopfield networks directly in script `gaOpfield`. After `nTs=200` asynchronous updates starting from each pattern at half strength, the script stores the stable state for each pattern `pat` in array YSS

MATLAB® BOX 13.4   This script uses the genetic algorithm to optimize the Hopfield rule.

```
% gaOpfield.m

nUnits=20; % set number of units in network
nPats=3; % set number of patterns
YSS=zeros(nPats,nUnits); % define stable-state output array
probA=0.5; % set actual probability that any pattern element is a 1
nTs=200; % set number of asymmetric updates for networks
popSize=5; % set the population size
pow=fliplr(0:popSize-1); % set powers for decoding
pw2=2.^pow'; % find powers of two for decoding genes
POP=rand(popSize)>0.5; % randomize initial population
chromL=5; % set length of each chromosome
numGen=30; % set the number of generations
muRate=0.01; % set mutation rate
probEvec=zeros(1,popSize); % estimated probability hold vector
DiffVec=zeros(1,popSize); % define difference hold vector
meanprobE=zeros(1,numGen); % mean estimated probability hold vector
meanDiff=zeros(1,numGen); % define mean difference hold vector

for gen=1:numGen % for each generation
    probEpre=probEvec; % store previous estimated probability vector
    probEvec=0.01+(0.49/31)*POP*pw2; % decode chroms into probabilities
    P=rand(nPats,nUnits)<probA; % pattern elements are 1 with probA
    for chrom=1:popSize % for each chromosome in the population
        if probEvec(chrom)~=probEpre(chrom) % if chromosome has changed
            probE=probEvec(chrom); % set estimated probability to chrom
            OP=(P'-probE)*(P-probE); % make optimal Hopfield matrix
            MSK=(ones(nUnits)-eye(nUnits)); % make mask matrix
            OP=OP.*MSK; % zero diagonal of connectivity matrix
            for pat=1:nPats, % for each pattern
                y=(P(pat,:)*0.5)'; % start state at half strength
                for t=1:nTs, % for each iteration
                    rindx=ceil(rand*nUnits); % random index
                    q=OP(rindx,:)*y; % find weighted input
                    y(rindx)=q>0; % apply threshold of 0
                end; % end asychronous updates
                YSS(pat,:)=y'; % save stable state in output array
            end % end loop over patterns
            DiffVec(chrom)=sum(sum(abs(P-YSS))); % difference on recall
        end % end change conditional
    end % end population loop
    meanprobE(gen)=mean(probEvec); % save mean estimated probability
    meanDiff(gen)=mean(DiffVec); % save mean difference
    if numGen==gen, break; end % do not change last generation
    if norm(DiffVec)==0, normDiff=DiffVec; % if norm is zero leave it
    else normDiff=DiffVec./norm(DiffVec); end % else normalize diff
    ranVec=rand(1,popSize); % generate a vector of random numbers
    normRan=ranVec./norm(ranVec); % normalize the random vector
    pertDiff=normDiff+normRan/3; % randomly perturb values for chroms
    [diffs,index]=sort(pertDiff); % sort chromosomes by perturbed value
    dad=POP(index(1),:); % dad has smallest perturbed value
    mom=POP(index(2),:); % mom has next smallest value
    coSite=ceil(rand*chromL); % choose a random crossover site
    son=[dad(1:coSite) mom(coSite+1:chromL)]; % generate son
    dtr=[mom(1:coSite) dad(coSite+1:chromL)]; % generate daughter
    POP(index(popSize-1),:)=son; % replace least fit by son
    POP(index(popSize),:)=dtr; % replace next least fit by dtr
    MUMX=rand(popSize)<muRate; % generate random mutation matrix
    POP=abs(POP-MUMX); % mutate the genome
end % end loop over generations
```

(A)

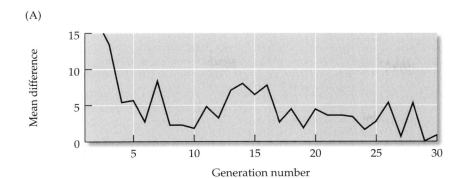

(B)

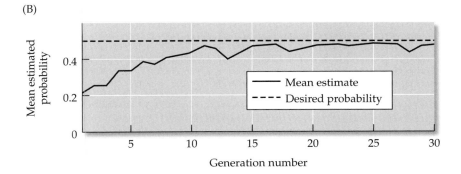

FIGURE 13.10   Using the genetic algorithm to find the optimal Hopfield covariation rule (A) The mean difference between desired and recalled patterns decreases over the course of the search. (B) The mean estimated pattern density probability moves closer to the actual pattern density probability over the course of genetic search.

using `YSS(pat,:)=y'`, and then finds the summed difference over all patterns using `DiffVec(chrom)=sum(sum(abs(P-YSS)))`.

Vector `DiffVec` holds the summed difference between the desired and recalled patterns for the Hopfield network encoded by each chromosome. Vector `normDiff` holds the normalized differences that are used to order the chromosomes according to their fitness. As in the speed-of-learning example, script `gaOpfield` evaluates the fitness of a chromosome only if its configuration was altered in progressing from the previous generation. Also, the degree of indeterminacy in selecting chromosomes for mating or replacement in the optimal Hopfield example is reduced by generating the perturbed ordering vector using `pertDiff=normDiff+normRan/3` in script `gaOpfield`.

We will do a run with the actual probability to be estimated set at `probA=0.5`. The mutation rate is set at `muRate=0.01`. The chromosomes are selected, recombined, replaced, and mutated as in the function minimization example. Script `gaOpfield` will store the population mean summed difference (error), and the population mean probability estimate, in arrays `meanDiff` and `meanprobE`, respectively. These means over the course of `numGen=30` generations of simulated evolution of the optimal Hopfield learning rule are shown for a representative run in Figure 13.10.

The population mean summed difference between the desired and recalled patterns decreases as the population progresses through the generations (see Figure 13.10A). This error measure is erratic but approaches and sometimes even reaches 0. The population mean probability estimate (estimate of p_d in Equation 13.2) over the generations is shown in Figure 13.10B. The population of Hopfield networks closely estimates the optimal p_d value of 0.5 and stays near it for many generations. By selecting the Hopfield networks with the smallest errors in pattern recall, the genetic algorithm indirectly selected the networks with the best estimates of the pattern density probability. In a similar way, it is easy to imagine how evolution could optimize the parameters of learning in organisms by selecting those that had the most accurate memories.

13.5 Evolving Connectivity Profiles for Activity-Bubble Neural Networks

The two neural network examples we have considered so far in this chapter involved a combination of evolution and adaptation. In the speed-of-learning example, the genetic algorithm determined the structure of the network by specifying the number of hidden units, but adaptation, in the form of back-propagation, was needed to train the network to accomplish the labeled-line transformation. In the optimal-Hopfield rule example, the genetic algorithm determined a parameter of the learning rule by specifying the pattern density probability, but adaptation, in the form of the Hopfield rule itself, was needed to train the network to store the patterns. While it is likely that many real neural systems are constructed through some combination of genetically determined development and/or learning rule and experience-dependent adaptation, it is also possible that some real neural systems are constructed through genetically specified mechanisms alone. We explore the latter possibility in the example in this section.

This example involves the use of the genetic algorithm to optimize the parameters defining the connectivity profile in activity-bubble networks. Like Hopfield networks, activity-bubble networks are attractor networks with stable fixed points, but the stable states of activity-bubble networks are contiguous, fixed-size subsets of active units completely surrounded by inactive units. Given a non-uniform input, the state of an activity-bubble network will grow to form a bubble centered at the location of the initially largest input. Activity-bubble networks are composed of nonlinear units that feed back on each other and on themselves, and the behavior of an activity-bubble network depends sensitively on its feedback (recurrent) connectivity profile. Activity-bubble networks can be constructed using feedback connectivity profiles that are the same for each unit. This uniformity suggests that the connectivity of an activity-bubble network could, in principle, be genetically pre-specified rather than learned. We will evolve activity-bubble neural networks in this example.

Simulated evolution of activity-bubble networks is implemented by script gaBubble, which is listed in MATLAB Box 13.5. The profile in this example

MATLAB® BOX 13.5   This script uses the genetic algorithm to optimize the connectivity profile of the activity-bubble network.

```
% gaBubble.m

nUnits=51; % set number of units in network
s=-25:25; % set space vector for network and input
V=eye(nUnits); % set input matrix (same for all)
signal=zeros(nUnits,1); % set input signal baseline
signal(25:27)=ones(3,1); % set input pulse
popSize=15; % set the population size
pow=fliplr(0:4); % set powers for decoding
pw2=2.^pow'; % find powers of two for decoding genes
POP=rand(popSize,popSize-1)>0.5; % randomize initial population
chromL=14; % set length of each chromosome
numGen=30; % set the number of generations
muRate=0.01; % set mutation rate
meanErr=zeros(1,numGen); % mean error hold vector
```

(Continued on facing page)

MATLAB® BOX 13.5   (continued)

```
for gen=1:numGen; % for each generation
    gsdVec=POP(:,1:4)*pw2(2:5); % decode narrow gaussian sd genes
    gsdVec(find(gsdVec==0))=0.001; % change 0s to small values
    dsdVec=POP(:,5:9)*pw2; % decode wide gaussian sd genes
    dsdVec(find(dsdVec==0))=0.001; % change 0s to small values
    dwtVec=POP(:,10:14)*pw2; % decode wide gaussian weight genes
    dwtVec=0.1+0.013*dwtVec; % scale wide gaussian weights
    error=zeros(1,popSize); % zero the error vector
    for chrom=1:popSize; % for each chromosome in the population
        g=gaussPro(s,gsdVec(chrom)); % make the narrow gaussian
        d=gaussPro(s,dsdVec(chrom)); % make the wide gaussian
        dog=g-(dwtVec(chrom)*d); % make connectivity profile (DOG)
        dog=[dog(26:51) dog(1:25)]; % shift DOG profile
        W=shiftLam(dog); % make connectivity matrix W from profile
        noise=rand(51,1); % make a new noise vector
        x=signal+noise; % add noise to signal to make input
        winnersTakeAll % find network responses for this input
        [nY,nTs]=size(y); % find the final response
        ySS=y(:,nTs); % take the final stable-state response
        error(chrom)=sum([(10-ySS(25:27)')*20 ... % compute
            ySS(1:24)' ySS(28:51)']); % the error
    end % end phenotype evaluation loop
    meanErr(gen)=mean(error); % save the mean error
    if numGen==gen, break; end % do not change last generation
    normErr=error./sum(error); % normalize errors
    ranVec=rand(1,popSize); % generate random vector
    normRan=ranVec./sum(ranVec); % normalize random vector
    pertErr=normErr+normRan; % randomly perturb errors
    [theErrs,index]=sort(pertErr); % sort by perturbed errors
    dad1=POP(index(1),:); % dad1 has smallest perturbed error
    mom1=POP(index(2),:); % mom1 has second smallest error
    dad2=POP(index(3),:); % dad2 has third smallest error
    mom2=POP(index(4),:); % mom2 has fourth smallest error
    permSites=randperm(chromL); % randomly permute sites
    coS1=permSites(1); % find crossover site for couple 1
    coS2=permSites(2); % find crossover site for couple 2
    son1=[dad1(1:coS1) mom1(coS1+1:chromL)]; % son 1
    dtr1=[mom1(1:coS1) dad1(coS1+1:chromL)]; % daughter 1
    son2=[dad2(1:coS2) mom2(coS2+1:chromL)]; % son 2
    dtr2=[mom2(1:coS2) dad2(coS2+1:chromL)]; % daughter 2
    POP(index(popSize),:)=son1; % replace least fit by son 1
    POP(index(popSize-1),:)=dtr1; % second least fit by dtr 1
    POP(index(popSize-2),:)=son2; % third least fit by son 2
    POP(index(popSize-3),:)=dtr2; % fourth least fit by dtr 2
    MUMX=rand(size(POP))<muRate; % random mutation matrix
    POP=abs(POP-MUMX); % mutate the chromosomes
end % end loop over generations
[minErr,indME]=min(error); % find chromosome with minimal error
```

is the familiar difference-of-Gaussians (DOG). The DOG profile is formed by subtracting a wider Gaussian curve with a smaller amplitude from a narrower Gaussian curve (see Chapter 3). Each curve, which is not precisely a density function, is of the form $f(x) = \exp[-1/2(x/\sigma)^2]$, where the domain of the function is symmetric about 0 and σ is equivalent to the standard deviation. To conform with script gaBubble we will use MATLAB (monotype) rather than mathematical notation to denote variable names in this example.

In script `gaBubble`, the DOG is constructed by subtracting a Gaussian d from a Gaussian g, after first weighting d by `dwt`. Each Gaussian is specified by its standard deviation, `gsd` for g and `dsd` for d. As in Chapter 3, the Gaussians are generated using the function `gaussPro` (see MATLAB Box 3.2). As such, they are not Gaussian probability density functions, but rather have amplitude 1 regardless of their width, and this facilitates their use in the construction of neural network connectivity profiles. The vector `s=-25:25` represents the spatial coordinate, and the Gaussians are generated using `g=gaussPro(s,gsdVec(chrom))` and `d=gaussPro(s,dsdVec(chrom))`, where `chrom` indexes the chromosomes. The DOG profile itself is then constructed using the command `dog=g(dwtVec(chrom)*d)`. Note that `gsdVec`, `dsdVec`, and `dwtVec` are vectors, indexed by `chrom`, that hold the narrow standard deviation `gsd`, the wide standard deviation `dsd`, and the difference weight `dwt` for each chromosome in the population.

The DOG is thus defined by three parameters: the standard deviations of the Gaussians g and d (`gsd` and `dsd`) and the weight of Gaussian d (`dwt`). Therefore, each chromosome must have three genes. Gaussian g always has a smaller standard deviation than Gaussian d (`gsd` < `dsd`), so `dsd` is represented as an integer from 0 to 31 using the same 5-bit gene used in the previous examples, but `gsd` is represented as an integer from 0 to 15 using a 4-bit gene. The weight `dwt` is represented as an integer between 0 and 31 using a 5-bit gene. These integer values for weight `dwt` (in vector `dwtVec`) are mapped into the 0.1–0.4 range using `dwtVec=0.1+0.013*dwtVec`. The three parameters together (`gsd`, `dsd`, and `dwt`) can be encoded by a bit string that is 14 elements long, and constitutes a 3-gene chromosome. Because each chromosome now has 3 genes, we will increase the population size to 15 chromosomes. The initial population can be generated as a 15-by-14 matrix in which each element is a 1 with probability 0.5. Each chromosome in the population is decoded to specify the parameters needed to construct an activity-bubble network. Note that the chromosomes must be separated into individual genes using subarray commands in order to be correctly decoded.

Activity-bubble networks have two layers of units: input and output. There is one input unit and one output unit for each of the 51 spatial coordinates specified by `s`. The DOG specifies the profile of the feedback (recurrent) connections in the output layer. After decoding each chromosome and generating the Gaussians, the DOG profiles are constructed as described above, then shifted to align the inputs and outputs, and the recurrent connectivity matrices are constructed from the DOGs using `W=shiftLam(dog)` (see MATLAB Box 3.1). Because the Gaussian is undefined for standard deviation equal to 0, script `gaBubble` replaces with a small value any standard deviations that are specified by the genes to be 0. The input–output connections are specified simply as the identity matrix `V=eye(nUnits)` where `nUnits=51`.

The input is the 51-element vector `signal` with a set of 3 contiguous 1s in the middle (elements 25–27) and 0s elsewhere. The input vector is corrupted by the uniform random noise vector `noise` using `x=signal+noise`. To make the adaptation robust, a new noise profile is added to the input before each individual network is evaluated. The output of each activity-bubble network is then computed using `winnersTakeAll` (see MATLAB Box 3.3), with feedback strength `rate=1`, cutoff `cut=0`, saturation `sat=10`, and number of time steps `nTs=20`. The unit state vector y after 20 time steps, which is presumed to be the stable-state output, is `ySS=y(:,nTs)`. The desired output is a contiguous set of 3 units that are fully active (state 10) while the rest are silent (state 0). This desired output is not represented explicitly. Instead the error is computed using a formula in which the desired output is implied: `error(chrom)=`

(A)

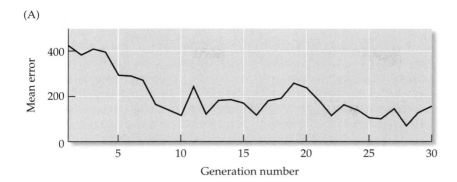

(B)

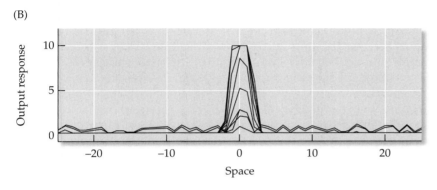

FIGURE 13.11 Using the genetic algorithm to optimize the connectivity of an activity-bubble network (A) The mean error between the ideal and actual (phenotypic) activity bubble decreases rapidly over the course of genetic search. (B) The activity-bubble network constructed from the difference-of-Gaussians (DOG) parameters of the fittest chromosome has a narrow activity bubble that is close to ideal.

`sum([(10-ySS(25:27)'*20 ySS(1:24)' ySS(28:51)'])`. Because only 3 of the 51 output units should be active, it is helpful to weigh the errors for the activity-bubble region (the central 3 units) more strongly than the flanking regions (the 48 units outside the ideal bubble). With this error measure, failure of the central 3 output units to achieve activity levels of 10 is weighted 20 times more heavily than failure of the flanking units to achieve activity levels of 0.

Vector `error` holds the error of the activity-bubble network encoded by each chromosome `chrom` and is used to order their fitness. Because this measure is an error, a scheme similar to the one used in the function minimization example can be used again here to order the networks, and their corresponding chromosomes, for selection for mating or replacement. Because there are three times as many individuals as before in the population, we will allow two pairs of chromosomes to mate, and another two pairs to be replaced by their offspring, on each generation. Again, the most fit (lowest error) chromosomes should be the most likely parents, and the offspring will most likely replace the least fit chromosomes. After mating and replacement, the chromosome population array is mutated at rate `muRate=0.01`.

Script `gaBubble` will store the population mean error in array `meanErr`. These mean values over the course of `numGen=30` generations of simulated evolution are shown for a representative run in Figure 13.11A. The population mean error decreases as the generations proceed. This decrease in population mean error had to be produced by changes in the parameters that define the DOG, because these are the only parameters that are manipulated by the algorithm. The solutions of the genetic optimization procedure are the values of those parameters for the fittest member of the final generation.

The fittest chromosome encodes a value of 1 for `gsd` and of 22 for `dsd`. The value of `gsd` is lower, while the value of `dsd` is higher, than the values of 3 and 15 that we assigned to these parameters in Chapter 3. By themselves, these changes represent a net loss of excitation that would eliminate activity bubble formation in the network. However, the weight of the Gaussian to be subtracted (`dwt`) is reduced from 0.3 (its value in Chapter 3) to around 0.2 for the fittest chromosome. This decrease in negative feedback effectively offsets the loss of positive feedback brought about by the decrease and increase in the standard deviations `gsd` and `dsd`, respectively. (Recall that the Gaussian curves generated by `gaussPro` are not probability density functions with normalized areas but have amplitude 1 regardless of their standard deviations, so a decrease in standard deviation causes a decrease in area, and conversely.) The narrower, positive Gaussian `g`, and the smaller weight `dwt` of the negative Gaussian, effectively sharpens the activity bubble without suppressing it. The activity bubble itself is shown in Figure 13.11B. It is indeed narrower and sharper that the activity-bubble we generated with hand-set DOG parameters in Chapter 3.

In this last example the genetic algorithm is used to specify not the numbers of units in a network, nor learning rule parameters, but the actual connection weights between the units. In the speed-of-learning and the optimal-Hopfield examples, the connection weights had to be learned. Learning clearly plays an important role in determining the weights of synaptic connections in many real neural systems, but it is possible that the connection weights in some neural networks could be specified directly by the genome. In the case of activity-bubble networks, it is at least reasonable to speculate that genes could encode proteins that mediate various process that would allow the network connections to develop the correct configuration and weighting without the need for learning.

For example, imagine an interspersed sheet of two sets of neurons, one set excitatory and the other inhibitory. The excitatory neurons make only short-range connections, while the inhibitory neurons make only long-range connections. Imagine further that the excitatory neurons can make synaptic contact with other excitatory neurons and with inhibitory neurons, but that the inhibitory neurons can make synaptic contact only with excitatory neurons. Then the excitatory neurons would excite their near neighbors, both excitatory and inhibitory. The inhibitory neurons would inhibit only more distant excitatory neurons. The net effect would be that the excitatory neurons would excite other excitatory neurons in their immediate vicinity, and inhibit more distant excitatory neurons, through the inhibitory neurons that are acting as interneurons. This local excitation with more distant inhibition could lead to DOG-type connectivity profiles and activity-bubble dynamics.

Rules that specify which neurons are excitatory and which inhibitory, and those governing allowable interconnections and length of projections, could in principle all be encoded by the genome. Other strategies are also possible, and suggest ways in which rules specified by the genome could play a direct role in the self-organization of the nervous system. While the genome cannot specify every synapse in the brain, it can set the parameters of developmental and adaptive processes, and it could provide initial structure in the form of pre-specified synaptic weights that are later modified through learning (see Chapter 7). Genetically specified molecular mechanisms are known to interact with activity-dependent mechanisms in development (Huberman et al. 2008), but it is at least possible that the genome could directly specify mature synaptic weight values in structures having regular, lattice-like connectivity patterns. In any case, research in the area of genetic neuroscience is active (e.g., Tonegawa et al. 2003), and appreciation for the importance of genetically specified molecular mechanisms in determining the structure and function of the nervous system, as indicated initially by the work of Rodger Sperry (1963), continues to grow.

Exercises

13.1 We used the genetic algorithm in script `gaHidden` (see MATLAB Box 13.2) to optimize learning speed by evolving the number of hidden units in three-layered networks of sigmoidal units trained by back-propagation to associate the labeled-line patterns. We found that the number of iterations needed to train the networks decreased as the number of hidden units increased. Repeat this experiment but substitute the exclusive-or (XOR) patterns for the labeled-line patterns: `InPat=[0 0; 1 0; 0 1; 1 1]` and `DesOut=[0; 1; 1; 0]`. Is the same relationship between required number of iterations and number of hidden units, which we observed using the labeled-line patterns, also borne out using the XOR patterns? How do the absolute numbers of required iterations compare between networks optimized on XOR versus labeled-line? Why should this difference exist?

13.2 We used the genetic algorithm in script `gaOpfield` (see MATLAB Box 13.4) to optimize the covariation learning rule by searching for an estimate of the pattern density probability, which is the probability that any pattern element in the desired, binary patterns is a 1. In the example, we optimized on the basis of the errors in recall of three patterns by a network of 20 units at an actual probability of 0.5. With a pattern density probability of 0.5, the optimal rule is a scaled version of the Hopfield rule (see Chapter 4). Change the actual probability to 0.05. At this low pattern density probability the optimal rule should be more like the Hebb rule (see also Chapter 4). Does the genetic algorithm converge on the correct pattern density probability when it equals 0.05? Now change the probability back to 0.5 but decrease the number of units in the network to 5. Does the algorithm perform as well with 5 as with 20 units? If not, why not?

13.3 We used the genetic algorithm in script `gaBubble` (see MATLAB Box 13.5) to optimize the parameters of difference-of-Gaussian (DOG) profiles to give us narrow bubbles in activity-bubble networks. Genes encoding the narrow and wide Gaussians, and the scale factor for the wide Gaussian (which is subtracted from the narrow Gaussian to make the DOG), were encoded by three-gene chromosomes. Our ideal activity bubble was only three units wide. The error measure was derived from the difference between the ideal and the actual (phenotypic) activity bubble, and the fittest chromosome had the smallest error. Try using an even "skinnier" ideal bubble. Change the error measure to `error(chrom)=sum([(10-ySS(26))*20 ySS(1:25)' ySS(27:51)'])`. This ideal bubble is only one unit wide. Does this higher, even more demanding ideal improve the performance of the genetic algorithm on this problem?

13.4 In Exercise 2.4 of Chapter 2 we implemented a nonlinear version of Wilson's model of the locust flight central pattern generator (CPG). This network is composed of four, recurrently connected sigmoidal units that represent the two sides of the CPG: units 1 and 2 on the left and units 3 and 4 on the right. Units 2 and

3 can be considered as motoneurons. They receive the input to, and provide the oscillatory output from, the network. They are reciprocally connected to each other, and each one inhibits itself through a leaky integrator on its same side: unit 2 through unit 1, and unit 3 through unit 4. We set up a step input using `x=zeros(1,nTs)`, and `x(fly:land)=ones(1,land−fly+1)`, where `fly=51`, `land=450`, `tEnd=500`, and `nTs=tEnd+1`. We set the feedforward weights as `V=[0 12 11.9 0]'` and the feedback (recurrent) weights as `W=[1 3 0 0;−12 1 −6 0;0 −6 1 −12;0 0 3 1]`. We defined the output array as `y=zeros(4,nTs)`, and for each time step we computed the weighted input sum as `q=W*y(:,t−1)+V*x(t−1)` and then made the unit responses nonlinear using the squashing function: `y(:,t)=1./(1+exp(−q))`. This model produced the desired performance, which was an oscillation that began and ended with the "fly" command from `x`, but we set the weights by hand. See if you can "evolve" a set of weights for the nonlinear version of the Wilson CPG model using the genetic algorithm. To make it simpler, keep the input weight matrix `V` the same, and fix the 1 and 0 values of `W`, and just evolve the values of `W` that are not 1 or 0. Because of the bilateral symmetry of the network, you need only evolve the values of three weights: the motoneuron-integrator weight, the integrator-motoneuron weight, and the reciprocal weight. The absolute value of each weight can be encoded using a 5-bit gene that is divided by 2 after decoding to give a value between 0 and 15.5. For this purpose you can use a modified version of `gaBubble` (listed in MATLAB Box 13.5), where each chromosome has three 5-bit genes. (Recall in `gaBubble` that each chromosome also had three genes, and the first two were 5-bit but the third was only 4-bit). On each generation, decode the chromosomes, set up the corresponding CPG networks, and determine the activity of the units during the "fly" interval. To find the error function, set a desired oscillation frequency (in cycles per time step) of `df=0.145`, set a time base `tb=1:land−fly+1`, and make a normalized sine and cosine at this frequency using `dsin=sin(2*pi*df*tb)`, `dcos=cos(2*pi*df*tb)`, `dsin=dsin/norm(dsin)`, and `dcos=dcos/norm(dcos)`. To determine the error of the network encoded by each chromosome `chrom` in the CPG population, take the output of network unit 2 during the fly interval, subtract its mean, and normalize it using `cpg=y(2,fly:land)`, `cpg=cpg−mean(cpg)`, and `cpg=cpg/norm(cpg)`. Then the error for each chromosome (CPG network) is `error(chrom)=1−norm([cpg*dsin' cpg*dcos'])`. Note that the term `norm([cpg*dsin' cpg*dcos'])` is roughly the normalized "power" of the CPG output at the desired frequency. Subtracting it from 1 gives us the error for each chromosome, and the genetic algorithm procedures we used in this chapter can also be used to evolve the nonlinear version of the Wilson CPG. Can you evolve connection weights for the CPG network that endow it with better performance than the hand set weights?

References

Anastasio TJ, Gad YP (2007) Sparse cerebellar input can morph the dynamics of a model oculomotor neural integrator. *Journal of Computational Neuroscience* 22: 239–254.

Berridge MJ, Rapp PE (1979) A comparative survey of the function, mechanism and control of cellular oscillators. *Journal of Experimental Biology* 81: 217–279.

Blalock TJ (2003) The frequency changer era—interconnecting systems of varying cycles. *IEEE Power and Electric Magazine* 1: 72–79.

Chen C, Tonegawa S (1997) Molecular genetic analysis of synaptic plasticity, activity-dependent neural development, learning, and memory in the mammalian brain. *Annual Review of Neuroscience* 20: 157–184.

Dowling JE (1992) *Neurons and Networks: An Introduction to Behavioral Neuroscience. Second Edition*. Belknap Press, Cambridge.

Friesen WO, Stent GS (1978) Neural circuits for generating rhythmic movements. *Annual Review of Biophysics and Bioengineering* 7: 37–61.

Goldberg DE (1989) *Genetic Algorithms in Search, Optimization, and Machine Learning*. Addison-Wesley, Boston.

Holland JH (1975) *Adaptation in Natural and Artificial Systems: An Introductory Analysis with Applications to Biology, Control, and Artificial Intelligence*. MIT Press, Cambridge, MA.

Huber AB, Kolodkin AL, Ginty DD, Cloutier JF (2003) Signaling at the growth cone: Ligand-receptor complexes and the control of axon growth and guidance. *Annual Review of Neuroscience* 26: 509–563.

Huberman AD, Feller MB, Chapman B (2008) Mechanisms underlying development of visual maps and receptive fields. *Annual Review of Neuroscience* 31: 479–509.

Inatani M (2005) Molecular mechanisms of optic axon guidance. *Naturwissenschaften* 92: 549–561.

Jacobson M (1991) *Developmental Neurobiology. Third Edition*. Plenum Press, New York.

Schaffer JD, Caruana RA, Eshelman LJ (1990) Using genetic search to exploit the emergent behavior of neural networks. *Physica D* 42: 244–248.

Selverston AI, Moulins M (1985) Oscillatory neural networks. *Annual Review of Physiology* 47: 29–48.

Sperry RW (1963) Chemoaffinity in the orderly growth of nerve fiber patterns and connections. *Proceedings of the National Academy of Sciences* 50: 703–710.

Tonegawa S, Nakazawa K, Wilson MA (2003) Genetic neuroscience of mammalian learning and memory. *Philosophical Transactions of the Royal Society of London* B 358: 787–795.

Watson JD, Baker TA, Bell SP, Gann A, Levine M, Losick R (2008) *Molecular Biology of the Gene. Sixth Edition*. Benjamin Cummings, San Francisco.

Wilson DM (1961) The central nervous control of flight in a locust. *Journal of Experimental Biology* 38: 471–490.

Yao X (1999) Evolving artificial neural networks. *Proceedings of the IEEE* 9: 1423–1447.

14

Future Directions in Neural Systems Modeling

In the future, neural systems models will become increasingly complex and will span levels from molecular interactions within neurons to interactions between networks

The ability immediately and flexibly to follow and apply explicit rules is a hallmark of cognitive function (Bunge 2004). No model yet exists that can plausibly simulate the neural mechanisms that underlie that ability. Meanwhile, an active area of artificial intelligence research concerns the development of procedures for extracting rules from the pattern associations learned by neural networks (Andrews et al. 1995; Sentino 2000; Tsukimoto 2000). This is ironic. Rules are embedded in the representations that neural networks can learn, over many iterations, but could not flexibly apply, while humans, who could not necessarily discern the rules directly from the training patterns, could apply them immediately and flexibly once they were extracted from neural networks.

This irony underscores the differences between real brains and artificial neural networks. Apparently, artificial neural networks can learn pattern associations of which brains are not capable, and from which humans would like to extract the rules. In contrast, certain cognitive functions are still beyond the reach of computer simulation. Neural systems modeling paradigms, such as those we have considered in this book, are successful in describing certain aspects of neural function in specific neural structures. However, they fail to simulate larger-scale processes that require the coordinated activity of various brain regions mediating heterogeneous functions, such as the flexible application of rules, or thinking in general. One of the great challenges for the future is to use modeling paradigms, like the ones we have considered, as components of larger models that attempt to simulate brain function on a higher level and on a larger scale. Neural systems models that combine two or more paradigms are currently being developed. We will discuss some of those in this chapter.

Learning is fundamental to brain function and to neural systems models as well. In many cases it is simply not possible to derive analytically the connection weight values that would give a neural network its desired function, and there is no alternative but to train it using a learning algorithm. While back-propagation and related algorithms are indeed powerful and useful in constructing models of neural systems, their neurobiological implausibility restricts their applicability. All of the old-standby, neurobiologically acceptable learning mechanisms are Hebbian. Unfortunately, their ability to train neural networks is meager (see Chapter 6). It is hard to imagine that the real nervous system would be limited to such a rudimentary form of learning. One of the great advantages to be anticipated from progress in neuroscientific research is a deeper understanding of the mechanisms of neural plasticity. In the future, an improved description of the molecular processes within neurons and synapses will extend the learning that is possible in neural systems models that use plausible adaptive mechanisms. This research has also already begun, and we will discuss some examples in this chapter.

While scientists tend to limit themselves to one level of phenomena (ion channels, for example, or single cells or a specific brain region), the brain operates holistically, with processes occurring on all levels simultaneously, and with many regions throughout the brain working together in a coordinated fashion. It is likely that brain function cannot be fully understood without taking a multilevel, integrated approach. Models of the future may be composed of networks of networks of complex neural units, which themselves may contain models of molecular interaction networks. We will refrain from active simulation in this chapter. Instead, we will speculate on several new areas that hold promise for the future development of neural systems modeling. We will begin our discussion of future trends with studies of the molecular basis of long-term potentiation.

14.1 Neuroinformatics and Molecular Networks

While the Hebb rule may seem simple in theory, activity-dependent changes in synaptic strength are quite complicated in reality. Perhaps the best known example of Hebbian learning in the real nervous system is long-term potentiation (LTP), which is an activity-dependent strengthening of the synapses onto hippocampal pyramidal neurons (Bliss and Lomo 1973). Research reveals that LTP is mediated by an extensive molecular interaction network. (For review, see Miyamoto 2006.) Part of this network is schematized in Figure 14.1.

The induction of LTP begins when the neurotransmitter L-glutamate is released from the pre-synaptic neuron, and binds and thereby activates N-methyl-D-aspartate (NMDA) glutamate receptors, which allow calcium ions (Ca^{2+}) to enter the post-synaptic neuron. A protein known as calcium-calmodulin-dependent kinase II (CaMKII) is activated by Ca^{2+} in the presence of calmodulin. CaMKII phosphorylates, and thus activates, another kind of

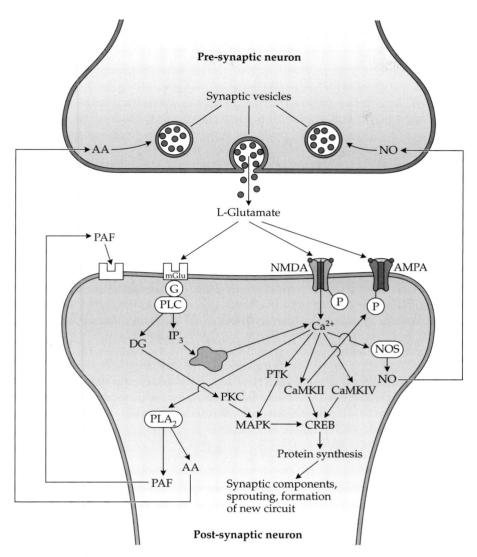

FIGURE 14.1   Some of the cellular signaling mechanisms involved in long-term potentiation (LTP) of synapses onto hippocampal pyramidal neurons Most of these occur in the post-synaptic neuron, but molecular feedback to the pre-synaptic neuron also takes place. NMDA, N-methyl-D-aspartate glutamate receptor; AMPA, alpha-amino-3-hydroxy-5-methyl-4-isoxazoleproprionic acid glutamate receptor; Ca^{2+}, calcium ion; PKC, protein kinase C; PTK, phosphotyrosine kinase; CaMKII and CaMKIV, calcium calmodulin kinase II and IV; MAPK, mitogen-activated protein kinase; CREB, cyclic adenosine monophosphate response element binding protein. See Miyamoto (2006) for other abbreviations. (After Miyamoto 2006.)

glutamate receptor known as the alpha-amino-3-hydroxy-5-methyl-4-isox-azoleproprionic acid (AMPA) receptor. Activated AMPA receptors produce larger post-synaptic responses when bound with glutamate, thereby produc-ing LTP. This rapid induction of potentiation is complemented by maintained potentiation that requires gene expression. (See Chapter 13 for a brief dis-cussion of gene expression and the role of gene products in learning.) Two other kinases, CaMKIV and mitogen-activated protein kinase (MAPK), are also activated during the induction of LTP, in part through activation of other protein kinases such as protein kinase C (PKC). CaMKIV and MAPK in turn activate gene expression, possibly by binding the gene transcription factor known as cyclic adenosine monophosphate response element binding (CREB) protein. The proteins resulting from CREB-activated gene expression produce structural changes such as increased density of AMPA receptors in existing synapses, and the sprouting of new synapses, possibly leading to the development of new connections between neurons.

The molecular pathways for LTP induction and maintenance sketched out above are but a rough outline of the highly complex cellular processes that underlie this form of synaptic plasticity in real neurons. As indicated in Figure 14.1, the processes involve many molecular species interacting in intricate and overlapping pathways. To better understand them, several studies have simulated the cellular processes that underlie LTP (e.g., Bhalla and Iyengar 1999; Smolen et al. 2006). These studies illustrate how molecular interactions occurring within hippocampal (and other) neurons could process signals, including those required for learning. For example, they show how repeated pre-synaptic activation can produce the kinds of sustained post-synaptic levels of PKC, MAPK, and CaMKII that have been associated with LTP in hippocampal neurons (Bhalla and Iyengar 1999; Nicoll 2003). What makes these molecular interactions even more complicated is that induction and maintenance of LTP does not occur in isolation but must be integrated with other cellular processes. Studies in neuroinformatics have begun to explore entire molecular networks in cells including hippocampal neurons.

Neuroinformatics is an emerging area of computational neuroscience that draws information from vast databases to construct highly complex models that can be explored using a variety of computational techniques (Arbib and Grethe 2001; Koslow and Subramanian 2005). A notable example is the analysis by Ma'ayan and colleagues (2005) of the cellular signaling pathways in hippocampal pyramidal neurons. They used information from the literature to construct a molecular-interaction network model having 545 nodes and 1259 connections (links), where each node represents a molecular species and each connection represents a chemical interaction. They used the model to analyze the signal flow through this cellular signaling system that would follow the binding of a ligand, such as an ion, neurotransmitter, hormone, or neural growth factor, to a cell surface receptor. The molecular signals would then regulate cellular processes such as gene expression, ion channel conductance, and cell secretion and motility (Figure 14.2A).

An initial indication of the complexity of this hippocampal cell signaling network is illustrated in Figure 14.2B, which shows the number of active links following binding of a ligand to a receptor. The independent variable is step number, where a ligand binding a receptor is the first step, the receptor activating the first node in its pathway is the second step, and so on. Although some pathways engage additional links faster than others, the graph shows that practically all of the links are active after about ten steps into the network, regardless of the ligand that initiates the signaling cascade. This modeling result suggests that there is an extremely high degree of interaction between molecular signaling pathways in hippocampal neurons.

To get more specific information, Ma'ayan and colleagues (2005) analyzed the types of regulatory motifs that are formed as signals propagate through the molecular interaction network following receptor binding. They focused on three of the ligands that are known to be important for plasticity in hippocampal neurons: glutamate (Glu), norepinephrine (NE), and brain-derived neurotrophic factor (BDNF). Motifs can be though of as sub-networks having characteristic connectivity patterns, such as feedback or feedforward. (Note that, in the context of neuroinformatics, feedforward motifs are also called feedforward loops when they describe a pattern of divergence and convergence that forms a closed boundary, even though actual recurrence does not

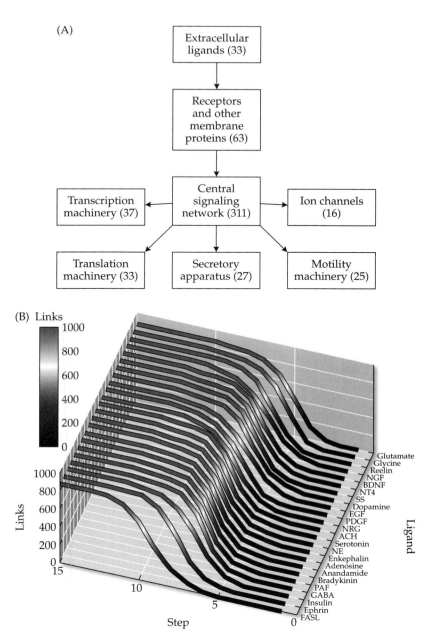

FIGURE 14.2   Analyzing the connectivity in the molecular signaling network of a hippocampal pyramidal neuron The cell signaling (molecular interaction) network model (not shown) has 545 nodes and 1259 links. Each node is a different molecular species. Links between the nodes represent chemical interactions. The network is analyzed either by following signals (sequences of links) in the complete model, or by reconstituting the model by sequentially adding back nodes of increasing connectivity. (A) Diagram illustrating the direction of signal flow. The numbers of nodes of each type are indicated in parentheses. (B) The number of links as a signal moves in steps (one link at a time) downstream from various ligands, such as neurotransmitters, hormones, and nerve growth factors. NGF, nerve growth factor; BDNF, brain-derived neurotrophic factor; ACH, acetylcholine; NE, norepinepherine; GABA, gamma-aminobutyric acid. For other abbreviations see Ma'ayan et al. 2005. (After Ma'ayan et al. 2005.)

FIGURE 14.3 **The number of feedback and feedforward loops that are progressively engaged following ligand binding in the hippocampal cell signaling network** (A) The number of three- and four-node feedback loops (positive and negative) increases in steps starting from the binding of ligands Glu, NE, and BDNF. (B) The number of three- and four-node feedforward loops also increases starting from binding of Glu, NE, and BDNF. Glu, glutamate; NE, norepinephrine; BDNF, brain-derived neurotrophic factor. (After Ma'ayan et al. 2005.)

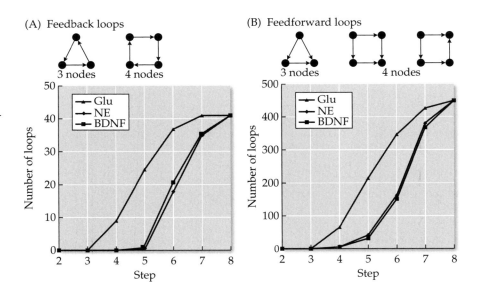

(A) Feedback loops

(B) Feedforward loops

occur.) The analysis shows that the number of feedback (Figure 14.3A) and feedforward (Figure 14.3B) motifs (loops) comprising three or four nodes increases faster following binding of Glu than of NE or BDNF. This is consistent with the different functional roles played by these ligands. Glu is involved in rapid changes in synaptic strength (LTP induction). In contrast, NE and BDNF are involved in slower, modulatory and structural changes. Figure 14.4 shows that negative feedback loops outnumber positive feedback loops early in each pathway, but that positive feedback loops outnumber negative feedback loops later in each pathway. This finding suggests that early processing may mediate selection, while later processing may bring about signal amplification once a cell is committed to a certain regulatory course.

Another way to analyze a cellular signaling network model is essentially to reconstruct it, and to examine the sub-networks that are formed as nodes of increasingly higher connectivity are added. Figure 14.5 shows that the number of "islands," which are isolated clusters of interconnected nodes that

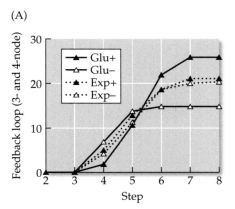

(A)

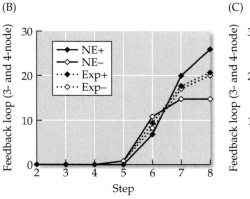

(B)

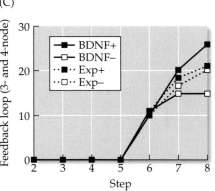

(C)

FIGURE 14.4 **Comparing the number of actual and expected feedback loops engaged following ligand binding in the hippocampal cell signaling network** The ligands are Glu (A), NE (B), and BDNF (C). The feedback loops can be positive (+) or negative (–), and actual (solid curves) or expected (Exp, dotted curves). Expectations for loops are based on the statistical properties of the signaling network. Glu, glutamate; NE, norepinephrine; BDNF, brain-derived neurotrophic factor. (After Ma'ayan et al. 2005.)

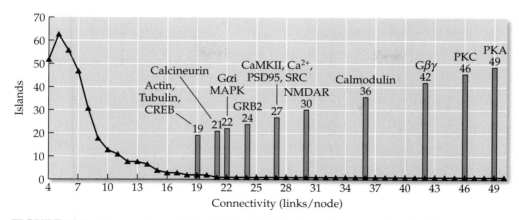

FIGURE 14.5   The number of islands (isolated clusters of connected nodes) decreases as the hippocampal cell signaling model is reconstituted by sequentially adding back nodes of increasing connectivity The labels on the vertical bars identify nodes (specific molecular species) in the hippocampal cell signaling network. The bar heights are proportional to the connectivity of each molecular species in terms of the number of links it has to other nodes. (After Ma'ayan et al. 2005.)

lack paths between them, decreases rapidly as nodes of increasingly higher connectivity are added to the network. When all of the nodes with up to 21 connections are added, the entire cellular signaling network forms a single island, indicating that every node in the network is involved. This result provides another indication that the degree of interaction between the signaling pathways in hippocampal neurons is extremely high.

The set of nodes with more than 21 links, which were not needed to bring the network to fully active connectivity, includes some of the molecular species identified as regulators of LTP, such as PKC, MAPK, and CaMKII. To explore the regulatory mechanisms of such highly connected nodes, Ma'ayan and colleagues (2005) analyzed the numbers of specific motifs that are engaged as nodes of increasingly higher connectivity are added during reconstitution of the signaling network model. Some of the motifs they examined were the feedforward and feedback motifs they had already explored in the signal propagation analysis (see Figure 14.3). Some of the other types of motifs they examined are illustrated in Figure 14.6A, and include scaffolds, which are three nodes interconnected with neutral links, and bifans, in which two upstream nodes connect to each of two downstream nodes. As shown in Figure 14.6B–E, the numbers of motifs of different types increase rapidly as nodes of increasingly higher connectivity are added, but they continue to increase over the range of node connectivity. This result suggests that, although the cellular signaling pathways are highly interconnected, they still exhibit some degree of specificity.

The computational analysis of cellular signaling networks is a new field that will yield new insights into the functions of the molecular systems inside individual neurons and synapses. Even at this early stage it feels safe to conclude that molecular networks are capable of various forms of signal processing (Bhalla and Iyengar 1999; Katz and Clemens 2001). It seems likely that the signal processing capabilities of individual synapses exceed those required for simple learning rules, such as the classic Hebb rule (see Chapters 4 and 6 for a discussion of Hebbian learning rules). A new avenue for neural systems modeling involves exploring the ways in which signal processing at the level of individual synapses can expand the adaptive capability of neural networks. In the next section we review a model in which "smart synapses" allow a neural network to be trained to produce the exclusive-OR transformation without back-propagation.

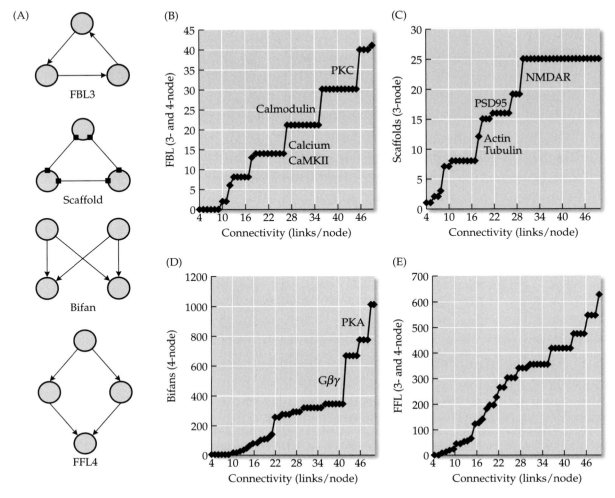

FIGURE 14.6   Types and abundance of motifs connecting nodes in the hippocampal cell signaling network (A) Motif types include the FBL3, feedback loop among three nodes; Scaffold, involving neutral binding (neither activating nor inactivating) between three nodes; Bifan, fully connected feedforward projection from two nodes to two other nodes; FFL4, feedforward loop involving four nodes. (B–E) As nodes with increasing connectivity are added in reconstituting the model, the number of motifs of specific types continues to increase. (After Ma'ayan et al. 2005.)

14.2 Enhanced Learning in Neural Networks with Smart Synapses

In the realm of neural systems modeling the exclusive-OR (XOR) transformation, reproduced in Table 14.1, is canonical because it is a component of many other input–output transformations, but it cannot be performed, or learned, by neural networks with fewer than three layers. The XOR transformation was used in the classic demonstration of the power of back-propagation to train multilayered networks of nonlinear units (Rumelhart et al. 1986). As discussed in Chapter 6, the power of back-propagation as a tool for constructing models of neural systems comes at the cost of its neurobiological implausibility as a learning mechanism. The main complaint about back-propagation is that its update to a weight onto a unit in a hidden (internal) layer requires that error signals be back-propagated to that unit from all of the units to which it

TABLE 14.1   **The logical exclusive-OR (XOR), and the winner-take-all version of the XOR used to train and test the smart-synapse network**

The logical exclusive-OR (XOR)		Winner-take-all version of XOR	
XOR input	XOR output	Input pattern	Desired output
0 0	0	0 0 1	0 1
1 0	1	1 0 1	1 0
0 1	1	0 1 1	1 0
1 1	0	1 1 1	0 1

In the network, the third input serves as a bias input. The hidden and output layers are winner-take-all so that only one hidden and output unit can be active on any network cycle.

projects. This neurobiological implausibility has lead to various alternatives to back-propagation. One of these, perturbative reinforcement learning, we explored in Chapter 7 and will revisit in Section 14.4.

Another alternative to back-propagation, due to Klemm and co-workers (2000), also employs a reinforcement signal, but instead of perturbation it exploits the potential of molecular networks within individual synapses to process signals. The use of smart synapses allows the XOR transformation to be learned without back-propagation. Like perturbative reinforcement learning (see Chapter 7), but unlike back-propagation (see Chapter 6), all of the connection weights in the smart-synapse network are updated in the same way. To emphasize that fact, and for completeness, the state and weight update equations are presented both for hidden and output units in the smart-synapse network, despite the structural similarities of these equations.

The network for learning XOR using local rules and smart synapses is schematized in Figure 14.7. It has three input units x_j ($j = 1, 2, 3$), three hidden units y_i ($i = 1, 2, 3$), and two output units z_k ($k = 1, 2$). The input–hidden weights are denoted as v_{ij}, and the hidden–output weights as u_{ki}, according to the same convention we followed in Chapters 6 and 7. As for all of the units we have considered so far in this book, each unit in the smart-synapse network also computes the weighed sum of its inputs as in Equations 14.1 and 14.2:

$$q_i = \sum_j v_{ij} x_j \tag{14.1}$$

$$q_k = \sum_i u_{ki} y_i \tag{14.2}$$

where q_i and q_k are the weighted input sums to the hidden and output units, respectively. Unlike the units we have considered so far (except for some in Chap-

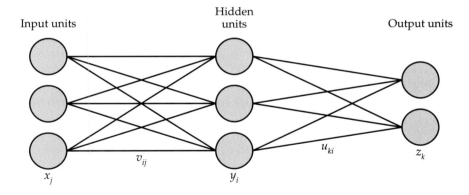

Input units   Hidden units   Output units

FIGURE 14.7   A three-layered network that can learn the exclusive-OR using local learning rules, reinforcement, and smart synapses Input units x_j ($j = 1, 2, 3$) project to hidden units y_i ($i = 1, 2, 3$) over weights v_{ij}, and hidden units y_i project to output units z_k ($k = 1, 2$) over weights u_{ki}.

ter 8), the units in the smart-synapse network are stochastic. Specifically, the binary (0 or 1) states of the units in the smart-synapse network depend probabilistically on their weighted input sums according to Equations 14.3 and 14.4:

$$p_i = \frac{\exp(\beta q_i)}{\sum_i \exp(\beta q_i)}$$ **14.3**

$$p_k = \frac{\exp(\beta q_k)}{\sum_k \exp(\beta q_k)}$$ **14.4**

where p_i and p_k are the activation probabilities associated with the hidden y_i and output z_k units, respectively. The hidden and output layers are modeled as winner-take-all, so only one hidden and one output unit can be active on any cycle. Thus, in this stochastic network, the p_i and p_k are, respectively, the probabilities that each hidden y_i and output z_k unit will be the single, winning unit in its layer.

The parameter β can loosely be thought of as the inverse of the temperature $\beta = 1/T$ in a physical system, and is inversely proportional to the amount of random noise in the network. This parameter regulates the extent to which the activation probabilities of all the units are determined by their weighted input sums. When the temperature is very high, the parameter β is very low, and $\exp(\beta q) \approx \exp(0) = 1$, so that $p_i = 1/3$ and $p_k = 1/2$ for all the hidden and output units, respectively, regardless of their weighted input sums. When the temperature is very low the parameter β is very high. In the case of very high β, the activation probability of each hidden and output unit depends sensitively on its weighted input sum, and each layer functions as a deterministic winner-take-all layer. Klemm and co-workers (2000) considered the stochastic case more realistic than the deterministic winner-take-all, and they set $\beta = 10$ for their learning simulations.

The particulars of the smart-synapse network require that the XOR be represented in an unusual way. The input and desired output patterns for the network are also shown in Table 14.1. Note that the third input unit serves as a bias unit and is always active. We used a similar method to represent the XOR input patterns with a bias unit in our studies of the delta rule in Chapter 6. Because only one of the binary units in each layer (including the output layer) can be active on any given network cycle in the smart-synapse network, the XOR output of 1 is encoded as output pattern [1 0], while the XOR output of 0 is encoded as output pattern [0 1].

The smart-synapse learning mechanism involves a combination of synaptic signal processing, the classic Hebb rule, and reinforcement learning. Basically, each weight is incremented on each learning cycle, but specific weights can be decremented by penalty δ if a certain condition is met. That condition involves storage and signal processing by the smart synapses. On each training cycle, the actual output is compared with the desired output, and the reinforcement signal $r = +1$ if they match but $r = -1$ if they do not match. Each synapse is also associated with a variable m_{ij} or m_{ki} that serves as an error counter, which can also be thought of as the "memory" of each smart synapse. The memory counter for a synapse is updated on network cycle c if the units pre-synaptic and post-synaptic to that synapse are both active. Because memory-counter updates depend on simultaneous pre-synaptic and post-synaptic activity, the smart-synapse learning rule is considered Hebbian.

The reinforcement signal is broadcast to all synapses in the network (as in Chapter 7) and updates the memory counter of each active synapse according to Equations 14.5 and 14.6:

$$m_{ij}(c+1) = \begin{cases} \Theta, & m_{ij}(c) - r > \Theta \\ m_{ij}(c) - r, & \Theta \geq m_{ij}(c) - r \geq 0 \\ 0, & 0 > m_{ij}(c) - r \end{cases} \qquad \textbf{14.5}$$

$$m_{ki}(c+1) = \begin{cases} \Theta, & m_{ki}(c) - r > \Theta \\ m_{ki}(c) - r, & \Theta \geq m_{ki}(c) - r \geq 0 \\ 0, & 0 > m_{ki}(c) - r \end{cases} \qquad \textbf{14.6}$$

Note for each option that reinforcement r is subtracted from the current value of a memory counter. Since $r = -1$ when the network is in error, the memory counters of all synapses that are active when the network is in error are incremented (positive direction). Thus, each memory counter counts the number of times its synapse was active when the output of the network was in error. If a counter m_{ij} or m_{ki} exceeds the threhsold Θ (which occurs whenever $m_{ij}(c) - r > \Theta$ or $m_{ki}(c) - r > \Theta$), then the counter is set to the threshold value and the corresponding weight is penalized, as shown in Equations 14.7 and 14.8:

$$v_{ij}(c+1) = v_{ij}(c) - \delta \qquad \textbf{14.7}$$

$$u_{ki}(c+1) = u_{ki}(c) - \delta \qquad \textbf{14.8}$$

To summarize the smart-synapse algorithm, all weights are incremented by a small amount on each training cycle c, but each synapse counts the number of times it contributes to network error and its weight is decremented by δ each time its memory counter m exceeds the threshold Θ.

Learning begins by randomizing all weight values and setting all counters m_{ij} and m_{ki} to 0. As for training with back-propagation, the XOR patterns are presented repeatedly and in random order. All weights grow slowly but are penalized according to Equations 14.5–14.8 when their error memory counter exceeds the threshold. The results with penalty $\delta = 1$, inverse temperature $\beta = 10$, and thresholds of $\Theta = 0$, 1, or 2 are shown in Figure 14.8.

With $\Theta = 0$, a weight is penalized each time it is associated with units that are active when the actual output is in error. In other words, with $\Theta = 0$ no averaging takes place, and the results show that no learning takes place either (i.e., network error is not reduced). The outcome is radically improved with $\Theta = 1$ or $\Theta = 2$, with even more rapid learning (reduction of error) at the higher threshold. The results can be explained by noting that the immediate weakening of all synapses associated with an erroneous output for a certain pattern wipes out successful learning on other patterns. This problem is avoided if a weight is penalized only if it is repeatedly associated with erroneous network performance. The memory of the smart synapse allows it to keep track of its errors over one or more pattern presentations.

The smart-synapse learning algorithm described here is also capable of training input–output transformations that are more complex than the XOR (Klemm et al. 2000). The use of a common, broadcast reinforcement signal and the otherwise local nature of the learning rule lend it neurobiological plausibility. As argued above, the complexity and potential computational power of molecular interaction networks suggest that having a memory to count the errors associated with individual synapses is not unrealistic. The idea of smart synapses will recur later in this chapter. In the next section we consider

FIGURE 14.8 Learning curves for the network that learns the exclusive-OR using local rules, reinforcement, and smart synapses When internal synaptic memory capacity is zero ($\Theta = 0$) the error is not decreased by learning. Networks with one-step synaptic memory ($\Theta = 1$) learn quickly, and those with two-step synaptic memory ($\Theta = 2$) learn even more quickly. Each learning curve is an average of 10,000 separate runs of the simulation. (After Klemm et al. 2000.)

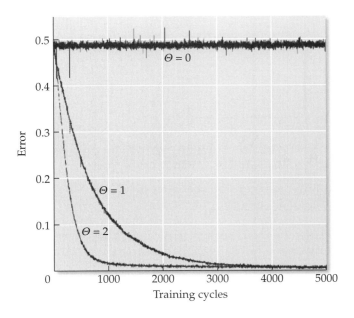

the other new direction in neural systems modeling, that of combining two or more network-level paradigms in the same model. In Section 14.4 we consider a model that combines both smart synapses and multiple network-level paradigms.

14.3 Combining Complementary Network Paradigms for Memory Formation

The neural systems modeling paradigms we have explored in previous chapters are each capable of simulating an isolated aspect of neural computation, but the nervous system operates holistically, with many different processes participating in a coordinated fashion. Another new avenue for neural systems modeling involves exploring the ways in which two or more different types of neural networks could work together. Many of these multi-network models are considered in the context of memory formation.

One example involves a model of working memory, which is the active memory involved in tasks that require the representation and manipulation of several items simultaneously. Hazy and coworkers (2006) proposed a model of working memory having three components: a posterior cortex system (comprising cortical regions located behind the central sulcus) that learns iteratively to produce input–output transformations, a hippocampal system that is capable of rapid (one-trial) learning of arbitrary patterns, and a prefrontal-cortex/basal-ganglia system that uses reinforcement learning to bias ongoing processing in the cortex. The modeling paradigms used to simulate these components are roughly similar to those we have studied in previous chapters in this book. The posterior cortex system is modeled using multilayered feedforward neural networks (see Chapter 6), the hippocampal system using recurrent, auto-associative networks (see Chapter 4), and the basal ganglia system using reinforcement learning (see Chapter 7). This model is capable of simulating a wide range of working-memory tasks by having the hippocampal system draw patterns from the posterior cortex system under the guidance of the basal ganglia system.

14.4 Smart Synapses and Complementary Rules in Cerebellar Learning

The cerebellum is situated behind the cerebrum in the vertebrate brain (Butler and Hodos 1996). Its function is most closely associated with movement (motor) control. Rather than produce movement commands itself, the cerebellum regulates ongoing movements and improves their accuracy and perhaps also their efficiency. Critical to its function is a capability for learning that allows the cerebellum to make adaptive changes in its regulation of movement. Most models of cerebellar learning, including many of the most recent, trace their origin back to a theory proposed by David Marr (1969).

David Marr, pictured neo-impressionistically in Figure 14.12, is considered by many to be the founder of the field of computational neuroscience. We have already encountered him in several places in this book. In Chapter 3 we discussed Marr's spatial filter (Marr 1982), which resembles the receptive fields of many visual neurons and acts as an edge extractor and contrast enhancer. In Chapter 4 we discussed Marr's model of memory (Marr 1971), which was a progenitor of auto-associative neural networks including Hopfield networks. In Chapter 9 we invoked Marr's three levels, those on which neural systems could be described. His brilliant career ended tragically when he died of leukemia at age thirty-five, but his work has had a profound influence on many neural systems modelers (including the author). His first major publication was actually the one describing his theory of cerebellar learning (Marr 1969). No other paper has had a bigger impact on thinking in this area. Many of the ideas he expressed in it have stood the test of time. It still stands as a singular achievement in the modeling of motor systems but, after forty years, some aspects of it might be up for revision.

The theory of cerebellar learning originated by Marr was later elaborated by James Albus (1971). In essence, the Marr/Albus paradigm posits the existence of a dedicated error signal, and treats cerebellar learning as a form of supervised learning. Because supervised learning is robust (see Chapter 6), cerebellar learning models based on the Marr/Albus paradigm are success-

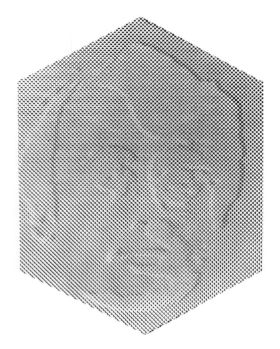

FIGURE 14.12   A portrait of David Marr by Nicholas Wade
This portrait could be described as a pointillist version of the output of a Marr filter given an image of Marr as input. (See Chapter 3 for a description of the Marr filter.)

(A)

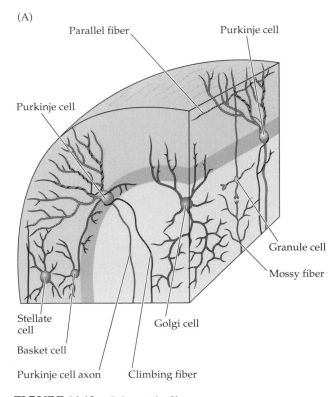

FIGURE 14.13 Schematic diagram of the Purkinje cell and its connections with neurons of other types in the cerebellum Purkinje cells receive excitatory input from parallel fibers and climbing fibers. The latter are so called because they "climb" the dendrites of the Purkinje cells. Parallel fibers arise from granule cells, which receive input from mossy fibers. Stellate, basket, and Golgi cells also receive parallel fiber input. Stellate and basket cells inhibit Purkinje cells, while Golgi cells inhibit granule cells. Purkinje cells regulate ongoing motor behavior by inhibiting neurons in the cerebellar deep nuclei and vestibular nuclei. (After Butler and Hodos 1996.)

(B)

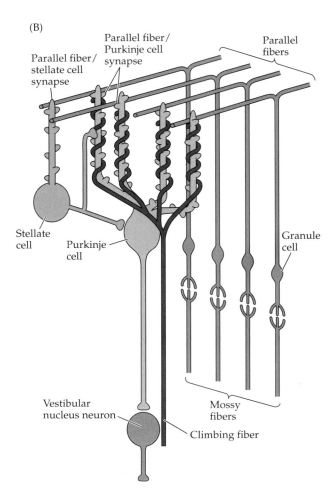

ful in simulating motor learning. However, the existence of an error signal capable of guiding cerebellar learning has not been established uneqivocally (Kitazawa and Wolpert 2005). This leaves room for an alternative to the Marr/Albus paradigm. The model we will consider in this section, called the input minimization (InMin) algorithm (Anastasio 2001), provides an alternative view of cerebellar learning.

The neural circuitry of the cerebellum is depicted in Figure 14.13. It is centered on the Purkinje cell, which is the principle cell type in the cerebellum (Butler and Hodos 1996). Purkinje cells receive excitatory input from two sources: parallel fibers, which originate from cerebellar granule cells, and climbing fibers, which originate from neurons in the inferior olive. Each Purkinje cell receives input from 100,000 to 200,000 parallel fibers but from only one climbing fiber. According to the Marr/Albus paradigm, the synapses of the parallel fibers onto the Purkinje cells are trained according to error signals carried by climbing fibers (Marr 1969; Albus 1971). However, climbing fibers are known to fire action potentials at a low average rate of about one spike per second, and with a temporal pattern that is mostly random (Keating and Thach 1995). Evidence that the climbing-fiber signal is an error signal is far from conclusive, and many alternative theories of climbing-fiber function exist (Kitazawa and Wolpert 2005).

Cerebellar granular cells, which give rise to parallel fibers, receive input from mossy fibers. Mossy fibers originate from many regions throughout the brain. Thus, the parallel fibers carry a diversity of signals including sensory, motor, and error signals (Miles et al. 1980). The InMin model is based on the idea that the error signals that guide cerebellar learning are those carried by the parallel fibers themselves. Due to the abundance of parallel fibers, the information that they could transmit concerning any signals, including error signals, is potentially very high (see Chapter 8). Because parallel fibers carry error as well as other types of signals, overall parallel-fiber activity should decrease as error decreases. The InMin algorithm produces adaptive behavior essentially by minimizing the parallel fiber input to model Purkinje cells. More specifically, InMin uses overall parallel-fiber activity as a (negative) reinforcement signal, and combines reinforcement learning with unsupervised learning and smart synapses to train a network of model Purkinje cells to reduce error by minimizing overall parallel-fiber activity. The InMin algorithm has been used to simulate adaptation by the cerebellum of the vestibulo-ocular reflex (VOR). We will briefly review this model.

The function of the VOR is to stabilize the retinal image during head movement by making eye rotations that counterbalance head rotations (see Chapter 2 for a discussion of the VOR). The cerebellum can adapt the amplitude of the VOR up or down, and VOR adaptation is associated with adjustments in the response amplitudes of Purkinje cells (Watanabe 1985). Purkinje-cell response amplitude is a function of the weights of the inputs to Purkinje cells from parallel fibers and from cerebellar inhibitory interneurons. The latter include stellate, basket, and Golgi cells. Stellate and basket cells inhibit Purkinje cells while Golgi cells inhibit granule cells. Only stellate cells are found in all vertebrates (Butler and Hodos 1996), so basket and Golgi interneurons can be ignored in models of basic cerebellar function. The Purkinje cells control VOR amplitude through direct inhibition of the neurons in the vestibular nuclei that mediate the VOR (see Chapter 2 for more details on VOR anatomy).

The architecture of the InMin model is based on cerebellar anatomy, as shown in Figure 14.14. The input to the model represents the input to the VOR and cerebellum from the vestibular semicircular canal primary afferents. For simplicity, the vestibular input is a sinusoid about a zero baseline. A constant offset is added to the input to simulate the background activity of vestibular nucleus neurons, which provide the motor command that drives the VOR. To simulate the diversity of mossy-fiber inputs to the cerebellum, the vestibular input signal carried by them is subjected to several phase shifts. Each mossy fiber contacts several granule cells. The granule cells have a diversity of response thresholds. Thus, the parallel-fiber inputs to the Purkinje cells are diverse, both in phase and in threshold. The stellate cell also receives input from the parallel fibers. The response of each model Purkinje cell is the weighted sum of its parallel-fiber inputs, and this sum is divided by an amount proportional to the weight of the connection to the Purkinje cell from the stellate cell, which acts as a shunting inhibition (Mitchell and Silver 2003).

Cerebellar Purkinje cells regulate the VOR by inhibiting vestibular nucleus neurons. To represent the influence of the Purkinje cells on the VOR, the responses of the Purkinje cells are summed and then subtracted from the vestibular nucleus neuron signal to form the actual output of the model. The actual output is compared with the desired output to form an error. This error is known as retinal slip error, and it is the error signal that ultimately arrives at the Purkinje cells via the parallel fibers.

Because the function of the VOR is to stabilize the visual image on the retina during head movement, a VOR error will result in slippage of the visual image over the retina. This retinal slip error signal is detected by visual motion sensitive neurons in the retina (and possibly in other parts of the visual system as well).

FIGURE 14.14 Diagram illustrating the architecture of the input minimization (InMin) model of cerebellar learning The phase-shifted input and delayed error signal are carried by mossy fibers, which send divergent projections to granule cells. Granule cells send parallel fibers to Purkinje and stellate cells. Stellate cells and climbing fibers also contact Purkinje cells. The summed Purkinje cell output is subtracted from the offset input to form the actual output of the model. The difference between the desired and actual output forms the error signal. (After Anastasio 2001.)

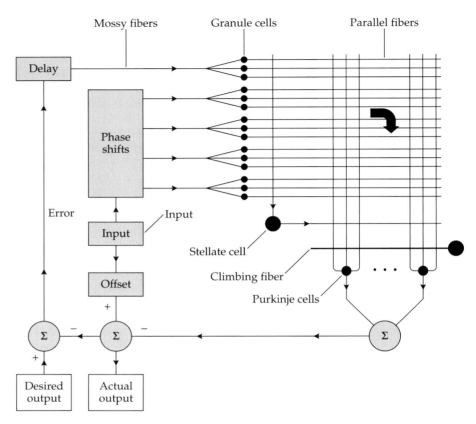

As such, it is subject to the retinal processing delay of about 0.1 second. For this reason, the retinal slip error signal is delayed before it is sent to the Purkinje cells over the mossy-granule-parallel-fiber pathway. The delay between Purkinje-cell adjustments of motor behavior and the error feedback associated with those adjustments poses a challenge for models of cerebellar learning.

Regardless of which fibers carry the retinal slip error signal or how it is used, any model of cerebellar adaptation of the VOR must take the retinal processing delay into account. For example, for the Marr/Albus paradigm, which is based on supervised learning, the correct weight update is proportional to the product of the delayed error at the current time and the input that occurred one delay interval in the past. One way to delay the input is by means of an "eligibility trace." The eligibility trace can be used essentially to store the input value over the delay interval until the corresponding error signal is available. Such an eligibility trace has been used, and assumed to be mediated by cellular signaling mechanisms, in a model of cerebellar adaptation of smooth pursuit eye movements that is based on the Marr/Albus paradigm (Kettner et al. 1997). An eligibility trace plausibly could be implemented by a smart synapse. An eligibility trace is one of the mechanisms that is implemented by smart synapses in the InMin model.

The InMin algorithm is based on unsupervised learning, perturbative reinforcement learning, and smart-synapse mechanisms. The (negative) reinforcement signal is the overall activity of the parallel fibers, some of which carry error signals. The climbing fibers do not carry error signals, but instead fire spikes at random intervals that average to one second. For the purpose of deriving a prediction (see later in this section) all the Purkinje cells in this version of the model receive input from the same, single climbing fiber. Climbing-fiber spikes serve to synchronize learning events in InMin, and they initiate the processes of unsupervised and reinforcement learning. The smart-synapse mechanisms are associated with the reinforcement learning component of InMin. These processes are summarized in Figure 14.15 and described in more detail in what follows.

Each climbing-fiber spike initiates a cycle of unsupervised learning of the weights of the parallel fibers onto the Purkinje cells. Specifically, a climbing-fiber spike sets off a competition among the Purkinje cells that selects the one with the largest response to the parallel fiber (granule cell) input. The parallel-fiber weights of the winning Purkinje cell and its neighbors are then updated according to the self-organizing map (SOM) unsupervised learning rule (see Chapter 5). Training by the SOM causes each model Purkinje cell to represent and respond to its own specific temporal segment of the parallel-fiber input. Since the parallel fibers carry vestibular signals that have a realistic diversity of phases, each model Purkinje cell becomes specialized for a different phase of the vestibular signal, and so has its own unique phase relationship with the VOR.

Each climbing-fiber spike also initiates one cycle of perturbative reinforcement learning of the stellate input weight onto the winning Purkinje cell. It does this by triggering four smart-synapse functions. The climbing fiber spike causes the winning Purkinje cell to initiate its eligibility trace, randomly perturb the weight of its stellate input connection, store the value of the perturbation, and remove the perturbation on the next time step. The reaching of eligibility triggers two more smart-synapse functions. The Purkinje cell detects the change in its overall parallel-fiber input, and it restores the perturbation of the stellate weight if that input decreases (that is, if the negative reinforcement signal decreases). What these mechanisms essentially accomplish is adaptation of the VOR, and it does this through regulation of model Purkinje cell response amplitude.

Perturbative learning adjusts the stellate input weight to the Purkinje cell, which in turn adjusts the sensitivity of the Purkinje cell to its parallel-fiber (granule cell) inputs. This changes the amplitude of the response of the Purkinje cell, which in turn changes its influence on the VOR. Basically, if the perturbation of its stellate input weight causes an improvement in the VOR, then the model Purkinje cell keeps the perturbation. The admittedly complicated synaptic and network mechanisms that InMin employs to make that

---

◆ Set numbers of neural elements; set the input and desired output; set the error delay and phase shifts; set granule cell thresholds; initialize the parallel-Purkinje and stellate-Purkinje weights; set learning rates.
◆ For each time step, Do
    ◆ Activate each granule cell whose input exceeds its threshold
    ◆ Compute the weighted sum of parallel fiber inputs to each Purkinje cell
    ◆ Divide weighted input sum by stellate weight to find Purkinje-cell response
    ◆ Sum the Purkinje-cell responses to find the total output of the cerebellum
    ◆ Compute actual output as offseft vestibular signal minus cerebellar output
    ◆ Compute error as difference between desired and actual output and delay it
    ◆ If the climbing fiber fires, then
        ◆ Find Purkinje cell with the maximum response to parallel fiber input
        ◆ Update its parallel-Purkinje weights (and its neighbors) using SOM
        ◆ Initiate the eligibility trace of the winning Purkinje cell
        ◆ Perturb the stellate-Purkinje weight of the winning Purkinje cell
        ◆ Store and remove the perturbation on the next time step
    ◆ If a Purkinje cell becomes eligible, then
        ◆ Detect change in number of active parallel fibers due to perturbation
        ◆ If number of active parallel fibers decreases, then restore perturbation
◆ End

FIGURE 14.15   Pseudo-code for the input minimization (InMin) algorithm Cerebellar Purkinje cells regulate the vestibulo-ocular reflex by inhibiting vestibular nucleus neurons. InMin uses unsupervised and perturbative reinforcement learning to tune this regulation. The unsupervised component trains Purkinje cells to represent and respond to their parallel-fiber (granule cell) inputs. The reinforcement component adjusts the stellate cell weights to Purkinje cells, which controls Purkinje-cell response amplitude. The (negative) reinforcement signal is the total number of active parallel fibers. (Some parallel fibers carry error signals.) Purkinje cells perturb their stellate weights and keep the perturbation if the number of active parallel fibers decreases.

FIGURE 14.16 Using InMin to simulate cerebellar adaptation of vestibulo-ocular reflex (VOR) amplitude to normal, low, or high levels (A) Actual output matches desired output in all cases. (B–D) Thin lines show the responses of all 24 model Purkinje cells. Dots mark the responses of the same model Purkinje cell at the three different VOR amplitude levels. (B) Model Purkinje cells develop temporally specific responses that cover the whole range of phase relationships with the vestibular input signal. (C) Down-adaptation (to low-amplitude VOR) increases and decreases Purkinje-cell responses that are respectively in-phase and out-of-phase with the vestibular input signal. (D) The opposite occurs for up-adaptation (to high-amplitude VOR). (After Anastasio 2001.)

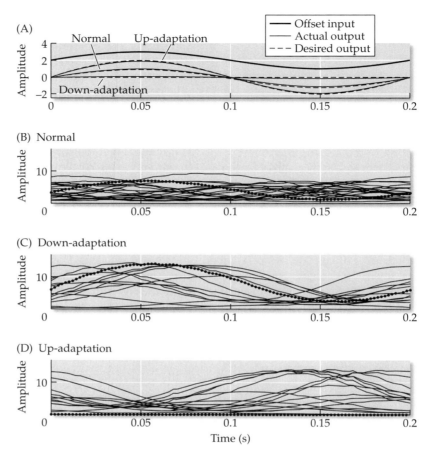

happen are needed to overcome the error signal delay. Equally importantly, they are needed to allow the Purkinje cells to decode multiplexed signals from their parallel fiber inputs, and use them both to drive their vestibular responses, which the Purkinje cells use to control the VOR, and to guide reinforcement learning of their stellate weights. Note that perturbative reinforcement learning of stellate weights occurs one Purkinje cell at a time in the original version of InMin described here (Anastasio 2001), but all stellate weights are updated in parallel over many Purkinje cells simultaneously in more recent versions (Rothganger and Anastasio, in review; see also Chapter 7). We will further scrutinize InMin as an algorithm after we examine the results it produces.

The results of the InMin learning procedure are illustrated in Figure 14.16. The model is trained to produce a normal VOR, or to down-adapt it (decrease its amplitude) or to up-adapt it (increase its amplitude). Figure 14.16A shows that InMin achieves accurate VOR adaptation in all cases. Because of the unsupervised component of InMin learning, each Purkinje cell becomes specialized for a different phase of the vestibular input, as shown in Figure 14.16B. This diversity of the phases of model Purkinje-cell responses matches the diversity actually observed for real Purkinje cells (Miles et al. 1980; Watanabe 1985). The model simulates VOR adaptation most directly through the perturbative reinforcement component of InMin learning, which allows individual Purkinje cells to adjust the amplitudes of their responses. Because the Purkinje cells inhibit the vestibular nucleus neurons, down-adaptation requires that Purkinje cells with responses that are in-phase with the vestibular input increase their amplitudes, while those with responses that are out-of-phase with the vestibu-

(A) Down-adaptation (B) Up-adaptation

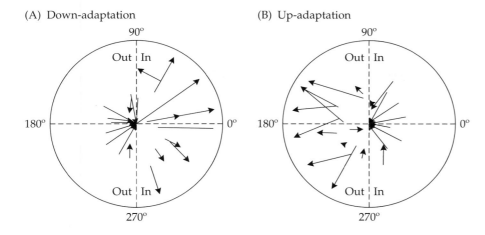

FIGURE 14.17 Polar plots showing the amplitude and phase of model Purkinje-cell responses before and after VOR adaptation The polar plots provide an alternative way to view the data that are shown as functions of time in Figure 14.16. The center of each circle corresponds to an amplitude of 0 and the outer edge to the maximal amplitude of 16. The base of each line segment marks normal amplitude and phase while the arrowhead marks adapted amplitude and phase. (A) Down-adaptation increases or decreases the amplitudes of model Purkinje-cell responses that are in-phase or out-of-phase with the vestibular input signal, respectively. (B) The opposite occurs for up-adaptation. (After Anastasio 2001.)

lar input decrease their amplitudes. Up-adaptation of the VOR requires the opposite pattern. The InMin algorithm produces the required adjustments in Purkinje-cell response amplitude, as shown in Figure 14.16C and D.

To compare the changes in model Purkinje-cell responses produced by InMin with those that are observed for real Purkinje cells as a result of VOR adaptation, the amplitude and phase data are redrawn using polar plots in Figure 14.17. In a polar plot, the amplitude of a response is represented as the distance of a point from the origin, while the phase is represented by the radial position of the point in degrees moving counterclockwise from the positive horizontal axis. The model Purkinje-cell response data in Figure 14.16C are re-plotted in polar coordinates in Figure 14.17A, where the beginning of each line segment represents the amplitude and phase for the normal VOR, and the arrowhead represents the amplitude and phase after down-adaptation of the VOR. Figure 14.17A shows clearly that down-adaptation causes in-phase and out-of-phase model Purkinje cells to increase and decrease their amplitudes, respectively. The opposite pattern pertains for model Purkinje cells following up-adaptation, as shown in Figure 14.17B. The patterns of amplitude change exhibited by Purkinje cells in the InMin model are very similar to those observed for real Purkinje cells following down- or up-adaptation of the VOR (Watanabe 1985), as shown in Figure 14.18A and B, respectively.

These results demonstrate that InMin is capable of accurately simulating VOR adaptation, and in so doing, to simulate the associated changes in response properties that are observed for real Purkinje cells. Furthermore,

(A) Down-adaptation (B) Up-adaptation

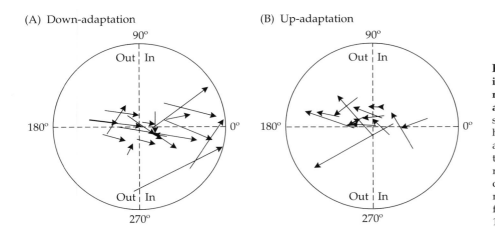

FIGURE 14.18 Polar plots showing the amplitude and phase of real Purkinje-cell responses before and after VOR adaptation The same plotting conventions are used here as in Figure 14.17. (A) Down-adaptation increases or decreases the amplitudes of real Purkinje-cell responses that are in-phase or out-of-phase with the vestibular signal, respectively. (B) The opposite occurs for up-adaptation. (After Watanabe 1985.)

InMin does this using climbing fibers that fire realistically at a low and random rate, and it avoids the weakly supported assumption that climbing fibers carry error signals. Admittedly, InMin is a complicated algorithm. It combines unsupervised learning (see Chapter 4) and perturbative reinforcement learning (see Chapter 7), but both of these mechanisms are plausible, and it is realistic to suppose that real neural systems employ multiple learning mechanisms (see previous section). The most speculative aspect of InMin concerns the functionality of its smart synapses, but these are also plausible.

Altogether, the smart synapses in InMin are capable of six functions. With the exclusion of the eligibility trace, which has already been attributed to cellular signaling mechanisms (Kettner et al. 1997), the smart-synapse functions in InMin can all be broken down into storage, addition, and subtraction of signals. These simple functions are well within the signal processing capabilities that have been hypothesized for molecular networks (Katz and Clemens 2001). Furthermore, Purkinje cells abound in cellular signaling pathways (Ito 2000). The parallel-Purkinje synapse is capable both of long-term potentiation (LTP) and long-term depression (LTD). Part of the molecular network thought to underlie LTD is shown schematically in Figure 14.19. The richness and complexity of this network certainly leave open the possibility for a substantial degree of molecular computation within Purkinje-cell synapses.

Like all of the models presented in this book, InMin is a hypothesis that needs to be tested experimentally. Particularly useful tests are those that serve to distinguish between alternative hypotheses. Appropriately, an experimental test that will distinguish InMin learning from Marr/Albus learning can be derived (Rothganger and Anastasio, in review). Because weight updates due to supervised learning are based on the correlation between any input signal and the error, the Marr/Albus paradigm predicts that all Purkinje cells that

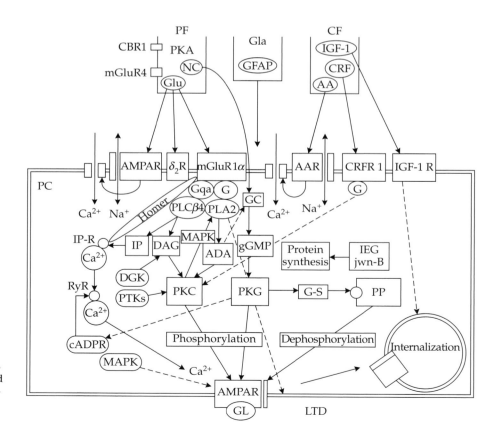

FIGURE 14.19 **The cell signaling pathways thought to underlie long-term depression (LTD) in the cerebellum** The diagram illustrates that cerebellar Purkinje cells abound in molecular interaction (cell signaling) pathways. See Ito (2000) for abbreviations. (After Ito 2000.)

Index

Citations in *italics* refer to information in a table or illustration.